T0292696

Methods in Neuronal Modeling

Methods in Neuronal Modeling
From Ions to Networks

second edition

edited by Christof Koch and Idan Segev

A Bradford Book
The MIT Press
Cambridge, Massachusetts
London, England

This book was set in Times New Roman on the Monotype "Prism Plus" PostScript Imagesetter by Asco Trade Typesetting Ltd., Hong Kong.

Library of Congress Cataloging-in-Publication Data

Methods in neuronal modeling : from ions to networks / edited by
Christof Koch and Idan Segev. — 2nd ed.
     p.   cm.
   Includes bibliographical references and index.
   ISBN 978-0-262-11231-4 (hc. : alk. paper) — 978-0-262-51713-3 (pb. : alk. paper)
   1. Neural networks (Neurobiology) 2. Nervous system—Computer
simulation. 3. Neurons—Computer simulation. I. Koch, Christof.
II. Segev, Idan.
QP363.3.M46   1998
573.8'01'13—DC21   97-17166
                                                       CIP

Throughout all his existence man has been striving to hear the music of the spheres, and has seemed to himself once and again to catch some phrase of it, or even a hint of the whole form of it. Yet he can never be sure that he has truly heard it, nor even that there is any such perfect music at all to be heard. Inevitably so, for if it exists, it is not for him in his littleness.
—"Last and First Man"
Olaf Stapledon

Contents

Computational neuroscience is an approach to understanding the information content of neural signals by modeling the nervous system at many different structural scales, including the biophysical, the circuit, and the systems levels. Computer simulations of neurons and neural networks are complementary to traditional techniques in neuroscience. This book series welcomes contributions that link theoretical studies with experimental approaches to understanding information processing in the nervous system. Areas and topics of particular interest include biophysical mechanisms for computation in neurons, computer simulations of neural circuits, models of learning, representation of sensory information in neural networks, systems models of sensory-motor integration, and computational analysis of problems in biological sensing, motor control, and perception.

Terrence J. Sejnowski
Tomaso A. Poggio

Preface

Nine years have passed since the publication of the first edition of this handbook. The success of the first edition has been due in part to the growing realization that to understand the brain, new interdisciplinary research methodologies must be developed that combine bottom-up experimental with top-down computational and modeling approaches.

The second edition reflects the various directions taken by computational neuroscience in the last decade, and has a clear bias toward theoretical developments and techniques whose importance in elucidating the brain's computational processes needs no further justification. These theoretical advances have been incorporated into many laboratories and represent a visible and vibrant contribution to modern neuroscience.

New interdisciplinary research programs, centered on understanding how the brain computes, stores, and represents information, have been inaugurated in universities and research facilities across the globe (e.g., the Sloan Centers for Theoretical Neuroscience at the Salk Institute, the California Institute of Technology, Brandeis University, the University of California at San Francisco, and New York University in the United States; the Institute for Neuroinformatics in Zürich, Switzerland, and the Center for Neural Computation at the Hebrew University in Israel). These research centers encourage interdisciplinary collaborations by theoretical and experimental researchers focusing on how information is processed in nervous systems, from the level of individual ionic channels to large-scale neuronal networks and from "simple" animals, such as sea slugs or flies, to cats and primates. The fruits of these collaborations are at the core of the second edition. They also serve as the inspiration for the "Methods in Neuronal Modeling" summer course at the Marine Biological Laboratory in Woods Hole, Massachusetts, which in its tenth year continues to attract outstanding students, and from which the first edition evolved. In 1996 a European counterpart to the Woods Hole summer course was established, the "Crete Course in Computational Neuroscience"; again, with great success.

Given the frenetic pace of late-twentieth-century science, eight years is a long time, and the second edition of this book is therefore very different from its predecessor. A general, and important, trend throughout this book is the tightening relationship between analytical/numerical models and the associated experimental data. Indeed, the available empirical database is gargantuan (and includes information from molecular biology, anatomy, biophysics, pharmacology, neurophysiology, and behavior) and continues to expand at breathtaking speed. Close connections between models and data, between prediction and experiment, find expression in all chapters of this edition.

A second trend is the broadening of modeling methods, both at the subcellular level (ions, channels, and receptors; see chapters 1 and 6) and at the level of large neuronal networks, where cellular models are no longer based on simple and very abstract units but incorporate key biophysical properties of neurons (in particular, multiple membrane conductances that give rise to spiking; see chapters 3, 12, and 13). Yet another novel development is reflected in chapter 8, which attempts to organize the wealth of knowledge gained by physical emulation of the components of the nervous system, cells, and networks with the aid of very-large-scale integrated (VLSI) electronic circuit technology.

We would here like to note, with great sadness, the premature death of Dr. Misha Mahowald in Zürich. She was one of the founders of the young field of *synthetic neurobiology*. Her chapter gives testimony to why she was so influential. Although young in years, she was attuned to much in life beyond science.

Finally, there is a healthy tendency—which complements a trend toward ever more detailed and complex models—to simplify complex models while retaining the essential elements of the behavior being modeled, based on a thorough understanding of the conditions under which this simplification can be carried out (see chapters 3, 5, 10, and 12). This is a crucial step towards understanding, and enables us to extract the significant parameters in a model from the wide range of parameters less relevant to the behavior under study; without it, researchers may well end up with a model as complex as the reality one wishes to understand.

Half of the chapters in this edition are completely new, covering developments that were either unknown or only in their infancy in 1989. We have added chapters on a general kinetic scheme for describing synaptic transmission (chapter 1), modeling dendritic excitability (chapter 5), calcium dynamics in dendrites and spines (chapter 6), fabrication of "silicon" neurons using analog VLSI circuit technology (chapter 8), information-theoretical approaches toward spike train analysis (chapter 9), evolution of small neural networks (chapter 10), and an analytical approach to modeling local cortical circuits (chapter 13).

We have eliminated five chapters from the first edition and revised the remaining seven. In cable theory, new developments for analyzing passive signals in dendritic trees (e.g., the morphoelectrotonic transform and method of moments) have been incorporated in chapter 2. The compartmental modeling approach has been extended, in chapter 3, to cover highly sophisticated and popular simulation tools such as NEURON and GENESIS (also discussed in chapter 12), as well as analytical methods for better understanding the performance of a particular model. The treatment of qualitative, phase-space analysis of simple networks, very popular in the first edition, has been substantially expanded in chapter 7. Chapters 11 and 12, on simulation of realistic biological systems, have been updated and more closely connected to biological data. Even the fundamental chapter on numerical methods in neuronal simulations (chapter 14) has undergone changes and includes the newest numerical techniques together with additional explanatory notes and examples. Finally, chapter reference lists have been combined at the end of the handbook in a master bibliography, and a comprehensive index assembled.

In order to bring this book up to date with state of the art communications many chapters invite readers to take advantage of interactive tutorials, simulation programs, and packages. We believe that such a dynamic learning method represent the most successful way to disseminate and complement the more static material in this book. All programs can be accessed via the Internet at http://www.klab.caltech.edu/MNM.

We hope that this new edition will be instrumental in raising a new generation of neuroscientists, equally at ease with theory and experiments. Enjoy it!

We wish to thank the far-seeing institutions that supported the field of neuronal modeling when it was less popular than today, and that made the writing of both editions of this book possible: the Office of Naval Research, the Alfred P. Sloan Foundation, the National Science Foundation, and the National Institute of Mental Health. We would also like to thank Michael (Miki) London for his careful help in processing the LaTeX files from which this edition emerged.

Idan Segev, Jerusalem
Christof Koch, Pasadena

Methods in Neuronal Modeling

1 Kinetic Models of Synaptic Transmission

Alain Destexhe, Zachary F. Mainen, and Terrence J. Sejnowski

1.1 Introduction: The Kinetic Interpretation of Ion Channel Gating

The remarkably successful quantitative description of the action potential introduced by Hodgkin and Huxley (1952) is still widely used over forty years since its introduction. The classical Hodgkin-Huxley description was not only accurate, it was also readily extensible to many other voltage-dependent currents. More recent single-channel recording techniques (Sakmann and Neher 1995) have been used to prove that voltage-dependent currents arise from populations of individual ion channels undergoing rapid transitions between conducting and nonconducting states. The macroscopic behavior of the currents can be accurately captured using kinetic models that describe the transitions between conformational states of these ion channels. This class of models, of which the Hodgkin-Huxley model is an instance, are commonly known as "Markov models."

Kinetic models not only provide good descriptions of voltage-dependent ionic currents but are general enough to describe almost all processes essential to neurophysiology. We will focus in this chapter on synaptically gated currents of all kinds, including neuromodulators, which are readily modeled by Markov kinetics. Moreover, many important biochemical reactions, including second-messenger systems, synaptic release, and enzymatic cascades can also be described by kinetic schemes. As a consequence, kinetic models provide the means to build coherent neural models in which subcellular, cellular, and network properties are described within the same formalism (see Destexhe, Mainen, and Sejnowski 1994b).

Kinetic models are inherently flexible in their level of detail, ranging from the most detailed and biophysically realistic gating models to highly simplified representations. Some detailed models determined from voltage clamp studies have more than a dozen states (e.g., Raman and Trussell 1992); others have been found for the gating of receptors by neurotransmitters and intracellular second messengers such as calcium. These models accurately describe the behavior of synaptic channels as measured by single-channel or macroscopic current recordings, and are appropriate for simulating patch clamp experiments.

The essential properties of ion channel activation can be captured by simplified kinetic models with just two states. The simplest kinetic models for the gating of different classes of ion channels are illustrated in table 1.1. For synaptic currents (Destexhe, Mainen, and Sejnowski 1994a) as for voltage-dependent currents (Destexhe, Mainen, and Sejnowski 1994b; Destexhe 1997), simplified kinetic models provide an efficient way to incorporate their basic properties, such as the time course of

Table 1.1
Most simple kinetic schemes to represent the gating of different classes of ion channels

Voltage-dependent gating (Hodgkin-Huxley)	$C \underset{\beta(V)}{\overset{\alpha(V)}{\rightleftharpoons}} O$
Calcium-dependent gating	$C + nCa_i \underset{\beta}{\overset{\alpha}{\rightleftharpoons}} O$
Transmitter gating	$C + nT \underset{\beta}{\overset{\alpha}{\rightleftharpoons}} O$
Second-messenger gating	$C + nG \underset{\beta}{\overset{\alpha}{\rightleftharpoons}} O$

Voltage-dependent channels: the channel is assumed to have opened (O) and closed (C) states modulated by voltage-dependent transition rates (α and β). *Calcium-dependent channels:* the opening of the channel depends on the binding of one or several intracellular Ca^{2+} ions (Ca_i). *Transmitter-gated channels:* molecules of neurotransmitter (T) are released transiently and bind to the channel, leading to its opening. *Second messenger-gated channels:* the opening of the channel is provided by the binding of one or several intracellular second messengers (G). Kinetic equations allow us to describe all these processes, which underlie electrophysiological properties and synaptic interactions, using the same formalism (see also chapter appendix A).

rise and decay and their summation behavior, in simulations that do not require the level of detail described above. Typical examples of this kind are simulations of networks of neurons where the most salient features of ion channel interactions must be represented with maximal computational efficiency.

In this chapter, we focus on models of synaptic interactions. We start with an overview of relatively detailed kinetic models for synaptic release (section 1.2) and for representative types of synaptic currents and receptors (section 1.3). We then review simplified models for these types of synaptic interactions (section 1.4). Although these simplified models have fewer states than detailed kinetic representations, they exhibit essential properties of synaptic currents, such as the summation of postsynaptic currents. Finally, the simplified models are used to simulate a small network of interacting neurons that exhibit complex behavior (section 1.5). These simplified models are computationally efficient (chapter appendix C) and may therefore prove useful in accurately representing synaptic transmission in large network simulations.

1.2 Presynaptic Mechanisms of Transmitter Release

We focus first on the mechanisms underlying the release of transmitter when an action potential arrives at the presynaptic terminal. A kinetic model of the intracellular reactions leading to ejection of transmitter by the presynaptic terminal is presented, and the results are compared with more simplified models.

1.2.1 Model of Transmitter Release

The exact mechanisms whereby Ca^{2+} enters the presynaptic terminal, the specific proteins with which Ca^{2+} interacts, and the detailed mechanisms leading to exocytosis represent an active area of research (e.g., Schweizer, Betz, and Augustine 1995). It is clear that an accurate model of these processes should include the particular clustering of calcium channels, calcium diffusion and gradients, all enzymatic reactions involved in exocytosis, and the particular properties of the diffusion of transmitter across the fusion pore and synaptic cleft. For our present purpose, we use a simple model of calcium-induced release inspired by Yamada and Zucker 1992. This model of transmitter release assumed that (a) upon invasion by an action potential, Ca^{2+} enters the presynaptic terminal due to the presence of a high-threshold Ca^{2+} current; (b) Ca^{2+} activates a calcium-binding protein, which promotes release by binding to the transmitter-containing vesicles; (c) an inexhaustible supply of "docked" vesicles are available in the presynaptic terminal, ready to release; (d) the binding of the activated calcium-binding protein to the docked vesicles leads to the release of n molecules of transmitter in the synaptic cleft. The latter process is modeled here as a first-order process with a stoichiometry coefficient of n (see details in Destexhe, Mainen, and Sejnowski 1994b).

The calcium-induced cascade leading to the release of transmitter was described by the following kinetic scheme:

$$4\,Ca^{2+} + X \underset{k_u}{\overset{k_b}{\rightleftarrows}} X^* \tag{1.1}$$

$$X^* + V_e \underset{k_2}{\overset{k_1}{\rightleftarrows}} V_e^* \xrightarrow{k_1} nT. \tag{1.2}$$

Calcium ions bind to a calcium-binding protein, X, with a cooperativity factor of 4 (see Augustine and Charlton 1986; and references therein), leading to an activated calcium-binding protein, X^* (eq. 1.1). The associated forward and backward rate constants are k_b and k_u. X^* then reversibly binds to transmitter-containing vesicles, V_e, with corresponding rate constants k_1 and k_2 (eq. 1.2). The last step of this reaction, governed by rate constant k_3, represents the (irreversible) release of n molecules of transmitter, T, from the activated vesicles into the synaptic cleft. The values of the parameters in this reaction scheme were based on previous models and measurements (Yamada and Zucker 1992).

The concentration of the liberated transmitter in the synaptic cleft, $[T]$, was approximated as follows. $[T]$ was assumed to be uniform in the cleft and cleared by processes of diffusion outside the cleft (to the extrajunctional extracellular space), uptake, or degradation. These contributions were modeled by the first-order reaction

$$T \xrightarrow{k_c} \cdots,\qquad(1.3)$$

where k_c is the rate constant for clearance of T. The values of rate constants were $k_b = 10^5\,\text{sec}^{-1}\,\text{mM}^{-4}$, $k_u = 100\,\text{sec}^{-1}$, $k_1 = 10^6\,\text{sec}^{-1}\,\text{mM}^{-1}$, $k_2 = 100\,\text{sec}^{-1}$, $k_3 = 4{,}000\,\text{sec}^{-1}$, $V_e = 0.01\,\text{mM}$, $k_c = 10^4\,\text{sec}^{-1}$ with a maximal concentration of calcium-binding proteins of 0.001 mM, and the number of transmitter molecules per vesicle was $n = 10{,}000$ (see Destexhe, Mainen, and Sejnowski 1994b).

Figure 1.1 shows a simulation of this model of transmitter release associated to a single compartment presynaptic terminal containing mechanisms for action poten-

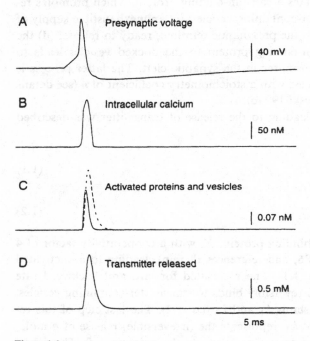

Figure 1.1
Kinetic model of presynaptic release. (A) A presynaptic action potential was elicited by injection of a 0.1 nA current pulse lasting 2 msec in the presynaptic terminal. (B) Intracellular Ca^{2+} concentration in the presynaptic terminal. A high-threshold calcium current was also present and provided a transient calcium influx during the action potential. Removal was provided by an active calcium pump. (C) Relative concentration of activated calcium-binding protein X^* (solid line) and vesicles V_e^* (dotted line). (D) Concentration of transmitter in the synaptic cleft. Modified from Destexhe, Mainen, and Sejnowski 1994b.

tials, high-threshold calcium currents, and calcium dynamics (see Destexhe, Mainen, and Sejnowski 1994b for details). Injection of a short current pulse into the presynaptic terminal elicited a single action potential (figure 1.1A). The depolarization of the action potential activated high-threshold calcium channels, producing a rapid influx of calcium. The elevation of intracellular $[Ca^{2+}]$ (figure 1.1B) was transient due to clearance by an active pump. Figure 1.1C shows that the time course of activated calcium-binding proteins and vesicles followed closely the time course of the transient calcium rise in the presynaptic terminal. This resulted in a brief (≈ 1 msec) rise in transmitter concentration in the synaptic cleft (figure 1.1D). The rate of transmitter clearance was adjusted to match the time course of transmitter release estimated from patch clamp experiments (Clements et al. 1992; Clements 1996) as well as for detailed simulations of the extracellular diffusion of transmitter (Bartol et al. 1991; Destexhe and Sejnowski 1995).

1.2.2 Further Simplification of the Release Process

The above-described release model would be computationally very expensive if it had to be used in simulations involving thousands of synapses. Therefore, for simulating large-scale networks, simplification of the release process is needed.

The first alternative is to use a continuous function to transform the presynaptic voltage into transmitter concentration (Destexhe, Mainen, and Sejnowski 1994b). This approach assumes that all intervening reactions in the release process are relatively fast and can be considered in steady state. The stationary relationship between the transmitter concentration $[T]$ and presynaptic voltage was fit to

$$[T](V_{pre}) = \frac{T_{max}}{1 + \exp[-(V_{pre} - V_p)/K_p]}, \tag{1.4}$$

where T_{max} is the maximal concentration of transmitter in the synaptic cleft, V_{pre} is the presynaptic voltage, $K_p = 5\,\text{mV}$ gives the steepness, and $V_p = 2\,\text{mV}$ sets the value at which the function is half-activated. One of the main advantages of using eq. 1.4 is that it provides a very simple and smooth transformation between presynaptic voltage and transmitter concentration. This form, in conjunction with simple kinetic models of postsynaptic channels, provides a model of synaptic interaction based on autonomous differential equations with only one or two variables (see also Wang and Rinzel 1992).

The second alternative is to assume that the change in the transmitter concentration occurs in a brief pulse (Destexhe, Mainen, and Sejnowski 1994a). This procedure is considered in more detail in section 1.4.

1.3   Markov Models of Postsynaptic Currents

Conventional synaptic transmission in the central nervous system is mediated by excitatory and inhibitory amino acid neurotransmitters, glutamate and GABA, respectively. Glutamate activates AMPA/kainate receptors, responsible for most fast excitatory transmission, and NMDA receptors, whose activation is both much slower than that of AMPA/kainate receptors and whose voltage dependence may be involved in synaptic plasticity. GABA also activates two classes of receptors, $GABA_A$ receptors, which have relatively fast kinetics, and $GABA_B$ receptors, which are much slower and involve second messengers.

It is important to note that there exists a considerable range of physiological subtypes within a given receptor class that arise from the exact molecular composition of the receptor. Most important, it has been shown that various properties of receptors are altered by variations in the particular subunits that make up a receptor. For example, NMDA receptor properties depend on the NR2 subunit type (A, B, C, or D), which alters the Mg^{2+} sensitivity and kinetics of the channel (Monyer et al. 1994). Similarly, the presence of the GluR-B subunit determines the Ca^{2+} permeability of AMPA receptors (Jonas et al. 1994), while the GluR-B and GluR-D subunits affect their desensitization (Mosbacher et al. 1994). It has been shown that interneurons and principal cells express AMPA receptor channels with distinct subunit composition and hence distinct properties—interneurons express faster, more Ca^{2+}-permeable AMPA receptors (Geiger et al. 1995). The subunit composition of receptors in different cell types and brain regions is currently the subject of intense study (see reviews by McKerran and Whiting 1996; Huntley, Vickers, and Morrison 1994; Molinoff et al. 1994; Zukin and Bennett 1995). Although the results of these molecular studies will undoubtedly continue to shape our understanding, for the purposes of this chapter, we will focus on the general classes of receptors and their prototypical properties.

Study of central synapses is hampered by inaccessibility, rapid kinetics, the difficulty of measuring or controlling the time course of neurotransmitter, and the electrotonically remote location of synapses from somatic recording sites. Nevertheless, progress in understanding the gating of these receptors has been made through the fast perfusion of transmitter to excised membrane patches containing receptors (Franke, Hatt, and Dudel 1987). With these and other methods, it has been shown that the time course of neurotransmitter in the synaptic cleft is very brief (Clements et al. 1992; Clements 1996) and that the kinetics of the postsynaptic receptor are responsible for the prolonged time course of the slower synaptic currents (Lester et al. 1990).

Detailed models of synaptic currents based on activation by a very brief increase in transmitter concentration must capture three main aspects of receptor gating kinetics:

• *Activation/binding.* The time course of the rising phase of the synaptic current can be determined either by the rate of opening after transmitter is bound to the receptor or, at low concentrations, by the amount of transmitter present. The rising phase can be delayed (made more sigmoidal) by requiring more than one transmitter molecule to be bound (analogous to the gating of the "delayed-rectifier" potassium channel).

• *Deactivation/unbinding.* The time course of decay can be determined by either deactivation following transmitter removal or desensitization (see below). The rate of deactivation is limited either by the closing rate of the receptor or, typically, by the rate of unbinding of transmitter from the receptor.

• *Desensitization.* Synaptic receptor-gated channels can be closed by entering a "desensitized" state analogous to the "inactivated" states of voltage-gated channels. Desensitization decreases the fraction of channels that open during a synaptic response and can affect the synaptic time course in several ways, including prolonging the decay time and shortening the rise time.

Because there are a finite number of channels at the postsynaptic membrane and they may have multiple closed and desensitized states, the dynamics that occur during a sequence of rapid activations can be complex:

• *Priming.* Due to slow activation kinetics, a pulse of neurotransmitter may bind to but not open a channel; this can prime the receptor for response to a subsequent pulse. For $GABA_B$ responses, this priming can occur through G-proteins on the K^+ channels (Destexhe and Sejnowski 1995; see section 1.3.4).

• *Desensitization.* A response that leads to significant desensitization may leave many receptors unable to open when neurotransmitter is released again shortly thereafter, causing a progressive decline in responsivity.

• *Saturation.* When a large fraction of receptors are bound by an initial pulse of neurotransmitter, subsequent pulses can produce greatly diminished responses because most channels are already open.

Thus receptor kinetics are important not only in determining the time course of individual synaptic events but also in the temporal integration during a sequence of synaptic events. In the following subsections, we review detailed kinetic schemes for the main receptor types mediating synaptic transmission in the central nervous system.

1.3.1 AMPA/Kainate Receptors

AMPA/kainate receptors mediate the prototypical fast excitatory synaptic currents in the brain. In specialized auditory nuclei, AMPA/kainate receptor kinetics may be extremely rapid with rise and decay time constants in the submillisecond range (Raman, Zhang, and Trussell 1994). In the cortex and hippocampus, responses are somewhat slower (e.g., Hestrin, Sah, and Nicoll 1990). The 10%–90% rise time of the fastest currents measured at the soma (representing those with least cable filtering) is 0.4 to 0.8 msec in cortical pyramidal neurons, while the decay time constant is about 5 msec (e.g., Hestrin 1993). It may be worth noting that inhibitory interneurons express AMPA receptors with significantly different properties. First, they are about twice as fast in rise and decay time as those on pyramidal neurons (Hestrin 1993), and second, they have a significant Ca^{2+} permeability (Koh et al. 1995). The latter property appears to be conferred by the lack of the GluR-B subunit in these receptors.

The rapid time course of AMPA/kainate responses is thought to be due to a combination of rapid clearance of neurotransmitter and rapid channel closure (Hestrin 1992). Desensitization of these receptors does occur but is somewhat slower than deactivation. The physiological significance of AMPA receptor desensitization has not been well established. Although desensitization may contribute to the fast synaptic depression observed at neocortical synapses (Thomson and Deuchars 1994; Markram and Tsodyks 1996), a study of paired-pulse facilitation in the hippocampus suggested a minimal contribution of desensitization even at 7 msec intervals (Stevens and Wang 1995).

A Markov kinetic model that accounts for these properties was introduced by Patneau and Mayer (1991; see also Jonas, Major, and Sakmann 1993) and had the following state diagram:

$$C_0 \underset{R_{u_1}}{\overset{R_b T}{\rightleftharpoons}} C_1 \underset{R_{u_2}}{\overset{R_b T}{\rightleftharpoons}} C_2 \underset{R_c}{\overset{R_o}{\rightleftharpoons}} O$$
$$R_d \big\Updownarrow R_r \qquad R_d \big\Updownarrow R_r \qquad\qquad (1.5)$$
$$D_1 \qquad\qquad D_2,$$

where the unbound form of the receptor C_0 binds to one molecule of transmitter T, leading to the singly bound form C_1, which itself can bind another molecule of T leading to the doubly bound form C_2. R_b is the binding rate, and R_{u_1} and R_{u_2} are unbinding rates. Each form C_1 and C_2 can desensitize, leading to forms D_1 and D_2, with rates R_d and R_r for desensitization and resensitization, respectively. Finally, the

Figure 1.2
Best fits of detailed kinetic models to averaged postsynaptic currents obtained from whole-cell recordings. (A) AMPA/kainate-mediated currents (obtained from Xiang, Greenwood, and Brown 1992; recorded at 31° C). (B) NMDA-mediated currents (obtained from Hessler and Malinow 1993; recorded at 22°–25° C in Mg^{2+}-free solution). (C) GABA$_A$-mediated currents. (D) GABA$_B$-mediated currents (data in panels C–D recorded at 33°–35° C by Otis, De Koninck, and Mody 1992, 1993). For all graphs, the averaged recording of the synaptic current (noisy trace) is represented with the best fit obtained using the models (continuous trace). Models are described in the text; transmitter release was modeled as in figure 1.1. Panel D modified from Destexhe and Sejnowski 1995; fitting procedures described in chapter appendix B.

doubly bound receptor C_2 can open, leading to the open form O, with opening and closure rates of R_o and R_c, respectively. This model was simulated with the mechanism for transmitter release described in section 1.2.1, and its parameters were optimized by direct fitting of the full model to whole-cell recorded AMPA currents (see chapter appendix B). The fitting procedure gave the following values for the rate constants (figure 1.2A): $R_b = 13 \times 10^6\,\mathrm{M}^{-1}\,\mathrm{sec}^{-1}$, $R_{u_1} = 5.9\,\mathrm{sec}^{-1}$, $R_{u_2} = 8.6 \times 10^4\,\mathrm{sec}^{-1}$, $R_d = 900\,\mathrm{sec}^{-1}$, $R_r = 64\,\mathrm{sec}^{-1}$, $R_o = 2.7 \times 10^3\,\mathrm{sec}^{-1}$, and $R_c = 200\,\mathrm{sec}^{-1}$.

The AMPA current is then given by

$$I_{AMPA} = \bar{g}_{AMPA}[O](V - E_{AMPA}), \tag{1.6}$$

where $\bar{g}_{AMPA}$ is the maximal conductance, $[O]$ the fraction of receptors in the open state, V the postsynaptic voltage, and $E_{AMPA} = 0\,\mathrm{mV}$ the reversal potential. In

neocortical and hippocampal pyramidal cells, measurements of miniature synaptic currents (10–30 pA amplitude; see McBain and Dingledine 1992; Burgard and Hablitz 1993) and quantal analysis (e.g., Stricker, Field, and Redman 1996) lead to estimates of maximal conductance around 0.35 to 1.0 nS for AMPA-mediated currents in a single synapse.

1.3.2 NMDA Receptors

NMDA receptors mediate synaptic currents that are substantially slower than AMPA/kainate currents, with a rise time of about 20 msec and decay time constants of about 25 msec and 125 msec at 32° C (Hestrin, Sah, and Nicoll 1990). The slow kinetics of activation is due to the requirement that two agonist molecules must bind to open the receptor, as well as a relatively slow channel opening rate of bound receptors (Clements and Westbrook 1991). The slowness of decay is believed to be due primarily to slow unbinding of glutamate from the receptor (Lester and Jahr 1992; Bartol and Sejnowski 1993). The open probability of an NMDA channel at the peak of a synaptic response has been estimated to be as high as 0.3 (Jahr 1992), raising the possibility that significant saturation of synaptic NMDA receptors may occur during high-frequency stimulus trains.

A unique and important property of the NMDA receptor channel is its sensitivity to block by physiological concentrations of Mg^{2+} (Nowak et al. 1984; Jahr and Stevens 1990a, 1990b). The Mg^{2+} block is voltage-dependent, allowing NMDA receptor channels to conduct ions only when depolarized. The necessity of both presynaptic and postsynaptic gating conditions (presynaptic neurotransmitter and postsynaptic depolarization) makes the NMDA receptor a molecular coincidence detector. Furthermore, NMDA currents are carried partly by Ca^{2+} ions, which have a prominent role in triggering many intracellular biochemical cascades. Together, these properties are crucial to the NMDA receptor's role in synaptic plasticity (Bliss and Collingridge 1993) and activity-dependent development (Constantine-Paton, Cline, and Debski 1990).

Several kinetic schemes have been proposed for the NMDA receptor (Clements and Westbrook 1991; Lester and Jahr 1992; Edmonds and Colquhoun 1993; Clements et al. 1992; Hessler, Shirke, and Malinow 1993). These models were essentially based on the same state diagram:

$$C_0 \underset{R_u}{\overset{R_b T}{\rightleftharpoons}} C_1 \underset{R_u}{\overset{R_b T}{\rightleftharpoons}} C_2 \underset{R_c}{\overset{R_o}{\rightleftharpoons}} O$$
$$R_d \big\updownarrow R_r$$
$$D.$$

$$(1.7)$$

This kinetic scheme is similar to that of AMPA receptors (eq. 1.5), with only one desensitized form of the receptor (D) and a single unbinding rate R_u. Direct fitting of this model to whole-cell recorded NMDA currents (in free Mg^{2+}; see below) gave the following values for the rate constants (figure 1.2B): $R_b = 5 \times 10^6 \, M^{-1} \, sec^{-1}$, $R_u = 12.9 \, sec^{-1}$, $R_d = 8.4 \, sec^{-1}$, $R_r = 6.8 \, sec^{-1}$, $R_o = 46.5 \, sec^{-1}$ and $R_c = 73.8 \, sec^{-1}$.

The NMDA current is then described by

$$I_{NMDA} = \bar{g}_{NMDA} \, B(V) \, [O] \, (V - E_{NMDA}), \tag{1.8}$$

where $\bar{g}_{NMDA}$ is the maximal conductance, $B(V)$ the magnesium block (see below), $[O]$ the fraction of receptors in the open state, V the postsynaptic voltage, and $E_{NMDA} = 0 \, mV$ the reversal potential.

Miniature excitatory synaptic currents also have an NMDA-mediated component (McBain and Dingledine 1992; Burgard and Hablitz 1993), and the conductance of dendritic NMDA channels has been reported to be a fraction of AMPA channels, between 3% and 62% (Zhang and Trussell 1994; Spruston, Jonas, and Sakmann 1994), leading to estimates of the maximal conductance of NMDA-mediated currents at a single synapse around $\bar{g}_{NMDA} = 0.01\text{–}0.6 \, nS$.

The magnesium block of the NMDA receptor channel is an extremely fast process compared to the other kinetics of the receptor (Jahr and Stevens 1990a, 1990b). The block can therefore be accurately modeled as an instantaneous function of voltage (Jahr and Stevens 1990b):

$$B(V) = \frac{1}{1 + \exp(-0.062V)[Mg^{2+}]_o / 3.57}, \tag{1.9}$$

where $[Mg^{2+}]_o$ is the external magnesium concentration (1 to 2 mM in physiological conditions).

1.3.3 GABA$_A$ Receptors

Most fast inhibitory postsynaptic potentials (IPSP$_s$) are mediated by GABA$_A$ receptors in the central nervous system. GABA$_A$-mediated IPSPs are elicited following minimal stimulation, in contrast to GABA$_B$ responses, which require strong stimuli (see section 1.3.4). GABA$_A$ receptors have a high affinity for GABA and are believed to be saturated by release of a single vesicle of neurotransmitter (see Mody et al. 1994; Thompson 1994). GABA$_A$ receptors have at least two binding sites for GABA and show a weak desensitization (Busch and Sakmann 1990; Celentano and Wong 1994). However, blocking uptake of GABA reveals prolonged GABA$_A$ currents that last for more than a second (Thompson and Gähwiler 1992; Isaacson,

Solis, and Nicoll 1993), suggesting that, as with AMPA/kainate receptors, deactivation following transmitter removal is the main determinant of the decay time.

We used the kinetic model introduced by Busch and Sakmann (1990) for GABA$_A$ receptors based on the following state diagram:

$$C_0 \underset{R_{u_1}}{\overset{R_{b_1}T}{\rightleftharpoons}} C_1 \underset{R_{u_2}}{\overset{R_{b_2}T}{\rightleftharpoons}} C_2$$

$$R_{o_1} \Updownarrow R_{c_1} \quad R_{o_2} \Updownarrow R_{c_2}$$

$$O_1 \qquad O_2 \tag{1.10}$$

Here, the transmitter GABA (T) binds to the unbound form C_0, leading to singly bound C_1 and doubly bound form C_2, with binding and unbinding rates R_{b_1}, R_{u_1}, R_{b_2} and R_{u_2} respectively. Both singly and doubly bound forms can open, leading to O_1 and O_2 forms with opening and closure rates of R_{o_1}, R_{c_1}, R_{o_2}, and R_{c_2}, respectively. Direct fitting of this model to whole-cell recorded GABA$_A$ currents gave the following values for the rate constants (figure 1.2C): $R_{b_1} = 20 \times 10^6\,\mathrm{M^{-1}\,sec^{-1}}$, $R_{u_1} = 4.6 \times 10^3\,\mathrm{sec^{-1}}$, $R_{b_2} = 10 \times 10^6\,\mathrm{M^{-1}\,sec^{-1}}$, $R_{u_2} = 9.2 \times 10^3\,\mathrm{sec^{-1}}$, $R_{o_1} = 3.3 \times 10^3\,\mathrm{sec^{-1}}$, $R_{c_1} = 9.8 \times 10^3\,\mathrm{sec^{-1}}$, $R_{o_2} = 10.6 \times 10^3\,\mathrm{sec^{-1}}$, and $R_{c_2} = 410\,\mathrm{sec^{-1}}$.

The current is then given by

$$I_{GABA_A} = \bar{g}_{GABA_A}([O_1] + [O_2])(V - E_{Cl}), \tag{1.11}$$

where $\bar{g}_{GABA_A}$ is the maximal conductance, $[O_1]$ and $[O_2]$ the fractions of receptors in the open states, and $E_{Cl} = -70\,\mathrm{mV}$ the chloride reversal potential. Estimation of the maximal conductance at a single GABAergic synapse from miniature GABA$_A$-mediated currents (Ropert, Miles, and Korn 1990; De Koninck and Mody 1994) leads to $\bar{g}_{GABA_A} = 0.25–1.2\,\mathrm{nS}$.

1.3.4 GABA$_B$ Receptors

In the three types of synaptic receptors discussed so far, the receptor and ion channel are both part of the same protein complex. In contrast, other classes of synaptic response are mediated by an ion channel that is not directly coupled to a receptor, but rather is activated (or deactivated) by an intracellular "second messenger" that is produced when neurotransmitter binds to a separate receptor molecule. This is the case for GABA$_B$ receptors, whose response is mediated by K$^+$ channels that are activated by G-proteins (Dutar and Nicoll 1988).

Unlike GABA$_A$ receptors, which respond to weak stimuli, responses from GABA$_B$ responses require high levels of presynaptic activity (Dutar and Nicoll 1988; Davies,

Davies, and Collingridge 1990; Huguenard and Prince 1994). This property might be due to extrasynaptic localization of $GABA_B$ receptors (Mody et al. 1994), but a detailed model of synaptic transmission on GABAergic receptors suggests that this effect could also be due to cooperativity in the activation kinetics of $GABA_B$ responses (Destexhe and Sejnowski 1995; see "Priming" in section 1.3). Typical properties of $GABA_B$-mediated responses in hippocampal and thalamic slices can be reproduced assuming that several G-proteins bind to the associated K^+ channels (Destexhe and Sejnowski 1995), leading to the following scheme:

$$R_0 + T \rightleftharpoons R \rightleftharpoons D \tag{1.12}$$

$$R + G_0 \rightleftharpoons RG \longrightarrow R + G \tag{1.13}$$

$$G \longrightarrow G_0 \tag{1.14}$$

$$C_1 + nG \rightleftharpoons O \tag{1.15}$$

Here the transmitter, T, binds to the receptor, R_0, leading to its activated form, R, and desensitized form, D. The G-protein is transformed from an inactive (GDP-bound) form, G_0, to an activated form, G, catalyzed by R. Finally, G binds to open the K^+ channel, with n independent binding sites. If we assume quasi-stationarity in (1.13) and (1.15), and consider G_0 in excess, then the reduced kinetic equations for this system are

$$\frac{d[R]}{dt} = K_1[T](1 - [R] - [D]) - K_2[R] + K_3[D] \tag{1.16a}$$

$$\frac{d[D]}{dt} = K_4[R] - K_3[D] \tag{1.16b}$$

$$\frac{d[G]}{dt} = K_5[R] - K_6[G] \tag{1.16c}$$

$$I_{GABA_B} = \bar{g}_{GABA_B} \frac{[G]^n}{[G]^n + K_d} (V - E_K), \tag{1.16d}$$

where $[R]$ and $[D]$ are, respectively, the fraction of activated and desensitized receptor, $[G]$ (in μM) the concentration of activated G-protein, $\bar{g}_{GABA_B} = 1\,nS$ the maximal conductance of K^+ channels, $E_K = -95\,mV$ the potassium reversal potential, and K_d the dissociation constant of the binding of G on the K^+ channels. This model accounted accurately for both the time course and the properties of $GABA_B$ responses. Direct fitting of the model to whole-cell recorded $GABA_B$ currents gave the following values (figure 1.2D; Destexhe and Sejnowski 1995): $K_d = 100 \, \mu M^4$, $K_1 = 6.6 \times 10^5 \, M^{-1} \, sec^{-1}$, $K_2 = 20 \, sec^{-1}$, $K_3 = 5.3 \, sec^{-1}$, $K_4 = 17 \, sec^{-1}$, $K_5 = 8.3 \times 10^{-5} \, M \, sec^{-1}$, and $K_6 = 7.9 \, sec^{-1}$, with $n = 4$ binding sites.

As discussed above, $GABA_B$-mediated responses typically require high stimulus intensities to be evoked. Miniature GABAergic synaptic currents indeed never contain a $GABA_B$-mediated component (Otis and Mody 1992; Thompson and Gähwiler 1992; Thompson 1994). As a consequence, $GABA_B$-mediated unitary IPSPs are difficult to obtain experimentally and the estimation of the maximal conductance of $GABA_B$ receptors in a single synapse is difficult. A peak $GABA_B$ conductance of around 0.06 nS was reported using release evoked by local application of sucrose (Otis, De Koninck, and Mody 1992).

1.3.5 Other Neuromodulators

Neurotransmitters including glutamate (through metabotropic receptors), acetylcholine (through muscarinic receptors), norepinephrine, serotonin, dopamine, histamine, opioids, and others have been shown to mediate slow intracellular responses. These neurotransmitters induce the intracellular activation of G-proteins, which may affect ionic currents as well as the metabolism of the cell. As with GABA acting on $GABA_B$ receptors, the main electrophysiological target of many neuromodulators is to open or close K^+ channels (see Brown 1990; Brown and Birnbaumer 1990; McCormick 1992). The model of $GABA_B$ responses could thus be used to model these currents, with rate constants adjusted to fit the time courses reported for the particular responses. However, the data available presently are not precise enough to allow the development of detailed models of these responses. If they are similar in their kinetics to $GABA_B$, then the same model may apply as in eqs. 1.16a–d.

1.4 Simplified Models of Postsynaptic Currents

It is possible to simplify the receptor kinetic models in the previous section to make them computationally more efficient while retaining the most important qualitative properties. It is also possible to greatly simplify the release process that determines the transmitter concentration T.

Voltage clamp recordings in excised membrane patches showed that 1 msec pulses of 1 mM glutamate reproduced PSCs that were quite similar as those recorded in the intact synapse (Hestrin 1992; Colquhoun, Jonas, and Sakmann 1992; Standley, Ramsey, and Usherwood 1993). Assume that the transmitter, either glutamate or GABA, is released according to a pulse when an action potential invades the presynaptic terminal. Then, a two-state (open/closed) kinetic scheme, combined with such a pulse of transmitter, can be solved analytically (Destexhe, Mainen, and Sejnowski 1994a). The same approach also yields simplified algorithms for three-state and higher schemes (Destexhe, Mainen, and Sejnowski 1994b). As a consequence, extremely fast algorithms can be used to simulate most types of synaptic receptors (see also chapter appendix C).

1.4.1 AMPA/Kainate Receptors

The simplest model that approximates the kinetics of the fast AMPA/kainate type of glutamate receptors can be represented by the two-state diagram:

$$C + T \underset{\beta}{\overset{\alpha}{\rightleftharpoons}} O, \tag{1.17}$$

where α and β are voltage-independent forward and backward rate constants. If r is defined as the fraction of the receptors in the open state, it is then described by the following first-order kinetic equation:

$$\frac{dr}{dt} = \alpha[T](1 - r) - \beta r, \tag{1.18}$$

and the postsynaptic current I_{AMPA} is given by

$$I_{AMPA} = \bar{g}_{AMPA} r (V - E_{AMPA}), \tag{1.19}$$

where $\bar{g}_{AMPA}$ is the maximal conductance, E_{AMPA} the reversal potential, and V the postsynaptic membrane potential.

The best fit of this kinetic scheme to whole-cell recorded AMPA/kainate currents (figure 1.3A) gave $\alpha = 1.1 \times 10^6 \, \text{M}^{-1} \, \text{sec}^{-1}$ and $\beta = 190 \, \text{sec}^{-1}$, with $E_{AMPA} = 0 \, \text{mV}$.

1.4.2 NMDA Receptors

The slower NMDA type of glutamate receptors can be represented with a two-state model similar to AMPA/kainate receptors, with a voltage-dependent term representing magnesium block (see section 1.3). Using the scheme in eqs. 1.17 and 1.18, the postsynaptic current is given by

$$I_{NMDA} = \bar{g}_{NMDA} B(V) r (V - E_{NMDA}), \tag{1.20}$$

where $\bar{g}_{NMDA}$ represents the maximal conductance, E_{NMDA} represents the reversal potential, and $B(V)$ represents the magnesium block (same equation as eq. 1.9).

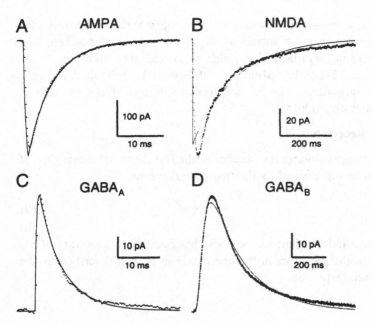

Figure 1.3
Best fits of simplified kinetic models to averaged postsynaptic currents obtained from whole-cell recordings. (A) AMPA/kainate-mediated currents. (B) NMDA-mediated currents. (C) GABA$_A$-mediated currents. (D) GABA$_B$-mediated currents. For all graphs, averaged whole-cell recordings of synaptic currents
(noisy traces; identical description as in figure 1.2) are represented with the best fit obtained using the
simplest kinetic models (continuous traces). Transmitter time course was a pulse of 1 mM and 1 msec duration in all cases. Panel A modified from Destexhe, Mainen, and Sejnowski 1994b; panel C modified from
Destexhe et al. 1994; panel D modified from Destexhe et al. 1996; fitting procedures described in chapter
appendix B.

The best fit of this kinetic scheme to whole-cell recorded NMDA currents (figure
1.3B) gave $\alpha = 7.2 \times 10^4 \, \mathrm{M}^{-1} \, \mathrm{sec}^{-1}$ and $\beta = 6.6 \, \mathrm{sec}^{-1}$, with $E_{NMDA} = 0 \, \mathrm{mV}$.

1.4.3   GABA$_A$ Receptors

GABA$_A$ receptors can also be represented by the scheme in eqs. 1.17 and 1.18, with
the postsynaptic current given by

$$I_{GABA_A} = \bar{g}_{GABA_A} r (V - E_{GABA_A}), \tag{1.21}$$

where $\bar{g}_{GABA_A}$ is the maximal conductance and E_{GABA_A} the reversal potential.

The best fit of this kinetic scheme to whole-cell recorded GABA$_A$ currents (figure
1.3C) gave $\alpha = 5 \times 10^6 \, \mathrm{M}^{-1} \, \mathrm{sec}^{-1}$ and $\beta = 180 \, \mathrm{sec}^{-1}$ with $E_{GABA_A} = -80 \, \mathrm{mV}$.

1.4.4 GABA_B Receptors and Neuromodulators

The stimulus dependency of GABA$_B$ responses, unfortunately, cannot be handled correctly by a two-state model. The simplest model of GABA$_B$-mediated currents has two variables and was obtained from eqs. 1.16a–d:

$$\frac{dr}{dt} = K_1[T](1 - r) - K_2 r \tag{1.22a}$$

$$\frac{ds}{dt} = K_3 r - K_4 s \tag{1.22b}$$

$$I_{GABA_B} = \bar{g}_{GABA_B} \frac{s^n}{s^n + K_d}(V - E_K), \tag{1.22c}$$

where all symbols have the same meaning as in eqs. 1.16a–d, with $r = [R]$ and $s = [G]$. Fitting of this model to whole-cell recorded GABA$_B$ currents (figure 1.3D) gave the following values: $K_d = 100\,\mu M^4$, $K_1 = 9 \times 10^4\,M^{-1}\,sec^{-1}$, $K_2 = 1.2\,sec^{-1}$, $K_3 = 180\,sec^{-1}$ and $K_4 = 34\,sec^{-1}$, with $n = 4$ binding sites.

The main difference between this model and eqs. 1.16a–d is the absence of a desensitized state for the receptor. We found that the desensitized state was necessary to account accurately for the time course of GABA$_B$ currents (figure 1.2D) but had little influence on the dynamical properties of GABA$_B$ responses (see Destexhe et al. 1996).

1.5 Implementation

In this section, we consider the implementation of simplified release processes together with the kinetic models of postsynaptic receptors described in section 1.4. Connecting presynaptic and postsynaptic compartments can be accomplished either by using functions that approximate the release process, such as eq. 1.4, or by using pulses of transmitter. In the first case, the network will be described by autonomous differential equations, which has potentially many applications for mathematical analyses. However, the drawback of this approach is that each synaptic contact gives rise to additional differential equations.

Using pulses of transmitter provides a good alternative if computational efficiency is an important concern. Typically, a pulse of transmitter is triggered at each time the presynaptic voltage crosses a given threshold (0 mV in the present examples). Taking advantage of the pulse, the equations can be solved analytically (see chapter appendix C, "Single Synapse"; Destexhe, Mainen, and Sejnowski 1994a). Therefore, no additional differential equation needs to be solved for postsynaptic currents. In appendix C, "Multiple Synapses," we present an algorithm that allows simulations of models with many synapses on the same compartment to be greatly expedited (Lytton 1996).

1.5.1 Synaptic Summation

The summation of postsynaptic potentials (PSPs) and postsynaptic currents (PSCs) is an important aspect of synaptic signaling. Although alpha functions are often used to represent PSCs in models, these template functions were originally introduced to fit a single PSP (Rall 1967) and consequently are inappropriate for modeling summated postsynaptic events, where they prove computationally inefficient because several waveforms substantially overlap. Kinetic models, on the other hand, provide a natural way to handle summation because receptors properly integrate successive releases of neurotransmitter.

The summation behavior of simple kinetic models is shown in figure 1.4 for the simple models of the four receptor types described in section 1.4. The three transmitter-gated receptor types (AMPA, NMDA, and $GABA_A$) showed PSP amplitudes proportional to the number of presynaptic spikes. In this case, the membrane potential always stayed far from the reversal potential, resulting in a relatively linear summation. However, for $GABA_B$ receptors, the situation is radically different: a single presynaptic spike cannot activate enough G-protein to evoke detectable currents. On the other hand, $GABA_B$-mediated currents are reliably evoked when a burst of ten presynaptic spikes occurs. This nonlinear stimulus dependency is typical of $GABA_B$ receptors (see Destexhe and Sejnowski 1995 for more details).

1.5.2 Connecting Networks

The main application of the simplified kinetic models described in section 1.4 is to build network simulations. Simple kinetic models may not be able to adequately simulate the finest details of synaptic currents, but they can provide a good approximation to some of their features, such as rise, decay, voltage dependence, and summation properties, while maintaining computational efficiency.

We present here an example of a simulation of thalamic oscillations that used the models described in section 1.4 together with presynaptically triggered pulses of transmitter (Destexhe et al. 1996). The occurrence of spindle oscillations depends critically on both intrinsic properties of cells and the types of synaptic receptors present in the circuitry (see Steriade, McCormick, and Sejnowski 1993). The minimal model for these oscillations is shown in Figure 1.5. Two types of cells were present, thalamocortical (TC) relay cells and thalamic reticular (RE) cells. Both thalamic

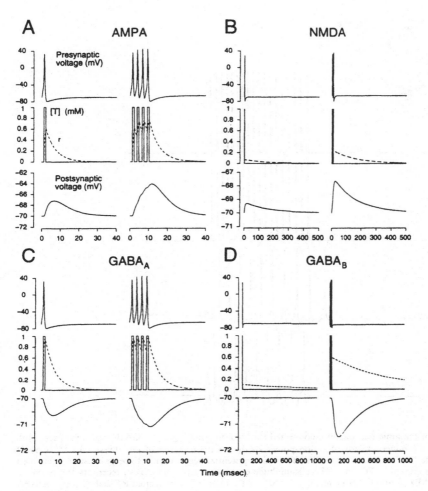

Figure 1.4
Summation of postsynaptic potentials in simplified kinetic models of different receptors. A single-compartment model (10 μm diameter, 10 μm length, 0.2 mS/cm² leak conductance, and −70 mV leak reversal) was provided with postsynaptic receptors (A) AMPA/kainate receptors. (B) NMDA receptors. (C) GABA$_A$ receptors. (D) GABA$_B$ receptors. In all cases, the behavior with one presynaptic spike (left panels) is compared with that of a burst of presynaptic spikes at high frequency (300–400 Hz; 4 spikes in Panels A, B, C; 10 spikes in Panel D). All synaptic conductances were of 0.1 nS; other parameters as in section 1.4.

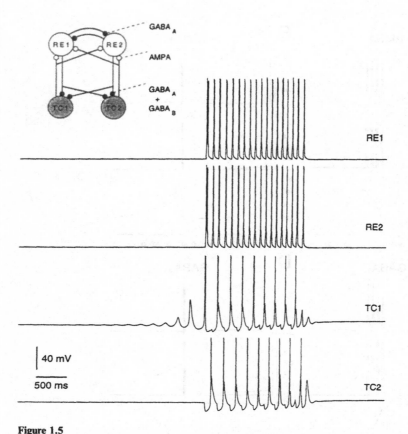

Figure 1.5
Simple circuit of thalamic neurons interconnected through glutamatergic and GABAergic synapses. Both types of neurons produced bursts of action potentials due to the presence of low-threshold Ca^{2+} current and had also Na^+/K^+ currents responsible for action potential generation; a hyperpolarization-activated current (I_h) was present in TC cells. RE cells inhibited each other through $GABA_A$ receptors and provided a mixture of $GABA_A$- and $GABA_B$-mediated IPSPs in TC cells. TC cells excited RE cells through AMPA receptors. This example was taken from a modeling study of thalamic oscillations (Destexhe et al. 1996) and was based on voltage clamp and current clamp data obtained in thalamic slices (Bal, von Krosigk, and McCormick 1995a, 1995b). Oscillations occurred spontaneously in this system and were critically dependent on the kinetics of both intrinsic and synaptic currents. Models of the Hodgkin-Huxley type were used for voltage-dependent currents, and pulse-based kinetic models for synaptic receptors (see section 1.4). All simulations were simulated with NEURON; figure modified from Destexhe et al. 1996.

neurons displayed bursts of action potentials due to the presence of a low-threshold calcium current. Connecting these neurons with AMPA, $GABA_A$, and $GABA_B$ receptors can give rise to oscillations in the network. These behaviors could be simulated using simplified kinetic models for synaptic currents, together with models of the Hodgkin-Huxley type for voltage-dependent currents. The various properties of these oscillations, including the frequency and phase relationships between cells, were within the range of experimental measurements only when realistic values were used for the rise and decay times of synaptic currents (Destexhe et al. 1996).

It must be noted that more complex synaptic interactions can be captured by simplified models involving more than two states. For example, fast synaptic depression of excitatory connections between pyramidal cells (Markram and Tsodyks 1996) can be captured phenomenologically using a three-state kinetic scheme that includes a desensitized state (Destexhe, Mainen, and Sejnowski 1994b). Such a scheme is also analytically solvable, and therefore could also be used as the basis for network simulations that include fast synaptic depression.

Acknowledgments

This research was supported by the Medical Research Council of Canada, Fonds de la Recherche en Santé du Québec, Howard Hughes Medical Institute, Office of Naval Research, and the National Institute of Mental Health. We thank T. Brown, Y. De Koninck, N. A. Hessler, R. Malinow, I. Mody, T. Otis, and Z. Xiang for providing whole-cell recordings.

Appendix A: Kinetic Models of Gating Mechanisms

This appendix formally describes state diagrams for different types of gating, presents the corresponding kinetic equations, and explains how to relate them.

Generally, kinetic models are written as state diagrams

$$S_1 \rightleftharpoons S_2 \rightleftharpoons \cdots \rightleftharpoons S_n, \tag{1.23}$$

where $S_1 \cdots S_n$ represents the various states of the channel. The transition between any pair of states can be written as

$$S_i \underset{r_{ji}}{\overset{r_{ij}}{\rightleftharpoons}} S_j, \tag{1.24}$$

where r_{ij} and r_{ji} are the rate constants that govern the transition between states S_i and S_j. The fraction of channels in state S_i, s_i, obeys the relation

$$\frac{ds_i}{dt} = \sum_{j=1}^{n} s_j r_{ji} - \sum_{j=1}^{n} s_i r_{ij}, \tag{1.25}$$

which is the conventional kinetic equation for the various states of the system.

In the case of voltage-dependent channels, the rate constants will depend on voltage:

$$S_i \underset{r_{ji}(V)}{\overset{r_{ij}(V)}{\rightleftharpoons}} S_j. \tag{1.26}$$

The voltage dependence of the rate constants can always be expressed as

$$r_{ij}(V) = \exp[-U_{ij}(V)/RT], \tag{1.27}$$

where $U_{ij}(V)$ is the free-energy barrier for the transition from state S_i to S_j, R is the gas constant and T is the absolute temperature. The exact form of $U_{ij}(V)$ is in general very difficult to ascertain, and may involve both linear and nonlinear components arising from interactions between the channel protein and the membrane electrical field (Stevens 1978). Assuming a linear dependence of U_{ij} on voltage leads to mono-exponential expressions for the rate constants, which is usually largely sufficient for modeling the voltage dependence of most types of ion channels.

In the case of ligand-gated channels, the transition between unbound and bound states of the channel depends on the concentration of ligand:

$$L + S_i \underset{r_{ji}}{\overset{r_{ij}}{\rightleftharpoons}} S_j. \tag{1.28}$$

Here, L is the ligand, S_i the unbound state, S_j the bound state (sometimes written S_iL), and r_{ij} and r_{ji} rate constants, as defined before. The same reaction can be rewritten as

$$S_i \underset{r_{ji}}{\overset{r_{ij}([L])}{\rightleftharpoons}} S_j, \tag{1.29}$$

where $r_{ij}([L]) = [L]r_{ij}$ and $[L]$ is the concentration of ligand. Written in this form, (1.29) is equivalent to (1.26). Ligand-gating schemes are generally equivalent to voltage-gating schemes, although the functional dependence of the rate constants on $[L]$ is simple compared to the voltage dependence discussed above. For gating processes depending on intracellular calcium, or second messengers such as G-proteins, the functional form is identical to (1.29).

All state diagrams described in sections 1.3 and 1.4 are analogues to eqs. 1.28–1.29 and the kinetic equations of the models are obtained using eq. 1.25. Either of these forms can be used to simulate the behavior of these receptors using NEURON (Hines 1993), which can handle state diagrams as well as differential equations.

It should be noted that the kinetic formalism is limited to the description of macroscopic phenomena, involving a large population of receptors and channels. In the case of smaller systems, in which a limited number of receptors or molecules are involved, a different formalism may be needed. For example, molecular interactions at a single release site may require to simulate the trajectories and binding of individual molecules in a three-dimensional model (Stiles et al. 1996). A general Monte Carlo simulation environment, called "MCELL" (Bartol et al. 1996), has been developed for exploring such models. MCELL focuses on the biochemistry of ligand-effector interactions on the time scale of microseconds to hundreds of milliseconds and the spatial scale of nanometers to tens of micrometers. It is complementary to other neurosimulation tools such as NEURON.

Appendix B: Fitting Kinetic Models to Experimental Data

This appendix briefly describes the methods used to fit the kinetic models to experimental data, as in figures 1.2–1.3.

For simplified kinetic models with two or three states, the time course of the current can be obtained analytically assuming that the transmitter time course follows a pulse (Destexhe, Mainen, and Sejnowski 1994a, 1994b; see appendix C, "Single Synapse"). It is then straightforward to fit this expression to experimental data using a simplex least squares fitting algorithm (see Press et al. 1986). The fitting then leads to very stable and unique values of the parameters from different initial conditions.

In the case of more complex models, the current was obtained by simulating the model and fit to experimental waveforms using the simplex algorithm. At each iteration of the simplex procedure, the model was run and the least square error calculated between model and experimental traces. The optimization procedures controlled and adjusted the model parameters at each iteration, until minimal error was reached. This procedure can be run using built-in features of the NEURON simulator (Hines 1993).

Several sets of initial parameter values must be used in order to check for uniqueness of the optimal values obtained after the fitting procedure. In some cases, the complexity of the models and the large number of parameters can make it impossible to obtain a unique set of values. This indicates that there are not enough constraints in the experimental data to estimate the value of all parameters. In such cases, uniqueness can be achieved when not all parameters are allowed to vary, for example when known parameters, such as the forward binding constant, are fixed. In these conditions, the optimal values for parameter must always be robust to changes in initial values, within a minimal error.

Appendix C: Optimized Algorithms

This appendix gives practical algorithms for calculating synaptic currents with high computational efficiency. These algorithms are applicable to two-state models of postsynaptic currents, such as that mediated by AMPA/kainate, NMDA, and GABA$_A$ receptors (cf. section 1.4).

Single Synapse

The use of a pulse of transmitter allows eq. 1.18 to be analytically solved during each phase of the pulse during which $[T]$ is constant (Destexhe, Mainen, and Sejnowski 1994a). In eq. 1.18, define the following two variables:

$$r_\infty = \frac{\alpha T_{max}}{\alpha T_{max} + \beta} \quad \text{and} \quad \tau_r = \frac{1}{\alpha T_{max} + \beta},$$

where T_{max} is the maximal concentration of the transmitter during the pulse ($T_{max} = 1$ mM here).

The analytical expression for the fraction of open receptors r for each phase of the pulse can be calculated as follows:

1. When the pulse is on ($t_0 < t < t_1$), $[T] = T_{max}$ and r is given by

$$r(t - t_0) = r_\infty + (r(t_0) - r_\infty) \exp[-(t - t_0)/\tau_r]; \tag{1.30}$$

2. When the pulse is off ($t > t_1$), $[T] = 0$, and r is given by

$$r(t - t_1) = r(t_1) \exp[-\beta(t - t_1)]. \tag{1.31}$$

In a backward Euler type of integration scheme, the update rule for each time step Δt is

$$r = r_\infty + (r - r_\infty) \exp[-\Delta t/\tau_r] \quad \text{if } [T] > 0$$
$$r = r \exp[-\beta \Delta t] \qquad\qquad\qquad \text{if } [T] = 0 \tag{1.32}$$

The computational advantage of two-state kinetic models of synaptic currents is therefore that (1) no differential equation needs to be solved; (2) at each time step Δt, only one exponential term is evaluated, independently of the number of spikes received by the synapse. This exponential term can be precalculated, leading to further increase in computational efficiency.

Multiple Synapses

Suppose that the same postsynaptic compartment receives N identical synaptic contacts from N different sources. The synaptic current at each individual contact is

$$I_i = \bar{g}_{syn} r_i (V - E_{syn}), \tag{1.33}$$

where r_i is the fraction of open receptors at synapse i.

Following eq. 1.32, the update rule for computing N synaptic currents at each time step Δt can be written as

$$
\begin{aligned}
r_i &= r_\infty + (r_i - r_\infty) \exp[-\Delta t / \tau_r] \quad &\text{if } [T]_i > 0; \\
r_i &= r_i \exp[-\beta \Delta t] \quad &\text{if } [T]_i = 0.
\end{aligned}
\tag{1.34}
$$

This update rule can be much optimized if all state variables r_i are merged together into two groups for active ($[T]_i > 0$) and inactive ($[T]_i = 0$) synapses, such that

$$R_{on} = \sum_i r_i \quad \text{(such that all } [T]_i > 0); \tag{1.35a}$$

$$R_{off} = \sum_i r_i \quad \text{(such that all } [T]_i = 0), \tag{1.35b}$$

and updated as

$$R_{on} = N_{on} r_\infty + (R_{on} - N_{on} r_\infty) \exp[-\Delta t / \tau_r]; \tag{1.36a}$$

$$R_{off} = R_{off} \exp[-\beta \Delta t], \tag{1.36b}$$

where N_{on} is the number of active synapses.

At each time a pulse of transmitter begins or ends, the variables R_{on} and R_{off} must be changed accordingly. This is easily done because the value of any r_i at any time can be calculated from its value at the time it last changed.

If a spike occurs at a synapse i, the following computations are performed:

$$r_i(t) = r_i(t_0) \exp[-\beta(t - t_0)]; \tag{1.37a}$$

$$R_{on} = R_{on} + r_i(t); \tag{1.37b}$$

$$R_{off} = R_{off} - r_i(t), \tag{1.37c}$$

where t_0 is the time of the preceding event that occurred at synapse i.

When the pulse of transmitter ends, the following computations are performed:

$$r_i(t) = r_\infty + (r_i(t_0) - r_\infty) \exp[-(t - t_0)/\tau_r]; \tag{1.38a}$$

$$R_{on} = R_{on} - r_i(t); \tag{1.38b}$$

$$R_{off} = R_{off} + r_i(t), \tag{1.38c}$$

where t_0 is the time at which the pulse of transmitter started.

This multisynapse algorithm was introduced by Lytton (1996) and allows considerable reduction of execution time for large numbers of synapses. Benchmarks (Lytton 1996) show that this algorithm is much faster than all other existing methods. Calculation of alpha functions, even when optimized (Srinivasan and Chiel 1993), would require at least one exponential to be calculated for each Δt for *each synapse*. For the present algorithm, at each time step Δt, many fewer exponentials are calculated, compared to the number of synapses.

Note that this algorithm can also be formulated for the case of multiple synapses with different conductances by introducing a multiplicative factor to each r_i in eq. 1.35a–b according to its conductance value (see details in Lytton 1996).

Appendix D: Tutorials for Implementing Network Simulations

We have developed tutorial simulations to illustrate the use of kinetic models for building network simulations. These tutorials can be obtained from the Internet at http://www.cnl.salk.edu/~alain/and are running on the publicly available NEURON simulator (Hines 1993; see also chapter 3, this volume).

Tutorial files are available for all models of synaptic currents described in this chapter, including the presynaptic release model, as well as detailed and simplified kinetic models for AMPA, NMDA, $GABA_A$, and $GABA_B$ receptors. Other tutorials illustrate how to implement these models to simulate network of neurons. The simulations provided reproduce some of the figures of published papers (Destexhe et al. 1994, 1996), in which a description of the biological background and the details of the ionic currents is given. A copy of these papers is also available on the Internet at the above address.

2 Cable Theory for Dendritic Neurons

Wilfrid Rall and Hagai Agmon-Snir

2.1 Background

The designation "cable theory" comes from the derivation and application of the cable equation for calculations essential to the first transatlantic telegraph cable, around 1855, by Professor William Thomson (later Lord Kelvin). Having mastered as a student in Paris the mathematical methods pioneered by Fourier, Thomson knew that his one-dimensional cable equation was formally the same partial differential equation (PDE) that Fourier had used to describe the conduction of heat in a wire or in a ring. In the 1870s, Hermann and Weber derived and applied a different PDE (including three-dimensional space in cylindrical coordinates) to the problem of electric current flow in and around a cylindrical core conductor (model of nerve axon); later, around 1900, Hermann and others explicitly recognized that when this core conductor equation is reduced to one spatial dimension, it becomes equivalent to Kelvin's cable equation. More detail and references to early contributions can be found in Brazier 1959, Taylor 1963, and Rall 1977. Experimental testing with single-fiber preparations in the 1930s (associated with the names of Cole and Curtis, Rushton, Hodgkin, Katz, Tasaki, and others) provided important evidence confirming the relevance of cable theory to nerve axons. Two classic papers, which presented derivations of the cable equation for nerve cylinders and included transient solutions as well as methods for estimating the values of key parameters, are Hodgkin and Rushton 1946 and Davis and Lorente de Nó 1947.

The application of cable theory to dendritic neurons began in the late 1950s, when it became necessary to interpret experimental data obtained from individual neurons by means of intracellular microelectrodes located in the neuron soma. Although Coombs, Eccles, and Fatt (1955a, 1955b) did consider current flow to the dendrites in their interpretation of measured input resistance, both they and Frank and Fuortes (1956) neglected the transient cable properties of the dendrites when calculating values for the membrane time constant (τ_m) from their transient data. This resulted not only in erroneously low values for τ_m but also led to complicated proposals designed to explain how synaptic potentials could decay more slowly than would be expected for a passive exponential decay governed by such low τ_m values. The recognition and correction of these errors and misinterpretations depended on the application of cable theory to dendritic neurons (Rall 1957, 1959, 1960). Valuable functional insights and guidance in the design of experiments followed from these cable theory results and from additional studies designed to explore the effects of different synaptic input distributions over the dendritic surface of a neuron (Rall

1962b, 1964, 1967, 1969a, 1969b, 1977; Jack and Redman 1971a, 1971b; Jack et al. 1975; also Rall and Shepherd 1968; Rall and Rinzel 1973; Rinzel and Rall 1974; Koch et al. 1982, 1983; Rall and Segev 1985, 1987; Holmes and Rall 1992a, 1992b; Holmes et al. 1992; Rall et al. 1992; Agmon-Snir and Segev 1993; Cao and Abbott 1993; Major et al. 1993a, 1993b; Agmon-Snir 1995).

Most of the analysis in this chapter is related to passive cables and dendrites (in which the membrane parameters are independent of voltage and time). Given the amount of evidence found for nonlinearities in dendrites, passive cable analysis might seem to be obsolete. However, such a conclusion would be erroneous: the intuition and the methods given by passive cable theory enhance our understanding of the integrative mechanisms even in excitable dendrites. The passive case is an important reference for the excitable case and helps us better understand the role of excitability. Moreover, the passive case is a useful approximation that, analyzed with powerful methods, gives rise to general rules concerning the role of the geometry of the dendritic tree and of the passive biophysical properties (see reviews in Mel 1994 and Segev 1995).

2.2 The Cable Equation

2.2.1 Definitions

The cable equation is a partial differential equation that neurophysiologists usually express as

$$\lambda^2(\partial^2 V/\partial x^2) - V - \tau(\partial V/\partial t) = 0 \qquad (2.1)$$

or, in terms of the dimensionless variables, $X = x/\lambda$ and $T = t/\tau$, as

$$\partial^2 V/\partial X^2 - V - \partial V/\partial T = 0. \qquad (2.2)$$

Here V represents the voltage difference across the membrane (interior minus exterior) as a deviation from its resting value (i.e., $V = V_i - V_e - E_r$), x the distance along the axis of the membrane cylinder, and λ the length constant of the core conductor (defined by eq. 2.13 or 2.14). Although both x and λ are expressed in centimeters or micrometers (cm or μm), their ratio $X = x/\lambda$, represents a dimensionless variable that is proportional to distance. Here also, t represents time and τ, the membrane time constant (sometimes also expressed as τ_m) of the passive membrane (defined by eq. 2.12). Although both t and τ are expressed in seconds or milliseconds (sec or msec), their ratio, $T = t/\tau$, represents a dimensionless variable that is proportional to time.

For a DC steady state, $\partial V/\partial t = 0$; the cable equation reduces to an ordinary differential equation (ODE) that can be expressed

$$d^2V/dX^2 - V = 0. \tag{2.3}$$

Many useful results, such as cable input resistance and steady-state voltage attenuation with distance, can be obtained most simply from solutions of eq. 2.3 for various boundary conditions (see section 2.3).

For AC (sinusoidal) steady states and for the Laplace transform domain, the cable equation becomes reduced to a somewhat different ODE, namely,

$$d^2\hat{V}/dX^2 - q^2\hat{V} = 0, \tag{2.4}$$

where $\hat{V}$ and q are both complex variables (with real and imaginary parts, implying a modulus and a phase angle). For AC steady states, $q^2 = 1 + j\omega\tau$, where $j = \sqrt{-1}$ and ω is the angular frequency $2\pi f$; solutions in this domain can be used to obtain expressions for AC admittance, impedance, and transfer functions (for examples, see appendices of Rall 1960; Rall and Rinzel 1973; Rall and Segev 1985). In the Laplace transform domain, $q^2 = 1 + \tau s$, where the complex variable s (sometimes called "complex frequency") is used to define the relation of $\hat{V}(X, s)$ in the Laplace transform domain to $V(X, t)$ in the time domain (for explanations, see the mathematical appendix of Jack et al. 1975 or a textbook on Laplace transforms; see also section 2.6.4); solutions in this domain can be used to obtain expressions or numerical algorithms for the solutions to various boundary value problems (Rall 1960; Rinzel and Rall 1974; Rall and Segev 1985; Jack and Redman 1971; Jack et al. 1975; Barrett and Crill 1974; Butz and Cowan 1974; Horwitz 1981, 1983; Koch and Poggio 1985; Holmes 1986; Agmon-Snir, 1995).

2.2.2 Assumptions and Derivation for Cable Equation

Nerve axons and dendrites consist of thin tubes of nerve membrane, often idealized as cylinders. They have been referred to as "core conductors" because both the intracellular cytoplasmic core and the extracellular fluid are ionic media that conduct electric current. What is important conceptually is that for short lengths (i.e., short compared with λ, but many times the cylinder diameter), the resistance to electric current flow across the membrane is much greater than the resistance along the interior core, or along the exterior; the electric current inside the core conductor therefore tends to flow parallel to the cylinder axis for a considerable distance before a significant fraction leaks across the membrane. When we formulate this concept mathematically, with a focus on only one spatial dimension, we are led to the cable equation.

Here we begin by assuming a uniform cylindrical core conductor having a length many times its diameter. That means uniform membrane properties (resistivity, capacitance, and electromotive force and a uniform intracellular resistance, r_i, per unit length of the core conductor. One key assumption of one-dimensional cable theory is that the intracellular voltage, V_i, is a function of only two variables, the time, t, and the distance, x, along the axis of the core conductor. A related key assumption is that the gradient of the intracellular potential can be expressed

$$\frac{\partial V_i}{\partial x} = -i_i r_i, \tag{2.5}$$

where i_i represents the intracellular current (core current), taken as positive when flowing to the right (in the direction of increasing values of x), and r_i is the intracellular resistance per unit length noted above. Note that eq. 2.5 can be obtained from panels A and B of figure 2.1, by taking the limit of $\Delta V_i / \Delta x$, as Δx approaches zero.

The assumption of a uniform core conductor, or uniform cable, implies that r_i is a constant, independent of x and t; consequently, when eq. 2.5 is differentiated with respect to x, we obtain

$$\partial^2 V_i / \partial x^2 = -r_i (\partial i_i / \partial x). \tag{2.6}$$

This second derivative of V_i with respect to x can be thought of as a one-dimensional Laplacian of V_i; its relation to the membrane current density is illustrated in figure 2.1C–D and described next. (1) If the core current remains unchanged over a length increment, Δx, then $\partial i_i / \partial x = 0$ and the Laplacian of V_i is zero; no current flows in or out across the membrane (along this Δx) because the core current into this core increment equals the core current out. (2) If the core current decreases over the length increment, Δx, then $\partial i_i / \partial x$ is negative and the Laplacian of V_i is positive; in this case, more core current flows in from the left than out to the right, implying that current must flow out across the membrane (unless this amount of current is drawn off by an electrode placed in the cylinder). (3) If the core current increases over the length increment, Δx, then $\partial i_i / \partial x$ is positive and the Laplacian of V_i is negative; in this case, more core current flows out to the right than flows in from the left, implying that current must flow in across the membrane (unless this amount of current is supplied by an electrode placed in the cylinder). In order words, when there is no current supplied by an intracellular electrode, continuity of current requires that the membrane current density, per unit length of cylinder (taken positive outward), be

$$i_m = -\partial i_i / \partial x. \tag{2.7}$$

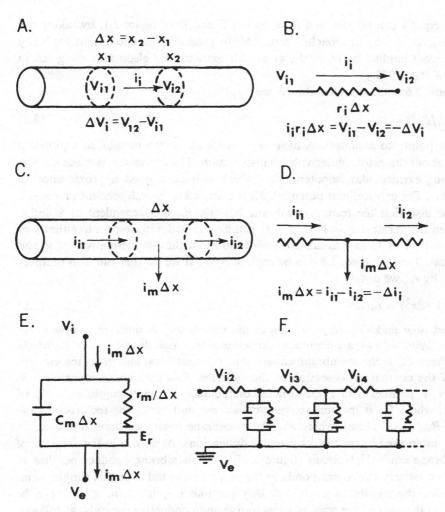

Figure 2.1
Diagrams related to cable equation derivation. Panels A and B illustrate core current flow along core resistance, with focus on the length increment, Δx, and the corresponding increment in intracellular voltage (see eq. 2.5). Panels C and D illustrate the relation of membrane current density to change in core current (see eqs. 2.6–2.7). Panel E shows equivalent electric circuit for membrane (see eq. 2.10). Panel F shows ladder network providing lumped parameter approximation to a continuous cable. From Rall 1977.

Note that eq. 2.7 can be obtained from panels C and D of figure 2.1, by taking the limit of $\Delta i_i / \Delta x$, as Δx approaches zero. (More general expressions that explicitly include current applied by intracellular and/or extracellular electrodes are given in figure 17 of Rall 1977.)

When eqs. 2.6 and 2.7 are combined, we have

$$(1/r_i)(\partial^2 V_i / \partial x^2) = i_m. \tag{2.8}$$

Up to this point, no assumptions have been made about the membrane equivalent circuit or about the extracellular voltage distribution. The derivation is made simpler by assuming extracellular isopotentiality (which is quite a good approximation in many cases). The extracellular potential, V_e, is assumed to be independent of x and t; we assume also that the resting membrane battery, E_r, is independent of x and t. Then, when the variable $V = V_i - V_e - E_r$ is differentiated with respect to either x or t, the derivatives of V_e and E_r are zero, with the result that the derivatives of V and V_i are equal. Thus V_i in eq. 2.8 can be replace by V. If we do this and also multiply both sides by r_m, we obtain

$$(r_m/r_i)(\partial^2 V / \partial x^2) = i_m r_m. \tag{2.9}$$

We must now make assumptions about the membrane. A uniform *passive* nerve membrane cylinder has a membrane capacitance per unit length, $c_m = C_m \pi d$ (in F/cm), where C_m is the membrane capacitance per unit area, and πd is the circumference of the circular cross section of the cylinder. This membrane capacitance is electrically in parallel with a membrane conductance per unit length, $g_m = G_m \pi d$ (in S/cm), where G_m is membrane conductance per unit area. The reciprocal, $r_m = (1/g_m) = R_m/\pi d$ (in Ω cm), where R_m, the membrane resistance times unit area (in Ω cm^2), is often used in spite of its peculiar dimensions. As shown in the diagram of the membrane equivalent circuit (figure 2.1E), the membrane conductance lies in series with a battery that corresponds to the resting potential. For this simple membrane model, the membrane current density per unit length, i_m (in A/cm), can be expressed as the sum of the parallel capacitative and conductive currents, as follows:

$$i_m = c_m(\partial V / \partial t) + (V_i - V_e - E_r)/r_m \tag{2.10}$$

or

$$i_m r_m = \tau_m(\partial V / \partial t) + V, \tag{2.11}$$

where we have made use of the definition of V and the constancy of V_e and E_r, and where τ_m represents the passive membrane time constant, defined as

$$\tau_m = r_m c_m = R_m C_m. \tag{2.12}$$

If we equate eqs. 2.9 and 2.11, the result is the cable equation (2.1), provided that we define λ as

$$\lambda = \sqrt{r_m/r_i} = \sqrt{(R_m/R_i)(d/4)}, \tag{2.13}$$

where r_m (in $\Omega\,$cm) is as defined above, and where $r_i = R_i/(\pi d^2/4)$ (in Ω/cm), R_i is the specific intracellular resistivity (in Ωcm) of the cytoplasm, and d is the diameter of the cylinder.

It should be noted that this expression for λ depends on assuming extracellular isopotentiality. When there is one-dimensional extracellular current flow through a restricted extracellular resistance, r_e, per unit length (in Ω/cm), a more general definition of λ should be used:

$$\lambda = \sqrt{r_m/(r_i + r_e)}. \tag{2.14}$$

This is appropriate for the thin layer of extracellular fluid that results when a non-myelinated axon is placed in oil (Hodgkin and Rushton 1946; see also equations 2.22–2.27 and 3.15–3.22 in Rall 1977). Similar considerations apply also to a population of simultaneously activated core conductors that are closely packed with their axes essentially parallel; then the effective value of r_e per core conductor can be significantly larger than r_i. The relative magnitudes of effective r_e and r_i are important to calculations of extracellular field potentials (see Rall and Shepherd 1968, 887–888; Rall 1970, 558–559; and also Klee and Rall 1977). However, when cable theory is applied to the branches of an individually activated neuron, it is advantageous (and usually justified) to set $r_e = 0$; then eq. 2.14 reduces to eq. 2.13, as it should, because zero extracellular resistivity implies extracellular isopotentiality.

If the value of r_i changes at some value of x (because of a diameter change, a branch point, or a cytoplasmic inhomogenity), then r_i does not have a zero derivative with respect to x, and eq. 2.6 is incomplete and must be replaced by

$$\partial^2 V_i/\partial x^2 = -r_i(\partial i_i/\partial x) - i_i(\partial r_i/\partial x). \tag{2.15}$$

This would complicate the derivation above, implying that the usual cable equation is strictly valid only for uniform stretches of cable. When two adjacent stretches of cable have different properties, they should be regarded as distinct uniform cable segments, each of which satisfies its cable equation along its length. To join these cables mathematically,we must state boundary conditions that provide for continuity of current and voltage (see section 2.2.3). It will be shown below that there exists a family of dendritic branching for which this difficulty disappears because such trees can be transformed to an equivalent cylinder. It should also be noted that when the one-dimensional Laplacian is used in the analysis of extracellular field potentials, an equation similar to eq. 2.15 (with subscript i replaced by subscript e) is applicable, which means that changes in the effective value of r_e must be taken into account, or spurious source (or sinks) may be inferred from experimental data.

2.2.3 Boundary Conditions for the Cable Equation

To solve the cable equation for a particular case, we need to specify the relevant boundary and initial conditions. Here we will formulate in brief the most useful boundary conditions.

A finite cable might have one or two of its ends sealed. The physical meaning of a *sealed-end boundary condition* is that there is no axial (core) current at this end. This implies that $\partial V(x, t)/\partial x = 0$ at this end point (see eq. 2.5).

Another type of condition is the *voltage clamp boundary condition*, formally written as $V(t) = V_C$ at the end point. Two useful cases are $V(t) = 0$ and $V(t) = -E_r$. The first case is usually called by engineers a "short-circuit boundary condition," and sometimes erroneously called a "killed-end boundary condition." Because we have defined $V = V_i - V_e - E_r$ (see section 2.2.1), $V(t) = 0$ implies that $V_i - V_e = E_r$, meaning that the membrane potential difference, $V_i - V_e$, is clamped to its resting value, E_r. In contrast, the second case, $V(t) = -E_r$, implies that $V_i = V_e$. For example, if the resting membrane potential difference is $-70\,\mathrm{mV}$ (interior minus exterior), then a true short circuit of the membrane would make $V(t) = +70\,\mathrm{mV}$.

The *leaky end boundary condition* is defined as $\pm(\partial V(x, t)/\partial x)/r_i = V(x, t)G_L$ at the end point. The physical meaning of this case is that a conductance load, G_L, connects the end of the cable to E_r, the resting potential; $\pm(\partial V(x, t)/\partial x)/r_i$ at the end point is the core current that flows to this point (eq. 2.5), and $V(x, t)G_L$ is the current that flows through the conductance load. The sign depends on whether x increases or decreases toward the end point. For a cable that extends from $x = 0$ to $x = \ell$, a plus sign will be used for a leaky end boundary condition at $x = 0$, and a minus sign will be used for a leaky end boundary condition at $x = \ell$. As we shall see in the next sections, the leaky end boundary condition is used in dendritic tree calculations.

If a current is injected at a sealed end of the cable, we get another type of boundary condition, defined as $\pm(\partial V(x, t)/\partial x)/r_i = I(t)$, where $I(t)$ is the current injected. In such a case the input current must equal the core current that flows from the end point. For a cable that extends from $x = 0$ to $x = \ell$, a minus sign will be used for a current injection at $x = 0$, and a positive sign will be used at $x = \ell$.

Complex boundary conditions can be formulated by combining some of the above boundary conditions. For example, a current can be injected at a leaky end, and the appropriate boundary condition can be easily formulated. Another theoretical, but rather important, boundary condition is used for infinite cables. A popular model is a cable of "semi-infinite" length that extends from $x = 0$ to $x = +\infty$ (this is distinguished from a "fully" or "doubly" infinite length, which extends also to $-\infty$). The *infinite end boundary condition* simply requires that $V(t)$ remain bounded as x approaches ∞. A similar boundary condition is used for a fully infinite cable when x approaches $-\infty$.

When two or more cables are connected at a branch point, the relevant boundary conditions provide for continuity of voltage and conservation of current. If n cables are connected at the branch point, $n - 1$ boundary conditions are used to state that the voltage at the joined ends of the cables is the same. Thus, for three cables, one boundary condition states that $V_{1,end}(t) = V_{2,end}(t)$ (where $V_{j,end}(t)$ is the voltage at the relevant end of cable j), and a second that $V_{2,end}(t) = V_{3,end}(t)$. Another boundary condition states that the sum of the currents from the cables to the branch point is 0 (the current to the branch point from cable j is $\pm(\partial V_j(x_j, t)/\partial x_j)/r_{i,j}$ at the branch point, where $V_j(x_j, t)$ is the voltage along cable j, and $r_{i,j}$ is the intracellular resistance per unit length of cable j). All together, we get n boundary conditions for a branch point of n cables. Usually, a dendritic branch point connects three cables, while a soma might connect any number of cables. In the case of a soma at the branch point (i.e., an isopotential structure), the sum of the currents from the cables to the branch point should be equal to the current that enters the soma, that is, $C_{soma}(\partial V(t)/\partial t) + V(t)G_{soma}$, where C_{soma} and G_{soma} are the capacitance and the conductance of the soma membrane and $V(t)$ is the voltage at the soma (i.e., at the branch point).

2.3   Steady-State Solutions for a Passive Uniform Cable

2.3.1   The Importance of the Steady-State Case

Because the synaptic input is transient, we are most interested in transient analysis of the voltage response in a passive structure. The steady-state case is an important step toward it. First of all, in electrophysiological experiments, long current pulses and voltage clamps are very useful and the analysis of these cases is based partially on the steady-state analysis. Second, in some realistic cases, the synaptic inputs arrive in high frequency; their input can be simulated as a steady current. Third, even for the analysis of a "real" transient input, the insights gained from the steady-state analysis are an important reference. Also, the tools for analyzing the transient case are mainly an extension of steady-state analysis tools. Finally, some of the results of the steady-state case are directly applicable to some properties of the transient case (as the zeroth moment, see section 2.6.5). Hence, the understanding of the tools and results of the steady-state analysis are crucial for understanding the voltage response to a more complicated transient inputs.

2.3.2 General Solution of Ordinary Differential Equation

For DC steady states obtained with steady applied current or voltage, we use mathematical solutions of the ordinary differential equation given above as eq. 2.3. This ODE is homogeneous, linear, and of second order, with constant coefficients. It can have only two linearly independent solutions; its general solution is composed of two such linearly independent solutions, with two arbitrary constants. For any specific application, two boundary conditions are needed to determine the values of the arbitrary constants, and thus provide a unique solution of that particular problem.

The general solution of eq. 2.3 is well known, and can be expressed in several alternative but equivalent forms, as follows:

$$V(X) = A_1 e^X + A_2 e^{-X} \tag{2.16}$$

$$V(X) = B_1 \cosh(X) + B_2 \sinh(X) \tag{2.17}$$

$$V(X) = C_1 \cosh(L - X) + C_2 \sinh(L - X), \tag{2.18}$$

where $\cosh(X) \equiv (e^X + e^{-X})/2$ and $\sinh(X) \equiv (e^X - e^{-X})/2$. Also, L is a constant used to express the electrotonic length, $L = \ell/\lambda$, where ℓ is the actual length of a cable. The hyperbolic functions are very useful for certain boundary conditions. Like the trigonometric cosine, the hyperbolic cosine is an even function that has zero slope and unit magnitude at the origin. Like the trigonometric sine, the hyperbolic sine is an odd function that has unit slope and zero magnitude at the origin. The derivative of $\cosh(X)$ is $\sinh(X)$, and the derivative of $\sinh(X)$ is $\cosh(X)$. Readers may find it a useful exercise to verify that eqs. 2.16–2.18 are indeed solutions of eq. 2.3; some may also wish to verify the following relations between the different pairs of arbitrary constants:

$$2A_1 = B_1 + B_2 = (C_1 - C_2)e^{-L}$$

$$2A_2 = B_1 - B_2 = (C_1 + C_2)e^{+L}.$$

2.3.3   Steady-State Solutions for Different Boundary Conditions

The various boundary conditions for the cable equation are described in section 2.2.3. Here the steady-state solutions are found for some important cases. A good reference case is the semi-infinite cable that extends from $X = 0$ to $X = +\infty$. Suppose, as one boundary condition, a voltage clamp maintains $V = V_0$ at $X = 0$. Suppose also, that our cable is uniform and that it may have recording electrodes but has no current or voltage applied anywhere between $X = 0$ and $X = +\infty$. Then, by the infinite end boundary condition, V remains bounded as X approaches ∞, and thus $A_1 = 0$ in eq. 2.16. The first boundary condition implies that $A_2 = V_0$, and the unique solution of this problem can be expressed simply as

$$V(X) = V_0 e^{-X} = V_0 e^{-x/\lambda}. \tag{2.19}$$

This mathematical result expresses the fact that for a semi-infinite length of uniform cable, the steady-state value of V (departure from resting value) decrements exponentially with distance along the cable (see curve E in figure 2.2). For this semi-infinite case, the length constant, λ, represents the distance over which the voltage decrements to $1/e$ (i.e., $V(x + \lambda)/V(x) = V(X + 1)/V(X) = 1/e$, or about 0.368), and this holds true anywhere along the cable. Given a number of data points, we could plot $\log_e(V/V_0)$ versus x, to fit a straight line whose slope should be $-\lambda$ with respect to x. Although we never actually have a semi-infinite length of cylinder, it may be noted that when a termination is more than four times λ distant from a point of observation, there is negligible difference from the semi-infinite case.

For finite lengths of cable, we must specify both the length and the terminal boundary condition. A sealed end boundary condition at point ℓ is written formally $dV/dx = 0$ at $x = \ell$, or $dV/dX = 0$ at $X = L$. This condition favors the use of eq. 2.18 because the zero slope at $X = L$ implies that $C_2 = 0$. The other boundary condition, usually $V = V_0$ at $X = 0$, then implies that $C_1 = V_0/\cosh(L)$, and the unique solution to this problem is

$$V(X) = \frac{V_0 \cosh(L - X)}{\cosh(L)}, \quad \text{for } dV/dX = 0 \text{ at } X = L. \tag{2.20}$$

In figure 2.2, curves F, H, and J illustrate this solution for three different values of L, 2.0, 1.0, and 0.5, respectively. Note that the sealed end causes all three of these curves to remain above reference curve E. Intuitively, we can view the sealed end as a dam against onward current flow.

This analysis can help us also for the excitable membrane case. We can predict that as an action potential approaches a sealed end, the membrane current density

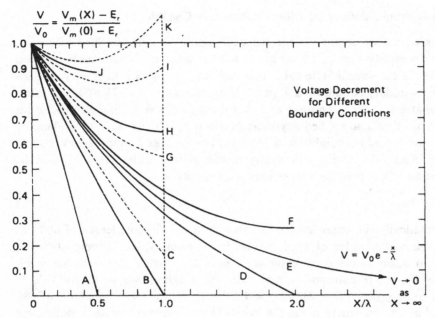

Figure 2.2
Examples of how steady voltage decrement with distance depends on the distal boundary condition. The applied voltage at $X = 0$ is normalized to 1.0 for all curves. Curve E shows an exponential decrement (eq. 2.19) for a semi-infinite length. Curves A, B, and D show steeper decrement (eq. 2.21) obtained when the most distal membrane is clamped to the resting potential, implying that $V = 0$ at $X = L$ for the different L values, 0.5, 1.0, and 2.0, respectively. Curves F, H, and J show less decrement (eq. 2.20) obtained for a sealed-end boundary condition, $dV/dX = 0$ at $X = L$, for the same three L values. Curves C and G both correspond to a leaky boundary condition at $X = 1$, see eq. 2.25 and associated text. Curves I and K both have a voltage-clamped boundary condition at $X = 1$; see eq. 2.22 and associated text. From Rall 1981.

becomes increased, the spike height increases, and the propagation velocity increases with approach to the terminal (see Goldstein and Rall 1974; see also Agmon-Snir and Segev 1993 for analysis of signal propagation in passive structures and its implications for the excitable case). It should be noted that the approach of an action potential to a sealed end is the same as its approach to a collision with an equal and oppositely propagating action potential; the point of collision satisfies the zero slope condition, $dV/dx = 0$.

On the other hand, curves A, B, and D in figure 2.2 correspond to a voltage clamp boundary condition, in this case to the resting potential $(V = 0)$ at $X = L$. This boundary condition implies that $C_1 = 0$ in eq. 2.18; if the other boundary condition is $V = V_0$ at $X = 0$, the unique solution is

$$V(X) = \frac{V_0 \sinh(L-X)}{\sinh(L)}, \quad \text{for clamped } V = 0 \text{ at } X = L, \tag{2.21}$$

which does satisfy the ODE, with $V = V_0$ at $X = 0$, and $V = 0$ at $X = L$. If the voltage clamp at $X = L$ is set to some other voltage, V_L at $X = L$, we must add to eq. 2.21 a solution that is zero at $X = 0$ and equals V_L at $X = L$ (this superposition of solutions is valid because eq. 2.3 is a linear ODE). This can be achieved by setting $B_1 = 0$ in eq. 2.17 and by setting $B_2 = V_L/\sinh(L)$. Combining this solution with eq. 2.21, we obtain

$$V(X) = \frac{V_0 \sinh(L-X) + V_L \sinh(X)}{\sinh(L)}, \tag{2.22}$$

which is the unique solution for the pair of voltage-clamped boundary conditions, $V = V_0$ at $X = 0$, and $V = V_L$ at $X = L$. This solution is illustrated by curves I and K in figure 2.2, for $L = 1$, with $V_L = 0.9V_0$ for curve I, and $V_L = 1.1V_0$ for curve K. Both of these curves exhibit a slope that changes sign because both values of V_L were set above curve H, which has zero slope at $X = L$.

Curves C and G of figure 2.2 differ from the others; they correspond to a leaky boundary condition at $X = L$. The leakage current is assumed proportional to the value of V at $X = L$ and is expressed as $V \cdot G_L$ at $X = L$, where G_L represents the leak conductance at $X = L$. This leak conductance can be larger or smaller than the reference conductance, G_∞ (see section 2.3.4), which corresponds to semi-infinite extension of the same cable (curve E). In figure 2.2, curve C corresponds to $G_L/G_\infty = 4$, while curve G corresponds to $G_L/G_\infty = 1/4$. The solution satisfying such boundary conditions is

$$V(X)/V_L = \cosh(L-X) + (G_L/G_\infty)\sinh(L-X), \tag{2.23}$$

from which it follows that

$$\begin{aligned} V_0/V_L &= \cosh(L) + (G_L/G_\infty)\sinh(L) \\ &= \cosh(L)(1 + (G_L/G_\infty)\tanh(L)) \end{aligned} \tag{2.24}$$

and that

$$\begin{aligned} V(X)/V_0 &= \frac{\cosh(L-X) + (G_L/G_\infty)\sinh(L-X)}{\cosh(L) + (G_L/G_\infty)\sinh(L)} \\ &= \frac{\cosh(L-X)}{\cosh(L)}\left(\frac{1 + (G_L/G_\infty)\tanh(L-X)}{1 + (G_L/G_\infty)\tanh(L)}\right). \end{aligned} \tag{2.25}$$

This type of solution has been very useful in the cable analysis of dendritic trees (see eq. 2.42; chapter 3, this volume).

2.3.4 Input Conductance and Input Resistance

From Ohm's law, the input resistance, R_{in}, at any point of the cable is equal to the ratio of the steady voltage (at that point) to the steady current supplied by the electrode; while the input conductance, G_{in}, is the reciprocal of the input resistance. At the origin of a semi-infinite cable, the input current can flow in only one direction (to the right is the usual convention); the ratio of this steady current to the steady voltage at the origin is known as G_∞, the reference input conductance for a uniform semi-infinite cable. In the case of a doubly infinite cable (extending to $+\infty$ and to $-\infty$), an equal amount of input current flows in both directions away from an input electrode. Thus, for any given steady input voltage, the input current must be twice that for the semi-infinite case, and the input conductance must be twice G_∞. (For nonsymmetric cases, where unequal currents flow to left and right, see Rall 1977, 72–74.)

When current flows only to the right at $X = 0$, the input current at this point must equal the core current that flows to the right at $X = 0$ (see section 2.2.3):

$$I_0 = (1/r_i)(-dV/dx)|_{x=0}. \tag{2.26}$$

For the semi-infinite case, we refer to eq. 2.19, differentiate it with respect to x, substitute in eq. 2.26, and obtain

$$I_0 = (1/\lambda r_i)V_0. \tag{2.27}$$

However, by definition, $I_0 = G_\infty V_0$ for the semi-infinite cable. Hence, $G_\infty = 1/\lambda r_i$. We can rewrite eq. 2.26 now in a very useful way:

$$I_0 = G_\infty(-dV/dX)|_{X=0}. \tag{2.28}$$

Note that eq. 2.28 holds not only for the semi-infinite case but also for other cases, such as those illustrated in figure 2.2. Based on the relation $G_\infty = 1/\lambda r_i$ and eq. 2.13, several equivalent definitions of both R_∞ and G_∞ can be expressed as follows:

$$R_\infty = \lambda r_i = (r_m r_i)^{1/2} = r_m/\lambda$$
$$= (2/\pi)(R_m R_i)^{1/2}(d)^{-3/2} = R_m/(\pi\lambda d) \tag{2.29}$$

and

$$G_\infty = (\lambda r_i)^{-1} = (g_m/r_i)^{1/2} = \lambda g_m$$

$$= (\pi/2)(G_m/R_i)^{1/2}(d)^{3/2} = G_m \pi \lambda d. \qquad (2.30)$$

Useful physical intuition (going back at least to Rushton in the 1930s) may be found in the fact that R_∞ is equal to a λ length of core resistance and that G_∞ is equal to the parallel membrane conductance for an area of membrane equal to a λ length of the cylinder. This should be tempered, however, by the knowledge that the steady-state core current is not constant along this λ length of core, nor is the membrane current density uniform along this λ length of membrane cylinder.

By inspection of the initial slopes of the curves in figure 2.2, we know which cases have input conductances larger or smaller than the reference value provided by G_∞. All of the curves above curve E have initial slopes that are less steep than for the reference case. From eq. 2.28 it follows that their input current values are less than the semi-infinite case and that the input conductance values for these cases are less than G_∞. For example, curves F, H, and J all correspond to sealed ends, for which it is easy to understand that the input conductance must be less than for the reference case. Similarly, all of the curves beneath curve E in figure 2.2 must correspond to cases with input conductance values greater than G_∞.

For the sealed end boundary condition at $X = L$, we refer to eqs. 2.20 and 2.28 and find that $I_0 = G_\infty V_0 \tanh(L)$. From this it follows that the boundary condition at $X = 0$ can be specified either as the applied current or as the applied voltage, because, in the steady state, each implies the other. This also implies the following expressions for input conductance and resistance at $X = 0$:

$$G_{in} = G_\infty \tanh(L), \quad \text{for a sealed end at } X = L \qquad (2.31)$$

and

$$R_{in} = R_\infty \coth(L), \quad \text{for a sealed end at } X = L. \qquad (2.32)$$

When we present input conductance expressions for several different cases, we are confronted with the problem of how to distinguish between them, whether to use identifying subscripts (e.g., in Rall 1977) or to use explicit qualifying words, as done here.

In contrast, for a voltage clamp to resting potential ($V = 0$ at $X = L$), we refer to eqs. 2.21 and 2.28 and get $I_0 = G_\infty V_0 \coth(L)$, which implies

$$G_{in} = G_\infty \coth(L), \quad \text{for clamped } V = 0 \text{ at } X = L \qquad (2.33)$$

and

$$R_{in} = R_{\infty} \tanh(L), \quad \text{for clamped } V = 0 \text{ at } X = L. \tag{2.34}$$

For more general voltage-clamping, at $X = L$, we refer to eqs. 2.22 and 2.28 to get

$$G_{in}/G_{\infty} = \coth(L) - \frac{V_L}{V_0 \sinh(L)} \tag{2.35}$$

for clamped $V = V_L$ at $X = L$, which is relevant to curves I and K of figure 2.2.

For the leaky boundary condition at $X = L$, we refer to eqs. 2.25 and 2.28 to get

$$G_{in}/G_{\infty} = \frac{\tanh(L) + G_L/G_{\infty}}{1 + (G_L/G_{\infty}) \tanh(L)}, \tag{2.36}$$

for leak current, $G_L V_L$ at $X = L$; the expression for R_{in}/R_{∞} is the inverse of this. It may be noted that one limiting case ($G_L = 0$) makes eq. 2.36 become equivalent to eq. 2.31, as it should because $G_L = 0$ is like a sealed end. Also, the other extreme ($G_L = \infty$) makes eq. 2.36 become equivalent to eq. 2.33, as it should because $G_L = \infty$ would clamp $V = 0$ at $X = L$. A third special case ($G_L = G_{\infty}$) makes G_{in}/G_{∞} equal unity, which means that any uniform membrane cylinder of finite length will have the same input conductance as for a semi-infinite length if it is terminated with a leak conductance equal to G_{∞}.

Eq. 2.36 can also apply to the origin ($X = 0$) of the trunk cylinder of a dendritic tree, provided that G_L corresponds to the sum of the input conductances of the branches that arise from this trunk at $X = L$. Note that here (in eqs. 2.23–2.25 and 2.36; also in figure 2.6A, but not in figure 2.6B) we use L to represent the ℓ/λ value of only this trunk, and not the electrotonic length of a dendritic tree, as is often done elsewhere. Below, we use L_D for dendritic trees that are reducible to an equivalent cylinder and L_N for some dendritic neurons.

2.4 Steady-State Solutions for Passive Dendritic Trees

2.4.1 Definitions and Concepts

A dendritic tree can be idealized by treating all branches as cylinders with uniform membrane properties; these cylinders can have different lengths and diameters and different uniform membrane properties. If we also assume extracellular isopotentiality then the ODE of eq. 2.3 holds for each of these cylinders, although the value of λ and of G_{∞} can be different in each cylinder. If R_m and R_i are the same for all cylinders, then λ is proportional to $d^{1/2}$, and G_{∞} is proportional to $d^{3/2}$. The boundary conditions described in section 2.2.3 are used to connect the cylinders and to define the sealed ends of the terminal branches.

As defined above with respect to a single cable, when a steady current input is injected at point x_1 in a tree, the *input resistance* at this point, $R_{in}(x_1)$, is the ratio between the steady voltage at point x_1 and the current input. A more general concept, the *transfer resistance*, $R_{tr}(x_1, x_2)$, is defined as the ratio between the voltage at a given location in the structure (x_2) and the current input at the injection point (x_1). If the current flows in the structure from point x_1 to point x_2, the *attenuation factor* between these points, $A(x_1, x_2)$, is the ratio between the voltage at point x_1 and the voltage at point x_2 (note that $A(x_1, x_2) \geq 1$ in passive structures). It is easy to verify that when a current is injected at point x_1, $R_{tr}(x_1, x_2) \cdot A(x_1, x_2) = R_{in}(x_1)$.

The Concept of Directional Properties at a Point   Several properties can be associated with a point in a dendritic tree. $G_{in}(x_1)$ and $R_{in}(x_1)$, the input conductance and the input resistance at point x_1 in a passive structure, are examples for such properties. $\lambda(x_1)$, the length constant, is another example of a point property; using it, we can define the electrotonic distance between two points in the dendritic tree, x_1 and x_2 as,

$$\int_{x_1}^{x_2} \frac{dx}{\lambda(x_1)} \tag{2.37}$$

where the integral is along the path from x_1 to x_2. On the other hand, some properties are attributes of a point in a structure and a given direction from it. Such properties are called here directional properties, and they are denoted by an arrow above their symbol (these are *not* vectors!!). If we consider, for example, a branch point x_1 in a dendritic tree, there are three available directions for current flow from this point. For every such direction, the directional input conductance, denoted by $\vec{G}_{in}(x_1)$, is defined as the input conductance of the structure (subtree) in this direction (when this structure is isolated). The mathematical relation between $G_{in}(x_1)$ at the branch point and the directional input conductances is $G_{in}(x_1) = \vec{G}_{in,1}(x_1) + \vec{G}_{in,2}(x_1) + \vec{G}_{in,3}(x_1)$, where $\vec{G}_{in,1}(x_1), \vec{G}_{in,2}(x_1), \vec{G}_{in,3}(x_1)$ are the various directional input conductances at point x_1 (see below, the *input conductance property*). In the case of an isopotential structure ("soma") connected to a cylinder, there are two directional input conductances at the soma point: one is the input conductance of the soma alone and the second is the input conductance of the cylinder at the connection point.

We will also use the *attenuation rate* of the voltage at point x_1 in a given direction, $\vec{A}_r(x_1)$, defined as the relative rate of the change in the voltage at this point, when the voltage attenuates in this given direction:

$$\vec{A}_r(x_1) = \left| \frac{\frac{dV(x)}{dx}}{V(x)} \right|_{x=x_1} = \left| \frac{d \ln V}{dx} \right|_{x=x_1}, \tag{2.38}$$

where the derivative is in the direction of interest. Using eq. 2.5 and the definition of $\vec{R}_{in}$, we can show that

$$\vec{A}_r(x_1) = \left| \frac{r_i(x)}{\vec{R}_{in}(x)} \right|_{x=x_1}, \tag{2.39}$$

where the directional input resistance is the input resistance of the structure in the given direction and the intracellular resistance (per unit length) refers to the cylinder connected in the given direction.

2.4.2 Properties of the Steady-State Voltage in Passive Dendritic Trees

The idealized dendritic tree described above can be viewed as a system, whose inputs are current injections and whose output is the voltage response at all the points of the tree. When the differential equations of this system are linear with constant coefficients and with the boundary conditions described, this system is identified as a "continuous time-invariant linear system." Another view of this idealized dendritic tree is as an electrical circuit. The electrical circuit of a cable is described in section 2.2.2, and the connections between the cables are also electrical. Hence, the whole dendritic tree may be viewed as an electrical RC circuit.

These two views of the dendritic tree imply many important properties of the voltage response in the tree. In this section, we describe the properties of the steady-state voltage response (with some notes about the time-dependent case).

Linearity Property   If $V_1(x)$ is the response to a steady current, I_1, injected at a given point x_1 in the tree, and if $V_2(x)$ is the response to a steady current, I_2, injected at a given point x_2 in the tree, then the voltage response when the two currents are injected is $V_1(x) + V_2(x)$. Here $V_1(x)$, $V_2(x)$ are functions of x that assign a steady voltage to every point in the dendritic tree. This result, based directly on the linearity of the dendritic tree, also holds in the transient case. If $V_1(x, t)$ is the response to a current, $I_1(t)$, injected at a given point x_1 in the tree, and if $V_2(x, t)$ is the response to a current, $I_2(t)$, injected at a given point x_2 in the tree, then the voltage response when the two currents are injected is $V_1(x, t) + V_2(x, t)$.

Reciprocity Property   From the reciprocity of RC circuits, we conclude that for any two points in a passive dendritic tree, $R_{tr}(x_1, x_2) = R_{tr}(x_2, x_1)$. This nonintuitive result helps in proving other properties (see below). The reciprocity holds also for the transient case. If the response at point x_2 to a transient input $I(t)$ injected at x_1 is $V_1(x_2, t)$, then if the same current $I(t)$ is injected at x_2, the transient response at x_1, $V_2(x_1, t)$, will be equal to $V_1(x_2, t)$.

Attenuation Rate Property As a direct result from eq. 2.39, we can see that the (directional) attenuation rate in a given direction, $\vec{A}_r(x)$, depends only on the details of the structure in this direction (this is the "downstream" structure, the direction to which the voltage attenuates). Hence, the attenuation rate is independent of the other structures (that are in other directions from point x) and of the location and amplitude of the current injection points (provided that they are not located in the "downstream" structure).

Attenuation Factor Properties The relation between the *attenuation factor*, $A(x_1, x_2)$, and the *attenuation rate*, $\vec{A}_r(x)$, can be expressed

$$\ln(A(x_1, x_2)) = |-\ln(V(x_2)) - \ln(V(x_1))|$$
$$= \left| \int_{x_1}^{x_2} \frac{d\ln(V)}{dx}\, dx \right| = \int_{x_1}^{x_2} \vec{A}_r(x)\, dx. \tag{2.40}$$

This relation and the *attenuation rate property* provide the result that the attenuation factor, $A(x_1, x_2)$, does not depend on the structure "upstream" of point x_1 and of the amplitude and location of the inputs, provided that these are at or "upstream" of point x_1. Another result from eq. 2.40 is that if x_2 is on the path from x_1 to x_3, then $A(x_1, x_3) = A(x_1, x_2) \cdot A(x_2, x_3)$.

From the reciprocity property we can deduce that for two given points in a tree, x_1 and x_2, $R_{in}(x_1)/R_{in}(x_2) = A(x_1, x_2)/A(x_2, x_1)$. Because the input resistance is usually different for every point in the tree, we can conclude that, generally, $A(x_1, x_2)$ is *not equal* to $A(x_2, x_1)$. Practically, in a dendritic tree, the input resistance is much higher in distal points, compared to the input resistance near the soma (or the origin of the dendritic tree). The attenuation factor from a distal point to the soma is much larger than the attenuation factor to the other direction. (For some related intuitions, see section 2.5.4; and in Rall and Rinzel 1973.)

Input Conductance Properties By analogy of the dendritic tree to an electrical circuit, the input conductance at a point is the sum of the various directional input conductances at this point. For the steady-state analysis of a cable connected at one of its ends to a dendritic tree with no current or voltage sources, the boundary condition at the "dendritic" end of the cable can be replaced by a leaky end boundary condition; the leak conductance would be the input conductance of the dendritic tree connected at this end. Input conductance properties will be used in the algorithms described below.

Attenuation Cost and Voltage Clamp Properties That the attenuation factor from a distal point to the soma is larger than the attenuation factor in the other direction may lead to an erroneous conclusion that a distal steady-state current injection has a minor effect on the voltage response at the soma, compared to an identical proximal input. The way to analyze this case correctly is to compare the voltage response at the soma (point s) when the steady current injection is at a dendritic point x_1 to the somatic voltage response when the same current injection is at the soma. The ratio between these voltage responses is $R_{tr}(x_1, s)/R_{in}(s)$. Using the reciprocity property, this ratio becomes $R_{tr}(s, x_1)/R_{in}(s)$, which is $1/A(s, x_1)$. Hence, the effect of a steady current injection on the somatic response is related to the attenuation factor from the soma to the injection point! When this attenuation factor is small (close to 1, as is usually the case for many realistic dendritic trees), the cost of placing the input current at a dendritic point instead of directly at the soma is small. The *attenuation cost* for placing the current injection at a dendritic point x_1 instead of placing it at the soma is defined by $1 - R_{tr}(x_1, s)/R_{in}(s) = 1 - 1/A(s, x_1)$. For example, if $A(s, x_1) = 1.5$, we get attenuation cost of $1/3$, which means that $1/3$ of the voltage response at the soma (relative to the resting potential) is lost when the input is located at x_1 instead of directly at the soma.

Another interesting case is when the soma is voltage clamped to the resting potential (by an electrode). When a steady current I is injected at point x_1, the voltage response at the soma (when there is *no* voltage clamp) is $R_{tr}(x_1, s) \cdot I$. Under the voltage clamp (V-clamp) conditions, the somatic electrode injects a current that will prevent this change in the somatic voltage. This current is $I_s = -(R_{tr}(x_1, s) \cdot I)/R_{in}(s)$. Rearranging, we get $I_s/I = -R_{tr}(x_1, s)/R_{in}(s) = 1/A(s, x_1)$. Thus, if the attenuation from the soma to the dendrites is small, the V-clamp current will be comparable to the current injected at a distal input point (see Rall and Segev 1985). Using the results in section 2.6.5, we find that for transients, the ratio between the total injected charge at the dendritic location and the total charge taken by the V-clamp electrode is equal to the steady-state attenuation factor from the soma to the dendritic point. In the above numerical example, the total charge taken by the V-clamp electrode will be $2/3$ of the total injected charge at the dendritic location.

2.4.3 Calculating the Input Conductance and Attenuation in a Dendritic Tree with Arbitrary Branching

To obtain the mathematical solution for the tree, the two arbitrary constants in the general solution for each branch must be determined from the boundary conditions (discussed in section 2.2.3); these include continuity of V and the conservation of core current at every branch point, plus a specification of the boundary condition at the distal end of every terminal branch, and of the applied voltage or applied current at the electrode location.

There are two different procedures for satisfying all of these boundary conditions. One is an iterative/recursive method (Rall 1959) that begins with the terminal branches and works back to the electrode location, which is often set at $X = 0$ of the tree trunk; the other method involves solving simultaneously a set of linear equations for the $2N$ arbitrary constants in the N general solutions (eqs. 2.16–2.18) for N branches of the dendritic tree. The first method will be sketched here; the second is a special case of a more general procedure described and used by Holmes (1986). All the algorithms described are justified mathematically using the properties listed in section 2.4.2.

Input Conductance at the Origin of a Dendritic Tree   We will start with the algorithm for computing the steady-state input conductance at the origin of a dendritic tree, based on Rall 1959. This algorithm can be implemented as a *recursive algorithm* or as an *iterative algorithm*.

This recursive implementation of the algorithm is sketched in figure 2.3. For understanding the algorithm, let us assume that the dendritic tree is in the form depicted in (3), that is, a cylinder connected to a subtree (T_1) at its far end. For computing the input conductance at the origin of the full tree, we should first compute the input conductance at the origin of T_1 (when T_1 is isolated). Then we can compute the input conductance at the origin of the full tree, using the equation

$$G_{in} = \frac{G_\infty \tanh(L) + G_L}{1 + (G_L/G_\infty)\tanh(L)},$$

(2.41)

which is based on eq. 2.36. Here $G_\infty = (\lambda r_i)^{-1}$, where λ and r_i are of the root cylinder (often called "trunk cylinder" or "primary branch"), L is the electrotonic length of the root cylinder ($L = \ell/\lambda$), and G_L is the input conductance of T_1. In the graphical representation of figure 2.3, this is shown by replacing T_1 by an equivalent conductance, and then using (2) to replace the resultant cable by another conductance.

We were left with the problem of calculating the input conductance at the origin of T_1. This tree is in the form depicted in (4), that is, two subtrees connected at their origin. T_1 of (3) is now the full tree in (4), and its two subtrees are denoted T_2 and T_3. After computing the input conductance at the origin of T_2 and T_3 (when they are isolated from each other), we can compute the equivalent input conductance at the origin of the full tree (which is T_1 of the original dendritic tree). This is done by using the input conductance properties in section 2.4.2. Because T_2 and T_3 are in the form depicted in (3), we can compute the input conductance at their origin in exactly the same way we computed it for the original tree. This is the recursive part of the algorithm.

48   Rall and Agmon-Snir

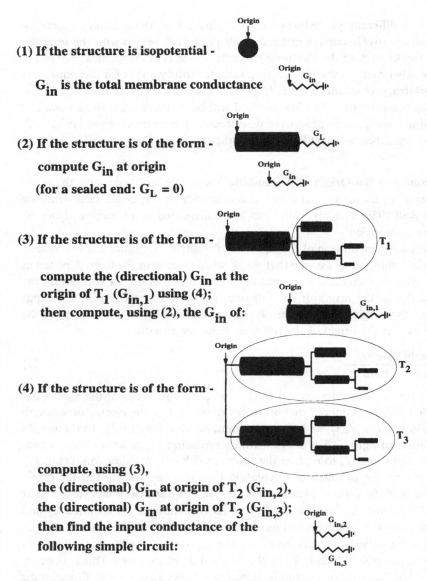

(1) If the structure is isopotential -

   G_{in} **is the total membrane conductance**

(2) If the structure is of the form -
   compute G_{in} **at origin**
   (for a sealed end: $G_L = 0$**)**

(3) If the structure is of the form -

   compute the (directional) G_{in} **at the**
   origin of T_1 **(**$G_{in,1}$**) using (4);**
   then compute, using (2), the G_{in} **of:**

(4) If the structure is of the form -

   compute, using (3),
   the (directional) G_{in} **at origin of** T_2 **(**$G_{in,2}$**),**
   the (directional) G_{in} **at origin of** T_3 **(**$G_{in,3}$**);**
   then find the input conductance of the
   following simple circuit:

Figure 2.3
Recursive algorithm for computing R_{in} at the origin of passive dendritic tree (see section 2.4.3). The calculation of (2) is based on eq. 2.41. The computation time of this algorithm scales linearly with the number of branches in the tree. Every point in a dendritic tree can be considered the "origin" of the tree for this algorithm, and then the R_{in} at this point can be computed. Modified from Agmon-Snir 1995.

The recursion is stopped when we get to the distal tips. At the most distal branch points we encounter structures of the form depicted in step 4, but T_2 and T_3 are just sealed cylinders. To compute the input conductance at the origin of these cylinders, we use eq. 2.31, which is equivalent to eq. 2.41 for $G_L = 0$.

The recursive implementation of the algorithm helps in the "bookkeeping" of the computations along the tree. The resultant code is shorter and clearer. If a software tool that does not support recursion is used (as FORTRAN), one can use the iterative implementation. The iterative algorithm starts at the terminals and proceeds towards the origin of the tree. First, the input conductance at the proximal (i.e., closer to the origin) side of every terminal branch is computed (when this branch is isolated from the tree). This is done using eq. 2.31. Then, at every branch point that connects two of these branches, the input conductance can be computed, using the input conductance properties in section 2.4.2. Next for the branch that is connected proximally to any of these branch points, the input conductance at its other end can be computed using eq. 2.41. This iteration continues until the input conductance at the origin of the tree is found.

If the model tree has a passive soma at its origin, the input conductance at the origin of the whole tree (including the soma) is $G_S + G_D$, where G_D is the input conductance of the tree (without the soma) and G_S is the total membrane conductance of the soma (see Chapter 3, this volume, for the use of this recursive computation).

Attenuation from the Origin of a Dendritic Tree   The second algorithm computes the attenuation factor from the origin of a passive dendritic tree to every point. This algorithm consists of two steps:

1. Compute G_{in} at the origin of the tree, using the algorithm just described. The important addition is that we keep the values of the directional input conductances found at the origins of all the subtrees in the structure. In other words, if our tree is of form depicted in step 3 of figure 2.3, we compute the input conductance at the origin of T_1 and save this value. Also, we keep the values computed for T_2 and T_3 for trees of the form depicted in step 4. Then we have, for each branch point, the input conductances its subtrees.

2. Compute attenuation factors along the branches of the dendritic tree for an input at the origin. Figure 2.4 shows a sample dendritic tree, and we assume an input at its origin, p_1. The origin branch b_0 is connected to a dendritic tree T_0. We know from the previous step the input conductance at the origin of the isolated T_0. Hence, we can compute the attenuation factor along b_0 using

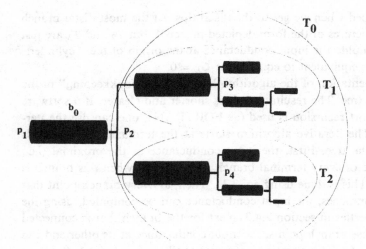

Figure 2.4
Schematic figure for the algorithms described in section 2.4.3. The structure in the figure consists of a cylinder denoted by b_0 and a dendritic tree denoted by T_0. T_0 consists of two subtrees, denoted T_1 and T_2; p_1 is the origin of the structure, and p_2, p_3, p_4 are branch points. Modified from Agmon-Snir 1995.

$$A(0, X) = \frac{\cosh(L) + (G_L/G_x)\sinh(L)}{\cosh(L - X) + (G_L/G_x)\sinh(L - X)}, \tag{2.42}$$

which is based on eq. 2.25. Point 0 is the proximal point of b_0 and X is the point that is at distance $X \cdot \lambda$ from point 0 (using the λ of this cylinder, of course). We continue recursively to subtrees T_1 and T_2, calculating the attenuation factor along their origin branches. At the end of the full recursive process, we have the attenuation factor along all the branches for an input at the origin of the tree.

Now we can compute the attenuation factor from the origin to any point in the structure by multiplying the attenuation factors along the branches on the path from the origin to the point. Moreover, as an outcome of the attenuation factor properties in section 2.4.2, one can compute the attenuation factor not only from the origin but from any point to any point *distal to it* by multiplying the attenuation factors along the path.

Algorithm That Computes Input Conductance at Every Branch Point and Attenuation Factor along All Branches From the attenuation factor property we can see that for every branch in the tree, there are just two possible values for the attenuation factor between its ends. One value is obtained when an input is located at the structure connected to one end of the branch, and the other value is obtained for an input in the structure connected to second end (if the input is located at some point along the branch, we should divide the branch at the input site).

This leads us to the third algorithm, which computes the input conductance at every branch point, as well as the attenuation factors along all segments (and in both directions) of the tree. For every dendritic point, we will distinguish between the *centripetal direction* from this point, which is the direction toward the origin of the tree, and the other or *centrifugal directions*. The first algorithm described above allows us to find, for each branch point, the input conductance of the subtrees that are centrifugal to every branch point. In other words, this algorithm finds, for each branch point, the directional input conductances in the centrifugal directions, although not the value of the directional input conductance in the centripetal direction. These centripetal input conductances of the branch points may be found using another recursive algorithm. To see that, we go back to figure 2.4. For the origin, p_1, there is no centripetal direction; thus all the directional input conductances are known. For p_2, we see that we have already the directional input conductances at this point in the direction of T_1 and T_2 (these are the centrifugal input conductances). The centripetal input conductance is easy to compute, as the structure in this direction is just a cylinder of the form depicted in (2) of figure 2.3 (hence, eq. 2.41 can be used).

Having all the directional input conductances at p_2, we can continue to points p_3 and p_4. For these points, the centrifugal input conductances were computed before. It is not hard to compute the centripetal input conductance of p_3. The structure in this direction is a cylinder with a dendritic load, knowing all the directional input conductances at p_2, we can calculate the input conductance of this dendritic load (in fact, we only need the centrifugal input conductance in the direction of T_2 and the centripetal input conductance; then we can add them to get the input conductance of the dendritic load). The same process can be applied to p_4, and we can continue recursively to distal points at the tree. After completing this step, we know the directional input conductances in all directions at every branch point and thus can compute the dendritic load at both ends of each branch. Therefore, using eq. 2.42, we can compute for every branch the attenuation factors along it in both directions (in fact, computing the centripetal input conductances and computing the attenuation factors can be done in the same pass over the tree).

Computation Time and Extensions of the Algorithms   The computation time of all the above algorithms scales linearly with the number of the branches in the structure (and independent of the length of the branches). After the calculations of the last algorithm, the attenuation factors between any two points in the tree can be easily found. Because the input conductances are computed for all branch points, the transfer resistances can also be found between any two branch points.

Although the first two algorithms make calculations with respect to the origin of the dendritic tree, every point in the tree can be regarded as the origin of a branching structure, and then these algorithms can apply to calculations with respect to this point. It is also not hard to extend the algorithms for dendritic models that include isopotential compartments (as a passive soma or a spine head). By using a special variant of a cable equation, the algorithms can be modified for tapering branches (see Rall 1962; Goldstein and Rall 1974; Holmes and Rall 1992a). As we shall see in section 2.6.5, these algorithms apply also for analysis of the time integral of transient current injections (see also Rinzel and Rall 1974 and Chapter 3, this volume).

2.4.4   The Effective Length Constant and the Morphoelectrotonic Transform

As shown above (see eq. 2.19), when a steady current is injected at the end of a semi-infinite length cylinder, the steady-state voltage is given by $V(X) = V_0 e^{-X} = V_0 e^{-x/\lambda}$, when V_0 is the voltage at the injection point. Hence, in this case, the attenuation rate $(\vec{A}_r(x))$ at every point is $1/\lambda$ (see eq. 2.38). We can generalize the concept of the length constant and define the *(directional) effective length constant*, $\vec{\lambda}_{eff}(x)$, as $1/\vec{A}_r(x)$. Using eq. 2.39 and eq. 2.29, we find that

$$\vec{\lambda}_{eff}(x) = \vec{\lambda}\, \frac{\vec{R}_{in}(x)}{\vec{R}_\infty(x)}, \tag{2.43}$$

where the directional input resistance is the input resistance of the structure in the given direction. $\vec{R}_\infty(x)$ and $\vec{\lambda}(x)$ are R_∞ and λ of the cylinder connected in the given direction. Using eq. 2.40, the relation between the *attenuation factor*, $A(x_1, x_2)$, and the *effective length constant* can be expressed

$$\ln(A(x_1, x_2)) = \int_{x_1}^{x_2} \frac{dx}{\vec{\lambda}_{eff}(x)}. \tag{2.44}$$

(Compare to eq. 2.37; see discussion of the effective length constant in Agmon-Snir and Segev 1993 and in Agmon-Snir 1995.)

The effective length constant may be used to obtain a transformed representation of a dendritic tree, in which each unit of distance represents an *e*-fold attenuation of voltage. Obviously, this transform depends on the site of current injection (and thus the direction of attenuation) in the tree. The transformation is done by scaling every infinitesimally small cylinder of length dx by the $\vec{\lambda}_{eff}$ that relates to the "downstream" direction of attenuation (i.e., the new length of this cylinder will be $dx/\vec{\lambda}_{eff}$. Practically, based on eq. 2.44, the length of each segment in the structure will be $\ln(A(x_1, x_2))$, where x_1, x_2 are the ends of the segment and the current injection point is assumed to be outside the segment (if it is inside the segment, the segment should be divided at the injection point). This transform, called an "attenogram," is one of a few *morphoelectrotonic transforms* (METs; Zador et al. 1995). Figure 2.5 demonstrates the use of the attenogram for a reconstructed dendritic tree; section 2.6.5 briefly discusses the use of the morphoelectrotonic transform for transients.

2.5 Family of Trees Related to an Equivalent Cylinder

2.5.1 Definition and Properties

We will use in this section the tree labeling scheme described in figure 2.6B. In this labeling scheme, a parent branch, identified by index j, extends from x_{j-1} to x_j and has a diameter d_j. Two daughter branches arise at x_j. One daughter, identified by index $k1$, extends from x_j to x_{k1} and has a diameter d_{k1}. The other daughter, identified by index $k2$, extends from x_j to x_{k2} and has a diameter d_{k2}. Corresponding to each diameter, there is a value of λ defined by eq. 2.13 and a value of G_∞ defined by equation 2.30. Although it is simplest to keep R_i and R_m constant, this is not necessary; we can specify different R_i and R_m values for each branch.

Many useful insights have resulted from the fact that an extensively branched dendritic tree can be represented as an equivalent cylinder, if several conditions are satisfied. The branching need not be symmetric, and all subdivisions of the tree need not contain the same number of orders of branching. The necessary conditions are

1. The values of R_m and R_i are the same in all branches.

2. All terminal branches end with the same distal boundary condition (usually taken to be the sealed end condition; see below for an explicit meaning of "same boundary condition").

3. All terminal branches end at the same electrotonic distance, L, from the trunk origin (i.e., L equals the sum of x/λ values along the path from $x = 0$ to the distal end of every terminal branch; this L is the electrotonic length of the tree and of the equivalent cylinder).

4. At every branch point, the diameters of the two daughter branches need not be equal but must satisfy the constraint that the sum of their 3/2 power values equal the 3/2 power of the parent branch diameter:

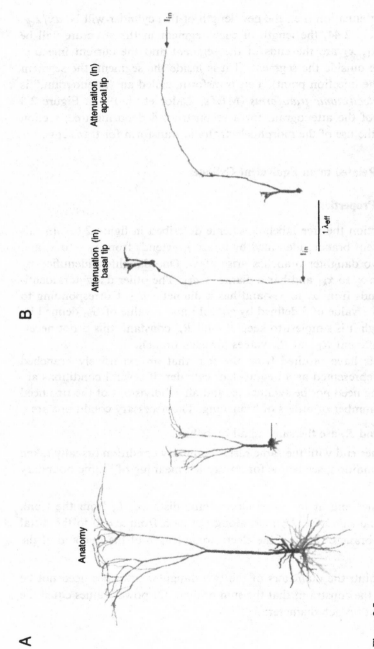

Figure 2.5
Demonstration of the morphoelectrotonic transform (see section 2.4.4). (A) *Attenogram* of a pyramidal cell from layer 5 of cat visual cortex (three-dimensional reconstruction made by R. Douglas; Douglas et al. 1991) is shown on right. This attenogram is for an input at the soma. The original anatomy of the cell is shown on left. (B) Attenograms of the same reconstructed cell, for dendritic input locations. Note the different scale. (C) Demonstration of the attenogram for other dendritic structures (input at the soma): a cerebellar Purkinje cell from the guinea pig (reconstructed by M. Rapp; Rapp et al. 1994) and a CA1 hippocampal cell from the rat (reconstructed by N. Ishizuka and D. Amaral; Ishizuka et al. 1995). The anatomical reconstructions are shown on left. In the middle column the attenograms are drawn to scale, while in the right column, the two structures are normalized to the same size, to emphasize the geometry. Based on steady-state analysis (section 2.4.2), as well as the method of moments (section 2.6.5 and Agmon-Snir 1995), those attenograms can be used for estimating attenuation costs, delay costs and attenuation and delays of current for the somatic V-clamp case (see details in Zador et al. 1995). Uniform biophysical parameters were used for all models in this figure: $R_m = 20\,k\Omega\,cm^2$, $R_i = 100\,\Omega\,cm$, and $C_m = 1\,\mu F/cm^2$. The algorithms for the morphoelectrotonic transform can be obtained from H. Agmon-Snir. Modified from Zador et al. 1995.

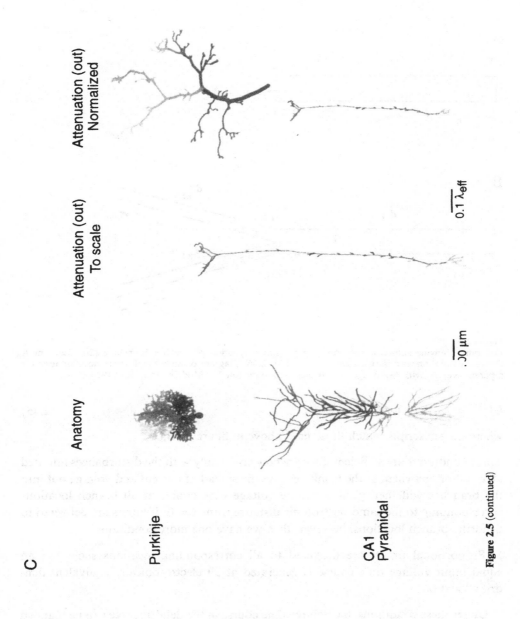

Figure 2.5 (continued)

A

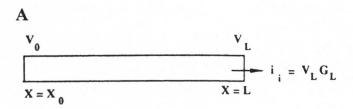

B

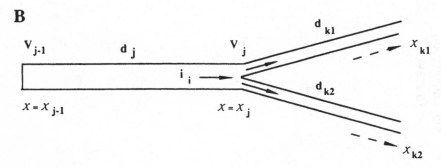

Figure 2.6
Diagrams showing subscript notation used for single cylinder (A) and for branching (B). Diagram A shows the notation used in eqs. 2.20–2.25 and 2.31–2.36. Diagram B shows the different notation used for a parent cylinder with two daughter branches used in section 2.5. Modified from Rall 1977.

$$(d_j)^{3/2} = (d_{k1})^{3/2} + (d_{k2})^{3/2}, \tag{2.45}$$

where the subscripts match those used above in figure 2.6B.

These conditions are sufficient if we are concerned only with the disturbances initiated at $x = 0$ or anywhere in the trunk because the spread of current and voltage out into the branches will then yield the same voltage time course at all branch locations corresponding to the same electrotonic distance from $x = 0$. If inputs are delivered to dendritic branch locations, however, then we have one more condition:

5. Proportional inputs are delivered to all corresponding locations such that an equal input voltage time course is generated at all electrotonically equivalent dendritic locations.

Under these conditions, the voltage time course in the dendritic tree can be mapped onto an equivalent cylinder by means of the electrotonic distance, X, measured from

$X = 0$. A method of solution, using the superposition approach, has been devised for the case of input to a single branch of a tree that is otherwise equivalent to a cylinder (the steady-state superposition is described and discussed in Rall and Rinzel 1973, while transient superposition is described and discussed in Rinzel and Rall 1974; see also sections 2.5.4, and 2.9.1).

It should be obvious that natural dendritic trees are unlikely to satisfy all these constraints on dendritic branching, which were presented, not as a law of nature, but by way of mathematical idealization to provide a valuable reference case. Nevertheless, it has been found that some natural dendritic trees do approximately satisfy the 3/2-power law constraint at individual branch points. For motoneurons of cat spinal cord, the major discrepancy results from the fact that many high-order branches are missing because their potential parent branches terminate at electrotonic distances (from the soma) significantly less than for terminal branches of higher order. The sum of $d^{3/2}$ for successively higher-order branches therefore decreases very significantly. Such dendritic trees are not equivalent to a cylinder but more nearly approximate a tapered core conductor or several cylinders of different length, placed electrically in parallel with a common soma. However, other neuron types have been reported to exhibit much less of this problem, with the result that they sustain a fairly constant sum of $d^{3/2}$ out to terminations at almost equal electrotonic distance from the soma (Bloomfield et al. 1987).

A different theoretical approach to dendritic trees equivalent to a cylinder derives the partial differential equation (PDE) for a hypothetical system with continuous taper and branching. By generalizing the concept of electrotonic distance, this approach transforms the PDE to a form that reduces to that for a cylinder when the taper parameter is set to zero (see Rall 1962a; Jack et al. 1975). Here, however, we merely demonstrate the effect that constraints 1–4 have on the input conductance at the tree origin and the voltage response for a steady-state current injected at the origin.

To justify the constraints, let us return to figure 2.6B and assume that $k1$ and $k2$ are two terminal branches. We will also assume that both branches have the same R_m and R_i values and the same *electrotonic* length, $L_k = L_{k1} = L_{k2}$ (but not necessarily the same real length because they might have different diameter; see eq. 2.13). Terminal branch $k1$ has a conductance leak G_{k1} at its distal end; terminal branch $k2$ has a conductance leak G_{k2} at its distal end. An additional important assumption is that the ratio $G_{k1}/G_{\infty,k1}$, which we shall denote by B, equals $G_{k2}/G_{\infty,k2}$, where $G_{\infty,k1}$ and $G_{\infty,k2}$ are the G_∞ values of these two branches. This assumption is the practical meaning of constraint 2 (note that if both ends are sealed, $B = 0$). The input conductance at the origin of a tree consisting of these two branches is (based on eq. 2.41)

$$G_{in} = (G_{\infty,k1} + G_{\infty,k2}) \cdot \frac{\tanh(L_k) + B}{1 + B\tanh(L_k)}, \tag{2.46}$$

which is equal to the input conductance at the origin of a cylinder with G_{∞} equal to $G_{\infty,k1} + G_{\infty,k2}$, with a conductance leak at its end equal to $B(G_{\infty,k1} + G_{\infty,k2})$, and with electrical length L_k. This cylinder is the equivalent cylinder for this small tree. Note that, from eq. 2.30, the diameter, d, of the equivalent cylinder does satisfy $(d)^{3/2} = (d_{k1})^{3/2} + (d_{k2})^{3/2}$. By examining eq. 2.25, we see that the voltage response along k_1, k_2, and the equivalent cylinder is the same for a steady input at the origin. In other words, the voltage will be the same at electrotonic distance X from the origin in $k1$, $k2$ and the equivalent cylinder.

Let us assume that the parent branch, j, of $k1$ and $k2$ has the same R_m and R_i values as $k1$ and $k2$ and that eq. 2.45 is satisfied. If we replace $k1$ and $k2$ by their equivalent cylinder, the whole structure becomes a uniform cylinder of length $L_j + L_k$. This is the equivalent cylinder for this structure. In a complicated tree that satisfies the constraints, this process can be continued iteratively to replace the whole tree by a uniform cylinder. Although we justified here the equivalence of dendritic trees satisfying the above constraints to an equivalent cylinder only for a steady-state input at the origin of the tree, this equivalence also holds for inputs at other points (satisfying the proportionality constraints) and for the PDE and its transient solutions.

2.5.2 Dendritic Surface Area and Input Conductance of Tree

A particularly useful property of dendritic trees satisfying the constraints for equivalence to a cylinder is that they have the same membrane surface area as that of an unbranched cylinder with the same diameter as the trunk of the tree and with the same electrotonic length, L_D, as the whole dendritic tree (note that $L_D = L_j + L_k$ in the simple example above). This result for membrane area was deduced as a part of the general treatment of the PDE presented in Rall 1962a, 1962b; here, however, we show it for the example above. The surface area of the parent (trunk) branch equals $\pi d_j \ell_j$, where $\ell_j = x_j - x_{j-1}$. The surface areas of the two daughter branches are $\pi d_{k1}\ell_{k1}$ and $\pi d_{k2}\ell_{k2}$, respectively. Although the diameters and lengths of these daughter branches are usually different, we know that these two daughters have the same electrotonic length, $L_k = \ell_{k1}/\lambda_{k1} = \ell_{k2}/\lambda_{k2}$. We also know that $\ell_k = \lambda_j L_k$ represents the length that must be added to the parent trunk to get the equivalent cylinder for the tree (note that this physical length is larger than that of either daughter branch for the usual case where both daughter branches have smaller diameters and λ-values than the trunk). What we need to show is that the surface area, $\pi d_j \ell_k$, added to the trunk is exactly equal to the sum of the areas of the two daughter branches. We note that each λ is proportional to $d^{1/2}$ (because the underlying resistivities are held constant), and that the three ℓ values (for subscripts k, $k1$, and $k2$) are proportional to their corresponding λ values (because the value of L_k is the same in all three cases). Consequently, for each subscript, the value of surface area, $\pi d \ell$, must be proportional to $d^{3/2}$. It follows that the surface areas match when

$$(d_j)^{3/2} = (d_{k1})^{3/2} + (d_{k2})^{3/2},$$

which is exactly the constraint (eq. 2.45) for equivalence to a cylinder. In other words, this constraint ensures that the dendritic surface area remains the same for few or many orders of branching, when constraints 1 and 3 are also satisfied.

Now we can appreciate the usefulness of a relation between the input conductance, G_D, of a dendritic tree, its membrane surface area, A_D, and its electrotonic length, L_D:

$$G_D = G_m A_D \frac{\tanh(L_D)}{L_D}, \tag{2.47}$$

which holds exactly for all dendritic trees that satisfy the equivalent cylinder constraints with a sealed end at $X = L_D$ of all terminal branches. This expression follows from eq. 2.31, together with the rightmost part of eq. 2.30, and from $A_D = \pi \ell d = \pi L_D \lambda d$. When we know the value of G_m (either in a simulation or in a favorable experimental situation), eq. 2.47 provides a valuable relation between dendritic surface area and dendritic input conductance. In experimental situations, however, we must beware of complications that may result from soma shunting caused by microelectrode penetration of the membrane (considered explicitly in eq. 2.50).

It is illuminating to contrast the effects of very short and very long dendritic length on the value of the correction factor, $\tanh(L_D)/L_D$. When L_D is very small, this correction factor is unity, which simplifies eq. 2.47 to $G_D = G_m A_D$. Because there is negligible voltage decrement in a very short dendritic tree, the dendritic membrane is essentially isopotential, which is why the input conductance is simply the product of the surface area and the membrane conductance per unit area. On the other hand, for large values of L_D, the dendritic membrane is clearly nonisopotential (there is very significant steady-state voltage decrement with distance). Note that for very large values of L_D, the value of $\tanh(L_D)$ is unity and the correction factor is simply $1/L_D$. Also, because $A_D/L_D = \pi \lambda d$, eq. 2.47 becomes simplified to $G_D = G_m \pi \lambda d = G_\infty$, as it should because the voltage decrement with distance is essentially the same for very large lengths (greater than four times λ). For intermediate L_D values of 0.5, 1.0, and 1.5, the nonisopotentiality correction factor has the values 0.924, 0.762, and 0.603, respectively. These values are less than 1.0 by amounts clearly related to the non-isopotentiality of the dendritic membrane potential during a steady-state input conductance measurement.

Although eq. 2.47 is strictly valid only for dendritic trees that are equivalent to a cylinder, the physically intuitive understanding provided in the preceding paragraph suggests that a somewhat similar, more generalized correction factor must result also from departure from isopotentiality in dendritic trees whose branching does not satisfy the equivalent cylinder constraints. This can be explored for different types of neurons. For the cat spinal cord, Burke and colleagues (see table 1 of Rall et al. 1992) provided a carefully studied sample of six type-identified motoneurons; here we found an average value of 0.71 as the generalized correction factor for this sample of nonideal branching (some branches terminate at shorter electrotonic distances than others).

This generalized correction factor can be defined by the expression

$$G_D = G_{md} A_D F_{dga},\tag{2.48}$$

where G_{md} represents dendritic membrane conductivity per unit area, and F_{dga} represents an empirical factor that can be determined for any given branching type. We already know that, for the idealized reference case of trees equivalent to a cylinder, eq. 2.47 provides an exact expression for F_{dga}, that is, the factor $\tanh(L_D)/L_D$. After finding the empirical value of F_{dga} for a given dendritic tree (using eq. 2.48 and the empirical/estimated values of G_{md}, G_D, A_D), we can solve numerically the equation $F_{dga} = \tanh(L_D)/L_D$ and obtain an "effective" electrotonic length, which corresponds to an ideal tree that has the same F_{dga} value as that for the nonideal given tree (see table 1 of Rall et al. 1992 for comparisons). Once these values are known for different neuron types, they can be used to make preliminary estimates for another neuron of the same type, even when the data for that neuron may be incomplete.

2.5.3 Input Conductance of a Neuron

Let us now consider a whole neuron composed of several dendritic trees attached to a common soma. When our focus is on the passive membrane properties of the soma and dendrites, we often omit an explicit axon. Some neuron types (such as granule cells of the olfactory bulb and amacrine cells of the retina) do not have axons; others (such as motoneurons and pyramidal cells) have axons whose dimensions and passive membrane properties make a relatively slight contribution to the input conductance of the whole neuron. However, under conditions where the nonlinear properties of axonal membrane become important (e.g., for an axon of large diameter), explicit addition of the axon to the model must be evaluated, according to the questions being asked.

Because the input conductances of the several dendritic trees are electrically in parallel with the soma membrane, the input conductance, G_N, of the whole neuron can be expressed

$$G_N = G_S + \sum_{j=1}^{n} G_{Dj} = (\rho + 1)G_S, \tag{2.49}$$

where G_S represents the soma input conductance, and the summation is for the input conductances of n dendritic trees. Note that the expression at the far right makes use of the parameter ρ used (Rall 1959) to represent the dendritic to soma conductance ratio, $\sum G_D/G_S$.

The soma input conductance, G_S, must now be made more explicit:

$$G_S = G_{shunt} + G_{ms}A_S = \beta G_{md}A_S, \tag{2.50}$$

where the shunt conductance caused by microelectrode penetration is included because it can be very large, A_S represents the soma surface area, and G_{ms} represents the soma membrane conductance per unit area (excluding the shunt conductance). G_{ms} could be different from G_{md}, the dendritic membrane conductance per unit area (here assumed constant for all of the dendrites). The expression at the far right constitutes a definition of β, which can be thought of as the soma shunting factor, or as the ratio of G_{md} to an apparent G_{ms} (implied by the shunt together with the actual G_{ms}). Note that the value of β could be as large as 1,000 when the shunt conductance is very large, or as small as 1 when $G_{ms} = G_{md}$ and the shunt conductance is zero.

It is important to understand that as the value of the soma shunt is increased, both the value of G_S and the value of the parameter $\beta = G_S/(G_{md}A_S)$ are increased. However, the value of the parameter $\rho = \sum G_D/G_S$ is decreased, such that the product, $\rho\beta$, remains constant because the value of G_S cancels, leaving

$$\rho\beta = \frac{\sum G_D}{G_{md}A_S} = \frac{\sum A_D F_{dga}}{A_S}, \tag{2.51}$$

where the subscript j, identifying different dendritic trees, has been suppressed only for the sake of less cumbersome expressions. The expression at the far right (making use of eq. 2.48) shows that the value of $\rho\beta$ is determined by membrane surface areas, together with the factor F_{dga}, whose value often lies between 0.7 and 0.9, depending upon the degree of nonisopotentiality of steady-state dendritic membrane potential. If all of the dendritic trees were to have the same effective electrotonic length, the value of F_{dga} would be the same for all of them, and this factor could be placed in front of the summation.

Using the results and notations above, we can now provide two useful alternative expressions for the ratio of whole-neuron input conductance to dendritic membrane conductivity:

$$G_N/G_{md} = A_S(\beta + \rho\beta) = \beta A_S + \sum_{j=1}^{n} A_{D_j} F_{dga_j}. \qquad (2.52)$$

These expressions are important in estimating the value of G_{md} from experimental measurements of G_N and the histological surface areas. Clearly, it is important to find good ways of estimating the value of the soma shunting factor, β, as well as those of the factor F_{dga}, for dendritic trees of different types (see comments made with eqs. 2.47 and 2.48).

2.5.4 Steady-State Decrement of Voltage with Distance

The quantitative results of several early computations led to qualitative insights that apply also to dendritic trees not fully satisfying equivalent cylinder constraints. These early computations, often done by hand (using a slide rule and math tables), can now be done easily with a handheld calculator that includes trigonometric and hyperbolic functions. In today's climate of powerful workstations and personal computers, we should remember that computer programs can have serious errors; it is wise to check a few key values by hand. The analytical solutions obtained for equivalent cylinders are especially useful for such calculations. In this section, we present results from equivalent cylinder computations that shed light on the steady-state voltage response even in dendritic trees not equivalent to a cylinder.

The belief that cable theory implies a simple exponential voltage decrement to $1/e$ for a λ distance is correct for a very long (many λ) cable that has uniform properties and is unperturbed (i.e., by any input, leak, short circuit, or voltage clamp). It is also correct for a finite length with one particular boundary condition that can be expressed as $G_L/G_\infty = 1$ at $X = L$, for example, in figure 2.2 and eq. 2.25. As that figure and that equation make clear, however, such a simple voltage decrement is a very special case. These theoretical results show that the general case of voltage decrement with distance depends upon both the length of uniform cable and the boundary condition at $X = L$. The special case $G_L = 0$ corresponds to the sealed-end boundary condition $dV/dX = 0$ at $X = L$. The special case $G_L = \infty$ corresponds to the voltage clamp $V = 0$ at $X = L$. For example, the attenuation factor

$V(X = 0)/V(X = L)$, expressed by eq. 2.24, is 1.54 for a sealed end at $X = L = 1.0$, meaning that the steady voltage decrements from 100% to about 65% in this case.

Although we have referred here only to one cylinder extending from $X = 0$ to $X = L$, these results apply also to dendritic trees equivalent to a cylinder, provided that the decrement is from the trunk into the branches. For inputs to dendritic branches, similar equivalent cylinder results apply only when all branches at the same electrotonic distance, X, receive their proportional share of the input, ensuring that $V(X)$ is the same in all of these branches. Thus, if a steady voltage were applied to all of the terminals of such a tree with $L = 1$, and if the trunk were sealed at $X = 0$, the decrement would be from 100% at the terminals to 65% at $X = 0$. The same decrement would also be expected from the dendritic terminals to the soma in an idealized neuron composed of several such trees coupled at $X = 0$ (assume no lumped soma, but a proximal bit of each trunk can be regarded as soma), provided that all dendritic terminals of all trees had the same steady voltage and the same value of L. In this case, the symmetry about $X = 0$ would cause all these trees to have $dV/dX = 0$ at $X = 0$, meaning that they would all have effectively sealed ends at $X = 0$, even though they were still connected to each other; in fact, this case can be represented by a single equivalent cylinder with voltage applied at $X = L$ and voltage decrement to a sealed end at $X = 0$.

In contrast to all of these cases, we would expect significantly greater attenuation if only one of these trees received input, while the others received none. For that case, and also for input to a single branch of one tree, the method described by Rall and Rinzel (1973) can be used to obtain results like those illustrated below in figure 2.7.

Figure 2.7 illustrates an idealized dendritic neuron consisting of six equal dendritic trees. Current is injected at a single branch terminal, here designated I; this input branch is distinguished from its sibling branch, S, and its first- and second-cousin branches, C-1 and C-2. The resulting steady voltage distribution in the various branches of the input tree (shown in figure 2.7) was computed from the general solution of this problem (Rall and Rinzel 1973), based on superposition methods and considerations of symmetry.

One noteworthy feature of these results is the contrast in voltage decrement in the input branch, compared with its sibling branch. Both branches have the same length and diameter in this idealized tree; the essential difference lies in the boundary conditions. The proximal end of the input branch is open to current flow into its parent branch; this permits a large flow of current along its cytoplasmic core, resulting in a steep voltage decrement along the length of the input branch. In contrast, the sealed terminal of the sibling branch allows zero current to flow out of that end and little

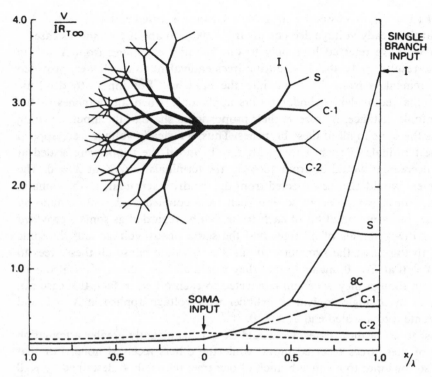

Figure 2.7
Diagram of idealized neuron model composed of six dendritic trees, and plot of steady-state voltage values for three different cases. Solid curve shows voltages computed for current input to a single distal branch terminal, designated *I* for input branch; in this case, the sibling branch, *S*, the first cousin branches, *C*-1, and the second-cousin branches, *C*-2, receive no input; they have sealed ends. Curve with long dashes (labeled 8*C*) corresponds to the same amount of input current divided equally among all eight terminal branches (cousins) belonging to the same tree. Curve with short dashes corresponds to the same amount of total input current applied at the soma. Modified from Rall and Rinzel 1973, which can be consulted for the mathematical statement and solution of this problem.

current to flow across the high resistance of the cylindrical branch membrane. With so little current flowing either in or out of this sibling branch, its voltage profile is almost isopotential. A similar contrast holds true also for the very small terminal branches known as "dendritic spines." When a spine head receives synaptic input there is significant attenuation along the spine stem, from a large membrane depolarization at the spine head to a smaller depolarization at the spine base and the parent dendrite where the spine stem is attached. For spines with excitable spine head membrane, the large depolarization at the spine head enhances the probability of reaching spike threshold. For an excitable spine not receiving synaptic input, the nearly isopotential spread of depolarization from the parent dendrite through the spine stem out to the spine head increases the probability such a spine may also reach spike threshold and thus contribute to a chain reaction that may result in the firing of clusters of excitable spines (Rall and Segev 1987).

Another feature of these results is the contrast in input resistance values when the distal input location is compared with a central input location (at the soma). In figure 2.7, the dashed curve shows the lower voltage values obtained when the same amount of current was injected at the soma as that previously injected at the distal branch. In this example, the distal input resistance is sixteen times larger than the somatic input resistance, and still larger factors can result from additional orders of branching (see Rall and Rinzel 1973), where it is also shown that the increased depolarization at a distal location cannot be more effective in its spread to the soma because steady-state voltage attenuation (from the distal input site to the soma) always exceeds the input resistance ratio. Nevertheless, the large local synaptic depolarization produced at distal dendritic locations is important for graded dendrodendritic synaptic interactions that depend on the local dendritic depolarization; it is also important to the attainment of threshold conditions in excitable dendritic spines located on distal dendritic branches. The relation between the attenuation along the dendrite and the differences in input resistances at various points is shown in section 2.4.2, as one of the attenuation factor properties.

2.6 Transient Solutions and Properties

2.6.1 Two Classes of Explicit Solutions

The cable PDE (eq. 2.2) has many solutions; the problem is to construct a solution that satisfies not only the PDE but also the boundary conditions and an initial condition. It is helpful to know that there are two rather different basic solutions from which the more complicated solutions are constructed.

One class of solutions comes from the classical method known as the "separation of variables." The solution $V(X, T)$ is assumed to be the product of two functions, one of which is a function of X but not of T, while the other is a function of T but not of X. Using this method, we find the following solution:

$$V(X, T) = (A \sin(\alpha X) + B \cos(\alpha X))e^{-(1+\alpha^2)T}, \tag{2.53}$$

where A and B are arbitrary constants, and α^2 is known as the separation constant. It is easy to verify, by partial differentiation, that this function satisfies the dimensionless cable equation (eq. 2.2); because this PDE is linear, any sum of solutions to it is also a solution (this sum is, obviously, not separable). For a cable of finite length with given initial and boundary conditions, the particular solution, which is a sum of solutions of the form given in eq. 2.53, can be determined. Each of the solutions in the sum has its own values of A, B, and α. Typically, α in the components of the sum is found to be restricted to a particular set of *eigenvalues*, or roots of the characteristic equation (an equation obtained by applying the boundary conditions to the PDE). An example of such a solution is provided below as eq. 2.55. In general, one can get the transient solution in any branching passive dendritic tree, by superposition of solutions of the form of eq. 2.53 (see Holmes et al. 1992a, 1992b; Major et al. 1993a, 1993b).

An alternative approach for solving eq. 2.2 uses a different class of solutions that can be constructed from what is variously called the "fundamental solution", "Green's function," "instantaneous point source solution," or "response function." This solution can be expressed

$$V(X, T) = C_o(\pi T)^{-1/2} e^{-(T+X^2/4T)}, \tag{2.54}$$

where X can extend from $-\infty$ to $+\infty$; the singularity (instantaneous point charge) is located at $X = 0$ when $T = 0$. If the amount of this charge is Q_o coulombs, then for a semi-infinite length (extending from $X = 0$ to $X = +\infty$), the value of C_o is $Q_o/(\lambda c_m)$, where λc_m represents the membrane capacitance of a λ length of cylinder (in farads), implying that C_o has the dimension of volts. This value for C_o can be confirmed by integrating the charge per unit length, $c_m V(X, T)$, from $X = 0$ to $X = \infty$, and showing that the total charge on the membrane is Q_o when $T = 0$. For the doubly infinite case, the charge spreads in both directions, and the value of C_o is half the above. Although this solution is most natural for infinite lengths, the method of images can be used to construct solutions for finite length and for any branching passive dendritic tree (e.g., Jack et al. 1975, 67–71; Cao and Abbott 1993). It is also useful to realize that even for finite lengths, eq. 2.54 provides a good approximation for very small values of X and T (i.e., for early times before the spread of charge can be influenced by a distant boundary condition).

2.6.2 Voltage Decay Transient for Cylinder of Finite Length with Sealed Ends

For a finite length with simple boundary conditions, Fourier first showed how to construct a solution that satisfies an arbitrary initial condition. Rall 1969a presents and discusses several examples of such solutions for application to experimental neurophysiology. A more general separation of variables for three-dimensional space and time can be found in Rall 1969b.

For a uniform cylinder of finite length, with two sealed-end boundary conditions ($\partial V/\partial X = 0$, at $X = 0$ and at $X = L$), coefficient A must be set to zero in eq. 2.53; the constant α can have infinitely many values, $\alpha_n = n\pi/L$, where n can be zero or any positive integer. Thus we can express a family of solutions in the form of a summation of infinitely many terms:

$$V(X, T) = \sum_{n=0}^{\infty} B_n \cos(n\pi X/L)e^{-[1+(n\pi/L)^2]T}, \tag{2.55}$$

where the coefficients, B_n, are known as "Fourier coefficients," which depend on the initial condition, $V(X, 0)$, as follows:

$$B_o = (1/L)\int_0^L V(X, 0)\,dX \tag{2.56}$$

and, for positive integer values of n,

$$B_n = (2/L)\int_0^L V(X, 0)\cos(n\pi X/L)\,dX. \tag{2.57}$$

A useful alternative expression of this result is the following:

$$V(X, T) = C_o e^{-t/\tau_o} + C_1 e^{-t/\tau_1} + C_2 e^{-t/\tau_2} + \cdots, \tag{2.58}$$

where $C_o = B_o$, τ_o equals the passive membrane time constant, $\tau_m = r_m c_m$ (because the membrane was assumed uniform and without a short circuit). Also

$$C_n = B_n \cos(n\pi X/L) \tag{2.59}$$

and the τ_n, called "equalizing time constants" for $n > 0$, are all smaller than τ_o, as shown by the following:

$$\tau_o/\tau_n = 1 + \alpha_n^2 = 1 + (n\pi/L)^2. \tag{2.60}$$

Useful physical intuition results from noting the effect of n on the harmonic status of the functions, $\cos(n\pi/L)$, that is associated with each exponential decay in eq. 2.55. Thus $n = 0$ associates the slowest decay time constant with a uniform voltage (corresponding to the average voltage along the finite length); this uniform component of charge decays only through the resting membrane conductance. In contrast, $n = 1$ associates the first equalizing time constant, τ_1, with decay and rapid equalization of charge between two half-lengths of the cylinder; note that $\cos(\pi X/L)$ is positive for values of X from 0 to $L/2$, and negative from $L/2$ to L). Similarly, $n = 2$ associates τ_2 with decay and even more rapid equalization of charge (over shorter lengths involving less core resistance) between the midregion and both ends of the cylinder; still larger values of n imply higher harmonics with more rapid equalization of charge over still shorter components of cylinder length.

It is important to note that while these time constants depend on L, they are completely independent of the initial condition or the point of observation. This means that the value of L can be calculated from a time constant ratio, using the expression

$$L = \frac{n\pi}{\sqrt{\tau_o/\tau_n - 1}}. \tag{2.61}$$

This useful theoretical result has been applied to experimental data from many neuron types. As explained in Rall (1969a), we can peel the slowest (τ_o) decay of an experimental or simulated passive decay transient (or of the transient response to an applied current step) and, provided that the coefficient C_1 is relatively large, obtain an estimate of τ_1, and thus of the ratio τ_o/τ_1, which we can then use (in eq. 2.61 with $n = 1$) to obtain an estimate of L. However, it is important to remember that eq. 2.61 is strictly correct for a uniform cylinder with two sealed ends. When this equation is applied to experimental data from neurons that deviate significantly from equivalence to a cylinder, we should not expect to get a valid estimate of L without evaluating the expected error (see also the comment at the end of section 2.6.3).

The coefficients C_n do depend on the initial condition (which determines B_n by eq. 2.57), and on the point of observation (which is X in eq. 2.59). An idealized initial condition (which serves as a useful reference case) is the case where $V(X,0)$ is proportional to the spatial delta function, $\delta(X = 0)$. This equals zero for all values of X except $X = 0$, where the delta function has infinite amplitude, while its integral over X from $X = 0$ to $X = L$ has unit value. Such an initial condition is proportional to an instantaneous point charge placed at $X = 0$ when $T = 0$. If the amount of such a charge is Q_o, the Fourier coefficients can be shown to reduce to

$$B_o = Q_o/(L\lambda c_m), \quad \text{and for } n > 0, \quad B_n = 2B_o, \tag{2.62}$$

where c_m represents the membrane capacitance per unit length of cylinder, $L\lambda = \ell$ the length of the cylinder and $L\lambda c_m$ the capacitance of the membrane cylinder. It may be noted that when the charge per unit length, $c_m v(X, T)$, is integrated from $X = 0$ to $X = L$, all terms for which $n > 0$ in eq. 2.55 yield zero integrals, and the term for $n = 0$ yields $B_o L = Q_o/(\lambda c_m)$, which equals the voltage expected if the same amount of charge were distributed uniformly along the length of the cylinder.

It is helpful to understand that the value of B_o is the same for any initial distribution of charge, Q_o, along the length of the cylinder, that the zero-order term, $C_o \exp(-t/\tau_o)$ of eq. 2.58, corresponds to the passive decay of this total charge, regardless of its initial distribution, and that the values of B_n, for $n > 0$, depend on the initial distribution. The higher-order decay terms, $C_n \exp(-t/\tau_n)$, result from rapid equalizing current flow (charge redistribution) between regions of higher and lower than average membrane potential; they are governed by the equalizing time constants, τ_n, which are smaller than τ_o (see eq. 2.60).

An instructive example has the initial condition proportional to $\delta(X = L)$, corresponding to an instantaneous point charge located at $X = L$. For this case, $B_n = 2(-1)^n B_o$, meaning that we have alternating signs: the values of B_n are negative for odd integer values of n, and positive for even integer values. Using eq. 2.59, we see that at $X = 0$, the value of $\cos(n\pi X/L) = 1$ for all n; thus the C_n have the same alternating signs as B_n (but note that at $X = L$, the C_n would all be positive). With alternating signs, such a sum can produce a smooth transient that resembles a synaptic potential (readers who have never summed such a series may find this an interesting example to compute).

Another instructive example has the initial condition proportional to $\delta(X = L/2)$, corresponding to an instantaneous point charge located at the midpoint, $X = L/2$. For this case, $B_n = 0$ for all odd integer values of n (because, in eq. 2.57, $\cos(n\pi X/L)$ becomes $\cos(n\pi/2)$, which is zero when n is odd). For even values of n, we have alternating signs, with negative values whenever $n/2$ is odd. In this case, although the symmetry leads us to expect the same transient (with alternating signs) at $X = 0$ and at $X = L$, at $X = L/2$, the values of C_n (for n even) are all positive.

A different example, roughly resembling an initial charge distributed over a lumped soma, has the initial charge distributed uniformly over a short length, from $X = 0$ to $X = A$, with a zero initial voltage everywhere beyond $X = A$ to $X = L$. Then eqs. 2.56–2.59 imply a coefficient ratio for the decay transient at any location X, which can be expressed

$$\frac{C_n}{C_o} = \frac{2 \sin(n\pi A/L)}{n\pi A/L} \cos(n\pi X/L). \tag{2.63}$$

The maximum value of this ratio is 2, which is obtained only in the limiting case where $A = 0$ and $X = 0$; this means that unless the initial condition is restricted to a point ($A = 0$) and the observation is made at the same point ($X = 0$), this coefficient ratio will be less than 2. For example, if A/L and X/L are both set equal to 0.1, this ratio is 1.87 for $n = 1$, and it is 1.51 for $n = 2$. This result provides a warning that parameter estimates based on the coefficient ratios found in experimental data should take this effect into consideration.

2.6.3 Lumped Soma Coupled to Cylinders

When a lumped soma is coupled to one or more equivalent cylinders, the mathematical solution of the PDE is more complicated. By losing the zero slope boundary condition at $X = 0$, we lose the earlier simple expressions for the eigenvalues α_n, the time constants τ_n, and the coefficients C_n. As explained in Rall 1969a, we now have to specify α_n as the roots of the transcendental equation

$$\alpha L \cot(\alpha L) = -\rho_\infty L, \tag{2.64}$$

where $\rho_\infty = G_\infty/G_S = \rho \coth(L)$ and ρ is defined in section 2.5.3; note that the equivalent cylinder could represent several dendritic trees, provided that they have the same value of L and satisfy the specified constraints. A figure showing how the resulting ratio of τ_o/τ_1 depends on the values of L was provided in Rall 1969a, but is not reproduced here. However, it is useful to know that these results can be approximated by the expression

$$\alpha_n \approx n\pi/L_N, \tag{2.65}$$

where L_N represents an effective L value for the whole neuron (soma plus dendrites); this L_N is greater than the L value of the dendritic equivalent cylinder, now labeled L_D. Intuitively, this means that the soma membrane (although isopotential) adds something to the apparent electrotonic length of the dendrites. Excluding very small values of ρ, it was found that useful approximations could be expressed

$$L_N/L_D \approx \sqrt{(\rho + 1)/\rho} \approx 1 + 0.5/\rho. \tag{2.66}$$

Here we include no details on the effect of soma coupling on the values of the coefficients C_n, or on the related sets of C_n obtained for an applied current step at $X = 0$ (see Rall 1977, 83, 84; see also Durand 1984, Kawato 1984, and Poznanski

1987, which consider the effect of a different soma membrane time constant, as would occur with significant soma shunting).

If there are k dendritic equivalent cylinders having different L_D values, these can be distinguished by an index, j, and the previous transcendental equation (eq. 2.64) becomes generalized to

$$\alpha = -\sum_{j=1}^{k} \rho_{\infty_j} \tan(\alpha L_{Dj}). \tag{2.67}$$

A useful numerical example (Rall 1969a) assumed the values $\rho_{\infty 1} = 3$, with $L_{D1} = 1$ for one dendritic equivalent cylinder, and $\rho_{\infty 2} = 5$, with $L_{D2} = 2$ for the other. Noting that $\alpha_0 = 0$ is a root, we find that $\alpha_1 \approx 1.10$, $\alpha_2 \approx 1.97$, and $\alpha_3 \approx 2.92$ are also roots of eq. 2.66. For $n > 3$, it was found that $\alpha_n \approx n\pi/3$; what makes this noteworthy is that it agrees with eq. 2.65, for $L_N = 3$, and in this example, $(L_{D1} + L_{D2}) = 3$. Furthermore, in view of the earlier approximation (eq. 2.66) that adds something for the soma, we could try $L_N \approx 3.2$. Using this, eq. 2.65 suggests α_n values of 1.96 and 2.94 for n of 2 and 3, respectively; these values are very close to the approximate values of α_2 and α_3 noted above. On reflection, this result is not difficult to understand; if the two ρ_∞ values were equal, the two cylinders would have the same diameter; their combined cylinder length would correspond to $L_D = 3$, and their combined value of $\rho = \rho_\infty(\tanh L_{D1} + \tanh L_{D2})$. A ρ_∞ value of 4 would then imply a combined ρ value of about 6.9, and eq. 2.66 would imply $L_N/L_D \approx 1.07$, or a value of about 3.2 for L_N. If ρ_∞ were very large, we would expect the soma to contribute negligible effective length. This kind of result has been verified with other examples.

It is important to emphasize that the voltage decay corresponding to τ_1 may not be apparent in experimental or simulated data because the coefficient associated with this time constant may be very small. In particular, when $L_{D1} = L_{D2}$, the eigenvalue $\alpha_1 = \pi/L_N = \pi/(2L_{D1})$ exists, but the corresponding coefficient, C_1, (for observation and input at the soma) is zero, which means that τ_2 but not τ_1 would be observed. If we were to apply eq. 2.61 knowing τ_o and this τ_2, we would get $L = L_N$. If, on the other hand, we did not know that the true τ_1 was absent from the data and we treated τ_2 as though it were τ_1, our application of eq. 2.61 would then yield $L = 0.5L_N = L_{D1} = L_{D2}$. The same result should be expected when the two cylinders differ slightly in their electrotonic lengths because then the value of C_1, although not zero, is still very small relative to C_0 and C_2. This insight can be extended to the case of a soma coupled to several dendritic cylinders, provided that their electrotonic lengths differ by less than 20% (Segev and Rall 1983).

2.6.4   Using the Laplace Transform for Analyzing the Transient Solution

An alternative approach for solving the PDE is to use the Laplace transform. The *Laplace transform* of a signal $f(t)$ is defined as

$$\tilde{f}(s) \equiv \int_{-\infty}^{\infty} e^{-st} f(t) \, dt, \tag{2.68}$$

where s is a complex number whose real part is nonnegative (in many practical uses, it is assumed that s is restricted to be a nonnegative real number). In many applied mathematics books, the Laplace transform is defined using 0 as the lower limit of the integral instead of ∞. This *right-sided* definition assumes that $f(t) = 0$ for $t < 0$. We are using the two-sided definition for generality. By a proper integration of the cable PDE (see the mathematical appendix of Jack et al. 1975 or other textbook on the Laplace transform), we get the cable equation in the Laplace domain (eq. 2.4), which is very similar to the steady-state cable equation. The boundary conditions can also be integrated in the same way. The analogy between the steady-state case and the Laplace domain case may be used in finding the transient solution of the cable equation. The methods used above for computations in the steady-state case can be used in the Laplace domain, and analytic results found. The main disadvantage is that, eventually, an inverse transformation to the time domain should be made, and this step involves nontrivial numerical calculations. Nonetheless, these methods can be found useful in some cases (see Butz and Cowan 1974; Horwitz 1981; Koch and Poggio 1985; Holmes 1986; van-Pelt 1992).

2.6.5   The Method of Moments

The *method of moments* is a general approach for characterizing and analyzing dendritic transients without solving the cable PDE explicitly. Rather than computing the whole time course of the voltage response, a few selected properties of the transient current and voltage response are computed analytically. These properties are defined using the moments of the transient signal. The *i*th *moment* of a transient signal $f(t)$, $m_{f,i}$ $(i = 0, 1, 2, \ldots)$ is

$$m_{f,i} \equiv \int_{-\infty}^{\infty} t^i f(t) \, dt. \tag{2.69}$$

For a detailed derivation of the method of moments, see Agmon-Snir 1995. In the present context, the basic ideas are explained in brief. The most important moments-based properties of a dendritic transient signal are depicted in figure 2.8:

• *Strength.*   Represented as $\hat{s}_f$, strength is defined as $m_{f,0}$, that is, the time integral of the signal

$$\int_{-\infty}^{\infty} f(t)\, dt.$$

For current signals, the strength is the total charge.

• *Characteristic time.*   Represented as $\hat{t}_f$, characteristic time is defined

$$\hat{t}_f \equiv \frac{m_{f,1}}{m_{f,0}} = \frac{m_{f,1}}{\hat{s}_f}, \tag{2.70}$$

where $\hat{t}_f$ has an interpretation of "center of gravity" (centroid) of $f(t)$ in the following sense:

$$\int_{-\infty}^{\infty} (t - \hat{t}_f) f(t)\, dt = 0. \tag{2.71}$$

• *Dispersion.*   Represented as $\hat{w}_f^2$, dispersion is defined

$$\hat{w}_f^2 \equiv \int_{-\infty}^{\infty} (t - \hat{t}_f)^2 \frac{f(t)}{\hat{s}_f}\, dt = \frac{m_{f,2}}{\hat{s}_f} - \hat{t}_f^2. \tag{2.72}$$

The definition of dispersion is similar to the definition of the variance in probability theory. It is a measure of the dispersion of the signal around the centroid. The *width* of the signal, $\hat{w}_f$, is defined as the square root of $\hat{w}_f^2$, similar to the definition of standard deviation in probability theory. It is another measure of the signal dispersion, with units of time.

We can also define other shape properties of the transient signal, such as *skewness* and *kurtosis*, based on higher moments.

The moments are closely related to the Laplace transform (eq. 2.68). Differentiating the Laplace transform i times with respect to s (when s is restricted to be real and nonnegative) and setting $s = 0$, we get the ith *moment* multiplied by $(-1)^i$. Hence, we can find the Laplace transform of the transient response, (discussed in section 2.6.4) and use straightforward differentiation to obtain the moments-based properties of the voltage response. As a result, the nontrivial transformation from the Laplace transform into the time domain can be avoided. In practice, there are technical shortcuts available; relatively simple algorithms, similar to those described in section 2.4 can be used to analyze the moments-based response in arbitrary-branched dendritic trees. The similarity between the mathematical analysis for the

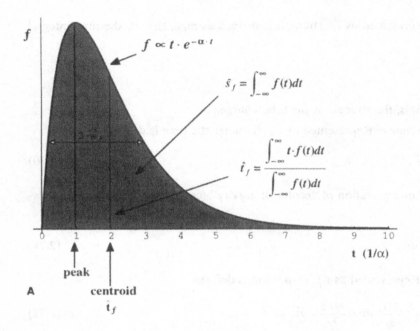

$$f \propto t \cdot e^{-\alpha \cdot t}$$

$$\hat{s}_f = \int_{-\infty}^{\infty} f(t)dt$$

$$\hat{t}_f = \frac{\int_{-\infty}^{\infty} t \cdot f(t)dt}{\int_{-\infty}^{\infty} f(t)dt}$$

peak

centroid
$\hat{t}_f$

A

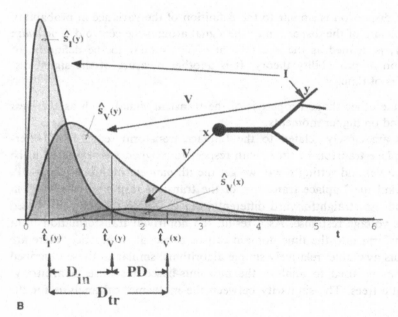

$\hat{s}_I(y)$

$\hat{s}_V(y)$

$\hat{s}_V(x)$

I

V

V

$\hat{t}_I(y)$ $\hat{t}_V(y)$ $\hat{t}_V(x)$

D_{in} PD

D_{tr}

B

steady-state case, for the Laplace transform of the transient response and for the moments-based properties of the transient response leads to many interesting results.

Strength Rinzel and Rall (1974) showed the similarity between the equations of the time integral (*strength*) of a transient voltage response in a passive structure and the steady-state cable equations (see also Jack et al. 1975, 187–188). This similarity holds for any time-invariant linear system. Specifically, in such a system, if the strength of the transient input is A and the strength of the output response is B, then if we apply a steady input of magnitude A to the system, we get a steady output of magnitude B. This important feature allows one to apply the same methods used for the steady-state analysis to the analysis of the strength of transients. Hence, when a transient current input is injected at point x_1 in a dendritic tree, the ratio between the strength of the transient voltage at point x_1 and the strength of the current input is equal to the (steady-state) *input resistance* at this point, $R_{in}(x_1)$ (see section 2.4.1). More generally, the ratio between the strength of the voltage response at a given location in the structure (x_2) and the strength of the current input at the injection point (x_1) is equal to the (steady-state) *transfer resistance*, $R_{tr}(x_1, x_2)$. If the transient signal propagates in the structure from point x_1 to point x_2, the ratio between the strength of the voltage at point x_1 and the strength of the voltage at point x_2 is equal to the (steady-state) *attenuation factor* between these points, $A(x_1, x_2)$. Similarly, the *attenuation rate* and the effective length constant (section 2.4.4), defined originally with respect to steady-state inputs, can be applied to the analysis of the strength of the transient response.

Moreover, the properties of the strength of the voltage response are easily derived from the properties of the steady-state response (section 2.4.2). An additional trivial outcome of the above discussion is the *shape invariance property*, stating that the transfer resistance and the attenuation factor between any two points in the passive

Figure 2.8
Definitions related to the method of moments. (A) Definitions of *strength, characteristic time,* and *width* of a signal. In this figure, a transient signal with a shape of an α-function, namely, $f(t) \propto t \cdot e^{-\alpha t}$, is depicted. The shaded area under the function is the signal strength, $\hat{s}_f$. The centroid of the signal is the signal characteristic time, $\hat{t}_f$. Because the signal width, $\hat{w}_f$, is analogous to the standard deviation in probability theory, $2\hat{w}_f$ is shown in the graph. The width is useful when comparing two signals. The peak point of the signal, which is classically used for characterizing the signal, is also shown as a reference. (B) Resistance, attenuation, and delays for transients (see section 2.6.5). In this scheme, a transient (α-function-shaped) current is injected at point y in a passive structure, and the voltage responses at y and at another location x are depicted. The shaded areas below the functions show the strengths of the various signals. The input resistance, $R_{in}(y)$, is equal to $\hat{s}_V(y)/\hat{s}_I(y)$; the transfer resistance, $R_{tr}(y, x)$, is $\hat{s}_V(x)/\hat{s}_I(y)$; and the attenuation factor, $A(y, x)$, is $\hat{s}_V(y)/\hat{s}_V(x)$. The vertical lines show the characteristic times of the various signals. The input delay, $D_{in}(y)$, is defined as $\hat{t}_V(y) - \hat{t}_I(y)$; the transfer delay, $D_{tr}(y, x)$, as $\hat{t}_V(x) - \hat{t}_I(y)$; and the propagation delay, $PD(y, x)$, as $\hat{t}_V(y) - \hat{t}_V(x)$. From Agmon-Snir 1995.

dendritic tree are independent of the shape of the injected transient current. Finally, the algorithms described in section 2.4.3 apply also to the analysis of the strength of the transient response, and attenograms made for the steady-state case (see section 2.4.4) can be used to analyze the attenuation of the strength of the transient response in dendritic trees.

Characteristic Time   Using the difference between the characteristic times of two signals, we can define delays. When a transient current input is injected at point x_1 in a dendritic tree, the *transfer delay* between the input at this point and the voltage at a given point x_2 is defined as $D_{tr}(x_1, x_2) = \hat{t}_V(x_2) - \hat{t}_I(x_1)$; the *input delay*, $D_{in}(x_1)$, is defined as $D_{tr}(x_1, x_1)$. The *propagation delay* is then defined as $PD(x_1, x_2) = \hat{t}_V(x_2) - \hat{t}_V(x_1)$, where x_1 and x_2 are points in the structure and the signal propagates from x_1 to x_2. Using the reciprocal of the derivative of $\hat{t}_V(x)$, the *velocity* of the signal is defined. These four definitions are analogous to the transfer resistance, input resistance, attenuation factor, and attenuation rate, respectively, for the steady-state case.

One of the properties of the characteristic time is the *shape invariance property*, stating that the transfer delay and the propagation delay between any two points in the passive dendritic tree are independent of the shape of the injected transient current (as a simple outcome, the input delay is independent of the shape of the injected current). Other important properties are analogous to the those of the steady-state response (section 2.4.2). Using the definition of the input delay, we can define an *effective time constant*, $\vec{\tau}_{eff}(x)$. It can then be shown that the velocity of the transient at a point x, as defined above, is $\vec{\lambda}_{eff}(x)/\vec{\tau}_{eff}(x)$ in the propagation direction. Finally, the algorithms described in section 2.4.3 can be extended to apply also to the analysis of delays, and another type of morphoelectrotonic transform, the *delayogram*, can be easily made for graphical representations of delays in dendritic trees (see section 2.4.4; Zador et al. 1995).

Similarly, using the *dispersion* of transient signals, we can define and analyze broadening with the help of analogous definitions, properties, and algorithms. Although the analysis can go further, to moments-based properties based on higher moments, most of the important information about the transient signal is to be found in the analysis of the first moments–based properties, and analysis of higher moments (which is harder computationally) is usually not required.

The method of moments is a tool for exploring the spatiotemporal integration properties in dendrites. It may provide answers for questions such as, what is the time delay for transient signals in arbitrary-shaped dendrites? How does this delay depend on the biophysical parameters of the tree? What is the width of the time window for synaptic integration or coincidence detection at various dendritic locations? What is the dendritic domain in which, the synapses may affect a target point in the dendrites? (For how the method of moments can be used to answer these questions, see Agmon-Snir and Segev 1993, 1996.)

2.7 Synaptic Input as a Conductance Change

2.7.1 Formal Representation of Synaptic Excitation and Inhibition

The membrane equivalent circuit used for synaptically mediated excitation and inhibition (Rall 1962a, 1964; see figure 2.9) is closely related to the models introduced by Fatt and Katz (1953) and by Coombs, Eccles, and Fatt (1955). The membrane capacity per unit area, C_m, is electrically in parallel with three conductance pathways per unit area. G_r represents the resting membrane conductance that lies in series with the resting battery, E_r (e.g., $-70\,\text{mV}$, interior relative to exterior); G_ε represents the synaptic excitatory conductance that lies in series with its reversal potential, E_ε (e.g., zero, interior relative to exterior); and G_j represents the synaptic inhibitory conductance that lies in series with its reversal potential, E_j (e.g., $-80\,\text{mV}$, interior relative to exterior). Following Kirchhoff's current law, the membrane current density across a space-clamped patch of uniform membrane can then be expressed

$$I_m = C_m(dV_m/dt) + G_r(V_m - E_r) + G_\varepsilon(V_m - E_\varepsilon) + G_j(V_m - E_j). \tag{2.73}$$

For time periods during which the membrane parameters remain unchanged and $I_m = 0$, this equation can be rearranged to the following form:

$$\tau dV/dt = -k^2(V - V^*), \tag{2.74}$$

where $\tau = R_m C_m = C_m/G_r$, $V = V_m - E_r$, V^* is the steady-state value of V (with $I_m = 0$), as shown by eq. 2.76 below, and k^2 is a factor defined by eq. 2.75. Equation 2.74 implies that V decays exponentially to V^* with a time constant equal to τ/k^2, where

$$k^2 = (G_r + G_\varepsilon + G_j)/G_r \tag{2.75}$$

and

$$V^* = \frac{G_\varepsilon(E_\varepsilon - E_r) + G_j(E_j - E_r)}{G_r + G_\varepsilon + G_j}. \tag{2.76}$$

For resting conditions, G_ε and G_j are both zero, $k^2 = 1$, and $V^* = 0$, meaning that V decays to zero with the resting time constant, τ. However, when $G_\varepsilon = 2G_r$ with zero

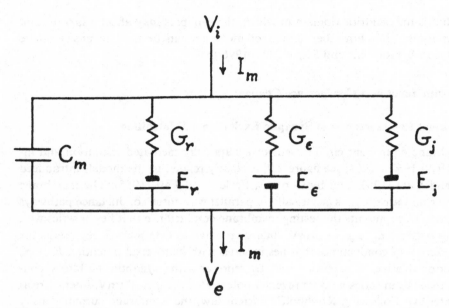

Figure 2.9
Equivalent electric circuit for membrane that can receive synaptic excitation and/or synaptic inhibition, based on Fatt and Katz 1953 and Coombs, Eccles and Fatt 1955. The membrane current, I_m, per unit area, can divide into four pathways: one capacitative, and three conductive. The resting conductance, G_r, per unit area, could be the sum of the resting conductance values for several ion species, and the reversal potential, E_r, could be a weighted sum of several different ionic reversal potentials. Both G_r and E_r are assumed independent of V and T. For resting conditions, both G_ε and G_j are zero. Synaptic excitatory input, increases G_ε (as a step, square pulse, or smooth alpha function); the reversal potential. E_ε, is often taken to be zero, relative to the resting potential, E_r. Synaptic inhibitory input increases G_j; its reversal potential, E_j, is constant that can be chosen to get minus 0.1 for the ratio $(E_j - E_r)/(E_\varepsilon - E_r)$.

G_j, then $k^2 = 3$ and $V^* = (2/3)(E_\varepsilon - E_r)$, meaning that V would decay to 0.67 (when V is normalized relative to $E_\varepsilon - E_r$) with an effective time constant that is $1/3$ the resting value. In figure 2.10A, the asymptote of the upper curve is less than 0.67 because this half cylinder was not space-clamped and there was a spread of current from the "hot" half to the "cold" half during the time that $G_e = 2G_r$ was kept on over half of the cylinder. If, instead, $G_\varepsilon = G_r$ over all of the cylinder, then $k^2 = 2$ and the normalized value of V^* would be 0.5, which would produce a transient similar to the middle curve of figure 2.10, but not identical. Why it would not be identical must be related to the effective value of λ^2 being reduced over the "hot" region while the synaptic conductance is on, which would upset the symmetry about the "midpoint." Although further details are omitted here, nonuniform synaptic inhibition was also explored by hand calculations summarized in figures 8 and 9 of Rall 1962a.

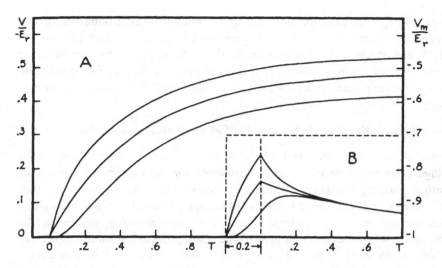

Figure 2.10
Transients of membrane depolarization at three locations in a dendritic tree or its equivalent cylinder (for $L = 1$), when a uniform synaptic excitatory conductance was applied to a half-length of the equivalent cylinder. The middle curves in A and B correspond to the midpoint ($X = 0.5$); the other curves correspond to the two ends ($X = 0$, or $X = 1.0$); the upper curves in A and B show the voltage transient at the "hot" end (i.e., end of the half-cylinder that received synaptic excitatory input), while the lower curve in A and B corresponds to the "cool" end of the equivalent cylinder. For A, the synaptic conductance ($G_\varepsilon = 2G_r$) came on as a step, when $T = 0$, and stayed on. For B, the on-step at $T = 0$ was followed by an equal off-step at $T = 0.2$; thus the input was a square conductance pulse over half of the membrane surface. The mathematical statement and solution of this problem are in Rall 1962a.

This theoretical paper provided useful analytical results; the hand calculations provided early insights about excitatory postsynaptic potential (EPSP) shapes for nonuniform synaptic input distributions, and about interactions of excitatory and inhibitory synaptic inputs. These were explored further in subsequent studies (Rall 1964, 1967, 1969a; Jack et al. 1975; Segev and Parnas 1983).

Although a square pulse of synaptic conductance was adequate for some computations, we often prefer to specify a brief smooth time course for the synaptic conductance. The function used for this purpose by Rall (1967), by Jack et al. (1971), and by others is a one-parameter function (often referred to as the "alpha function"):

$$G(T) = \alpha^2 T \exp(-\alpha T) = \alpha(T/T_p)\exp(-T/T_p), \tag{2.77}$$

where α and T are both dimensionless. This function is zero for $T = 0$, rises smoothly to a peak at a time $T_p = 1/\alpha$, and then falls somewhat more slowly back to zero. Halfway up, $T \approx 0.23\, T_p$, and halfway down, $T \approx 2.68\, T_p$, implying a half-width of 2.45 T_p. The peak amplitude equals α/e, and the area under this curve equals unity. Plots of this time course for α values of 10, 20, 40, and 100 can be found in Jack and Redman 1971 and Jack et al. 1975. Alternatively, the synaptic conductance is sometimes represented as a sum of two exponential functions. The alpha and the two-exponent representations are now built into several neuronal modeling tools.

2.7.2 Synaptic Excitation Distributed over Half of an Equivalent Cylinder

One early transient calculation (Rall 1962a) is summarized by figure 2.10, which shows voltage (membrane depolarization) transients for the case of an equivalent cylinder with a synaptic excitatory conductance distributed uniformly over one-half of its length. The excited half could represent either the proximal or the distal half of the dendritic surface area of a dendritic tree. The synaptic intensity, defined as the ratio of synaptic conductance per unit area to the resting membrane conductance per unit area, was set equal to 2, turned on at $T = 0$, and left on for the three curves shown in A of figure 2.1. For the three curves in B, however, the synaptic conductance was turned off at $T = 0.2$, implying a brief square on-off transient of synaptic conductance that generates a crude synaptic potential (EPSP). In both A and B, the middle curve was calculated at the midpoint ($X = 0.5$) of the cylinder, the upper curve was calculated at one end (the "hot" end belonging to the excited half of the cylinder), and the lower curve was calculated at the "cold" end of the cylinder.

There are several points to be noted about these results. One is the difference in the shapes of the transients in B. As noted in the original paper, "the transient at the 'hot' end rises and falls more rapidly. The transient at the 'cold' end begins very slowly, but it continues to rise after the conductance pulse is over; this is due to an equalizing flow of current between the two halves of the dendritic tree" (Rall 1962a, 1088). Considering an experimental EPSP to be recorded near the proximal end of a dendritic tree, we note that the upper curve shows the steeper rise to a larger peak, as well as the rapid early decay obtained for proximally located synaptic input, while the lower curve shows the slower rise to a later and more rounded peak (with no rapid early decay) of an EPSP produced by distally located synaptic input. These are the kinds of differences in EPSP shape that were pursued further with compartmental computations (Rall 1964, 1967), leading to shape indices defined as the half-width and the rise time (or time-to-peak) and to the shape index plot, which facilitated the comparison of theory and experiment (Rall et al. 1967) and helped to establish the importance of the dendritic location of a synaptic input (see figure 2.11).

Another point of interest is that the late decay, an exponential decay with the passive membrane time constant, is the same for all three curves, whereas the early decay is significantly modified by the rapid equalizing current flow between regions of unequal potential. The equalizing time constants governing this equalizing flow were implied by the eigenvalues γ_n^2 (Rall 1962a), and made explicit as τ_n in a later publication (Rall 1969a); see eqs. 2.58–2.60, which hold for passive decay to the resting potential). It is important to note that while the synaptic conductance is on, the perturbed membrane (the portion of membrane that receives this input) would have its local membrane conductivity tripled. An isolated patch of this perturbed membrane would have a time constant only 1/3 of that for passive resting membrane; however, the system composed of both regions of this cylinder has eigenvalues and time constants determined by equations 44–46 of Rall 1962a. Consequently, the rate of rise of the upper curves in A of figure 2.10 is much steeper than the rate of late decay in B; see equations 2.74 and 2.75, above, and see Rall 1962a for more details.

2.8   Insights Gained from Compartmental Computations

Compartmental modeling of a neuron was introduced in the 1960s. As explained in Rall 1964, this adaptation from compartmental modeling of metabolic systems was facilitated by interaction with the analytical and computational expertise of John Hearon and Mones Berman, Colleagues in the Mathematical Research Branch at the National Institutes of Health. A single compartment could correspond to a single dendritic branch, a group of branches, or just a segment of a trunk or branch element, according to the needs of a given problem. The region of the neuron represented by a single compartment is treated as isopotential; voltage differences between regions are represented as differences between compartments. Mathematically, the PDE of cable theory is replaced by a system of ODEs for which analytical and computational solutions are already available. The major advantage is flexibility: the membrane properties and the amount of synaptic conductance input or current injection can be different in every compartment; dendritic branching need not satisfy equivalent-cylinder constraints. It is possible to compute the consequences of any branching geometry and any spatiotemporal pattern of input that one chooses to specify.

The necessary equations explained and illustrated in Rall 1964 are also discussed in chapter 3, this volume, while chapter 14 presents efficient numerical methods for their solution. Here we point briefly to basic early results that were obtained using a simple chain of ten equal compartments. Because they were made equal, these compartments provide a lumped representation of an equivalent cylinder. As indicated by the diagram (upper right in figure 2.11), this ten-compartment model can represent the entire soma-dendritic extent of the neuron; compartment 1 can be regarded as the soma; compartment 2 represents the trunks of all dendritic trees belonging to this neuron; compartments 3 to 10 represent increasing electrotonic distance away from the soma to the dendritic terminals of all these trees. Each compartment represents an equal amount of membrane surface area available for synaptic input. Given this model, the focus in figure 2.11 is on the effect of input location on EPSP shape; the effect of spatiotemporal input pattern is shown in figure 2.12, and the effect of location of synaptic inhibition is shown in figure 2.13.

2.8.1   Effect of Synaptic Input Location on the Excitatory Postsynaptic Potential Shape at the Soma

The three voltage transients shown at lower right in figure 2.11 represent three different EPSP shapes computed for the soma compartment in response to brief synaptic excitatory conductance input to a single compartment for three different choices of input location. The EPSP amplitudes have been normalized; the input locations were compartments 1, 4, or 8, as indicated by the numbers inside the open triangles; the input conductance time course (shown as the dotted curve above them) was the same in each case. The reference EPSP (designated by the black triangle) resulted when the same input time course was applied uniformly to all ten compartments. It is apparent that the EPSP obtained with the most proximal input location (compartment 1) rises most steeply to the earliest peak; this is a sharp peak because of rapid early decay, which can be understood as due to rapid equalizing spread of depolarizing charge away from the soma to the dendritic compartments. The rapid rise and rapid early decay are responsible for a relatively short half-width (duration at half maximum). In contrast, the EPSP obtained at the soma in response to the distal input location (compartment 8) shows a delayed, slow rise to a later, more rounded peak; this can be understood as due to equalizing spread of depolarizing charge toward the soma from the distal dendritic input location. The slow rise and slow early decay are responsible for a relatively long half-width. The difference between these shapes resembles that seen in figure 2.10B, with essentially the same explanation.

To facilitate comparison of many experimental EPSP shapes with these theoretical EPSP shapes, the shape index plot was devised (Rall et al. 1967) illustrated at left in figure 2.11. This was particularly useful because the input locations for the experimental EPSPs were unknown. Hence the shape scatter of an experimental EPSP population was compared with the two theoretical shape index loci shown in figure 2.11. The solid line through the black triangle is the locus of shapes computed for uniform synaptic input to all ten compartments, when the input time course is

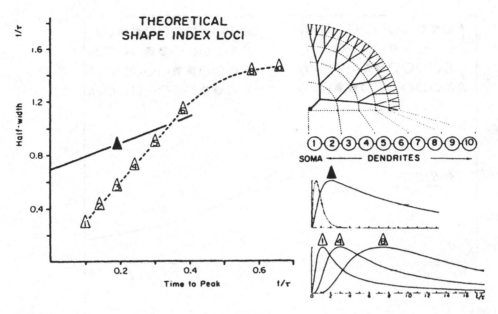

Figure 2.11
EPSP shapes and shape index loci. Somadendritic membrane (upper right) mapped into a chain of ten equal compartments. Four voltage transients (lower right) represent computed EPSPs at the soma; their shapes differ because of different synaptic input locations; the brief synaptic excitatory conductance transient (dotted curve with peak at $t = 0.04\tau$) was the same for all four cases. The upper EPSP (black triangle) resulted when the input was equal in all compartments; the three lower EPSP shapes are for synaptic input restricted to a single compartment (open triangles 1, 4, or 8, designate the input compartment for each case). These EPSP shapes are on the shape index plot (at left), of half-width versus the time-to-peak. Curve through open triangles represents a theoretical locus of EPSP shapes obtained by varying only the location of the single input compartment. Line through the solid triangle represents a theoretical locus of EPSP shapes obtained by varying only the input time course (i.e., the parameter α), for synaptic input distributed uniformly over the somadendritic surface. From Rall et al. 1967; tables of computed values and other details in Rall 1967.

changed by choosing different values of the parameter alpha in eq. 2.77. The dashed curve through the open triangles is the locus of shapes computed when the input was restricted to different choices of a single compartment, using the same input time course (i.e., $\alpha = 25$ in eq. 2.77) with each of these locations.

In the original paper by Rall et al. (1967) and in papers by Jack et al. (1971) and others, it was found that the variation in the shapes of EPSPs produced by single I_a afferent fiber input to motoneurons of cat spinal cord is in much better agreement with theoretical loci of the type shown in figure 2.11 by the dashed curve with the open triangles. It was concluded that these synapses are distributed over proximal

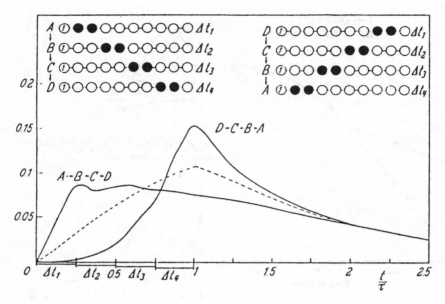

Figure 2.12
Effect of spationtemporal pattern of synaptic input on the resultant composite EPSP at the soma, computed with a ten-compartment model. The total amount of synaptic input was the same in each case. Diagram at upper left shows the synaptic input sequence, A-B-C-D, (proximal location first, distal location last); this produced the soma voltage transient labeled A-B-C-D at lower left. Diagram at upper right shows the opposite synaptic input sequence, D-C-B-A, (distal location first, proximal last); this produced a soma voltage transient, with delayed rise to a larger peak amplitude, labeled D-C-B-A. In both cases, the input compartments (shown filled) received a synaptic excitatory conductance pulse ($G_\epsilon = G_r$ for 0.25τ) during one of the four labeled time increments. The same total amount of synaptic input (when uniform over compartments 2 to 9 from $t = 0$ to $t = \tau$) produced the dashed curve. Modified from Rall 1964.

and distal dendritic locations, that unitary EPSP shapes can be accounted for by these locations, and that compound EPSP shapes can be accounted for by two or more input locations. Additional details can be found in the original papers; important experimental confirmation of the correlation of EPSP shape and synaptic location has been provided by the experiments of Redman and Walmsley (1983).

2.8.2 Effect of Spatiotemporal Pattern of Synaptic Input

The purpose of the computations summarized in figure 2.12 was to demonstrate that it should be possible to distinguish two synaptic inputs that are equal in amount and differ only in one aspect of their spatiotemporal pattern. This computation used the ten-compartment model, and the synaptic excitatory conductance input sequences,

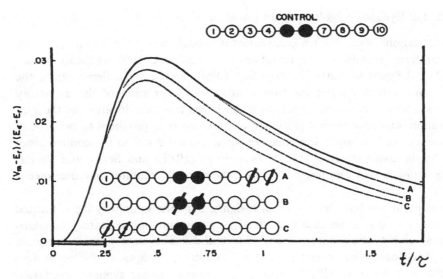

Figure 2.13
Effect of location of synaptic inhibition, computed with ten-compartment model. The control EPSP at the soma, shown as the solid curve, was produced by a synaptic excitatory conductance in compartments 5 and 6 (square pulse from $T = 0$ to $T = 0.25$, with $G_\varepsilon = G_r$). Dotted curves show effect of three inhibitory input locations (indicated by diagonal slash in compartmental diagrams); this inhibition was a sustained inhibitory conductance ($G_j = G_r$, with $E_j = E_r$; shunting inhibition). For curve A, the inhibitory input location was distal to the control input; this did not reduce the control EPSP amplitude at the soma. For curves B and C, the inhibitory input location was either proximal to or the same as the control input; both reduced the EPSP amplitude significantly. Larger reductions of EPSP amplitude would result from larger values of G_j and from hyperpolarized values for E_j. Modified form Rall 1964.

A-B-C-D and D-C-B-A, which were composed of equal square pulses of synaptic conductance (see figure legend and Rall 1964 for details). The resulting composite EPSPs are significantly different, and would be distinguished by a neuron whose spike threshold is 0.12 ± 0.02 in the normalized ordinate scale of this figure; such a difference could be exploited for motion detection, provided that the synapses are appropriately arrayed.

Each of these two spatiotemporal input patterns yields a result that can have functional value. The case A-B-C-D shows how one can obtain a quick rise to a subthreshold plateau; such a plateau provides a bias voltage that would poise the neuron to be ready to fire in response to a relatively small, sharp additional input. The case D-C-B-A shows that greater EPSP amplitude at the soma is attained when the distal input precedes the proximal input.

2.8.3   Effect of Synaptic Inhibitory Input Location

Other computations with the ten-compartment model were used to compare the effects of moderate sustained synaptic inhibitory conductance at three locations (see figure 2.13 and figure legend). The resulting EPSPs at the soma demonstrate the importance of inhibitory input location relative to the location of the excitatory input. The synaptic inhibition is effective when it has the same location as the synaptic excitation, and also when it is located at the soma (i.e., proximal to the control input location), but it is much less effective when located distal to the control input location. As discussed by Rall (1964), Jack et al. (1975), and Segev and Parnas (1983), the timing is also very important when the synaptic inhibitory conductance is brief.

These computations have led to useful insights. Synaptic inhibitory input located at the soma is nonspecific because it is effective against synaptic excitatory depolarization that spreads to the soma from any of several dendritic trees, as well as against excitatory input located at or near the soma. In contrast, synaptic inhibition at dendritic locations is more specific because it is effective against synaptic excitation located in the same dendritic tree, provided that the inhibitory input location is the same or proximal, but not distal to the excitatory input location (see Rall 1964, 1967; Jack et al. 1975; see also Koch et al. 1982, 1983).

2.9   Insights Gained from Other Cable Computations

2.9.1   Transients at Different Locations in a Dendritic Tree for Input to One Branch

The transients of figure 2.14 were computed for the same neuron model as was used in figure 2.7; the mathematical solution for the transient response to input restricted to one branch terminal (Rinzel and Rall 1974) was based on the same superposition concepts as were used for the steady-state problem. It may be noted that while this computation did not require a compartmental model, it did require computational convolution of the input current time course with several response functions. We can see the qualitative effects of electrotonic spread from the input branch toward the soma and into the other trees: the time of peak is increasingly delayed and the peak amplitude is increasingly attenuated. Quantitatively, these peak times and amplitudes, as well as those for the sibling and cousin branch terminals, are available in a table (Rinzel and Rall 1974, table I; also Rall 1977, table 5), which has been used to test a set of comparable compartmental computations (Segev et al. 1985). Discussion of many topics, including the relation between transient charge attenuation and

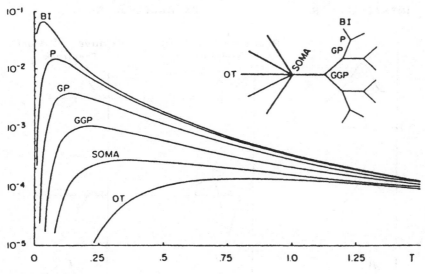

Figure 2.14
Semilog plot of voltage transients at several locations in an idealized neuron model (inset) in response to injection of a brief current to one branch terminal. BI designates the input branch terminal, while P, GP, and GGP designate the parent, grandparent, and great-grandparent nodes (branch points) along the main line from BI to the soma; OT designates the distal terminals of the other trees. This model had six equal dendritic trees (see figure 2.7); the input tree had three orders of branching, with each branch length equal to 1/4 of λ. Thus $L = 1$ for this tree, and also for the five other trees (here indicated by schematic equivalent cylinders). Additional details about this figure and about several related figures, including a table of peak times and amplitudes (for these and other locations), can be found in Rinzel and Rall 1974.

steady-state attenuation, the distribution of charge dissipation over different regions of the model, and the nonlinearities associated with synaptic conductance input, can be found in Rinzel and Rall 1974.

2.9.2   Computation of Field Potentials in Olfactory Bulb

The diagrams in figures 2.15 and 2.16 indicate how a compartmental cable model played a role in a theoretical reconstruction of extracellular field potentials generated by synchronous antidromic activation of the mitral cell population in the olfactory bulb (Rall and Shepherd 1968). Computing the intracellular voltage transients required only the compartmental model. To get extracellular potentials, it was necessary to model three-dimensional aspects of the mitral cell population. By assuming a spherical cortical layer with closed radial symmetry (not shown in either figure), we were able to compute the first set of extracellular potential transients shown in figure 2.15. Then, by considering the concept of punctured spherical symmetry and the

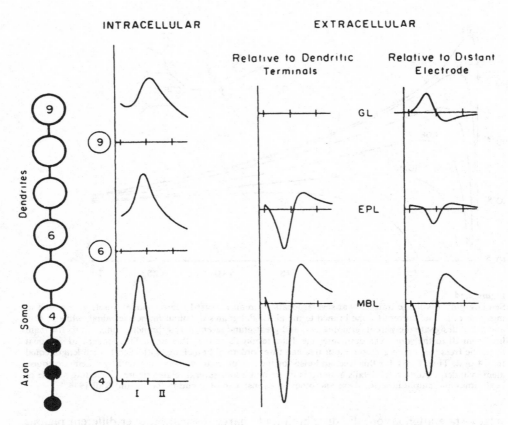

Figure 2.15
Computed intracellular and extracellular voltage transients in response to synchronous antidromic activation of the mitral cell population in a model of the olfactory bulb. Leftmost diagram shows a compartmental model of a simplified mitral cell; the three axonal compartments (shown filled) and the soma compartment had excitable membrane; the five dendritic compartments had passive membrane in this computation (but had excitable membrane in other computations). Computed voltage transients are shown only for compartments 4, 6, and 9, assumed to correspond to three depths (layers) in the olfactory bulb; as shown also in figure 2.16, these layers are the mitral body layer (MBL), the external plexiform layer (EPL), and the glomerular layer (GL). The intracellular voltage transients show the computed passive electrotonic spread, from an action potential at the soma. The extracellular potentials were computed by using the mathematical model of Rall and Shepherd 1968. Related insights are discussed also in Rall 1970, as well as in Klee and Rall 1977.

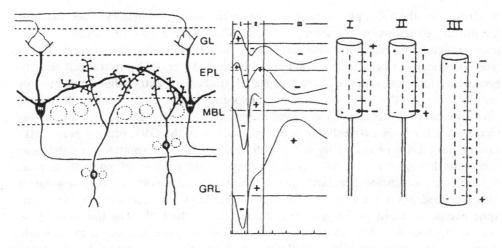

Figure 2.16
Diagram showing depth distribution of extracellular field potentials in time periods, I, II, and III, in relation to cortical layers in the olfactory bulb, and in relation to cable models that distinguish the granule cell population from the mitral cell population. Schematic diagram at left shows two mitral cells and two granule cells in relation to four cortical layers: the glomerular layer (GL), the external plexiform layer (EPL), the mitral body layer (MBL), and the granular layer (GRL). The voltage transients (at center) are field potentials recorded at depths corresponding to those four layers, relative to a distant reference electrode. The three equivalent cylinder models at right contrast the current flow and extracellular potential difference generated by the mitral cell population in periods I and II with that generated by the granule cell population during period III, according to our modeling and interpretation of the data. This contrast was crucial to our expectation of dendrodendritic synaptic interactions between mitral cells and granule cells (Rall et al. 1966; Rall and Shepherd 1968). Modified from Rall 1970.

distinction between the primary extracellular current (radial in the cortex) and the secondary extracellular current, which flows out of the cortex to ground and back through the puncture (see Rall and Shepherd 1968; Klee and Rall 1977 for a detailed explanation and validation of this concept), we obtained the second set of extracellular potential transients shown in figure 2.15. These theoretical results agree quite well with the early portion of the experimental records (designated periods I and II in the middle part of figure 2.16). However, it was important to notice that the field potentials of period III could not have been generated by activity in the mitral cell population, as explained next.

Figure 2.16 shows schematically how the cortical layers of the olfactory bulb are related to four depths at which field potentials were recorded; also, at the right of this figure, the primary extracellular current flow, and its associated field potential polarity, are shown for the mitral cell population (in periods I and II), and for the granule cell population (in period III). The axonless granule cell population extends dendrites over the full depth range shown, hence the long equivalent cylinder. Because the mitral cell axons (in the granular layer, GRL) have a core resistance per unit length much larger than their associated dendritic core resistance (for many dendrites lying electrically in parallel in the external plexiform layer, EPL), mitral cell activity generates much less radial current and radial gradient of extracellular potential in the GRL than in the EPL. This statement expresses our mathematical modeling explanation of what was actually observed in periods I and II; it also explains our conviction that the large extracellular potential gradient in the GRL (during period III) cannot have been produced by mitral cell activity. Our interpretation of the field potentials during period III (as caused by activity in the granule cell population) then required that membrane depolarization in the granule cells would have to be greatest for their dendrites in the EPL, not for those in the GRL; this suggested massive synaptic excitatory input to the granule cell dendrites in the EPL. The timing of these events, together with the proximity of the two sets of dendrites, led us to conclude there must be dendrodendritic synaptic interactions between the mitral cell dendrites and the granule cell dendrites in the EPL.

As explained more fully in the original papers (Rall et al. 1966; Rall and Shepherd 1968; see also Rall 1970), our theoretical predictions and the histological results of our collaborators, Tom Reese and Milton Brightman, converged on the recognition of reciprocal dendrodendritic synapses in the EPL. Our functional interpretation of these synapses was as follows: first, mitral dendritic depolarization activates mitral-to-granule excitatory synapses, and then, the resulting depolarization of the granule cell dendrites in the EPL activates granule-to-mitral inhibitory synapses that suppress the excitability of the mitral cells. It is noteworthy that neither of these synapses needs to be activated by an action potential, that both are dendrodendritic, that one of them is excitatory while the other is inhibitory, and that one cell type is axonless while the other has a conventional axon. These synapses provide a pathway for graded recurrent inhibition that could provide both lateral inhibition and self-inhibition. Lateral inhibition could contribute to olfactory discrimination. Both inhibitions could contribute to local damping of mitral cell excitability and to rhythmic activity of these two interacting cell populations. Thus a remarkable set of new facts and insights resulted from this interaction between theory and experiment.

2.9.3 Voltage Clamp at the Soma of a Dendritic Neuron

Many laboratories now have the ability to voltage-clamp a neuron soma, but they are confronted with uncertainty about how far the effect extends into the dendrites for steady conditions, for transient conditions, and for sinusoidal steady states. For any neuron whose specific geometry and membrane properties are known, this

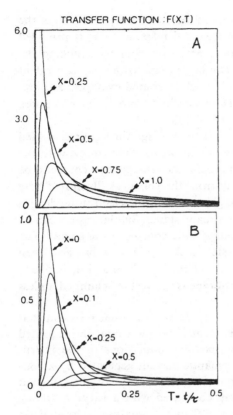

Figure 2.17
Transfer function (panel A) and its convolution (panel B) for voltage clamping at the soma of a passive soma-dendritic model with $L = 1.5$. Curves have two interpretations: (1) as the voltage transient, $V(X, T)$, at point X, in response to a voltage transient, $V(0, T)$, imposed by the voltage clamp at the soma, and (2) as the current transient, $I(0, T)$ detected by the voltage clamp at $X = 0$, for a synaptic current, $I_i(X, T)$, imposed at point X. In panel B, the imposed transient is the one labeled $X = 0$. In panel A, the imposed transient corresponds to a Dirac delta function. Details of equations and interpretations can be found in Rall and Segev 1985.

problem can be investigated with a compartmental model that incorporates all of the known complications. Nevertheless, a valuable idealized reference case is provided by assuming completely linear passive membrane properties and by assuming the soma to be isopotential, and that the dendrites can be represented by one equivalent cylinder. For this idealized case, analytical results and computed examples are presented and discussed in Rall and Segev 1985. Here we illustrate only the computed results shown in figure 2.17.

If a voltage clamp imposes at the soma $(X = 0)$ the voltage time course labeled $X = 0$ in panel B, then, by computational convolution of this time course with the transfer functions illustrated in panel A, we can predict the voltage time course to be expected at different electrotonic distances away from the soma, as illustrated here for $X = 0.1$, 0.25, 0.5, 0.75, and 1.0 in panel B, given a dendritic electrotonic length $L = 1.5$, together with the idealized assumptions already stated. Similar results can be computed for different examples of imposed voltage time courses at the soma. (The voltage decrement with distance, for a voltage step at $X = 0$, $T = 0$, has also been illustrated in figure 3 of Rall and Segev 1985 for $T = 0.1$, 0.2, 0.5, 1.0, and ∞.) These results make it clear that the dendritic membrane is not voltage-clamped, unless the value of L is very small.

Sometimes a voltage clamp at the soma is used to record a current transient that results from synaptic activity. If the synapse is located on the soma, the recorded current equals the synaptic current, except for possible limitations of the instrumentation, and with the qualification that the synaptic current generated by a conductance transient will be slightly different from normal because of the constant driving potential provided by the voltage clamp compared with a varying driving potential under normal (unclamped) conditions. When the synapse is located on a dendritic branch, a significant discrepancy can be expected between the synaptic current generated at the input site and the current transient detected by the voltage clamp at the soma. As demonstrated and discussed by Rall and Segev (1985), that discrepancy can be defined quantitatively by the same transfer functions and convolutions already illustrated in figure 2.17. Thus the curves in panel B (for each labeled value of X) give the predicted current transient at the somatic voltage clamp in response to synaptic current injected at each labeled value of X, assuming that the injected current time course is given by the curve labeled $X = 0$. These examples illustrate a theoretical basis for better experimental estimation of the synaptic current time course generated at dendritic synaptic locations. Theoretical expressions for sinusoidal steady states can also be found in Rall and Segev 1985.

3 Compartmental Models of Complex Neurons

Idan Segev and Robert E. Burke
Appendix by Michael Hines

3.1 Introduction

An understanding of information processing at the level of individual nerve cells requires detailed information about interactions between anatomical structure, physiological properties, and synaptic input. It is often very useful to embody such information in some type of formal model in order to explore ideas about current flows, voltage perturbations, and input-output relations. This chapter is focused on the use of compartmental models to employ such data sets. The main assumption in the compartmental approach is that small pieces of the neuron can be treated as isopotential elements, so that the essentially continuous structure of the neuron can be approximated by a linked assemblage of discrete elements. This not only simplifies the mathematics but also opens the possibility that individual compartments can possess nonuniform properties. Section 3.2 and chapter 2, this volume, provide an outline of cable theory as it applies to the development and justification of the compartmental model approach.

The choices of structural model and the level of detail at which such models are constructed are critical considerations. It is frequently the case that some aspects of the system are known in much greater detail than others. For example, intracellular injection of tracer substances such as horseradish peroxidase or neurobiotin permit quantitative reconstruction of the morphology of functionally identified neurons in exquisite detail (e.g., Birinyi et al. 1992; Cameron, Averill, and Berger 1985; Cullheim et al. 1987a; Moschovakis, Burke, and Fyffe 1991; Rose, Kierstead, and Vanner 1985). However, there is usually much less quantitative information about the types and spatial distributions of identifiable synaptic input systems on reconstructed neurons. The use of whole-cell patch clamp methods, and more recently the "perforated patch" technique, have greatly enlarged our information about the dynamics of voltage-sensitive and ligand-gated membrane channels, but the electrotonic isolation of the dendrites has again prevented characterization of membrane properties throughout the entire neuron (Spruston, and Johnston 1992; see also Stuart and Sakmann 1994; Magee and Johnston 1995; Hoffman et al. 1997). Thus choices, assumptions, and guesses about these incompletely defined areas are also an integral part of neuronal modeling (Mainen et al. 1995; Rapp, Yarom, and Segev 1996). These issues will be taken up in section 3.3.

3.2   Principles of Compartmental Neurons Models

3.2.1   Overview

The one-dimensional cable theory of neurons describes current flow in a continuous passive dendritic tree using partial differential equations (with the appropriate boundary conditions see chapters 2 and 14, this volume). These equations have straightforward analytical solutions for transient *current* inputs to an idealized class of dendritic trees that are equivalent to unbranched cylinders ("equivalent cylinder"; Rall 1959; Rall and Rinzel 1973; Rinzel and Rall 1974; Jack, Noble, and Tsien 1983; Segev, Rinzel, and Shepherd 1995). As noted below, this idealization requires strict constraints that are, in general, not matched by any real dendritic trees.

The solutions are more complicated for passive dendritic trees with an arbitrary branching structure. In such structures it is still possible to compute recursively the voltage trajectory in response to an arbitrary current injection (Butz and Cowan 1974; Horwitz 1981, 1983; Wilson 1984; Koch and Poggio 1985; Major, Evans, and Jack, 1993a, 1993b; Major 1993; Cao and Abbott, 1993; Agmon-Snir and Segev 1993; Agmon-Snir 1995; Steinberg 1996; see also chapter 2, this volume). However, these algorithms become more complex as well as computationally expensive when the system is perturbed by *synaptic* currents produced by conductance changes (Rinzel and Rall 1974; Poggio and Torre 1978; Koch, Poggio, and Torre, 1982; Holmes 1986; Tuckwell 1985, 1989). When the membrane properties are *voltage-dependent*, as is the case with membranes that show rectification or that support action potentials, the analytical approach using linear cable theory is no longer valid. As Rall pointed our early on, these complex cases must be dealt with using compartmental rather than analytical models (Rall 1964).

The compartmental approach replaces the continuous differential equations of the analytical model by a set of ordinary differential equations. Thus, if the continuously distributed system is divided into sufficiently small segments (or compartments), one makes a negligibly small error by assuming that each compartment is isopotential and spatially uniform in its properties. Nonuniformity in physical properties (e.g., diameter, specific electric properties) and differences in voltage occur *between* compartments rather than within them (Rall 1964; Perkel, Mulloney, and Budelli 1981; see also Holmes and Rall, 1992a).

A chain of three cylindrical dendritic segments that are sufficiently short to be considered isopotential is shown in figure 3.1A. Assuming the membrane is passive, these segments may be represented by the equivalent circuit of figure 3.1B. Focusing on the *j*th segment, one can see that the "resting" membrane channels are repre-

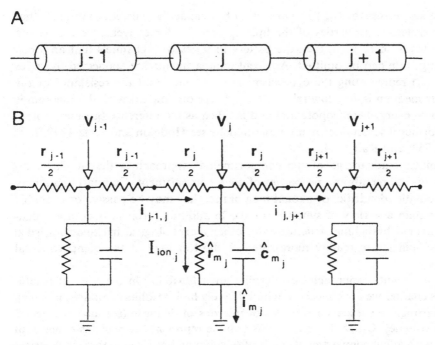

Figure 3.1
Equivalent circuit for a compartmental model of a chain of three successive small cylindrical segments of passive dendritic membrane. (A) The constant-diameter jth segment is assumed to be sufficiently short electrically that may be considered as isopotential. (B) The resting-membrane resistance and capacitance of that segment are lumped into one resistor, $\hat{r}_{m_j}$ and one capacitor, $\hat{c}_{m_j}$. The net ion current that flows via $\hat{r}_{m_j}$ is I_{ion_j}. The net current through the membrane is $\hat{i}_{m_j}$. The axial resistance of the segment, r_j, is split in half and the membrane R–C elements are placed in between. Membrane potential, V_j, is defined as the displacement from the resting potential. It is assumed that the resistivity of the extracellular medium may be taken as zero, hence the connection of the extracellular side of the membrane R–C to ground. For simplicity, the resting potential is taken as zero, eliminating the need for a battery in series with the membrane resistance. The term I_{ion_j} represents transmembrane ionic current in the jth compartment. Longitudinal resistance between compartment j and $j+1$ (denoted in the text as $r_{j,j+1}$) is the sum of half the longitudinal resistance of segment j and half the longitudinal resistance of segment $j+1$, that is, $r_{j,j+1} = (r_j + r_{j+1})/2$. The corresponding longitudinal current through this resistance is designated as $i_{j,j+1}$.

sented by a single resistor $(\hat{r}_{m_j})$ in parallel with a capacitive current path $(\hat{c}_{m_j})$ that models the dielectric properties of the lipid bilayer.[1] If for convenience the resting potential is taken to be zero, then the battery in series with channels that are open in the resting state can be omitted. Adjacent compartments are connected by series resistances (r_j) representing the cytoplasm. It is assumed that the resistance of the extracellular medium is very low relative to r_j. Therefore, the extracellular medium is assumed to be everywhere isopotential and is taken as the reference (ground) potential. (For further discussion of membrane models, see Hodgkin and Katz 1949; Fatt and Katz 1953; and Rall 1964.)

One significant advantage of the compartmental approach is that it places no restrictions on the membrane properties of each compartment. Compartments may represent somatic, dendritic, or axonal membrane; they may be passive or excitable and may contain a variety of synaptic inputs. In addition, arbitrarily complex dendritic and axonal branching structures and other morphological irregularities, such as dendritic spines, are readily represented in the topology of the compartmental connections.

The compartmental approach also permits great flexibility in the level of resolution. In this chapter we are concerned with relatively high-resolution models, in which each compartment represents a few tens of microns of dendrite (see also chapters 5 and 6, this volume). Other chapters in this volume represent the neurons either with a single or with a few compartments each of which may have very complex electrical structure (e.g., chapter 4).

While the compartmental approach has many advantages for neural modeling, it should be regarded as a complement to analytical models derived from Rall's cable theory (see chapter 2, this volume). Many insights about and initial evaluations of key parameters can be obtained by first applying the analytical approach to simplified and idealized approximations of the neuron or neurons under study. Based on these approximations, a subsequent, more detailed compartmental model can be constructed and used to refine the analytical results (see implementation of this combined analytic/numerical approach in Fleshman, Segev, and Burke 1988; Stratford et al. 1989; Nitzan, Yarom, and Segev 1990; Rall et al. 1992; Holmes and Rall, 1992a, 1992b; Rapp, Segev and Yarom, 1994; Major et al. 1994; and section 3.3).

3.2.2 Mathematical Formulation

As mentioned above, the mathematical consequence of compartmental models of neurons is a system of ordinary differential equations (or a corresponding set of difference equations), one for each compartment. Each equation is derived from Kirchhoff's current law, which states that in each compartment, j, the net current through the membrane, $\hat{\imath}_{m_j}$, must equal the longitudinal current that enters that compartment minus the longitudinal current that leaves it (figure 3.1B). For an unbranched region, where the jth compartment lies between the $(j-1)$th and the $(j+1)$th compartments, the membrane current is

$$\hat{\imath}_{m_j} = i_{j-1,j} - i_{j,j+1}, \tag{3.1}$$

where $i_{j-1,j}$ is the longitudinal current that flows from compartment $j-1$ to j and $i_{j,j+1}$ is the current that flows from compartment j to $j+1$ (figure 3.1B).

The equivalent circuit shows that the membrane current is the sum of capacitive current and the net ionic current (I_{ion}) that flows through the transmembrane resistive pathways ($\hat{r}_m$). For the jth compartment, the membrane current can be expressed as

$$\hat{\imath}_{m_j} = \hat{c}_{m_j} \frac{dV_j}{dt} + I_{ion_j}, \tag{3.2}$$

where V_j is the membrane potential measured with respect to the resting potential. For compartments that are stimulated by an external current source (e.g., an electrode), an additional term (I_{stim}) must be added to the membrane current. The longitudinal current can be described as the voltage gradient between directly connected compartments divided by the axial resistance between these compartments. Thus eqs. 3.1 and 3.2 can be rewritten as

$$\hat{c}_{m_j} \frac{dV_j}{dt} + I_{ion_j} + I_{stim_j} = \frac{V_{j-1} - V_j}{r_{j-1,j}} - \frac{V_j - V_{j+1}}{r_{j,j+1}} \tag{3.3}$$

or

$$\hat{c}_{m_j} \frac{dV_j}{dt} + I_{ion_j} + I_{stim_j} = (V_{j-1} - V_j)g_{j-1,j} - (V_j - V_{j+1})g_{j,j+1}, \tag{3.4}$$

where $r_{j-1,j}$ (or $1/g_{j-1,j}$) is the axial resistance (conductance) between the $(j-1)$th and the jth compartments. For the parent compartment at a branch point, current flow into the two daughter branches is represented by adding a second expression identical to the right-hand side of eqs. 3.3 and 3.4, with appropriate subscripts to identify the daughter branches (figure 1 of Parnas and Segev 1979). For the first and last compartments in a chain, only the first term for the longitudinal current appears on the right-hand side of the equations.

The transient solution of eqs. 3.3 and 3.4 (i.e., the values of $V_j(t)$ for $j = 1, \ldots, N$, where N is the number of compartments in the model) depends critically on the description of I_{ion}. This term can embody the properties of the many types of channels

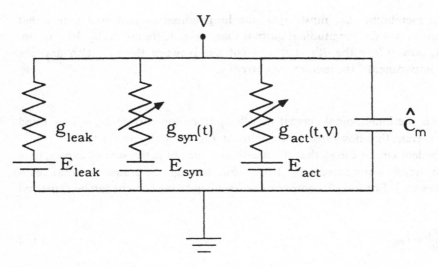

Figure 3.2
Equivalent circuit model of isopotential patch of nerve membrane that consists of the three basic classes of transmembrane channels. The leftmost branch represents ohmic leak channels in the patch. It consists of a constant conductance, g_{leak}, in series with a constant battery (E_{leak}) through which the passive ionic current flows. synaptic (chemically gated) channels are represented by the middle time-varying branch ($g_{syn}(t)$) which is in series with a battery (E_{syn}), representing the reversal potential of the synaptic processes. Active channels are represented by the rightmost resistive branch. A time- and voltage-dependent resistor ($g_{act}(t, V)$) is in series with a battery (E_{act}) whose value is the equilibrium potential of the ionic species involved (Na^+, K^+, Ca^{2+}, etc.). The capacitance of this membrane patch is denoted by $\hat{c}_m$.

in neural membranes and may have a mathematical description that ranges from simple to very complex. The following section divides ion channels into three distinct classes and presents their general formal description together with the corresponding membrane models. (More detailed descriptions can be found in chapters 4, 5, and 6, this volume).

3.2.3 Membrane Models

The conductive branches in figure 3.2 summarize the three basic classes of ionic channels that are found in nerve membrane: *passive* or *leak*, *synaptic*, and *active* channels. From a modeling viewpoint, the simplest class of membrane channels is the passive channels. Passive membrane is electrically represented by a constant (time- and voltage-independent) transmembrane conductance (g_{leak}; left branch in equivalent circuit of figure 3.2) in series with a fixed voltage source (E_{leak}) that designates the reversal potential of the passive channels. The ionic current through this branch obeys Ohm's law and can be expressed simply as

$$I_{leak} = g_{leak}(V - E_{leak}). \tag{3.5}$$

Other membrane channels may be controlled by external or internal chemical agents (e.g., neurotransmitters or second messengers). Synaptic channels change their conductance to a certain ion or ions when the appropriate chemical stimulus binds to the receptor associated with these channels. Synaptic membrane is most simply modeled as a time-dependent, but voltage-independent, conductive pathway ($g_{syn}(t)$) in series with a constant voltage source (E_{syn}), which is the reversal potential of the ionic species involved (Rall 1964, 1967).[2]

One convenient expression for such a time-varying conductance change is based on the "alpha function" (Rall 1967; Jack et al. 1983) and has the form $g_{syn}(t) = \alpha T e^{-\alpha T}$, where $\alpha = \tau_m/t_{peak}$, $T = t/\tau_m$, τ_m is the membrane time constant (see below), and t_{peak} is the time-to-peak of the conductance transient. In some cases the sum of two exponentials approximates more accurately the time-varying synaptic conductance change while still using a simple expression. The middle conductive branch of figure 3.2 shows the electrical representation of this class of channels. The synaptic current that flows through this (nonlinear) branch is

$$I_{syn}(t) = g_{syn}(t)(V(t) - E_{syn}). \tag{3.6}$$

Although both the AMPA- and GABA-mediated synaptic conductance are well approximated by a purely time-varying conductance change, the NMDA-mediated synaptic conductance is more complicated because it is both time- and voltage-dependent and, therefore, belongs to the category of voltage-gated (active) conductances. (Chapter 1, this volume, provides a detailed scheme for modeling AMPA-, GABA-, and NMDA-mediated conductances.)

The class of voltage-dependent channels is represented by the rightmost conductive branch in figure 3.2. This branch consists of a voltage source (E_{act}) in series with a *voltage-* and *time-dependent* conductance, $g_{act}(t, V)$, through which the active current flows. The equation describing this current has the same form as the synaptic current in eq. 3.6, with g_{act} and E_{act} replacing g_{syn} and E_{syn}, respectively. Depending on the description of g_{act}, this class of nonlinear channels may produce membrane responses that mimic various sorts of subthreshold membrane rectification or action potential (see Hodgkin and Huxley 1952; Nagumo, Arimoto, and Yoshizawa 1962; FitzHugh 1969; Gutfreund, Yarom, and Segev 1995; and chapters 4 and 5, this volume).

The total membrane current through a patch of membrane that has all three types of ionic channels is the sum of all those currents plus the capacitative current:

$$\hat{i}_m = \hat{c}_m \frac{dV}{dt} + g_{leak}(V - E_{leak}) + g_{syn}(V - E_{syn}) + g_{act}(V - E_{act}). \tag{3.7}$$

Combining this equation with eq. 3.4 for the jth compartment (without the stimulus current) and rearranging, the following general form is obtained for the system of differential equations associated with compartmental models:

$$\hat{c}_m \frac{dV_j}{dt} = g_{j-1,j}V_{j-1} - (g_{leak_j} + g_{syn_j} + g_{act_j} + g_{j-1,j} + g_{j,j+1})V_j + g_{j,j+1}V_{j+1}$$

$$+ g_{leak_j}E_{leak_j} + g_{syn_j}E_{syn_j} + g_{act_j}E_{act_j}. \tag{3.8}$$

Note that within each of the basic classes of channels there may be several subtypes, for example, active channels that carry Na^+ or K^+ or Ca^{2+} ions, each with its own voltage and time dependencies (see chapter 4, this volume, and Hille 1992 for a summary of the properties of different channels).

3.2.4 Methods and Approaches

We have demonstrated that the mathematical consequence of a compartmental approach to nerve cell models is a set, or matrix, of coupled, first-order differential equations of the form given by eq. 3.8. They can also be written as a matrix differential equation of the form

$$\dot{V} = A\vec{V} + \vec{b}, \tag{3.9}$$

where $\vec{V} = \text{col}(V_1, V_2, \ldots, V_N)$ is the unknown vector of membrane potentials of the different compartments, $\dot{V}$ is the time derivative of V, A is a matrix composed of the coefficients, and $\vec{b}$ is a column vector consisting of the products of batteries and conductances. For constant coefficients (i.e., passive channels), a linear system of equations is obtained and classical algebraic methods can be employed to invert matrix A and directly obtain the required transient solution (Hearon 1963; Rall 1964; Perkel, Mulloney, and Budelli 1981; Holmes and Rall 1992a, 1992b). Indeed, in this case the eigenvalues and eigenfunctions of A can be directly computed and the solution, (V_i, at any compartment, $i = 1, \ldots, N$) can be written as a sum of N decaying exponentials (time constants). Note that the solution for the corresponding continuous (cable) case is a sum of an infinite number of decaying exponentials (see chapter 2, this volume). As shown by Holmes and Rall (1992a; Holmes, Segev, and Rall 1992; Rall et al. 1992), this analytic solution for the compartmental model of a known morphology is very useful for estimating model parameters from experimental transients.

When the coefficients are not fixed, however, as is the case with synaptic perturbation and with active currents, matrix A and vector b change from instant to instant. For these cases, one usually replaces the matrix of differential equations with a corresponding matrix of difference equations and employs numerical methods (e.g., linearization, direct elimination, integration, etc.; for more details, see Rall 1964; Parnas and Segev 1979; and chapter 14, this volume). We would like to note that a common feature of all matrix representations of multicompartmental neuron models is that they are very sparse, that is, most of the matrix terms are zero. Thus any numerical approach to the solution should utilize sparse matrix algorithms that only store and operate on nonzero terms. This will increase the efficiency of the computation and allow solution of very large systems of equations.

There are two ways to approach the solution of such systems. One can write a computer program designed to solve a specific set of equations (see, for example, Perkel, Mulloney and Budelli 1981; Cooley and Dodge 1966; Rall and Shepherd 1968; Traub et al. 1991; Shelton 1985; Clements and Redman 1989) or one can use a more generalized equation-solving or modeling system (e.g., Rall 1964, using the SAAM program by Bergman, Shahn, and Weiss; Shepherd and Brayton 1979, using IBM-ASTAP; and see review in De Schutter 1992). The first approach allows one to tailor the program to the needs of the particular model, which could result in significant savings in computer resources. Furthermore, as noted above, for certain compartmental models it may be possible to obtain an analytical solution (see Perkel, Mulloney, and Budelli 1981; Holmes and Rall 1992a). In these cases, the behavior of the system can be understood in terms of the parameters that govern it, such as the time constants that determine transient response.

The use of more general-purpose computer programs in neural modeling will likely be less efficient than custom-designed programs in terms of computer time, but they offer at least three advantages. First, one does not have to write the program oneself. Second, because such programs are not designed with any specific model in mind, one can easily accommodate new data and ask new questions without having to rewrite and debug additional code. Third, a number of modeling packages are available that run on computer systems that range from PCs to workstations, minicomputers, mainframes, and even supercomputers. This makes it easier to share data and models and may allow one to take advantage of computer resources best matched to the complexity of the modeling problem.

As first suggested by Shepherd and Brayton (1979), it is natural to utilize computer programs that serve to test and design electrical circuits (e.g., NET2, ADVICE, ASTAP, SCEPTRE) for constructing compartmental models of nerve cells. Indeed, most of the early realistic compartmental models of neurons utilized these programs, in particular the very popular program SPICE (Bunow, Segev, and Fleshman 1985; Segev et al. 1985; Fleshman, Segev, and Burke 1988). Representing the morphology of the modeled tree by a set of interconnected electrical compartments, these programs can perform transient analysis, as one does experimentally, in which the time-domain response of the system is computed at discrete time steps, Δt, over a specified interval, $0, \ldots, T$. AC analysis may be also be used to describe model behavior in the frequency domain (e.g., see Rall and Segev, 1985).

In recent years, several very popular computer software packages have been specifically developed for simulating signal processing in nerve cells. These simulators implement the compartmental modeling approach and can typically simulate both chemical (e.g., ion diffusion) and electrical signals in large and complicated trees (or in networks of neurons). They have powerful graphical tools for representing and manipulating the modeled structure, and for depicting the simulation results in colors. Examples include NEURON (Hines and Carnevale, 1997; and see chapter appendix) and GENESIS (Bower and Beeman 1995; see chapter 12, this volume), both run on UNIX machines and also on personal computers, and NODUS (De Schutter 1992), which runs on Macintosh computers. For single-neuron modeling, the typical input of these computer programs is a data set that represents the morphology of the neuron to be modeled, as well as a set of biophysical parameters (electrical or chemical) that characterize elements in the modeled structure (see below). Finally, input to the model (e.g., a current step to the soma or transient synaptic conductance change at some dendritic location) is also specified. The resultant mathematical model is a system of differential equations, as in eq. 3.9, which is then solved numerically by the computer program. (Information about these and other software packages, such as SWIM, NEMOSIS, AXON-TREE, and SABER can be found in De Schutter 1992.)

3.3   Embodying Neuronal Morphology in Compartmental Models

Every neuron model must begin with a structural framework, either assumed or based on an actual neuronal morphology. The seminal equivalent cylinder model introduced by Rall (1959) was based in part on observations of Golgi-stained motoneurons in the cat, which, while not quantitative, appeared to be consonant with the constraints required to collapse the complex branched dendrites of a neuron into a single "equivalent cylinder" (see chapter 2, this volume, and below). This approach made it possible to develop analytical expressions derived from cable theory and to apply this theory to various type of neurons. It revealed critical relations between the cable structure of the dendritic tree, the location and time course of the synaptic input and the properties of the synaptic potential at the output site (soma). Indeed, this theory remain the basis for our current thinking about the way in which neurons process synaptic information (see chapter 2, this volume; Segev, Rinzel, and Shepherd 1995; and Segev 1995).

3.3.1 Encoding Neuron Structure

Compartmental neuron models are embodied in computer files that encode the physical dimensions of the individual segments (compartments), along with some identification scheme that uniquely specifies the location of each compartment in the electrical circuit representing the topology of the original neuron. As noted above, the advent of intracellular injection of tracer substances has permitted visualization and quantitative reconstruction of the morphology of functionally identified neurons. The use of horseradish peroxidase (HRP) and neurobiotin as tracers has shown that the earlier work with radioactive (Lux Schuhert and Kreutzberg 1970) and fluorescent tracers such as lucifer yellow (Barrett and Crill 1974) did not reveal the full extent of the dendritic (and axonal) trees of large neurons like motoneurons. Recent advances in optical techniques (e.g., confocal microscopy, infrared differential interface contrast videomicroscopy) and the introduction of new intracellular dyes should permit increasingly reliable reconstruction of neurons of various sizes in both invertebrates and vertebrates.

Virtually all such reconstructions are done using light microscopy because of the physical size of the neurons involved (for using electronmicroscopy, however, see White and Rock 1980; and Anderson et al. 1992, 1994). Quantitative neuronal reconstruction is as much art as science. There are two tasks: (1) mapping the labeled structure into a linked list of discrete geometric elements (segments) with a coding system that uniquely specifies the relative position of each element in the structure; and (2) measuring the dimensions of each cell element. Some neurons can be reconstructed from whole-mount preparations, but large cells such as spinal motoneurons and cortical pyramidal cells usually require reconstruction from serial sections. Serial section reconstruction requires elaborate precautions to ensure that the labeled pieces in one section are matched with their appropriate continuations in the neighboring section. There are now a number of commercial reconstruction systems that use computer interfaces in order to accomplish this purpose and to tabulate the measurements.

Neuronal somata are usually approximated as spheres or oblate spheroids for modeling purposes. The choice of exact shape is not critical because it is difficult to define transition points between "soma" and "dendritic trunks." From the electrotonic standpoint, the soma is a compartment that can reasonably be regarded as isopotential. Many neuron models omit consideration of the axon's initial segment and the axon itself. Although the myelinated axon is assumed to present a negligible passive load to the soma, this assumption deserves additional systematic study (see Major et al. 1994; Mainen et al. 1995; Rapp, Yarom, and Segev 1996).

Quantitative mapping of a dendritic tree involves approximating these sinuous and complex structures with linked sequences of discrete cylinders having appropriate lengths and diameters, and in some cases also locations in three-dimensional space. The fidelity with which the reconstruction follows reality depends on technical factors such as microscope resolution and distortion in the imaging system and (certainly not least) the skill of the operator. In general, the fidelity of reconstruction varies inversely with the size of the pieces chosen for measurement. Increasing fidelity rapidly increases the data file size, which can tax even powerful computer resources. In practice, it is usually necessary to reach some compromise between anatomical correctness and the level of detail needed for the proposed use of the data.

The length of linear elements in a microscope field represents the projected image of three-dimensional structures often having tangential trajectories within the depth of the section or whole mount. This can be taken into account by encoding microscope focus, calculating the Pythagorean length of the actual structure, and correcting for the large shrinkage that usually occurs in section thickness in dehydrated serial sections. Estimating the diameters of linear elements also presents a number of problems. For example, the apparent diameters of neuronal dendrites vary along their length, with fine branches frequently showing "beads" that may or may not be artifactual. Because it is very difficult to devise generally accepted rules to handle such problems, the operator must use careful judgment when measuring dendritic trees. Finally, most neuron reconstructions are plagued by the limited resolution of light microscopes, which makes it difficult to estimate diameters of less than $1.0\,\mu m$ accurately.

Adding to the list of problems, many central neurons (e.g., cerebellar Purkinje cells and cortical pyramidal cells) have virtually innumerable dendritic spines with varying shapes and dimensions. The numbers and densities of these important structures significantly increase the total dendritic area (by about 75% in Purkinje cells and by 25%–40% in cortical pyramids). Therefore, spines must be taken into account in compartmental models in some global way rather than by modeling each and every one explicitly (see section 3.4.3).

Conventional methods for the preparation of serial sections for light microscopy introduce variable amounts of tissue shrinkage, particularly in section thickness (z plane). It is important to estimate total section thickness in the preparation at hand, again using the microscope focus, in order to correct the Pythagorean estimates by the fractional shrinkage from the original thickness where the sections were cut. Moreover, large, air-dried sections can exhibit some degree of "waviness" from one part to another, which requires continued attention and recalibration. Because of these problems, it is necessary to use relatively high magnification with objectives of high numerical aperture to map neurons. It is also important to take into account shrinkage in the X-Y plane. This can be estimated by comparing the dimensions of fixed tissue blocks with those of the sections after cutting and mounting (Cullheim et al. 1987a), and is usually found to be much less than the shrinkage in section thickness. Of course, all "corrections' for shrinkage must assume that it occurs isotropically, which is not necessarily the case. Indeed, neurons labeled with a reaction product may be "stiffer" than the surrounding tissue and may shrink less than the tissue as a whole.

Figures 3.3A and 3.3B show an example of the process of decomposing a stained neuronal structure into geometrical subunits. A camera lucida drawing of the two-dimensional projection of a three-dimensional HRP-filled dendrite and soma of a guinea pig vagal motoneuron is shown in figure 3.3A. Dendritic lengths were corrected for the thickness of the histological sections using the Pythagorean rule; diameters were measured at the midpoint of each segment (see also Cullheim et al. 1987b). Because, as shown, dendrite diameters were not necessarily uniform between branch points, it was necessary to choose a criterion for segmenting the dendrites. In the example illustrated, whenever the diameter of a dendritic segment changed by more than $0.2\,\mu m$, it was replaced by two segments (segmentation is shown by crossing lines on dendrite in panel A). Using this sampling rule, twelve segments were needed to represent the relatively simple dendrite of figure 3.3A, and one more was used for the soma. The continuous cable representation of this structure by geometrical entities (cylinders and an ellipsoid) is shown in panel B; the corresponding equivalent electrical circuit (compartmental model) of this anatomical segmentation, in panel C.

As noted above, the data entries for length and diameter of each linear element in a neuron data file must be accompanied by a unique identifier that specifies the location of that element within the original structure. Of the various coding systems that can be used to accomplish this purpose, most take advantage of the general rule that neuronal dendrites branch dichotomously. For example, Cullheim and coworkers (1987b) used a binary nomenclature for dendrites in which each element is identified by four integers: dendrite number, order, branch, segment. The numbering of branch order begins at the soma with the trunk coded as order $= 0$ and branch $= 1$. Branch codes for any tree will vary between 0 and $2^{m-1} - 1$, where m is branch order. Successive daughter branches are numbered according to the parent branch number, k,

A. Physiologically & morphologically characterized neuron

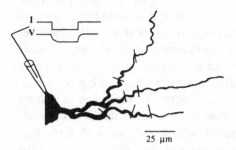

B. Cable model

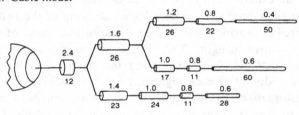

C. Compartmental model

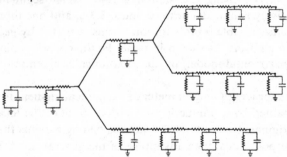

Figure 3.3
Stages in abstraction from an anatomical dendritic tree to an electrical circuit analogue. (A) Two-dimensional projection of part of the soma and one dendrite of a vagus motoneuron in the guinea pig (Nitzan, Segev, and Yarom, 1990). Points at which unbranched dendrites were broken into successive cylindrical segments are indicated by lines. Cable parameters are estimated from the somatic transient voltage response to a current pulse injected to the soma (inset). (B) Continuous (cable) representation of the same dendrite as a branched system of cylindrical segments, indicating the length (below) and diameter (above) of each dendritic segment (in μm). Diameters are not drawn to the same scale as the lengths, but both are in the correct proportions. The motoneuron soma (shown partially) had a maximum diameter of 20 μm and minimum diameter of 15 μm. (C) Discrete (compartmental) representation of cable model in panel B, with each cylindrical segment modeled by a lumped circuit analogue (see figure 3.1).

as k and $k + 1$; successive elements or segments making up a given branch are numbered from 1 to n. This system allows the topology of the tree to be easily specified from an examination of the codes for terminating segments. Because all coding schemes must contain the same information, it is relatively easy to develop computer algorithms to interconvert data files to accommodate input files for different neuronal modeling packages. The NEURON, GENESIS, and NODUS software packages have built-in translators for different coding schemes.

3.3.2 Neuron Simulation

Because each model compartment is, by definition, regarded as an isopotential element, its dimensions must be chosen to minimize the computational error introduced by this assumption. Spherical elements such as the neuron soma are, with considerable assurance, regarded as isopotential (Rall 1959). Linear elements like dendrites and axons, however, should have physical lengths that conform to a relatively small fraction of the characteristic length, λ. Although this fraction should be small (e.g., $<0.1\lambda$) when the element in question is at or near the site of a voltage perturbation, such as a synaptic input, it can be safely relaxed when the element is electrotonically distant from the perturbation site (Segev et al. 1985). Some recent modeling systems have adopted algorithms that permit compartments to be dynamically expanded and collapsed depending on the flow of electrical signals within the structure (Manor, Koch, and Segev 1991). Of course, calculation of λ requires estimates of membrane and cytoplasmic specific resistivities (R_m in $\sim\text{cm}^2$ and R_i in $\sim$cm, respectively), which are usually unknown when the neuron is being digitized. It is therefore generally wise to err on the side of more rather than less detail during the reconstruction process, consistent with considerations of file size as discussed above. One can always compact data later on, if necessary (see below and chapter 12, this volume).

3.3.3 Estimation of Passive Membrane Parameters

The problem of estimating membrane and cytoplasmic electrical constants (the "inverse estimation" problem; Holmes and Rall 1992a) conveniently illustrates some general principles in the way compartmental models can be used. This problem has great generality because informed estimates for R_m, R_i, and C_m are essential to any neuron-modeling project. It also illustrates some of the serious limitations inherent in the available approaches, including the effects of various assumptions and the issue of nonunique results (Stratford et al. 1989; White, Manis, and Young 1992).

Various approaches have been used to tackle the inverse estimation problem, ranging from simple to quite elaborate (see, for example, Barrett and Crill 1974; Holmes and Rall 1992a; Durand 1984; Fleshman, Segev, and Burke 1988; Clements and Redman 1989; Nitzan, Segev, and Yarom 1990; Major et al. 1994; Rapp, Segev, and Yarom 1994; Evans, Major, and Kember 1995; Ulrich, Quadroni, and Lüscher 1994; and references there in). All have the same purpose, which is to reconcile the electrophysiological responses of an actual neuron with the electrical behavior of a neuron model embodying its anatomical structure (see review in Rall et al. 1992). These approaches usually begin with basic assumptions about the boundary condition at dendritic terminations (usually "sealed-end") and negligible extracellular resistance (Rall 1959, 1977). Most inverse parameter estimations make two further assumptions: (1) the neuronal membrane is passive (at least within the range of voltage perturbations modeled); and (2) the electrical behavior of the axon can be ignored. The former is almost certainly wrong, and the latter requires more attention than it has received so far. Even though there is evidence of active membrane properties in dendrites (Haag and Borst 1996; Hoffman et al. 1997; Markram, Helm, and Sakmann 1995; Rapp, Yarom, and Segev 1996; Stuart and Sakmann 1994; Stuart and Spruston 1995; and Wilson and Kawaguchi 1996; see also chapter 5, this volume), the passive membrane assumption remains the essential starting point for more complex models with active membranes (Stratford et al. 1989; Major et al. 1994; Rall et al. 1992).

Although there is no general agreement as to what experimental data are most useful (or least misleading; see Rall et al. 1992 and references cited above), all inverse estimations involve the introduction of voltage or current perturbations at the soma. The responses are usually recorded using computer averaging in order to maximize signal-to-noise ratio. At minimum, the neuron model under test should exhibit the same steady-state input resistance, R_N, as the actual cell, and similar behavior during transient perturbations. Because it is computationally expensive to simulate transients for all possible combinations of R_i, R_m and C_m, it is often advisable to begin by narrowing the possibilities using a steady-state calculation, which requires only choices for R_i and R_m (the value of C_m is irrelevant at this stage), and which proceeds very rapidly on desktop computers, even for models with hundreds or thousands of compartments (see step 1 in figure 3.5).

3.3.4 Current Flow in Cylindrical Compartments: Normalized Conductance Ratios

It is quite easy to calculate the steady-state value of R_N at any point in a compartmental neuron model of arbitrarily complex morphology, using the iterative technique involving normalized (dimensionless) conductance ratios introduced by Rall (1959, 1977; and see chapter 2, this volume). These ratios represent the actual conductance at a given point, G_i, divided by the input conductance, G_∞, of a semi-infinite cylinder with the same (constant) diameter, d_i, and electrical parameters:

$$B = \frac{G_i}{G_\infty},$$

(3.10)

where

$$G_\infty = \frac{\pi}{2} \frac{d_i^{3/2}}{\sqrt{R_i R_m}}.$$

(3.11)

In a sequence of membrane cylinders ordered according to the direction of current flow and with equal diameters, d, the normalized output conductance for the jth cylinder, $B_{out,j}$, is equal to the normalized input conductance of the next cylinder, $B_{in,j+1}$:

$$B_{out,j} = B_{in,j+1}.$$

(3.12)

In order to accommodate the realistic possibilities that dendrites taper (usually simulated as a sequence of membrane cylinders with unequal diameters; see figure 3.3, top) and may have unequal specific membrane resistivities (Fleshman, Segev, and Burke 1988), this equation can be expanded to

$$B_{out,j} = \frac{B_{in,j+1} \left(\frac{d_{j+1}}{d_j} \right)^{3/2}}{\sqrt{\frac{R_{m,j+1}}{R_{m,j}}}}.$$

(3.13)

The value of the input conductance for current flowing *into* the jth membrane cylinder depends on its output conductance, $B_{out,j}$, and its electrotonic length, X_j:

$$B_{in,j} = \frac{B_{out,j} + \tanh X_j}{1 + B_{out,j} \tanh X_j},$$

(3.14)

where

$$X_j = \frac{\ell_j}{\lambda} = \frac{\ell_j}{\sqrt{d_j}} \sqrt{\frac{4R_i}{R_m}}$$

(3.15)

and ℓ_j is the physical length of the cylinder.

At a branching point, the output conductance of the parent branch is the sum of the input conductances of the two daughter branches, weighted by the ratios of daughter to parent diameters:

$$B_{out,par} = B_{in,dau1}(d_{dau1}/d_{par})^{3/2} + B_{in,dau2}(d_{dau2}/d_{par})^{3/2}.$$

(3.16)

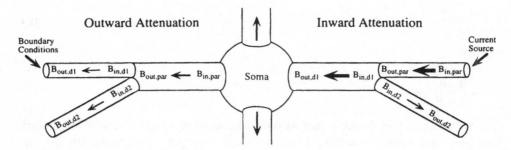

Figure 3.4
Diagram to show the relation of dimensionless input (B_{in}) and output (B_{out}) conductances (see text), in relation to the direction of current flows (arrows) in a simple cable model with a soma and four dendrites. Note that boundary conditions are defined at the terminations to *which* current is flowing (i.e., farthest from the source of current). Calculation of the conductances begins at these terminations and proceeds toward the source of current.

In order to allow for the possibility of different R_m values, this equation expands to

$$B_{out,par} = \frac{B_{in,dau1}\left(\frac{d_{dau1}}{d_{par}}\right)^{3/2}}{\sqrt{\frac{R_{m,dau1}}{R_{m,par}}}} + \frac{B_{in,dau2}\left(\frac{d_{dau2}}{d_{par}}\right)^{3/2}}{\sqrt{\frac{R_{m,dau2}}{R_{m,par}}}}. \tag{3.17}$$

3.3.5   Steady-State Input Resistance of Dendrites and Neurons

The input conductance at any point in an arbitrarily complex compartmental model of dendritic tree can be calculated using these normalized conductance ratios in an iterative procedure. For the case of currents flowing from the soma into the dendrites (as is the case for determination of the neuron input resistance, R_N) the desired quantity is the input conductance from the soma into the stem dendrite (the "outward attenuation" limb in figure 3.4). The calculation begins by assuming values for R_m and R_i, and a boundary condition for the conductance at the *terminations* of the tree (i.e., the termination values B_{out}). The usual assumption of sealed-end conditions gives $B_{out} = 0$ at all dendritic terminations. The computation then proceeds *backward* toward the soma, in the direction opposite to the current flow, beginning with any terminating segment and proceeding down that branch toward the soma, using eqs. 3.13 and 3.14. On reaching a branch point, the input conductance of the other daughter branch is similarly calculated and then eq. 3.17 is used to calculate the output conductance of the parent segment. This iteration continues until the input conductance of the stem segment, $B_{in,stem}$, is obtained. The actual input conductance, G_{stem}, can then be calculated by

$$G_{stem} = B_{in,stem}G_\infty = \frac{\pi}{2}\frac{B_{in,stem}d_{stem}^{3/2}}{\sqrt{R_iR_{m,stem}}}.$$ (3.18)

The whole-neuron input conductance, G_N, (excluding any contribution by the axon) is simply the sum of the input conductance of the soma plus the input conductances for all n dendrites originating from it:

$$G_N = \frac{A_{soma}}{R_{m,soma}} + \sum_{j=1}^{n} G_{stem,j}.$$ (3.19)

With appropriate software, the iterative process of R_N calculation is quite rapid even for models with many hundreds of compartments. Of course, in a membrane parameter search, the calculation must be repeated for every new choice of R_m and/ or R_i in the trial-and-error search for values that produce the experimentally observed R_N (see figure 3.5, step 1). In general, it is relatively easy to develop an optimization program that will search the parameter space until an optimal best fit to the target parameter (e.g., R_N or even to the waveform of the experimental voltage transient) is obtained (see Stratford et al. 1989; and discussion in chapter 5, this volume).

3.3.6 Steady-State Attenuation

It should be noted that the normalized input conductances tabulated for the steady-state R_N calculation can also be used to calculate the steady-state attenuation for point source voltage perturbations (Rall 1977). This calculation is particularly useful for estimating the attenuation of synaptic currents flowing from dendritic sites to the soma. The attenuation of the charge flowing from dendritic sites to the soma is much less than the decrement in amplitudes of voltage transients such as postsynaptic potentials (PSPs; see examples in Burke, Fyffe, and Moschovakis 1994). Indeed with proper scaling for local input resistance, the steady-state attenuation of voltage is equal to the relative decrement of the temporally integrated current flowing from the input site to the site being measured (Redman 1973; Rinzel and Rall 1974).

Calculation of attenuation factors within a neuron model follows the same rule as given above; one defines the boundary conditions (B_{out} values) at the points farthest from the source of current and then proceeds toward it. The basic equation for the attenuation factor, AF_j, for a given membrane cylinder was defined by Rall (1977, in his equation 3.24) as

$$AF_j = \frac{V_{in}}{V_{out}} = \cosh(X_j) + B_{out,j}\sinh(X_j),$$ (3.20)

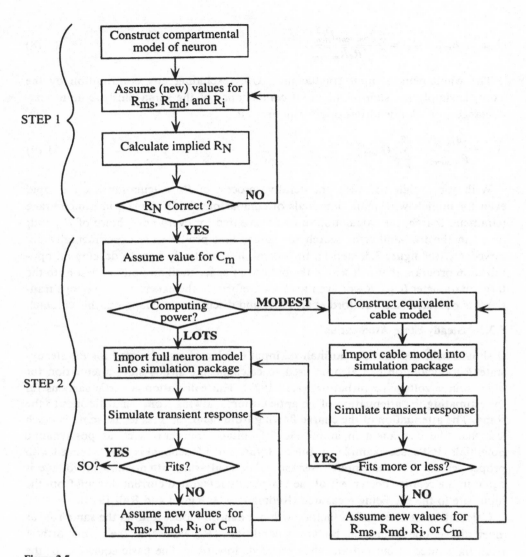

Figure 3.5
Flow diagram of one approach to estimating key electrotonic parameters (R_m, R_i, C_m) of an anatomically reconstructed neuron for which an experimental estimate of steady-state neuron input resistance (R_N) and records of transient responses to a somatic current pulse or step are available.

with V_{in} representing the voltage at the input site where current flows into the cylinder, and V_{out}, the voltage at the other end. In the case of current injected into the soma (outward attenuation), the iterative calculation proceeds in exactly the same way as that for calculation of dendritic input conductance described above. When the current source is located within a given dendrite, however (figure 3.4, inward attenuation), care must be taken because the "parent" branches at all branch points along the path from the voltage perturbation to the soma are the segments on that path, which is obviously different from their identification during outward current flow (see also Agmon-Snir 1995; Zador, Agmon-Snir, and Segev 1995; and chapter 2, this volume).

3.3.7 Matching Experimental and Simulated Transient Responses

The explicit calculation of steady-state R_N, although often quite useful, is not strictly necessary in the search for membrane parameters that reconcile electrophysiology and morphology; information about R_N is inherent in the transient responses that are the sine qua non of this process (see figure 3.5, step 2). For example, if one assumes that R_m and R_i are the same everywhere in the model neuron (spatial uniformity), a large number of value pairs will produce the same R_N. Limiting the range to biologically plausible values helps some, but not much, and the search can be constrained only by analyzing transient responses. The longest apparent time constant in the transient response is referred to as the "system time constant," τ_0. With passive membrane that is spatially uniform, $\tau_0 = \tau_m = R_m C_m$. Although this condition may not apply to real neurons (see below), it is possible to use the τ_0 extracted from voltage transients to limit the range of R_m and R_i pairs that may apply to a given parameter search. With a given morphology and any assumed values for C_m and R_i, there is only one value of spatially uniform R_m that will give the appropriate value for both τ_0 and steady-state R_N. The range of values for R_i in neurons that are biologically plausible is relatively restricted, ranging from about $70\,\Omega\text{cm}$ (Barrett and Crill 1974; Burke, Fyffe, and Moschovakis 1994) to 200–$300\,\Omega\text{cm}$ (Major et al. 1994; Ulrich, Quadroni, and Lüscher 1994). Happily, the acceptable range of C_m is more limited (between 0.7 and $2.0\,\mu\text{F/cm}^2$; see Cole 1968; Major et al. 1994; Ulrich, Quadroni, and Lüscher 1994), although the estimates of R_m are very sensitive to small changes in C_m (Burke, Fyffe, and Moschovakis 1994).

Unhappily, using values for R_i and C_m within these ranges often cannot explain the observed transient behavior of anatomically defined neurons. This has led to the conclusion that R_m may in fact not be spatially uniform (Iansek and Redman 1973; Durand 1984; Fleshman, Segev, and Burke 1988; Rose and Vanner 1988; Clements and Redman 1989; Burke, Fyffe, and Moschovakis 1994; Major et al. 1994). There is evidence that neurons, when penetrated with conventional "sharp" electrodes, develop (or at least manifest) increased conductance at the soma ("somatic shunt") that is functionally equivalent to a decreased specific membrane resistivity (Pongracz, Firestein, and Shepherd 1991; Staley, Otis, and Mody 1992; Spruston and Johnston 1992). Until recently, most work on the inverse estimation problem has been done using sharp electrodes. In modeling such neurons, one can deal with this possibility by introducing an explicit shunt conductance at the soma or by using a value of R_m on the soma (R_{ms}) that is lower than the value assumed for the dendrites (R_{md}). As a first approximation, R_{md} is usually assumed to be spatially uniform.

Simulation of a somatic shunt by a low effective value of R_{ms} emphasizes the fact that a somatic shunt creates a neuron with two membrane time constants. This situation changes the transient response of the cell in complex and interesting ways; in contrast to the uniform R_m case, when R_m is not uniform, current redistribution in the dendritic structure continues throughout the whole time course of voltage perturbation (see Fleshman, Segev, and Burke 1988). One very serious effect of continued current redistribution is that the "true" τ_0 of the system may contribute so little to the experimental transient response that it is experimentally undetectable (Rall et al. 1992; Burke, Fyffe, and Moschovakis 1994).

It should come as no surprise that the introduction of spatially nonuniform parameters greatly complicates the inverse estimation problem and adds to the already large number of possible nonunique solutions (Stratford et al. 1989; White, Manis, and Young 1992). No aspect of the model's transient response is predictable a priori, and it therefore must be simulated or computed, requiring initial estimates for four parameters; R_{ms}, R_{md}, R_i, and C_m. The critical test of the choice of parameter values is whether the neuron model will produce a transient response that matches the experimental record when supplied with a current pulse of the same duration and amplitude as used in the original experiment. Although other, computationally intensive approaches have recently become available (Stratford et al. 1989; Major 1993; Major and Evans 1994; Evans, Major, and Kember 1995), this trial-and-error simulation in compartmental models remains a practical and instructive way to proceed. The degree of match between actual and simulated responses guides refinement of the assumed values and illuminates the relative sensitivity of the system to changes in each parameter. Although, in principle, R_{ms}, R_{md}, R_i, and C_m are all free parameters, initial estimations are most efficiently done by assuming biologically plausible values for R_i and C_m based on previous data, and then exploring variations of R_{ms} and R_{md} that produce the require value of R_N. As noted above, model transients can be calculated using custom-made software (e.g., Clements and Redman 1989; Evans, Major, and Kember 1995) or simulated using general-purpose compartmental model packages that solve the required differential equations by a variety of standard methods (e.g., GENESIS, NEURON, NODUS, SABRE, SPICE, etc.; see De Schutter 1992).

Figure 3.5 shows a flowchart for one version of the trial-and-error process of refining parameter estimates (Burke, Fyffe, and Moschovakis 1994). Step 1, which involves only the steady-state calculations discussed above, attempts to narrow the ranges of possible values for R_i and R_m (R_{ms} and R_{md}). Step 2 searches through the R_i and R_m values for those producing model transients that match the experimental data when provided with an assumed value of C_m. There are two ways to proceed with this part. If the available computing resources are sufficiently large, it may be practical to use the full anatomical model of the cell for the trial-and-error process of transient fitting. Otherwise, it is often more practical to use a reduced "equivalent cable" model, which collapses all of the dendrites into a single cable structure of much less complexity than the original, fully branched structures (Clements and Redman 1989; Fleshman, Segev, and Burke 1988; Stratford et al. 1989). When combined with a spherical soma having the appropriate dimensions, a properly computed equivalent cable has approximately the same R_N, final time constant, τ_0, and total membrane area as the fully branched structure (see below).

The smaller and simplified matrices that represent equivalent cable models are solved much more quickly than the fully branched model, so that the trial-and-error search for suitable parameters can proceed relatively rapidly (Clements and Redman 1989; Burke, Fyffe, and Moschovakis 1994). As always, there is a price to pay for this convenience. The transients produced by the cable representation are *not* identical to those produced by the fully branched tree, for reasons discussed below. Hence parameter estimates derived using equivalent cables must be evaluated and then further refined using the fully branched representation (Clements and Redman 1989; Burke, Fyffe, and Moschovakis 1994).

3.4   Reduced Models of Neurons

The concept of complexity in neuron models can be considered by making a two-dimensional chart. One dimension would be membrane complexity, ranging from the simple case of a passive linear membrane, to that of postsynaptic membrane models with time-varying ion permeability (or conductance), and then to excitable membrane models, possibly with many different species of ion channels. The other dimension would be geometric complexity, ranging from the simple case of an iso-potential region of membrane (a soma or a space-clamped section of a cylinder) to complex dendritic trees attached to a soma. Which model to choose depends, in each case, upon the context. How much information do we already have about the neurons under consideration? What questions do we wish to explore?

For many questions, the neuron model used may be more complex than required to answer these questions. It is therefore advantageous in these cases to consider ways for reducing the complexity of the neuron model while retaining the essential input-output characteristics of the full model. As shown below, this can be done using the insights that were gained from Rall's cable theory. Such carefully reduced neuron models can then serve as the building block for large neuronal networks. The challenge remains however, to show that these biologically more realistic networks have an enriched computational capability, as compared to most of the current network models typically based on one-compartment neurons (see below; and chapters 5 and 12, this volume).

There are many ways to reduce the full-neuron model. One direction is to apply the principles of Rall's "equivalent cylinder" to derive a set of rules for replacing the full tree by a geometrically simpler structure, while attempting to map the electrical (and synaptic) properties from the full tree into its reduced geometrical representation. This approach is elaborated below; other related approaches are only briefly mentioned. Methods for reducing the *electrical complexity* of neuron models are also underway (Rinzel 1985; Mevnier 1992; Kepler, Abbott, and Marder 1992; Bush and Sejnowski 1991). These methods are briefly discussed below, using the insightful example of Pinski and Rinzel (1994) for a reduction of model complexity in both geometrical and electrical dimensions. Finally, we briefly discuss reduced-neuron models that incorporate a large number of dendritic spines and massive synaptic inputs.

3.4.1   Reducing Geometrical Complexity: "Equivalent Cables"

Rall's pioneering development of the idealized equivalent cylinder model for dendrites (1959) opened up the field of neuronal modeling that has given us a legacy of valuable insights, as well as a modus operandi, in studying information processing in complex neurons (see chapter 2, this volume; and Segev, Rinzel, and Shepherd 1995; Segev, 1995). The genius of the equivalent cylinder approach is that it provides an analytical solution of many aspects of the electrotonic behavior of complex branching dendrites. Rall presented his results in an easily understood way, providing powerful intuitive insights about dendritic function for two generations of neuroscientists, from cognoscenti to the mathematically illiterate.

Historically, equivalent cylinder models were used to explore the electrical behavior of neurons when current or voltage perturbations were introduced at the soma. The effect of branching on voltage distributions from voltage perturbations introduced elsewhere within dendrites was explored by Rall and Rinzel (1973; Rinzel and Rall 1974) using a passive tree with ideal symmetry. To represent a branching dendrite by a single membrane cylinder with constant diameter, a number of constraints should hold: (1) the sum of the diameters of daughter branches at each branch point, raised to the 3/2 power, must equal the parent branch diameter, also raised to 3/2 power (the "3/2 power rule"); (2) all dendritic terminations must be at the same electrotonic distance from the soma and have the same boundary conditions; and (3) R_m and R_i must be spatially uniform within the branching structure. In such an ideal branched structure, all points at a given electrotonic distance (X) from the soma will be at the same potential during centrifugal current flow and thus can be lumped together to produce the equivalent cylinder, whose diameter, raised to the 3/2 power, is the sum of all diameters at a given X, each diameter raised to the 3/2 power. Rall showed that, at the soma, the input resistance and transient responses in the full (ideal) tree are the same as in the corresponding equivalent cylinder.

It is now well recognized that the dendrites of real neurons almost never exhibit morphologies that conform to these strict constraints. Although the equivalent cylinder approximation continues to be useful for some simulations (Ulrich, Quandroni, and Lüscher 1994), there has been interest in developing an analogous simplification that would accurately represent the electrotonic behavior of actual dendrites, as viewed from the soma (e.g., Stratford et al. 1989; Douglas and Martin 1992; review in Segev 1992). Clements and Redman (1989) and Fleshman, Segev, and Burke (1988) introduced such a simplification to produce a single "equivalent dendrite" with a sequence of compartments of varying diameter, each representing the same increment of electronic length. We will refer to this structure more generally as an "equivalent cable," to conform to the analogy with the constant diameter "equivalent cylinder."

To construct this equivalent cable representation from the original neuron (figure 3.6), one begins by assuming values for R_{md} and R_i because (as is the case with the equivalent cylinder) the corresponding parts of the dendritic tree to be lumped together are those within increments of electrotonic distance, ΔX. At a given electrotonic distance, X_j, the diameter, d_{eq}, of the equivalent cable compartments within each successive ΔX window is calculated by summing the 3/2 power of the diameters of all n dendritic segments present within each ΔX window and taking the 2/3 root of the sum,

$$d_{eq}(X_j) = \left[\sum_{i=1}^{n} (d_i(X_j))^{3/2} \right]^{2/3}. \tag{3.21}$$

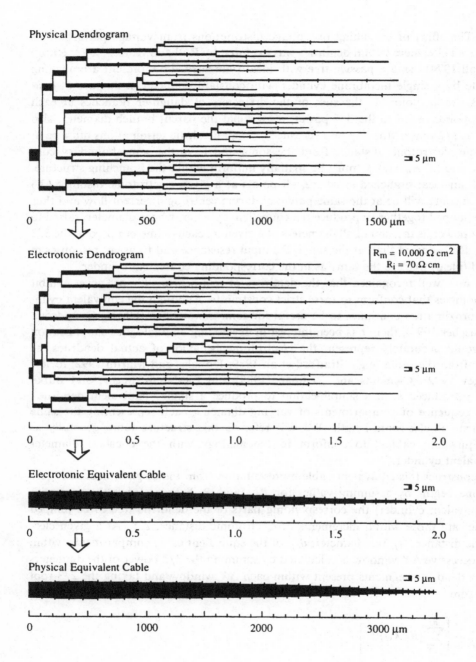

Physical Dendrogram

$R_m = 10,000\ \Omega\ cm^2$
$R_i = 70\ \Omega\ cm$

Electrotonic Dendrogram

Electrotonic Equivalent Cable

Physical Equivalent Cable

The physical length of each sequential cable compartment, j, can then be calculated using $d_{eq}(X)$ for that compartment and the selected value of ΔX:

$$\ell_j = \Delta X \lambda = \Delta X \sqrt{\frac{R_{md}}{4R_i}} \sqrt{d_{eq}(X_j)}. \tag{3.22}$$

In essence, this structure has the same membrane area in each ΔX, and thus the same total membrane area, as in the original fully branched tree. On the other hand, the input conductance is only approximately that of the fully branched tree because, as Clements and Redman (1989) point out, the distribution of steady-state voltages in the equivalent cable is *not* the same as the original branched structure, mostly because the cable neglects the end effects of dendritic paths of unequal electrotonic length. For the same reasons, the transient response produced in an equivalent cable model is similar, but *not* identical, to that produced by the fully branched neuron on which it is based, although both have the same "true" τ_0 (Clements and Redman 1989; Rall et al. 1992, figures 4, 5 and 7), provided that R_m is spatially uniform.

If R_{md} is assumed to be constant everywhere in the dendrites, it is possible to prepare a single file to represent the electrotonic structure of a neuron without prior specification of R_{md} and R_i (e.g., Major 1992). Using eq. 3.15, the electrotonic distance, X_j, between any point in the dendritic tree and the neuron's soma is given by

$$X_j = \sqrt{\frac{4R_i}{R_m}} \sum_{k=1}^{n} \left(\frac{\ell_k}{\sqrt{d_k}} \right), \tag{3.23}$$

where n is the number of cylindrical segments in the jth path between the selected compartment and the soma. Thus the electrotonic distance for each compartment can be represented by a tabulation of $\Sigma(\ell_{k,j} d_{k,j}^{-0.5})$ and calculated for arbitrary values of R_m and R_i (Burke and Glenn 1996).

Such reduced structures not only speed the calculation of voltage transients during parameter searches but also provide a simplified representation of the electrotonic architecture of individual neurons, enabling comparisons among different neurons

Figure 3.6
Steps in the transformation of a physical dendrogram (top panel) into a physical equivalent cable (bottom panel) by passing through two intermediate steps. In the first, the physical dendrogram is converted into an electrotonic dendrogram (second panel from top) with selecting values of (R_m) and (R_i). Then, for a given X value, the diameters of dendritic segments are raised to the 3/2 power, and summed (eq. 3.21). The 2/3 root of this sum then gives the diameters at successive ΔX increments in the electrotonic equivalent cable (third panel from top). In this example, $\Delta X = 0.05$ resulting in an equivalent cable that consists of forty compartments. Finally, the compartment lengths in the physical equivalent cable are calculated, using eq. 3.22.

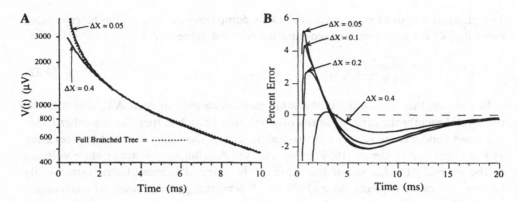

Figure 3.7
Comparison of voltage decay transients following brief somatic current pulses (5 nA, 0.3 msec duration) in models of a fully branched tree (see fig. 3.6, second panel from the top) and equivalent cables with ΔX of 0.05, 0.1, 0.2, and 0.4, each joined to a spherical soma with diameter 10 μm. All of the equivalent cables had the same total membrane areas as the full tree but exhibited slightly larger input conductances. (A) Comparison of the initial 10 msec in transients from the full tree model (dashed) and equivalent cables with ΔX of 0.05 and 0.4. Note that the coarser cable response diverges from the full tree response at times shorter than 2 msec, but thereafter both cable transients are very close to the transient generated in the full tree. (B) Calculation of the percentage error of transients produced by four equivalent cable models with ΔX of 0.05, 0.1, 0.2, and 0.4 during the initial 20 msec of the transients. Thereafter, all curves converged asymptotically to zero error. At times later than 3 msec, the error in all of the curves was less or equal to 2%, and that for the coarsest cable (ΔX of 0.4) was the smallest.

(Fleshman, Segev, and Burke 1988; Clements and Redman 1989; Burke, Fyffe, and Moschovakis 1994). Although the transient responses produced in equivalent cables are not identical to those generated by fully branched dendrites (Rall et al. 1992), when the cable representation is constructed carefully, the errors are relatively small and involve only the first portion of the transient response. Figure 3.7 shows an example using several equivalent cables from the branched tree depicted in figure 3.6, to which a spherical soma with diameter of 10 μm was added ($R_{ms} = R_{md} = 10{,}000\ \Omega\text{cm}^2$, $R_i = 70\ \Omega\text{cm}$, and $C_m = 1\ \mu\text{F/cm}^2$). Panel A illustrates superimposed records of the initial 10 msec of simulated voltage decay transients following injection of a 5 nA, 0.3 msec constant current pulse into the model soma for the fully branched tree (top panel in figure 3.6) and two curves from equivalent cables calculated with $\Delta X = 0.05$ and $\Delta X = 0.4$. The former had a total of forty compartments and took five times longer to run than the latter, which had only six compartments. For comparison, the fully branched tree plus soma, with 143 compartments, took almost twenty times longer than the six compartment model to produce the same duration transient (50 msec).

The transient curves in panel A diverged beyond the thickness of the lines only for times shorter than 2 msec. Curves of the percent error (panel B) between the full tree and cable transients showed that all of the curves were identical beyond about 25 msec but diverged at shorter times. Surprisingly, the model with the coarsest compartmental divisions ($\Delta X = 0.4$) showed the lowest percentage error between 2 msec and 25 msec. It appears that quite simple cables can be used to simulate somatic voltage transients.

Although equivalent cables are not perfect representations of branched dendrites, their relative simplicity has several advantages for neuronal model studies. Equivalent cables can serve in compartmental models as reasonable passive approximations for a portion of the dendritic trees of a neuron, while fully branched representations of one or more other dendrites can be used for detailed studies of synaptic action (e.g., Burke, Fyffe, and Moschorakis 1994). Equivalent cables can also be useful for examination of the effects of spatial distribution of various active membrane properties, if such active properties are assumed to vary in the same ways with electrotonic distance from the soma in all dendrites. Simulation of such conditions in a fully branched model with hundreds of compartments is not only costly in computer resources but very tedious to develop. Indeed, in a recent application of the equivalent cable approach, to model active propagation in branching axons, an algorithm was developed that permits dynamic expansion and collapse of compartments, depending on the location of the action potentials within the modeled axon (Manor, Koch, and Segev 1991). Other approaches to reducing the geometrical complexity of single-neuron models have been recently proposed (see Bush and Sejnowski 1993; Douglas and Martin 1992; and review in Segev 1992). Nevertheless, it seems clear that we need more systematic study of ways to reduce single-neuron model complexity for various passive and excitable cases.

3.4.2   Pinski and Rinzel Reduced Model for Hippocampal CA3 Neurons

A nineteen-compartment cable model for CA3 pyramidal cells dendrites of guinea pig hippocampus was developed by Traub et al. (1991). Experimentally based parameters were chosen for each compartment, using up to six active ionic conductances, and controlled by ten channel-gating variables. The network of model neurons could simulate several important aspects of the repertoire of experimental rhythmogenesis. Although Traub et al. recognized that their successful simulations depended on specifying significantly different ion channel densities for the soma and for the dendrites, the critical importance of this difference was made starkly clear by Pinsky and Rinzel (1994), who obtained essentially the same behavioral repertoire by using a network composed of only two compartments per pyramidal cell. One compartment, representing the soma and proximal dendrites, was equipped with ion channels for fast spiking currents (inward sodium, and delayed rectifier). The other compartment, representing the distal dendrites, contained the ion channels for the slower calcium currents (calcium-inward, and calcium-modulated currents). Pinsky and Rinzel's results showed that at least two compartments (but not necessarily more) are needed to simulate this behavior; a single lumped compartment, with all of the ion channels in parallel, could not produce the same behavior—especially not the rhythm, which basically involves an alternating flow of current between the two coupled compartments. Apart from its simplicity, the reduced (two-compartment) neuron model enables one to explore in an intuitive way how much the interesting behavior depends on the values of key parameters. The behavior of very large networks can be explored more efficiently using such a reduced-neuron model, although further study may show that the two-compartment model cannot match the fuller model in certain important tests. The two-compartment approach has also been successfully applied to neocortical pyramidal cells (Mainen and Sejnowski 1995; see also chapter 5, this volume).

3.4.3 Dendritic Spines and Massive Synaptic Inputs

Many central neurons are covered with a large number of dendritic spines (see reviews in Harris and Kater 1994; Shepherd 1996), which start with a narrow (0.1–0.5 μm) and short (0.1–2 μm) stem that ends with a bulbous head. The area of a typical spine is about 1.5 μm^2. Neocortical and hippocampal pyramidal cells bear 10,000 spines or more that in total constitute 25%–40% of the dendritic membrane area. An extreme example is the cerebellar Purkinje cell, where more than 100,000 spines (75% of dendritic area) cover the dendritic tree. Consequently, spines cannot be ignored in a faithful compartmental model of spiny neurons. Yet representing each spine by one (or more) compartments will unnecessarily and fatally overload most computer resources. Some global way for incorporating the spines into the neuron model is required.

The approaches that have been suggested for handling this problem are, again, based on insights gained from cable theory. For plausible values of R_m, C_m, and R_i when current flows *from the dendrite into the spine*, the spine base and the spine head membrane are essentially isopotential (i.e., they are, electrically, the same point; see Jack et al. 1983, Segev and Rall 1988), and the membrane area of the dendritic spines can therefore be globally incorporated into the membrane of the parent dendrite. This can be done by two *equivalent* methods. One can increase the physical dimensions (length, ℓ, and diameter, d) of the dendritic segment from which the spines arises (Stratford et al. 1989):

$$\ell' = \ell F^{2/3} \tag{3.24a}$$

$$d' = d F^{1/3}, \tag{3.24b}$$

and

$$F = (area_{dend} + area_{spines})/area_{dend}, \tag{3.25}$$

where $area_{dend}$ is the membrane area of the parent dendrite without spines and $area_{spines}$ is the membrane area of spines at that dendritic segment. Alternatively, one can adjust R_m and C_m by the factor F in eq. 3.25 as follows (Holmes and Rall 1992a; Rapp, Yarom, and Segev 1992):

$$R'_m = R_m/F \tag{3.26a}$$

$$C'_m = C_m F. \tag{3.26b}$$

Both methods are valid for the case where the spines and parent dendrite have the same specific membrane properties (R_m and C_m); the second method, however, can be extended also to nonuniform cases (Rapp, Yarom, and Segev 1992). Furthermore, both of these methods preserve the area, input and transfer conductances, membrane time constant, and effective electrotonic length of the spiny segment.

This global incorporation of spines is not valid, however, when the current is generate at the spine head membrane (e.g., from activation of synaptic input there) and the voltage transient at the spine head is of interest. In this situation there is a large voltage drop between the spine head membrane and the spine base. Thus spines receiving direct synaptic inputs (or spines that generate active currents) should be modeled in full (perhaps by a few compartments each).

Another situation that can be greatly simplified in neuron models is the case in which a large number of transient and asynchronous synaptic inputs bombard the whole dendritic tree. Indeed, dendritic trees of central neurons typically receive a large number of transient synaptic inputs, each input may be activated spontaneously a few times per second ("background synaptic activity"). Such a dendritic tree must experience an approximately steady conductance change. For any given type of synaptic input (e.g., AMPA-mediated) that impinges in a given dendritic segment (compartment) the *effective* conductance change, g_{steady}, can be approximated by

$$g_{steady} = Nf \int_0^\infty g_{syn}(t)\, dt, \tag{3.27}$$

where N is the number of (e.g., AMPA) synapses that contact this dendritic segment, $g_{syn}(t)$ the transient synaptic conductance changes, and f the frequency (in Hz) of (random) activation of each of these synapses (Bernander et al. 1991, Rapp, Yarom, and Segev 1992). The effective membrane resistivity, R_m^*, of this dendritic segment when it receives the background synaptic input is then

$$R_m^* = area_{seg} \bigg/ \left[\sum_i g_{steady}(i) + g_{rest} \right], \qquad (3.28)$$

where $area_{seg}$ is the total area of the dendritic segment (parent dendrite + spines), $g_{steady}(i)$ is the effective conductance change obtained from eq. 3.27 for the synapses of type i (e.g., AMPA, NMDA, GABA, etc.), and g_{rest} is the resting conductance of the dendritic segment without the synaptic input ($g_{rest} = area_{seg}/R_m$).

Using R_m^* from eq. 3.28, one can compute the impact of background synaptic activity on various cable parameters such as the input resistance, the voltage attenuation between two dendritic locations, and so on. The effective electrotonic structure of a dendritic tree before ($f = 0\,\text{Hz}$) and after ($f = 2\,\text{Hz}$) it is bombarded with spontaneous synaptic activity is graphically shown in figure 3.8. Finally, it should be emphasized that *transient* effects in the background synaptic activity (e.g., voltage fluctuations) cannot be computed using the above approach.

3.5 Discussion

In the last decade, compartmental modeling has proved to be a popular approach for simulating electrical and chemical activity in single neurons and neuronal networks. Its generality and flexibility enables one to examine ideas about signal processing at a wide range of levels, from receptors and ion channels through synapses and dendritic spines, and on to single neurons and neuronal networks. These advantages, plus the development of powerful and accessible computers, have stimulated the appearance of specialized neurosimulation software packages that implement the compartmental approach in a user-friendly way (review in De Schutter 1992). Indeed, it is likely that in the next few years these simulators will be further refined and adapted to new platforms (e.g., parallel machines), so that new and ever more sophisticated compartmental modeling projects can be undertaken (e.g., the Surf-Hippo software, written by Lyle Borg-Graham, information at http://www.cnrs-gif.fr/iaf/iaf9/surf-hippo.html).

Like many good things, ready access to powerful neurosimulators has a potential negative side. Unless one understands the constraints and assumptions inherent in

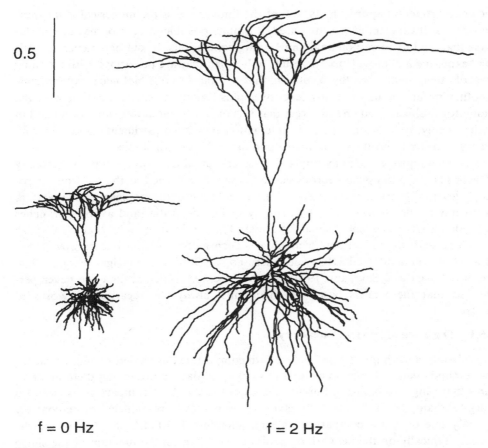

0.5

f = 0 Hz   f = 2 Hz

Figure 3.8
Effect of spontaneous background synaptic activity on the electrotonic structure of dendrites. In this
graph, the morphoelectrotonic transform, MET (Zador, Agmon-Snir, and Segev 1995; and figure 2.5) is
used to depict the *effective* electrotonic structure of the dendritic tree. Although in the absence of background synaptic activity ($f = 0\,\text{Hz}$), the neuron is electrically compact, when each of the 4,000 excitatory
and 1,000 inhibitory modeled synapses is activated randomly at $f = 2\,\text{Hz}$, the neuron is significantly extended. This MET is performed in the *centrifugal* direction. The scale bar corresponds to the distance over
which steady voltage attenuates by a factor of $e^{0.5}$ in an infinitely long cable. Modified from Bernanader et
al. 1991.

the compartmental approach, as well as the limitations of the numerical algorithms on which software simulators are based, it is quite possible to develop flawed simulations that lead to correspondingly misleading conclusions. In our experience, modeling "experiments" provide useful results only when they are performed with the same level of attention and healthy skepticism that is applied to real biological experiments. Another pitfall for users at any level of sophistication is that fascination with the simulator itself can lead one to forget that it is only a research tool and not an end in itself. Ideally, there should be close interaction between experiment, modeling, and theory in order to produce real understanding of the system studied.

New techniques are rapidly improving experimental data on the fine morphology of neurons (e.g., complete neurons can be now reconstructed at the electron microscope level). Electrical parameters of the membrane and cytoplasm, however, are much more difficult to obtain, particularly in fine dendritic (and axonal) branches (e.g., dendritic spines and axonal boutons). This problem is only beginning to be overcome with the aid of new technologies such as two-photon microscopy (Denk et al. 1996) and infrared DIC videomicroscopy (Dodt and Zieglgansberger 1994; see also Stuart and Sakmann 1994). In any case, experimental data are never perfect, so that the models based on them must always be regarded as works in progress.

3.5.1 The Issue of Model Complexity

This chapter and chapters 5 and 6 deal with compartmental models of single neurons that embody detailed anatomical and physiological data, representing them in structures that range from tens to hundreds or even thousands of compartments (see also Borg-Graham, 1997). In other chapters, single neurons are modeled more coarsely by only one or a few compartments each (chapters 4, 10, 12, and 13), where the focus is typically on the network dynamics rather than on the function of the single neuron. Indeed, as argued in this chapter, there is a wide range of choice in model complexity, from very simple to rather complex neuron models. As always, the choice of model complexity depends on the context—how much detailed information is available and what questions are to be asked.

When the anatomy and physiology of a particular neuron, or neuron class, is known in detail, preservation of the branching structure in at least some of the model dendrites may be important. This is particularly true when experimental data indicate that synapses and/or membrane properties are distributed nonuniformly within a given dendrite or in different dendrites. Nonuniform distribution of active channel densities of several ion channel types over the surface of the soma and dendrites can lead to vary interesting and potentially important functional consequences (e.g., De Schutter and Bower 1994; Pinski and Rinzel 1994; Mainen and Sejnowski 1996; see also chapter 5, this volume).

On the other hand, many network models assume that network properties depend primarily upon the connectivity between the neurons, rather than upon the interactions within individual cells. In such studies, simple one-compartment models are typically used to represent neurons, or even groups of neurons. Although such models can provide useful insights into network behavior, there is considerable evidence that neurons in actual biological networks perform functions that require more than one compartment for adequate simulation (Traub et al. 1991; Pinski and Rinzel 1994). It is obviously not necessary to include all known anatomical and physiological details; one simply should consider what level of complexity preserves the most significant regional specializations that could affect the outcome (e.g., nonuniform distributions of electrical properties, synapses, and ion channels). It can be very instructive to perform the same simulation at several levels of model complexity, in order to separate critical details from those which are not. There are valuable examples of this approach (see review by Borst and Egelhaaf 1994).

An important point emphasized throughout this book is that there is no a priori level of reduction of model complexity for a particular problem. Rather, the modeler needs to develop a deeper understanding about the critical parameters that govern the behavior of the system under study, which can only come from repeated simulation at different levels of resolution with various models of this system. Systematic reduction of model complexity while keeping the essential computational capability of the full model and of the system it represents is an excellent example of this process (see review in Segev 1992).

3.5.2 Passive versus Active Membrane

The discussion of detailed compartmental models of nerve cells presented in this chapter has dealt entirely with passive model systems. As noted above, there is abundant evidence that all neuronal membrane—dendritic as well as somatic—has nonlinear voltage-dependent conductances, many with time-dependent properties as well. Indeed, neurons would not be neurons without active membranes! One can reasonably ask, therefore, whether it is worthwhile to continue to use passive membrane models. The answer is, in our view, emphatically yes, for a number of compelling reasons (see also Rall et al. 1992; and chapter 5, this volume).

The most compelling (but not the most important) reason for at least starting out with passive models is that we have precious little quantitative information about the spatial distributions and densities of the many types of active channels known or believed to be present in neuron dendrites. One can, of course, make guesses, educated or not, on this matter, and many intuitive insights can be gained even in the absence of precise information. However, these insights are always made within a frame of reference established by a thorough understanding of the system as it behaves with *passive* membrane. This is clearly the most important reason to continue work with passive neuron models, which serve as the reference, or benchmark, systems, essential to understanding the sometimes exceedingly complex behavior of neuron models with nonlinear membrane (see, for example, Wilson, 1995). Indeed, initial estimates of key parameters like R_m, R_i, and C_m (all of which strongly affect the neuron dynamics also in the nonlinear case) can only be attempted using the passive membrane assumption. Once thoroughly understood, such reference models can then be refined by incorporating additional data or by relaxing one or more of the original constraints, while determining the effects of these changes on its performance (Bunow, Segev, and Fleshman 1985; Bernander et al. 1991; Rapp, Yarom, and Segev 1992, 1996; De Schutter and Bower 1994; Spruston, Jaffe, and Johnston, 1994; and see chapter 5, this volume). The usual outcome of such modeling exercises is the redirection of experimental work toward questions that will improve the model and, therefore, one's understanding of the underlying system.

3.5.3 Conclusions

The combination of cable theory and compartmental modeling studies has significantly deepened our understanding of the ways neurons process their chemical and electrical signals. One approach in the early theoretical studies, emphasized in this chapter, was to integrate the available morphological and physiological data in order to interpret experimental results (e.g., Rall et al. 1967). A second approach was to suggest different possibilities prior to experimental exploration (e.g., that some dendritic spines have excitable channels that may generate action potentials in the spine head; Shepherd et al. 1985). A third approach was to explore the computational roles of dendrites and dendritic spines, including (1) possible involvement in complicated input classification tasks (Rall and Segev 1987; Mel 1993); (2) logical AND-NOT–like operations (Koch, Poggio, and Torre 1982; Shepherd and Brayton 1987); (3) submillisecond coincidence detection (Segev and Rall 1988; Softky 1994; Yuste and Denk 1995); and (4) chemical compartmentalization for very localized plastic processes (see review in Denk et al. 1996; and chapter 6, this volume). We strongly believe that the parallel strands of experiment and modeling must interweave from time to time to enrich our understanding of the secrets of neurons, the elementary building blocks of the nervous system.

Acknowledgments

We thank Muki Rapp, Elad Schneidman, and Miki London for their help at various stages of this chapter. This work was supported by the US-Israel Binational Science Foundation and US Office of Naval Research grants to Idan Segev.

Appendix: The Neurosimulator NEURON

In this chapter we have used both NODUS and NEURON to perform the simulations described above. Information about NODUS can be found in De Schutter 1992. This appendix was written by Michael Hines, who developed NEURON, and is intended to highlight some basic principles of operation of this very popular simulator. More complete description and further information can be found in the NEURON manual at http://www.neuron.yale.edu, and in Hines and Carnevale 1997.

The NEURON program is intended to be a flexible framework for handling problems in which membrane properties are spatially inhomogeneous and where membrane currents are complex. The flexibility comes from a built-in object-oriented interpreter which is used to define the morphology and membrane properties of neurons, establish the appearance of a graphical interface, control the simulation, and plot the results. The default graphical interface is suitable for initial exploratory simulations involving the setting of parameters, control of voltage and current stimuli, and graphing variables as a function of time and position.

Simulation speed is excellent because the membrane voltage is computed via an implicit integration method optimized for branched structures (see also chapter 14, this volume). To maintain efficiency when membrane channels with complex kinetics are involved, user-defined membrane mechanisms are described by expressing models in terms of kinetic schemes (see chapter 1, this volume), differential equations, and sets of simultaneous equations (see above), which are then automatically translated into "C", compiled, and linked into the rest of NEURON.

While NEURON is a compartmental modeling program, it tries to separate the specification of neuron properties (shape and physiology) from the numerical issue of compartment size. The fundamental notion in NEURON that makes this possible is the "Section" which is intended to represent a continuous length of cylindrically symmetric cable. Although each section is ultimately discretized into segments (compartments), values that can vary with position along a section are specified in terms of a continuous parameter that varies from 0 to 1. In this way, section properties are discussed without regard to the number of segments (compartments) used to represent a particular section. Sections are created by declaring names for them using a "create" statement as in

```
create soma, axon, dendrite[3]
```

These sections are connected together to form a tree using statements like

```
connect axon(0), soma(1)

for i = 0,2 connect dendrite[i](0), soma(0)
```

where the first section name in the "connect" statement refers to the child and the second refers to the parent. The numbers in parentheses tell which end (0 or 1) of a child section is connected where on a parent section $(0 \leq x \leq 1)$[3]. The only limitation on connections is that they cannot form a loop because the numerical method for solving the branched cable equation is optimized for, and restricted to, trees.

Physical length (microns), diameter (microns), and compartmentalization of a section are specified using statements of the form

```
access soma

L = 40
```

```
diam = 30

nseg = 1

for i = 0,2 dendrite[i] { L = 1000 diam = 6 nseg = 10 }

axon.L = 5000

axon.diam = 4

axon.nseg = 50
```

using, somewhat artificially for demonstration purposes, the three syntactic forms (in order of increasing precedence) available for specifying which section is under discussion. One can obtain a simple view of the compartmental connectivity by executing the "topology( )" statement. With the above section declarations, connections, and compartmentalization, it prints:

```
|-|  soma(0-1)

  '--------------------------------------------------| axon(0-1)

  '---------| dendrite[0](0-1)

  '---------| dendrite[1](0-1)

  '---------| dendrite[2](0-1)
```

The number of dashes represents the number of segments in the section.

There are several statements that deal with collections of sections, but the typical iterator is illustrated by

```
forall Ra = 100
```

in which the axial resistivity (Ωcm) of all existing sections is assigned a constant value. (Ra is denoted by Ri in the body of the text).

Distributed membrane mechanisms such as Hodgkin-Huxley nonlinear conductances and passive conductances are inserted into sections using

```
soma {

    insert hh

    gnabar_hh=.5*.120

}

axon {

    insert hh

}

for i = 0,2 dendrite[i] {

    insert pas

    g_pas = .0001

    e_pas = -65

}
```

Inserting a membrane mechanism creates a separate set of parameters, states, and auxiliary variables for each segment in the section. These variables, which normally have a suffix indicating the name of the mechanism, are called "range variables" to stress that their values are generally functions of position. The units employed by distributed mechanisms are milliamperes per square centimeter (mA/cm^2) for membrane current, and siemens per square centimeter (S/cm^2) for membrane conductance.

A list of the parameters associated with the first segment of a section is printed with the "psection( )" command. For the soma specification up to this point the "psection" function prints:

```
soma { nseg = 1 L = 40 Ra = 100

    /* location 0 attached to cell 0 */

    /* First segment only */

    insert morphology { diam = 4 }

    insert capacitance { cm = 1 }

    insert hh { gnabar_hh = 0.06 gkbar_hh = 0.036 gl_hh = 0.0003 el_hh = -54.3}

    insert na_ion ena = 50

    insert k_ion ek = -77
}
```

Similar functions are used to display state variables such as "m_hh" and variables that are mere functions of state during a simulation such as the total sodium current, "ina."

Although, range variable parameters are most commonly specified as constants along the length of a section (as in the example above), they can also be specified as a piecewise linear function using syntax like

```
axon {

    diam(0 : .1) = 10 : 1
    diam(.1 : 1) = 1 : 1

}
```

where the argument range specifies the relative position along the section (.1 means one tenth of the length) and the diameter of segments within this range are assigned linearly interpolated values according to the colon separated expressions on the right-hand side.

One can also specify a value for a particular location as in

```
gkbar_hh(.5) = .018
```

but it is important to realize that this is for the segment that contains the value of "x" and the extent therefore depends on "nseg."

Retrieval of range variable values require a location argument (default is location .5). A common way to print all the values for a particular variable in a section is with

```
axon for (x) {

    print x, L*x, diam(x)

}
```

where the iteration variable, in this case "x," takes on all the values at the centers of segments (including position 0 and 1):

```
0 0 9.1
```

```
0.01 50 9.1

0.03 150 7.3

0.05 250 5.5

0.07 350 3.7

0.09 450 1.9

0.11 550 1

0.13 650 1

0.1

...

0.95 4750 1

0.97 4850 1

0.99 4950 1

1 5000 1
```

In contrast to distributed mechanisms, "point processes" such as electrodes and synapses are attached at a specific location and are dealt with using the interpreter's standard object syntax. For example, to stimulate the soma with a current pulse, one would say:

```
objref stim

stim = new IClamp( )

dendrite[0] stim.loc(.5)

stim.dur = .1 // millisec

stim.amp = 10 // nanoamps
```

The "stim" variable is declared as a generic object reference and is used as the label for a new instance of a current pulse mechanism with a duration of .1 msec and amplitude of 10 nA. (For point processes conductance is measured in microsiemens). The "loc" function specifies that the point process is to be inserted in the middle of the dendrite indexed by 0.

The stimulus can be moved to another location using a function call on the object reference such as

```
axon stim.loc(1)
```

which moves the stimulus to the distal end of the axon.

This completes a rough outline of how one specifies the physical properties of a cell with the NEURON program. One controls the time integration using functions for initialization of states and numerical integration of the equations associated with states and membrane potential. Initialization merely involves assigning values to all the states and voltages. This can be done in detail using an interpreted function or en masse with the generic function

```
finitialize(v_init)
```

which initializes all sections to a constant value of membrane potential and calls built-in initialization functions for each inserted mechanism. In the Hodgkin and Huxley case (1952), this sets the channel states, "m_hh," "h_hh," and "n_hh," to their steady-state values with respect to membrane potential.

Numerical integration from "t" to "t + dt" is carried out with the built-in function "fadvance." The kernel of any simulation run is thus

```
finitialize(v_init)

while (t < tstop) {

   fadvance()

}
```

which in practice will be elaborated with statements to print and graph variables and save them to a file.

Single-Compartment Simulations

Regardless of the ultimate degree of spatial complexity used to describe a neuron, the number of neurons, and the pattern of synaptic connections between them, it is crucial for the investigator to explore the behavior of the channels in the context of a space-clamped single compartment. This allows one both to verify correct functioning of a channel and to develop enough intuition about its behavior and interaction with other channels to be able to critically evaluate its contribution to the larger system. To make this concrete, the following section leads the reader through simulation of a Hodgkin-Huxley (HH) membrane (space-clamped) action potential elicited by a synapse whose conductance change follows an "α-function." The script used for single-compartment simulations is part of the standard interpreter library and basically consists of

```
create soma

access soma

{ diam = 10 L = 10/PI } // PI = 3.14...

load_proc("nrnmainmenu")

nrnmainmenu( )
```

Defining the soma as the "default section" makes unnecessary any further reference to the section name in specifying parameters and mechanisms. Setting the length and diameter so that the section area is $100\,\mu m^2$ is merely a convenience to relate point-process currents and distributed mechanism current density; thus $1\,mA/cm^2$ over $100\,\mu m^2$ is nA (nanoampere). The "load_proc" statement searches a standard set of directories for a file containing the indicated procedure and loads that file, in this case our standard run library. Executing the procedure pops up a menu from which a complete graphical control interface can be constructed. In particular, figure 3.9 was fashioned by selecting various menu items of "NEURON Main Panel" and arranging the resulting windows on the screen. After using the "Inserter" to create HH channels in the soma and using the "PointProcessManager" to specify a current clamp electrode along with stimulus parameters, the "RunControl" is used to carry out a simulation. The "Print and File Window Manager" was used to arrange itself and all the windows on a page for printing and save the graphical user interface specification for later retrieval.

Simulations of Three-Dimensional Reconstructed Cells

Three dimensional information about the shape of a section in NEURON is stored as a sequence of "x, y, z, diameter" coordinates ordered with respect to increasing arc length. Because all 3-D reconstruction file formats contain such data along with an "id field" and the parent "id," it is straightforward to read such files into NEURON directly or to use a filter to transform the raw data into a program that can be executed by the NEURON interpreter. It is important and useful to realize, however, that the number of 3-D points describing a section is completely independent of the number of segments, "nseg," used to simulate the section. Segment diameter, area, and axial resistance are computed via trapezoidal integration

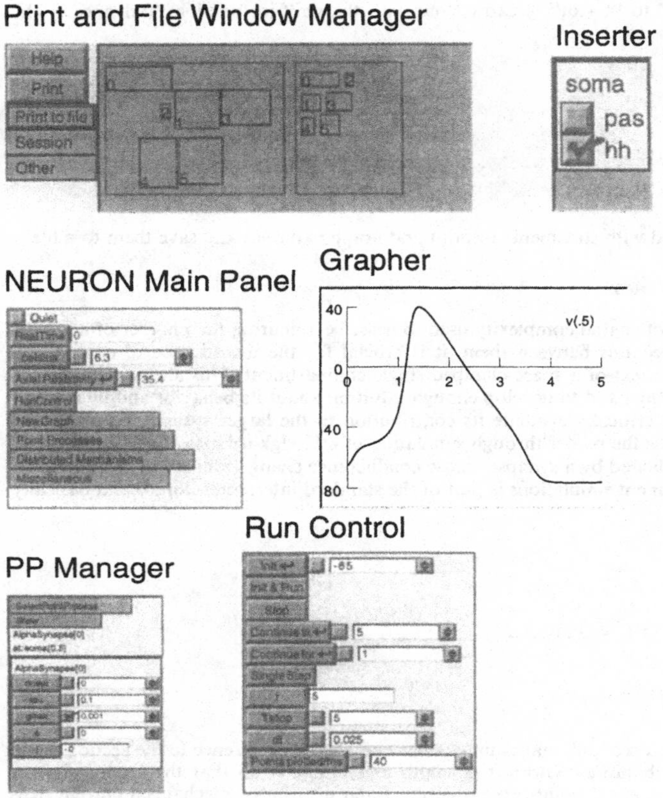

Print and File Window Manager

Inserter

NEURON Main Panel

Grapher

v(.5)

Run Control

PP Manager

Figure 3.9
Postscript output generated by the "Print and File Window Manager," PWM (window titles added separately). The PWM shows the arrangement of NEURON windows on the screen icon represented by wide rectangle. Window icons (small rectangles) are positioned and sized on the paper-shaped rectangle for printing. Notice that the overall arrangement of windows in the figure is the same as that on the paper icon. Menu items in the "NEURON Main Panel" are used to create the other windows on the display. Although not shown here, any variable that affects the simulation is easily viewed by creating a panel of field editors using the "NEURON Main Panel." The "Run Control" serves rudimentary "Oscilloscope level" simulations by providing single sweep runs and single stepping through a simulation. The "Point-Process Manager" places any kind of point process in a section and shows a panel of variables for viewing and assignment of values by the user. The "Inserter" adds and deletes density mechanisms in/from the indicated section by pressing the checkbox buttons. The "Grapher" here displays an *x-y* plot of voltage at the center of the soma.

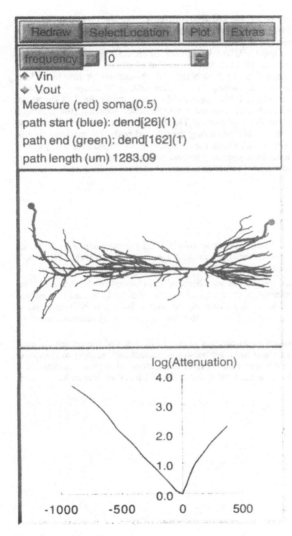

Figure 3.10
Voltage attenuation at the soma with respect to current injection along a path. On a computer screen the red, blue, and green dots as well as the red-colored path are clearly visible as such. For this gray-scale figure, the red path has been widened for clarity. See text for further explanation. This tool is invoked from the "NEURON Main Panel" by selecting the "Miscellaneous/Impedance/Path" menu item. In this simulation the cell membrane is passive, with $R_a = 200\,\Omega\text{cm}$, $R_m = 30,000\,\Omega\text{cm}^2$, and $C_m = 1\,\mu\text{F/cm}^2$.

over the overlapping 3-D points, and thus there is a great efficiency increase over the typical method of using one compartment per 3-D point. At the same time, displays of the cell shape make use of all the 3-D points to allow immediate orientation with regard to stimulus and measurement locations.

To illustrate the use of 3-D shape displays in the NEURON program, figure 3.10 shows a 3-D reconstruction of a hippocampal pyramidal cell (Claiborne 1992) and measurement of voltage attenuation at the soma with respect to current injection at each point along a path through the cell (thick line in middle frame). The tool shown was built by the interpreter from more primitive "Impedance," "Shape," "Graph," and "xpanel" components (Carnevale, Tsai, and Hines 1996). The middle panel shows the 3-D shape on which the user selects an injection/measurement path and a measurement/injection location (the meaning is determined by the selection of "Vin/Vout" in the top panel). The bottom graph shows the log of attenuation at the soma as a function of injection site distance along the selected path. The computation is performed with an "Impedance" class object which calculates the complex input impedance everywhere along with the complex transfer impedance between a specific location and all other locations (i.e., the diagonal and one row/column of the symmetric transfer impedance matrix) at a single frequency (see also figure 2.5).

Notes

1. The symbols $\hat{r}_m$, $\hat{c}_m$, $\hat{r}_i$, and $\hat{i}_m$ are used throughout the chapter to represent *per compartment* values, as distinguished from r_m, c_m, r_i, and i_m, which conventionally represent *per unit length* values. "Resting" channels are the channels that are open at the resting potential.

2. The assumption that E_{syn} is constant is valid only if the specificity of the channel to the different ions flowing through it is time-independent. For example, a channel that carries both sodium and potassium, that is, $g_{syn}(t) = g_{Na}(t) + g_K(t)$, can be modeled as a conductive branch with a fixed battery (whose value lies between the Nernst potential values of E_{Na} and E_K) only if the ratio $g_{Na}(t)/g_K(t)$ remains constant throughout the conductance change.

3. It is generally, though not always, more convenient to connect to one of the ends of the parent because the computation of membrane potential is guaranteed to be second-order correct with respect to compartment size. Connecting a child section (or point source of current) to the interior of a parent section at a position that does not correspond to the center of a segment reduces the accuracy to first-order in compartment size.

4 Multiple Channels and Calcium Dynamics

Walter M. Yamada, Christof Koch, and Paul R. Adams

4.1 Introduction

The cornerstone of modern neurobiology is the analysis by Hodgkin and Huxley (1952) of the initiation and propagation of the action potential in the squid giant axon. Their description accounted for two ionic currents: the fast sodium current, I_{Na}, and a delayed potassium current, I_K. Almost without exception, impulse conduction along axons can be successfully analyzed in terms of one or both of these ionic currents (see Parnas and Segev 1979; Waxman, Kocsis, and Stys 1995; and Weiss 1996 for examples of experimental and theoretical studies investigating action potential propagation in invertebrate and vertebrate axons with various branching patterns). When modeling active structures other than the squid axon, researchers have usually adopted Hodgkin and Huxley's system of coupled four-dimensional nonlinear differential equations because models more applicable to vertebrate neurons have not been fully developed. However, while the Hodgkin-Huxley formulation has been singularly important to biophysics, their equations do not describe a number of important phenomena such as adaptation to long-lasting stimuli or the dependency of some conductances on various ionic concentrations. Moreover, the transmission of electrical signals within and between neurons involves more than the mere circulation of stereotyped impulses. Impulses must be set up by subthreshold processes; the shape of these impulses is variable, reflecting the roles of voltage-dependent ion currents beyond those described by Hodgkin and Huxley.

In recent years, numerous ionic membrane currents have been described (see Hille 1992), which differ in principal carrier, voltage and time dependence, dependence on internal calcium, and susceptibility to modulation by synaptic input and second messengers. Our understanding of these currents and, to a lesser extent, the role they play in impulse formation, has been accelerated by various technical innovations such as single-cell isolation and patch clamping. To understand more completely how these currents determine membrane responses, however, we must develop empirical equations that approximate the behavior of the currents under physiological conditions and compare numerical simulations of these equations with the physiological preparation.

This chapter will focus on modeling the electrical properties of one particular neuron type whose various macroscopic currents have been described in detail, the bullfrog sympathetic ganglion "B"-type cell (see figure 4.1). Cells of this type are the largest in the ganglion, having a mean diameter of 35 μm (Honma 1984; for a

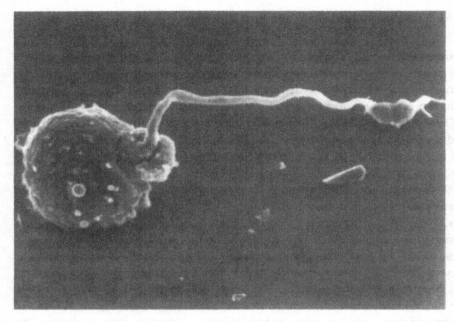

Figure 4.1
Electron micrograph of an isolated bullfrog sympathetic ganglion "B"-type cell (×1,600). The complete absence of dendritic processes, a single nonbranching axon, and the spherical shape of the soma, make this cell an excellent preparation for electrophysiological study. The diameter of the cell body is about 30 μm. Courtesy of Barry Burbach and Paul Adams.

scanning electron microscope study of the bullfrog sympathetic ganglion, see Baluk 1986). They receive inputs from rapidly conducting presynaptic axons, the terminals of which engulf the soma and axon hillock. There are several reasons why these cells have provend to be unusually favorable objects for research. They are indubitably neuronal. They can be studied in their fully mature form at various levels of simplification (within the intact ganglion, in explant cultures, or after complete dissociation) and using a variety of different techniques (two-electrode voltage clamp, single-electrode voltage clamp, whole-cell and single-channel patch recording, and intracellular injection). Because dendrites are absent and all synapses are formed on or near the cell body, these cells present few space clamp problems. Thus, the soma of these cells can be modeled accurately by a single spherical compartment. Finally, the voltage-dependent conductances of the cells are targets for various types of unusual "modulating" slow synaptic actions that are far more prevalent in the nervous system than originally suspected (Adams and Brown 1982; Kuffler and Sejnowski 1983;

Nicoll 1988). Thus the bullfrog sympathetic ganglion cells provide an ideal environment for studying cellular adaptation, slow synaptic transmission, and other such phenomena crucial for understanding information-processing operations that occur on time scales from milliseconds to many minutes.

Our aim in this chapter is to provide the reader with a complete model for these typical vertebrate cells, which are geometrically rather simple but electrically quite complex, and to describe the relevant numerical algorithms. Our approach is by now a common one: we attempt to dissect out or hold constant as many of the features of the system under study as possible and to describe the remaining features with empirical equations of sufficient detail to determine how they affect the behavior of the system as a whole. By allowing subsystems observed in isolation (e.g., channels recorded under patch clamp or currents measured in isolation by pharmacologically blocking other currents) to interact with the other components of the system, simulations serve not merely to display a system already described in detail but also to test the modelers' understanding of that system's integrative aspects. Furthermore, features of the system that are experimentally inaccessible or not easily controlled (e.g., the activation state of a given current) can easily be visualized with the aid of the computer.

Sections 4.2–4.4 present a rather detailed description of the various inward and outward currents using the rate constant formalism employed so successfully by Hodgkin and Huxley. Section 4.5 deals with the synaptic input, while section 4.6 treats calcium diffusion and buffering, a topic of ever-increasing importance. We then discuss how these ingredients can be incorporated into a single system, solved numerically, and show pertinent results. Chapter 5, this volume, extends the present approach to geometrically complex neurons.

4.2 Modeling Ionic Current Flow

In this section, we briefly review the general methodology used to describe ionic currents, focusing on one current found in the bullfrog, the fast sodium current (for a more detailed discussion, see Hille 1992). We begin by assuming that all ionic current flow occurs through channels or pores and that the instantaneous current-voltage relation is linear. The ionic current, $I(t)$, is then related to the voltage across the membrane, V, by Ohm's law:

$$I(t) = g(t, V) \cdot (V - E), \tag{4.1}$$

where E is the Nernst potential for the ionic current under study and $g(t, V)$ is the conductance associated with the channel. In general, this conductance depends on time and on the membrane potential but may also depend on various chemical mediators such as intracellular calcium. The use of Ohm's law is best justified by the results of past simulations that have successfully predicted membrane voltage responses (most notably, Hodgkin and Huxley original 1952 study). We should note, however, that the relationship between instantaneous current and voltage of most membranes is not linear but shows some degree of rectification: extracellular and intracellular ionic activity differences cause ionic current flowing in one direction to be preferred over the other.

The so-called Goldman-Hodgkin-Katz equations have been formulated to account for the unequal distribution of ions on both sides of the membrane and the associated rectification (Goldman 1943; Hodgkin and Katz 1949; Hille 1992). Whether the calcium current should be described by the linear Ohm's law or by the nonlinear Goldman-Hodgkin-Katz equation has never been carefully evaluated from an experimental point of view. Numerical models matching simulations against experimental records have used, variously, Ohm's law (Hudspeth and Lewis 1988; Traub and Miles 1991; McCormick, Hugenard, and Strowbridge 1992) and the Goldman-Hodgkin-Katz equation and variants thereof (Linás, Steinberg, and Walton 1981; Lytton and Sejnowski 1991; McCormick and Huguenard 1992; Borg-Graham 1998). In defense of the linear Ohm's model used in this chapter, it should be noted that—under physiological conditions—the cell spends almost all of its time at membrane potentials of less than $-40\,\text{mV}$, a region in which the current-voltage (I-V) relationship can be closely approximated by a linear one. Cells only briefly transgress to more positive potentials.

We assume that all ionic movement across the membrane is via channels permeable to a single ionic species and having two states, open or closed. The total conductance associated with any particular population of channels can then be expressed as the maximal conductance of the particular membrane patch under investigation, $\bar{g}$ (given by the conductance of a single channel in the open state times the channel density times the area of the membrane patch), times the fraction of all channels that are open. This fraction is determined by hypothetical activation and inactivation variables m and h raised to some integral power. In general, we have

$$g(t, V) = \bar{g} \cdot m(t, V)^i \cdot h(t, V)^j, \tag{4.2}$$

where i and j are positive integers. The dynamics of the variables m and h obey first-order kinetics of the form

$$\frac{dm(t, V)}{dt} = \frac{m_\infty(V) - m(t, V)}{\tau_m(V)}, \tag{4.3}$$

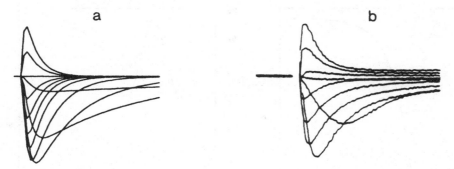

Figure 4.2
I_{Na} elicited by clamping the somatic potential to a fixed potential. The model (a) is compared with experimental data (b) taken from dissociated bullfrog cells with external Mn^{2+} used to block calcium currents (Jones 1987). Both traces are 5 msec long. The trajectories illustrate the sodium current elicited by voltage steps from -80 mV to $-30, -20, -10, 0, +10, +20, +30, +40, +50, +60$, and $+70$ mV. Inactivation leads to the complete reduction of I_{Na} after several milliseconds at most voltage values. I_{Na} becomes an outward current (positive current values) if the voltage is stepped beyond the Nernst potential for sodium (50 mV).

where the steady-state value of m, m_∞, and the time constant, τ_m, are defined functions of voltage. In the original Hodgkin and Huxley study, m_∞ and τ_m were expressed in terms of rate constants, α_m and β_m, that can be thought of as the forward and backward rates governing the transition of the channel between hypothetical "open" and "closed" states. The rates themselves depend on the potential across the membrane in a well-specified manner; for some currents, such as I_C and I_{AHP}, the rate constants depend as well (or solely) on the concentration of intracellular calcium. The rate constants, which ultimately specify the behavior of the current, must be measured experimentally on the basis of extensive voltage clamp experiments in conjunction with the application of pharmacological agents to block other currents.

Such data are shown in figure 4.2 for the case of the somatic fast sodium current recorded in dissociated cells. The axonal contribution of I_{Na} to the total current recorded at the soma is minimal in this preparation because the axon is dissociated from the cell body. However, in general, it is likely that the action potential is actually initiated out in the axon beyond the axon hillock and the initial segment and then propagates back into the soma (Colbert and Johnston 1996).

From these data we derive appropriate numerical values for the activation and inactivation variables (shown as a function of voltage in figure 4.3). In other words, the description of an individual current measured under voltage clamp conditions and in isolation provides the input data for our model. Note that the steady-state

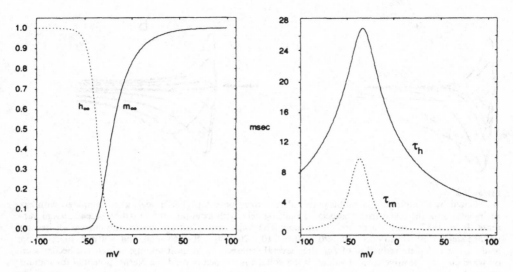

Figure 4.3
Times constants and steady-state values of the activation and inactivation variables for the fast sodium current I_{Na} as a function of voltage. This current is very similar to data published for the node of Ranvier (Frankenhaeuser and Huxley 1964), except that the curves for m_∞ and h_∞ are both shifted toward more depolarized values. The detailed equations are given in the chapter appendix.

variable (m_∞ in this case) for an activation variable is a monotonic *increasing* function of voltage, while any steady-state inactivation variables are monotonic *decreasing* functions of voltage. With the single exception of I_{Ca} inactivation, we will use this rate formalism to describe all currents present in the bullfrog sympathetic ganglion (a complete set of all equations can be found in the chapter appendix).

The Hodgkin and Huxley research program has been enormously important for the development of biophysics, linking the level of membrane potential in a quantitative and deterministic manner to the underlying level of macroscopic membrane conductances and rate constants. Although Hodgkin and Huxley offered a conceptual interpretation of these variables in terms of "gating particles" vacillating between open and closed states, their model is a phenomenological one, based on empirical equations describing currents resulting from the activity of membrane elements that at that time were still the object of much controversy. The advent of the patch clamp recording technique (Sakmann and Neher 1983) has revealed ionic channels to be all-or-nothing pores that behave very much in a probabilistic manner. Researchers have successfully addressed the issue of how action potentials can be constructed from the time- and voltage-dependent kinetics of stochastic single-channel currents (Strassberg and DeFelice 1993). In this interpretation, the macroscopic activation (or gating) particle, $m(t)$, is equivalent to the open-channel probability. If the channel is closed, the probability that a channel gate will remain closed for a time, T, is $e^{-\alpha T}$, and if it is open the probability that the channel will remain open is $e^{-\beta T}$. If several hundred or more channels are simulated in this manner around the resting potential consistency between the macroscopic and the microscopic domain can be demonstrated. For our purposes, however, this deterministic phenomenological description is quite sufficient.

4.3 Inward Currents

The ganglion cell bodies exhibit two rapidly activating inward currents, I_{Na} and I_{Ca}, which closely resemble those already described in a variety of axonal, glandular, or invertebrate preparations. Closer examination of I_{Na} reveals that it is the summation of several distinct sodium conductances, each of which can be distinguished by its sensitivity to various pharmacological agents (tetrodotoxin, cadmium) and by different activation thresholds and kinetics (Jones 1987; for an overview, see Barchi 1987 as well as Colbert and Johnston 1996). We restrict our model to the largest component of the sodium ionic current, I_{Na}. The peak sodium conductance increases sigmoidally with depolarization, having an effective threshold near $-20\,\text{mV}$. Both activation and inactivation seem to be shifted to more positive values than in the frog node of Ranvier (Frankenhaeuser and Huxley 1964). In intact cells, the threshold for initiating action potentials is more negative than the threshold in isolated cells, possibly due in part to this shift in activation and inactivation voltage dependence (Jones 1987). I_{Na} is described as

$$I_{Na} = \bar{g}_{Na} m_{Na}^2 h_{Na} \cdot (V - E_{Na}). \tag{4.4}$$

Both intra- and extracellular changes in sodium ion concentration are very small, justifying our assumption of a constant Nernst reversal potential, E_{Na}.

The calcium current, I_{Ca}, is smaller and slower than the sodium current, I_{Na}, and contributes little to the electric charge entering the cell during an action potential. However, it inactivates very slowly and thus dominates the inward current during long depolarizations (Adams, Brown, and Constanti 1982). Of the three types of calcium currents described by Nowycky, Fox, and Tsien (1983), it most closely resembles the L-form. Inactivation is primarily current rather than voltage-dependent and thus reflects channel block as a result of internal calcium accumulation in the space just below the cell membrane (Eckert and Chad 1984). Removal of inactivation (and thus presumably of internal calcium) takes several seconds following closure of the calcium channels. The voltage-dependent inactivation present in other calcium currents (Carbone and Lux 1984) is present to a much lesser extent in bullfrog sympathetic ganglion cells. The threshold for activation of I_{Ca} is about $-32\,\text{mV}$. Hyperpolarization to $-80\,\text{mV}$ does not reveal any rapidly inactivating low-threshold calcium current, unlike the situation in many other cells (Carbone and Lux 1984). I_{Ca} is described as

$$I_{Ca} = \bar{g}_{Ca} m_{Ca} h_{Ca} \cdot (V - E_{Ca}). \tag{4.5}$$

Activation is modeled as in eq. 4.3, and the equilibrium potential for calcium, E_{Ca}, is described in section 4.6.1. Inactivation is dependent on the concentration of intracellular calcium below the membrane by a mechanism that has yet to characterized. Therefore, we use the simplest Michaelis-Menten equation (Stryer 1995) to describe calcium current inactivation:

$$h_{Ca} = \frac{K}{K + [Ca^{2+}]_n}, \tag{4.6}$$

where the halfway inactivation concentration, K, is a constant and the concentration of free calcium in the shell just below the membrane, $[Ca^{2+}]_n$, is described in section 4.6.

4.4 Outward Currents

The remaining five ionic currents are potassium currents. A number of experimental limitations preclude detailed descriptions of these currents. They are much more difficult to separate than the inward currents because there exist no completely selective blockers. Two of these currents, I_C and I_{AHP}, are activated as a result of calcium influx. Though much progress is being made in developing kinetic schemes for both I_C and I_{AHP}, the exact time course of the calcium concentration changes within the cell during clamp steps or action potentials is uncertain, and so it is not yet possible to develop a detailed kinetic description for these currents (Moczydlowski and Latorre 1983; Gurney, Tsien, and Lester 1987). The remaining currents, I_M, I_K, and I_A, are controlled by membrane voltage alone, although varying external calcium may affect the size and kinetics of I_K (Lancaster and Pennefather 1987). Understanding the interplay of these currents is best accomplished via modeling.

The potassium currents fall into three functional groups. First, the large and fast currents, which can in principle rapidly change membrane potential, I_K and I_C. I_K closely resembles the delayed rectifier current of squid axon and amphibian node of

Ranvier (Frankenhaeuser 1963), showing a sigmoidal onset, very slow inactivation, and sensitivity to millimolar external tetraethylammonium (TEA). Unlike the node of Ranvier, however, I_K has little responsibility for the rapid repolarization of the cell to near resting potentials after depolarization during the spike. This role is served by I_C, which develops its maximum value within 3 msec during pulses that cause large calcium entry (e.g., to 0 mV). Repolarization to the resting potential quickly shuts off this conductance. This simple picture of I_C is consistent with its role in repolarizing the cell rapidly toward E_K and turning off immediately in readiness for another spike. I_K and I_C are described by the following equations:

$$I_K = \bar{g}_K m_K^2 h_K \cdot (V - E_K) \tag{4.7}$$

and

$$I_C = \bar{g}_C m_C \cdot (V - E_K), \tag{4.8}$$

where the activation variable for I_C, m_C, depends on both voltage and intracellular calcium concentration. We have chosen a particularly simple calcium dependency (see chapter appendix), in which binding to a single calcium binding site suffices to effect the transition from a closed to an open channel configuration. Although this is a gross oversimplification (see, for example, Moczydlowski and Latorre 1983 for more realistic, albeit more complex, transition schemes), it approximates the calcium dependency of I_C well enough for our purposes. Because the ratio of intracellular to extracellular potassium varies significantly during spiking activity in these cells, the Nernst potential for potassium, E_K, has to reflect this change and thus is continuously reevaluated throughout the simulation (see section 4.7).

If I_C was the only calcium-dependent current activated by a single spike, the spike afterhyperpolarization (AHP) would promptly return to rest with a time constant equal to the membrane time constant. However, healthy cells show a much slower decaying component of AHP, which reflects another calcium-dependent potassium conductance. It has been shown that this conductance is quite distinct from the fast calcium-dependent calcium conductance: it is small and is maximally activated by pulses of 1–2 msec duration, it deactivates very slowly following brief depolarizations, is not voltage-dependent, and is partially blocked by the bee venom toxin apamin.

I_{AHP} thus falls into the second functional group, small currents that can show prolonged activity at potentials between threshold and rest. The other member of this group is I_M, a small, slow, noninactivating potassium current almost completely inhibited by muscarinic receptor stimulation. Both I_M and I_{AHP} can best be thought of as subtracting from small suprathreshold applied current stimuli and can thus prevent spike firing. Both currents therefore contribute and control spike frequency adaptation but in different ways (see figure 4.8). The AHP (afterhyperpolarizing) and M (noninactivating muscarinic-sensitive) currents are modeled using the following equations:

$$I_{AHP} = \bar{g}_{AHP} m_{AHP}^2 \cdot (V - E_K), \tag{4.9}$$

where m_{AHP} is dependent solely on the internal calcium concentration, and

$$I_M = \bar{g}_M m_M \cdot (V - E_K). \tag{4.10}$$

The third type of outward current requires hyperpolarization for its activation. This is I_A, which in molluscan cells is largely responsible for generating good proportionality between firing rate and stimulus current even at very low firing frequencies (Connor and Stevens 1971). This current is present in bullfrog cells and can strongly affect responses to hyperpolarizing current injections, but does not appear to have a major physiological role because hyperpolarizing synaptic input is absent in bullfrog "B"-type sympathetic neurons. I_A is modeled using the following equation:

$$I_A = \bar{g}_A m_A h_A \cdot (V - E_K). \tag{4.11}$$

Finally, the passive voltage-independent leak current is described by

$$I_{leak} = g_{leak} \cdot (V - E_{leak}), \tag{4.12}$$

where both g_{leak} and E_{leak} are constants that partially reflect impalement damage.

4.5 Synaptic Input

Type "B" ganglion cells receive synaptic input from one (sometimes several) preganglionic axons arising from motoneurons in the spinal cord. Because bullfrog sympathetic ganglion cells possess no dendrites, all of the typical forty synaptic boutons made by the axon at the axon hillock and over the cell body (Sargent 1983) are located close to the recording electrode. These synapses release acetylcholine (ACh). Axonal stimulation of "B"-type cells in the bullfrog sympathetic ganglion results in a fast excitatory postsynaptic potential (EPSP), caused by ACh binding to nicotinic receptors, and a much slower EPSP, associated with a muscarinic receptor. The fast EPSP, usually triggering an action potential, is generated by a brief inward current lasting about 15–20 msec (Adams et al. 1986). We modeled this "conventional" synaptic input by a time-varying conductance, $g_{syn}(t)$, associated with a synaptic reversal potential, $E_{syn} = -10\,\text{mV}$:

$$I_{syn} = g_{syn}(t) \cdot (V - E_{syn}). \tag{4.13}$$

The time course of the synaptic induced conductance change is given by a standard alpha function that accurately describes the transient behavior of synaptic input for a number of preparations, such as nicotinic input to vertebrate sympathetic ganglion cells or the synaptic input mediated by the mossy fibers (Brown and Johnston 1983; Yamada, Koch, and Adams 1989; Williams and Johnston 1991):

$$g_{syn}(t) = \text{const} \cdot t \cdot e^{-t/t_{peak}}, \tag{4.14}$$

which reaches its maximum value, $\text{const} \cdot t_{peak} \cdot e^{-1}$, at $t = t_{peak}$. For $t_{peak} = 2.5\,\text{msec}$, the resulting time course of the inward current agrees well with experimental records (Kuba and Nishi 1979).

The second synaptic event begins rising 50–100 msec after the end of the fast EPSP, reaches a peak after 1–2 sec, and lasts about 1 min. The underlying inward current has a similarly slow time course. This small EPSP (several millivolts) is accompanied by a dramatic change in the response of the cell to long depolarizing test pulses. While normally the cells respond to extended suprathreshold current steps with only one or several action potentials, during the slow EPSP the cell responds much more vigorously to extended current stimuli. In other words, the cell has lost most of its adaptation to action potential firing. The underlying mechanism is the almost complete (90%) blockage of I_M current (indeed, the M in I_M stands for muscarine, the application of which leads to inhibition of this current) and the partial (less than 30%) blockage of I_{AHP}. We can reproduce this loss of adaptation by partially blocking these two currents. In hippocampal neurons, the role of I_{AHP} in controlling repetitive firing appears to be more striking than that of I_M. We did not explicitly model the time course of the slow EPSP (see, however, figure 4.8C).

4.6   Calcium Diffusion and Buffering

Any detailed description of neuronal excitability must take into account the behavior of certain ionic species inside and outside the cell, most notably calcium and potassium. The dynamics of free, intracellular calcium are of particular interest because the level of calcium controls activation of certain potassium conductances and is crucial for the initiation of phenomena believed to underlie synaptic plasticity. (For more details on calcium signaling in neurons, see Hille 1992; Ghosh and Greenberg 1995; and Clapham 1995; or the insightful review, Meyer and Stryer 1991; for further computational methods, such as pumping, more complex binding calcium-binding schemes, and so on, consult chapter 6, this volume.)

The most complex and sensitive aspects of this model are those involving the simulation of free intracellular calcium. Four processes that affect intracellular calcium concentration are modeled; (1) the entry of calcium into the cell via I_{Ca}; (2) the diffusion of calcium throughout the cell; (3) the action of intracellular calcium binding proteins (buffers); and (4) the efflux or uptake of calcium via the action of membrane-bound pumps. This list neglects the uptake and release of free intracellular calcium (which can be both voltage- and/or calcium-dependent) from intracellular organelles, in particular mitochondria and the endoplasmic reticulum. Because their relative contributions to the regulation of $[Ca^{2+}]$ are far from clear, we have neglected these processes in our model.

4.6.1 Calcium Current

The voltage-dependent calcium current discussed above, I_{Ca}, is the only direct liaison in our model between the membrane voltage and intracellular calcium. The change in intracellular calcium concentration due to the influx of calcium ions (carrying $2e$ charge per ion) is given by

$$\frac{\partial [Ca^{2+}]_n}{\partial t} = \frac{-I_{Ca}}{2FV_n},$$

(4.15)

where F is Faraday's constant ($9.649 \cdot 10^4$ coulombs per mole), $[Ca^{2+}]_n$ the calcium concentration in the shell just below the membrane, and V_n the volume of this shell. The value of the reversal potential for calcium is then determined by the Nernst equation

$$E_{Ca} = 12.5 \cdot \log \frac{[Ca^{2+}]_o}{[Ca^{2+}]_n},$$

(4.16)

where $[Ca^{2+}]_o$ is the constant extracellular calcium concentration ($4\,mM$).

4.6.2 Calcium Diffusion

Given the absence of dendrites and the near-spherical nature of the cell body, we solve the diffusion equation in spherical coordinates (for an introduction to the mathematics of diffusion, see Crank 1975). We neglect tangential components of diffusion, thus reducing the three-dimensional diffusion equation to a one-dimensional one. If $[Ca^{2+}]$ is the free calcium concentration and r is the distance from the center of the sphere, the diffusion equation (Crank 1975) can be written as

$$\frac{\partial r[\text{Ca}^{2+}]}{\partial t} = D \frac{\partial^2 r[\text{Ca}^{2+}]}{\partial r^2}, \tag{4.17}$$

where $D = 6 \cdot 10^{-6} \, \text{cm}^2 \text{sec}^{-1}$ is the diffusion constant of calcium in aqueous solution (Blaustein and Hodgkin 1969). Solving this equation requires discretization in both space and time. Because we are primarily interested in the action of calcium on the voltage trajectory of the cell, it is crucial to model the space just below the cellular membrane as accurately as possible because it is here that the binding of intracellular calcium to calcium-dependent potassium channels occurs. Our model assumes a relatively large, well-mixed central core compartment with a radius given by r_{core} (typically, $19 \, \mu\text{m}$), surrounded by a number of equally spaced shells (of thickness Δr; typically we use $n = 10$ shells with $\Delta r = 0.1 \, \mu\text{m}$). The last shell corresponds to the intracellular space just below the cell's membrane (see figure 4.4). This model bears some resemblance to an onion, with a large number of thin shells and a large core. Numerically, a more accurate model—but computationally more expensive, which is the reason it was not implemented in 1984, the year these computer simulations had their origin—would be to forgo the central, large core and to model the entire sphere using thin shells (as in Sala and Hernández-Cruz 1990).

Although we could use a simple, explicit forward Euler integration scheme that is stable and bound to converge for small enough Δx and Δt, to be able to exploit much larger values of Δt we use a mixed explicit-implicit scheme for solving eq. 4.17, first proposed by Crank and Nicolson (1947; for a more thorough discussion see chapter 6, this volume). Here the derivative of the function to be evaluated at t is replaced by half of the sum of the derivative at time t and the derivative at $t + \Delta t$. Eq. 4.17 then transforms into

$$\frac{r_i}{\Delta t}([\text{Ca}^{2+}]_{i,t+\Delta t} - [\text{Ca}^{2+}]_{i,t}) = \frac{D}{2\Delta r^2}((r_i + \Delta r)([\text{Ca}^{2+}]_{i+1,t+\Delta t} + [\text{Ca}^{2+}]_{i+1,t})$$

$$- 2r_i([\text{Ca}^{2+}]_{i,t+\Delta t} + [\text{Ca}^{2+}]_{i,t}) + (r_i - \Delta r)([\text{Ca}^{2+}]_{i-1,t+\Delta t}$$

$$+ [\text{Ca}^{2+}]_{i-1,t})), \tag{4.18}$$

where r_i is the radial distance between the center of the sphere and the midpoint of shell number $i, r_i = r_{core} + i\Delta r$. The central core corresponds to compartment $i = 0$, and the shell just below the membrane to $i = n$. The local truncation error of this scheme is quadratic in both Δr and Δt, while the straightforward, explicit Euler scheme is quadratic in Δr but only linear in Δt (Smith 1985).

To solve this partial differential equation, we need proper initial as well as boundary conditions. As initial conditions, we assume that intracellular free calcium is

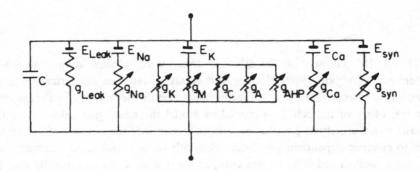

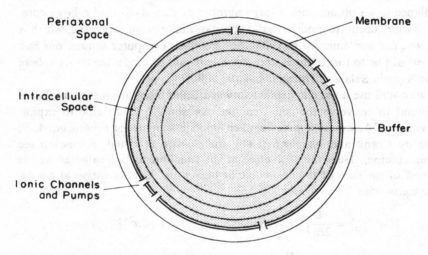

Figure 4.4
Basic structure of the model. The drawing at the top shows the equivalent electrical circuit of our model bullfrog sympathetic type "B" ganglion cell. The membrane conductances $g_{Na}, g_{Ca}, g_K, g_M, g_C, g_A, g_{AHP}$, and g_{syn} all depend on time. The first six conductances also depend on the membrane potential, and g_C and g_{AHP} depend on the calcium concentration $[Ca^{2+}]$ in the shell just below the membrane. The diagram at the bottom illustrates the underlying assumption for modeling the extracellular accumulation of potassium ions as well as the intracellular diffusion of calcium ions. Nondiffusible buffer is distributed inside the cell. Not drawn to scale.

distributed homogeneously across the cell with $[Ca^{2+}]_{initial} = 50$ nM. The boundary condition for the nth shell just below the membrane can be obtained by visualizing an imaginary $(n + 1)$th shell beyond the nth shell and then setting $[Ca^{2+}]_{n+1} = [Ca^{2+}]_n$. The boundary condition at the central core $(i = 0)$ is somewhat tricky because the geometry is nonhomogeneous. One way to obtain this condition is to assume another imaginary shell at $i = -1$ inside the central core, setting $[Ca^{2+}]_0 = [Ca^{2+}]_{-1}$, and recalling that the flux across the central sphere will be a factor of 3 greater than through any given shell. A different approach reverts back to Fick's first law underlying the diffusion equation (Crank 1975) for the innermost compartment. Both methods yield the same result in the limit as $\Delta r/r_{core} \to 0$. If the entire sphere is modeled in terms of thin shells, the boundary condition at the center will be slightly different (see Sala and Hernández-Cruz 1990).

4.6.3 Calcium Buffers

We now consider the change in calcium due to its binding to various calcium buffers, such as the ubiquitous protein calmodulin, with four separate calcium binding sites, or to paravalbumin, calbindin, calcineurin, and other buffers (McBurney and Neering 1987). Because we are interested only in the free calcium and not in the behavior of the buffer, however, our model assumes that calcium binds to a single binding site on a single buffer. Adapting the model to multiple binding sites is straightforward (Gamble and Koch 1987). We assume this buffer to be so large in terms of its molecular weight that diffusion of buffer molecules can be neglected at the time scale of interest to us. This will underestimate the true rate at which calcium diffuses (because there are now two sources of calcium mobility: direct diffusion of Ca^{2+} ions and diffusion of bound calcium riding "piggyback" along with the buffer; this effect can be surprisingly large; Sala and hernández-Cruz 1990).

The forward (f) and backward (b) rates of the binding reaction are 10^8 M^{-1}sec^{-1} and 100 sec^{-1} respectively ($K_D = b/f = 1$ μM). Furthermore, we assume that the total concentration of the buffer, that is, free buffer, $[B]_i$, plus calcium bound to the buffer, $[Ca\,B]_i$, is equal to $[B]_{i,Total}$, with $[B]_{i,Total} = 30$ μM in the shell just below the membrane $(i = n)$ and 3 μM everywhere else. These numbers are similar to those estimated for calcium buffering in the squid axon (Simon and Llinás 1985) and for calmodulin. We then have a second-order reaction (first-order in calcium) of the form

$$B + Ca^{2+} \underset{b}{\overset{f}{\rightleftharpoons}} Ca\,B. \tag{4.19}$$

It follows that

$$\frac{\partial[\text{Ca}^{2+}]}{\partial t} = \frac{\partial[B]}{\partial t} = b[\text{Ca } B] - f[\text{Ca}^{2+}][B], \tag{4.20}$$

as well as

$$[B] + [\text{Ca } B] = [B]_{Total}. \tag{4.21}$$

Because we are using a second-order numerical method to solve the diffusion equation, we are forced to use an equally accurate method to solve the buffering equation because any less accurate method, such as first-order Euler, will result in our losing any gain from the more accurate second-order scheme. Applying the Crank and Nicolson scheme (1947), we replace the differential in eq. 4.20 by the difference equation

$$\frac{[\text{Ca}^{2+}]_{i,t+\Delta t} - [\text{Ca}^{2+}]_{i,t}}{\Delta t} = b \cdot [B]_{i,Total} - \frac{b}{2}([B]_{i,t+\Delta t} + [B]_{i,t})$$

$$-\frac{f}{2}([B]_{i,t+\Delta t}[\text{Ca}^{2+}]_{i,t+\Delta t} + [B]_{i,t}[\text{Ca}^{2+}]_{i,t}). \tag{4.22}$$

Equation 4.22 is quadratic, that is, it contains terms in both buffer and calcium concentration. This nonlinearity is rather difficult to solve in a straightforward manner but can be circumvented by exploiting a slightly different mixed explicit-implicit integration scheme:

$$\frac{[\text{Ca}^{2+}]_{i,t+\Delta t} - [\text{Ca}^{2+}]_{i,t}}{\Delta t} = b \cdot [B]_{i,Total} - \frac{b}{2}([B]_{i,t+\Delta t} + [B]_{i,t})$$

$$-\frac{f}{2}([B]_{i,t+\Delta t}[\text{Ca}^{2+}]_{i,t} + [B]_{i,t}[\text{Ca}^{2+}]_{i,t+\Delta t}). \tag{4.23}$$

Using a Taylor expansion around i, t, one can show that eqs. 4.22 and 4.23 both have a local truncation error of the order of $(\Delta t)^2$, commensurate with the order of the numerical scheme we use to estimate the contribution of diffusion toward calcium dynamics. The equation for updating the buffer concentration $[B]$ is analogous to eq. 4.23:

$$\frac{[B]_{i,t+\Delta t} - [B]_{i,t}}{\Delta t} = b \cdot [B]_{i,Total} - \frac{b}{2}([B]_{i,t+\Delta t} + [B]_{i,t})$$

$$-\frac{f}{2}([B]_{i,t+\Delta t}[\text{Ca}^{2+}]_{i,t} + [B]_{i,t}[\text{Ca}^{2+}]_{i,t+\Delta t}). \tag{4.24}$$

We thus have $2n + 2$ linear equations for the entire sphere. As initial conditions for $[B]$, we compute the stationary value of eq. 4.24 for $[Ca^{2+}]_{initial} = 50\,nM$.

4.6.4 Calcium Pumps

Although the calcium-buffering system discussed above reduces the amount of free intracellular calcium, the remaining calcium ions must ultimately be removed from the cell if calcium homeostasis is to be maintained. Two major transport systems have been identified (DiPolo and Beauge 1983; McBurney and Neering 1987): a sodium-dependent Ca^{2+} efflux, in which the energy required for the extrusion of calcium ions is derived from the inward movement of Na^+ ions down their electrochemical gradient, and a calcium extrusion system that works independently of Na^+ and requires ATP as an energy source. The former extrusion system is a high-capacity but low-affinity system (half activated at $1\text{–}10\,\mu M$), while the ATP-driven pathway is active at lower values of $[Ca^{2+}]$ ($K_m = 0.2\,\mu M$) but has a smaller capacity. We neglect the Na^+-Ca^{2+} exchange system in our model and describe the ATP-driven pump by a first-order equation, with a voltage-dependent time constant so as to mimic the voltage trajectory of recovery from inactivation:

$$\frac{d[Ca^{2+}]}{dt} = \frac{[Ca^{2+}]_{equil} - [Ca^{2+}]_n}{\tau_{pump}(V)}, \tag{4.25}$$

where $[Ca^{2+}]_{equil}$ is the equilibrium concentration of the pump (50 nM), $[Ca^{2+}]_n$ the concentration of calcium in the shell just below the membrane, and $\tau_{pump}(V) = 17.7e^{(V/35)}$ msec the pump's time constant. The appropriate difference equation is

$$\frac{[Ca^{2+}]_{n,t+\Delta t} - [Ca^{2+}]_{n,t}}{\Delta t} = \frac{[Ca^{2+}]_{equil}}{\tau_{pump}(V)} - \frac{[Ca^{2+}]_{n,t+\Delta t} + [Ca^{2+}]_{n,t}}{2\tau_{pump}(V)}. \tag{4.26}$$

Note that these membrane-bound pump proteins have to move Ca^{2+} against an extremely large calcium gradient (five orders of magnitude).

4.7 Potassium Accumulation

A number of phenomena such as the magnitude of the repolarization phase of a spike cannot be properly understood without simulating the reduction of the potassium battery, E_K, due to extracellular accumulation of potassium. Potassium accumulation is handled by assuming the existence of a well-mixed shell (pericellular space) surrounding the neuron that corresponds to the anatomical space between the nerve cell membrane and the glial sheath (Frankenhaeuser and Hodgkin 1956). The dynamics of extracellular potassium $[K^+]_o$ are governed by the influx of potassium from inside the cell via the five potassium currents ($I_{K\,total}$) and the efflux of potassium by glial cell uptake as well as outward diffusion into the surrounding tissue. Faraday's law is used to convert the current due to the K^+ ions into a concentration change. The shell is assumed to lose its potassium load with a time constant $\tau_{K-diff} = 7\,\text{msec}$ and to be about 70 nm thick, based on electrophysiological and anatomical estimates (Taxi 1976; Lancaster and Pennefather 1987). Thus

$$\frac{d[K^+]_o}{dt} = \frac{I_{K\,total}}{V_{peri}F} - \frac{([K^+]_o - [K^+]_{rest})}{\tau_{K-diff}}, \tag{4.27}$$

where F is Faraday's constant ($9.649 \cdot 10^4$ coulomb per mole), V_{peri} is the pericellular volume, and $[K^+]_{rest}$ is the resting extracellular potassium concentration (2.5 mM). The value of the potassium reversal battery is given by the Nernst equation

$$E_K = 25 \cdot \log\frac{[K^+]_o}{[K^+]_i}, \tag{4.28}$$

where $[K^+]_i$ is the intracellular potassium concentration, which is held constant at 140 mM throughout the simulation because the relative size of the concentration change is too small to be significant. Only the small volume of the periaxonal space coupled with the much lower extracellular concentration requires us to take extracellular potassium accumulation into account.

4.8 Integration

We are now faced with the formidable task of integrating all seven conductances, described by eleven different rate constants, with the passive properties of the cell and the varying concentrations of calcium, calcium buffer, and potassium. Conceptually, the system can be dissected into two different subsystems: the seven membrane-bound ionic conductances (and potassium accumulation) governed mainly by voltage, V, and the calcium system throughout the cell, which includes calcium diffusion, buffering, and extrusion. The calcium subsystem is linked to the voltage subsystem via the calcium current, I_{Ca}, while linkage in the reverse direction is effected via the calcium-dependent currents, I_{Ca}, I_C, and I_{AHP}, and, to a much lesser extent, via the calcium battery, E_{Ca}. Solving this system requires the simultaneous solution of a set of highly nonlinear ordinary and partial differential equations in fifteen dimensions!

We simplify this problem by updating the two subsystems in series, that is, explicitly, rather than using an implicit simultaneous update. Specifically, when advancing the voltage by one time step to $V(t + \Delta t)$, we use the value of the calcium concentration at t. Subsequent to this step, we compute the new distribution of calcium throughout the cell at $t + \Delta t$ as an explicit function of $V(t + \Delta t)$. As rationale for this approximation, we note that the concentration of calcium and buffer changes on a slower time scale than the membrane conductances. Over the range of Δt values, we use (10–100 μsec), our approximation appears to be a good one. We will now discuss the two algorithms required to update both subsystems.

4.8.1 Voltage Update

We use the simplest possible second-order predictor-corrector scheme to solve both for the membrane potential and for the rate constants. For example, voltage is predicted using an explicit first-order Euler scheme,

$$V(t + \Delta t) = V(t) + \Delta t \frac{dV(t)}{dt}, \tag{4.29}$$

and corrected using the simplest possible second-order mixed explicit-implicit integration method to solve for both the membrane potential and the rate constants,

$$V(t + \Delta t) = V(t) + \frac{\Delta t}{2} \left(\frac{dV(t + \Delta t)}{dt} + \frac{dV(t)}{dt} \right). \tag{4.30}$$

These two voltage values are compared against each other. If they fall within a predetermined convergence criterion (here $7 \cdot 10^{-5}$ mV), the new voltage value is accepted. Otherwise, the new value is used to recompute a better approximation of voltage until the convergence criterion is satisfied. Within the range of Δt chosen, the algorithm converges after at most two such iterations. The rate constants are updated in a similar fashion using this mixed second-order method. The three calcium-dependent rate constants (inactivation of I_{Ca} and activation of both I_C and I_{AHP}) use the calcium concentration in the shell, $[Ca^{2+}]_n$, at time t. All the details are described by Cooley and Dodge (1966), who used the same scheme to numerically integrate the Hodgkin and Huxley equations in an unmyelinated axon. The potassium concentration, $[K^+]_o$, and battery, E_K, are updated using a straightforward first-order Euler scheme.

4.8.2   Calcium Update

The calcium update routine must simultaneously solve for calcium diffusion, buffering, pumping, and the influx of calcium current. This can simply be achieved by combining eqs. 4.15, 4.18, 4.23, and 4.26 into a single set of $n + 1$ simultaneous equations, based on the mixed explicit-implicit Crank and Nicolson method. Although, in principle, we must also evaluate the calcium influx due to the calcium current in a similar fashion, that is, in the form of $d[Ca^{2+}]_n/dt = -(I_{Ca}(t + \Delta t) + I_{Ca}(t))/(4FV_n)$, to our knowledge no technique is currently available to solve this implicit nonlinear equation efficiently. As stated above, we decouple the voltage and calcium systems by the use of eq 4.23. For the outermost shell, n, we have

$$\frac{1}{\Delta t}([Ca^{2+}]_{n,t+\Delta t} - [Ca^{2+}]_{n,t}) = \frac{D(r_n - \Delta r)}{2r_n\Delta r^2}([Ca^{2+}]_{n-1,t+\Delta t} + [Ca^{2+}]_{n-1,t}$$

$$- [Ca^{2+}]_{n,t+\Delta t} + [Ca^{2+}]_{n,t}) - \frac{I_{Ca}}{2FV_n}$$

$$+ b[B]_{i,total} - \frac{b}{2}([B]_{n,t+\Delta t} + [B]_{n,t})$$

$$- \frac{f}{2}([B]_{n,t+\Delta t}[Ca^{2+}]_{n,t} + [B]_{n,t}[Ca^{2+}]_{n,t+\Delta t})$$

$$+ \frac{[Ca^{2+}]_{equil}}{\tau_{pump}(V)} - \frac{[Ca^{2+}]_{n,t+\Delta t} + [Ca^{2+}]_{n,t}}{2\tau_{pump}(V)}. \tag{4.31}$$

The equation describing calcium concentration changes for the shells between the core and the membrane is

$$\frac{1}{\Delta t}([Ca^{2+}]_{i,t+\Delta t} - [Ca^{2+}]_{i,t}) = \frac{D}{2r_i\Delta r^2}((r_i + \Delta r)([Ca^{2+}]_{i+1,t+\Delta t} + [Ca^{2+}]_{i+1,t})$$

$$- 2r_i([Ca^{2+}]_{i,t+\Delta t} + [Ca^{2+}]_{i,t})$$

$$+ (r_i - \Delta r)([Ca^{2+}]_{i-1,t+\Delta t} + [Ca^{2+}]_{i-1,t}))$$

$$+ b[B]_{i,total} - \frac{b}{2}([B]_{i,t+\Delta t} + [B]_{i,t})$$

$$- \frac{f}{2}([B]_{i,t+\Delta t}[Ca^{2+}]_{i,t} + [B]_{i,t}[Ca^{2+}]_{i,t+\Delta t}). \tag{4.32}$$

The equation describing the calcium concentration change at the core is

$$\frac{1}{\Delta t}([Ca^{2+}]_{0,t+\Delta t} - [Ca^{2+}]_{0,t}) = \frac{3D}{2r^2_{core}}([Ca^{2+}]_{1,t+\Delta t} + [Ca^{2+}]_{1,t}$$

$$- [Ca^{2+}]_{0,t+\Delta t} + [Ca^{2+}]_{0,t}) + b[B]_{i,total}$$

$$- \frac{b}{2}([B]_{0,t+\Delta t} + [B]_{0,t})$$

$$- \frac{f}{2}([B]_{0,t+\Delta t}[Ca^{2+}]_{0,t} + [B]_{0,t}[Ca^{2+}]_{0,t+\Delta t}). \qquad (4.33)$$

The equation describing buffer concentration change from step to step is identical for all shells (see eq. 4.24):

$$\frac{[B]_{i,t+\Delta t} - [B]_{i,t}}{\Delta t} = b \cdot [B]_{i,Total} - \frac{b}{2}([B]_{i,t+\Delta t} + [B]_{i,t})$$

$$- \frac{f}{2}([B]_{i,t+\Delta t}[Ca^{2+}]_{i,t} + [B]_{i,t}[Ca^{2+}]_{i,t+\Delta t}). \qquad (4.34)$$

With the appropriate boundary conditions for $i = n$ and $i = 0$, we finally arrive at a set of $2n + 2$ linear equations in $2n + 2$ unknowns with constant coefficients. The simplest technique to solve this system is to substitute $[B]_{i,t+\Delta}$ (evaluated from eq. 4.34 as a function of $[B]_{i,t}$, $[Ca^{2+}]_{i,t+\Delta t}$, and $[Ca^{2+}]_{i,t}$) into eqs. 4.31–4.33, and to invert the resulting tridiagonal $n + 1$ by $n + 1$ matrix to arrive at the new value of $[Ca^{2+}]_i$ at time Δt. Efficient recursive algorithms are available for this purpose (e.g., Cooley and Dodge 1966; Press et al. 1992).

4.8.3 Variable Time Step

Until now, we have assumed that the time step Δt used to integrate the differential equations is fixed. During any particular simulation run, however, the dynamics of the system may first change very rapidly but later settle down to a more quiescent course (see the discussion on "stiffness" in the appendix to chapter 14). A typical example of this occurs during the application of long-lasting current stimuli. If the stimulus is above threshold, an action potential occurs, requiring a small value of Δt, due to the rapid change in the membrane currents, in particular I_{Na}, I_{Ca}, and I_C, and the large and rapid influx of calcium. A healthy cell will now show spike frequency adaptation (see figure 4.8A) and will fail to respond to the stimulus with any additional spikes. Because little change occurs during the adapted state, a large value of Δt can be used, substantially reducing the number of iterations required. We thus include a variable time step routine outside the main update loop (described above), which, given a time step Δt, advances the entire system (voltage and calcium) from time t to time $t + 2\Delta t$. Briefly, we advance the system in two steps from t to $t + \Delta t + \Delta t$ by computing the intermediate state at time $t + \Delta t$. Voltage and the value of calcium in the shell below the membrane are then compared against the same variables computed when advancing the system in a single step (using as the step size $2\Delta t$) from t to $t + 2\Delta t$. If the difference is below a given fixed lower threshold, the time step is increased and the system continues at time $t + 2\Delta t$. If the difference is above a given upper threshold, the time step is reduced and the system is reset to its state at time t. If the difference falls between the two thresholds, the system continues with its present value of Δt.

The speedup due to this simple procedure can be substantial, in the case of a simple Hodgkin and Huxley–like piece of squid membrane between one and two orders of magnitude. The increase in speed for partial differential equations is less noticeable because the system has to be evaluated at every node for every step. Moreover, in the case of the bullfrog soma with an added axon (Yamada, Koch, and Adams 1988), action potentials propagate from the cell body out into the axon. The system cannot therefore take advantage of the relatively slow rate of change at the soma following the action potential because compartments along the axon will be subject to large changes in potential and will thus require a small value of Δt.

To summarize, we decouple the system into two components, updating each one of the subsystems independently using a mixed explicit-implicit integration scheme with a local truncation error of the order of $(\Delta t)^2$ in time and $(\Delta r)^2$ in space. Superimposed onto these two algorithms is a routine determining the optimal value of Δt.

4.9 Results

Although the model contains numerous assumptions, it accurately predicts the observed voltage clamp responses of bullfrog sympathetic "B" cells. This accuracy is not surprising because the model is largely derived from experimental voltage clamp data (of the type shown in figure 4.2). It is now of great interest to see how successfully the model predicts independent current clamp data under various conditions. Two particular set of conditions are examined here: (1) single spikes elicited by large but very short current pulses; and (2) spike trains elicited by long-lasting but rather small current pulses. In each case we examined the effects of various pharmacological manipulations for which we have experimental data (for instance, the block of I_{Ca} via cadmium or the block of I_{AHP} via curare or apamin). The basic response of the standard model (fully described in the chapter appendix) is shown in the panoramas of figures 4.5 and 4.6.

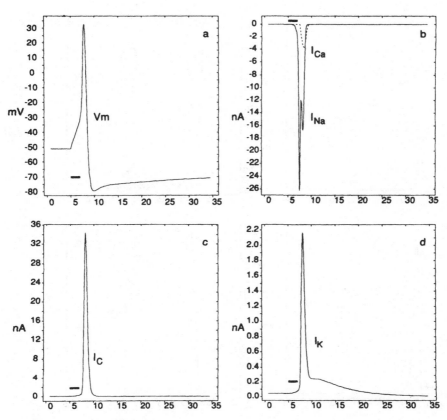

Figure 4.5
Response of quiescent system (at −51.26 mV for our standard parameters) to a brief (2 msec) current pulse of 1.75 nA amplitude applied at 5 msec (indicated in this and following figure by a black bar). This panorama depicts the fast components of the cell's response. The voltage trajectory is shown in panel a. Notice the fast and slow components of the afterhyperpolarization following the action potential. Panel b illustrates the two inward currents, I_{Na} and I_{Ca}. Only 9% of the incoming charge is carried by the Ca^{2+} ions. Panel c shows the fast, calcium-dependent potassium current I_C, and panel d, the delayed-rectified potassium current I_K. Because I_C is much larger than I_K, it is primarily responsible for recharging the cell's membrane potential back to rest.

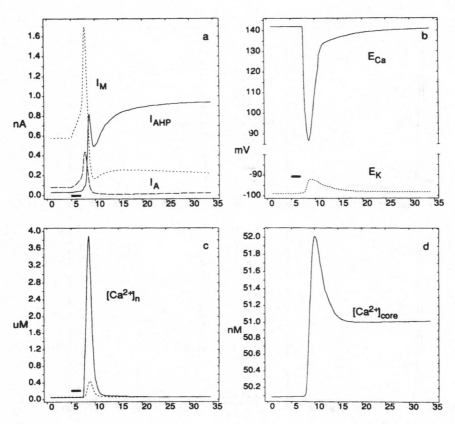

Figure 4.6
Response of system following same stimulus as in figure 4.5. The three small potassium currents, $I_A, I_M,$ and I_{AHP}, are plotted in panel a. I_{AHP} and, to a lesser extent I_M, are responsible for the slow phase of the AHP following action potentials (figure 4.5a). The change in the Nernst potential for Ca^{2+} and K^+ is illustrated in panel b. The rapid and slow components of increase in E_{Ca} reflect free intracellular calcium dynamics in the thin ($\Delta r = 0.1\,\mu m$) shell just below the membrane, $[Ca^{2+}]_n$ shown in panel c. Activation of I_{Ca} leads to a rapid influx of Ca^{2+}, which quickly becomes bound to the buffer. The slow decay results from calcium loss via the pump as well as diffusion toward the core of the cell. $[Ca^{2+}]$ for the tenth shell below the membrane is also illustrated in this diagram. The calcium concentration in the core ($19\,\mu m$) is shown in panel d.

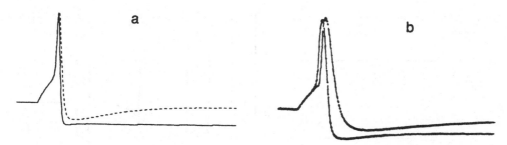

Figure 4.7
Effect of blocking calcium entry on simulated and observed action potentials. In panel a, computed action potentials are superimposed with normal (116 nS) and 5% normal value (5.8 nS) of the maximal calcium conductance, $\bar{g}_{Ca}$, during manual clamp to -60 mV. In panel b, experimental data recorded before and after application of cadmium to block I_{Ca} show a very similar time course. The peak depolarization is 98 mV. Both traces are 50 msec long.

The computed action potential, the individual ionic currents, the Nernst reversal potential for Ca^{2+} and K^+, and intracellular calcium all are displayed here. The somatic action potential in this vertebrate cell shares a number of similarities with the axonal action potential of the squid (an invertebrate). Threshold, afterhyperpolarization, and repolarization back to the resting potential are all evident in figure 4.5a. One noticeable difference to the shape of a Hodgkin and Huxley action potential is the second, long-lasting phase of the afterhyperpolarization, mediated by the calcium-activated voltage-independent potassium conductance I_{AHP}. Moreover, the peak of the fast, transient, calcium-dependent potassium current, I_C, is about ten times larger than the peak of the delayed rectifier current, I_K, and thus is largely responsible for repolarizing the potential following the excursion of the membrane potential to 0 mV and beyond. Thus the I_K of the squid giant axon is replaced by I_C in the bullfrog sympathetic ganglion.

The role of calcium influx, and therefore of I_{Ca}, in shaping the action potential is demonstrated in figure 4.7. Here the standard computed action potential elicited by a brief current pulse is superimposed onto the action potential elicited after reducing the membrane calcium conductance to 5% of its normal value. The rate of repolarization is reduced; the peak afterhyperpolarization occurs later, is smaller, and decays much more rapidly under these circumstances than in control conditions (because I_{AHP} is not being activated). Despite its being almost zero under these conditions, I_C has a significant effect on the rapid spike repolarization. This is because even minor spike broadening, due to slower repolarization, can recruit substantial increases in potassium current. The same phenomenon is seen in a real cell (figure 4.7b) exposed to the calcium current blocker cadmium.

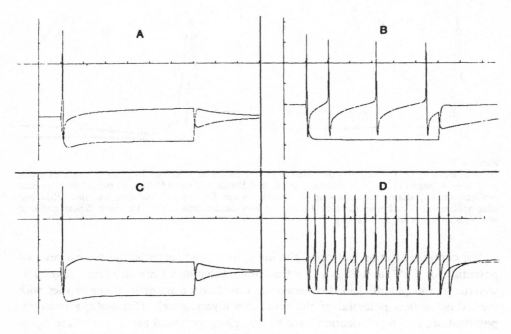

Figure 4.8
Roles of two potassium currents in controlling cellular adaptation. The response of our model cell during long-lasting (300 msec) injections of depolarizing (1.25 nA) and hyperpolarizing (−1.25 nA) current steps is shown. Panel A shows the response of the cell during its usual adapted state. In the next two panels, either I_M (panel B) or I_{AHP} (panel C) is blocked. Panel D shows that adaptation is practically absent if both of these currents are blocked simultaneously. Each horizontal tick corresponds 50 msec and each vertical 20 mV.

Figure 4.8 illustrates the predicted effects on action potential firing adaptation during various pharmacological manipulations. Figure 4.8A shows the control, highly adapting response in the absence of any synaptic or pharmacological blockers. Although a suprathreshold input (1.25 nA) is present for 300 msec, only a single spike is triggered. After blocking I_M, adaptation is reduced but still obvious (figure 4.8B). Blocking I_{AHP} by itself does not suppress adaptation but reveals the after-depolarization following the spike (figure 4.8C). Simultaneous blocking both I_M and I_{AHP} eliminates almost all of the adaptation, and the model cell responds as long as a suprathreshold stimulus is present (figure 4.8D). The synergistic role of these two currents in procuring efficient adaptation is also seen experimentally. This prominent spike frequency adaptation is characteristic of bullfrog sympathetic ganglion cells

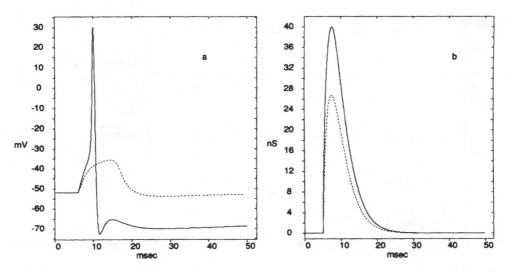

Figure 4.9
Modeling synaptic input. In panel a, the calculated ganglion cell response to a conductance increase is
shown to have the same time course as the fast nicotinic excitatory postsynapatic current (EPSC) observed
experimentally (Kuba and Nishi 1979). The two superimposed voltage records were obtained with two
different-sized conductance changes ($g_{peak} = 40\,nS$ and $27\,nS$), shown in panel b.

and, indeed, of a large class of vertebrate neurons in the CNS (Connors and Gutnick
1990). As pointed out in section 4.5, both currents are reduced under natural conditions by the release of acetylcholine from presynaptic terminals and their subsequent binding to muscarinc receptors on the sympathetic ganglion cell.

We have modeled nicotinic synaptic transmission in these cells by incorporating a
time-dependent conductance change into our model (figure 4.9). An action potential
can be initiated if the peak synaptic conductance change is 28 nS or larger. During a
train of synaptic inputs, only the first synaptic input triggers an action potential in
normal, adapted cells because this action potential recruits sufficient I_M and I_{AHP} to
induce adaptation. Following blockage of both of these currents, each synaptic input
can elicit an action potential.

Figure 4.10 shows the associated relationship between the frequency of the action
potentials generated and the injected current for these four different conditions. To
a first approximation, when blocking I_{AHP}, the current threshold for eliciting action
potentials remains constant (at about 0.63 nA), while the slope increases by a factor
of 2 (from 2.4 spikes to 4.7 spikes per nanoampere). Blocking only I_M leaves the
slope relatively unchanged while reducing the current threshold to 5% of its original

spikes

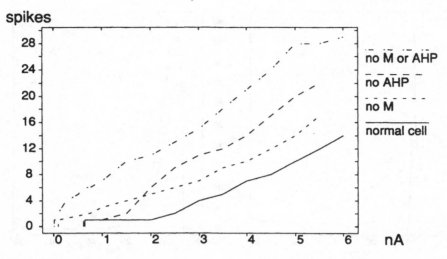

Figure 4.10
Firing behavior versus injected current. The number of calculated spikes during 200 msec current steps of variable amplitude in the adapted cell, after the complete simulated blockage of either I_{AHP} or of I_M, and after the simultaneous blockage of both I_{AHP} and I_M. Blocking I_{AHP} does not appreciably change the current firing threshold but increases the slope of the f-I curve, while blockage of I_M reduces the spiking threshold.

value, that is, to 0.03 nA. Blocking both conductances both lowers the threshold and increases the slope, leading to the dramatic removal of spike adaptation observed experimentally.

4.10   Discussion

The function of the large transient ionic currents, I_{Na}, I_{Ca}, I_C, and I_K, in the daily chores of our ganglion cell are obvious: the sodium current generates and carries the action potential, while the remaining three large currents ultimately subserve the patterning of the action potential discharge. In this view, the principal role of the calcium current, I_{Ca}, is to activate the calcium-dependent potassium currents–leading to a fast repolarization and spike frequency adaptation. Moreover, I_{Ca} provides the crucial link—via influx of calcium ions—between electrical activity and the initiation of metabolic events. In contrast, the role of I_{Ca} in depolarizing the cell body during the action potential is small. Oversimplifying, one may view the role of the small but persistent currents, I_M and I_{AHP}, as controlling the transmission of information through the cells by increasing the excitability of the cell (I_{AHP}) or reducing the spiking threshold (I_M). Because these currents can be blocked via synaptically released substances, they could be the neuronal substratum for neuronal operations such as sensory adaptation or routing messages selectively from a single neuron to different postsynaptic targets (Koch and Poggio 1987).

The seven currents discussed here are of relevance far beyond the bullfrog: very similar currents have been characterized in a host of other preparations, ranging from mollusc neurons to human neocortical neurons (for a review, see Llinás 1988). Indeed, CA1 and CA3 pyramidal cells express all seven currents found in bullfrog cells, as well as a sustained sodium current, a slow, noninactivating calcium current, and a small, mixed sodium-and-potassium current, I_Q, that is activated when the cell is hyperpolarized. The importance of individual currents may vary, though, from cell type to cell type. For example, blocking I_{AHP} in hippocampal pyramidal cells leads to a much more dramatic reduction in spike frequency adaptation than in bullfrog sympathetic cells (Madison and Nicoll 1984; Lancaster and Adams 1986). Nevertheless, the description of these currents in terms of activation and inactivation variables appears to remain relatively invariant across species and cell types (see chapter 5, this volume).

In the last three decades we have come to understand the electrical behavior and the integrative function of both nonmyelinated and myelinated axon, the cell body with its numerous currents and passive dendrites in the presence of massive synaptic inputs (see chapters 3 and 5, this volume). The daunting challenge facing us now is to extend this understanding to include the highly nonlinear electrical properties of dendrites (see chapter 5, this volume). The principal obstacle in this endeavor is that most neurons in the central nervous system possess a highly elaborate dendritic tree. Thus, events in the dendritic tree are electrically distant from the recording point, usually in the cell body. This lack of space clamp makes any quantitative evaluation of voltage-dependent currents exceedingly difficult (Rall and Segev 1985). It seems to us that only the judicious application of novel experimental techniques, combined with computer simulations such as described in this book, will enable us to understand the entire neuron as a computational entity.

Appendix: Modeling Bullfrog Sympathetic Ganglion Cells

Principal Equation

The principal equation describing the change in intracellular potential at the soma (given in absolute terms by $V(t)$) is

$$C_N \frac{d}{dt} V + I_{Input} + I_{Na} + I_{Ca} + I_k + I_M + I_A + I_C + I_{AHP} + I_{leak} + I_{syn} = 0$$

In the following pages, we will describe in detail the kinetics, voltage and calcium dependencies of these currents, in terms of Hodgkin and Huxley–like rate constants with first-order kinetics (all rate constants are normalized to 22° Celsius).

All variables have the following units:

Voltage	mV
Current	nA
Time	msec
Concentration	millimols per liter (mM)
Conductance	μS
Resistance	MΩ
Capacitance	nF
Volume	l

Fast Sodium Current

$$I_{Na} = \bar{g}_{Na} m^2 h (V - E_{Na}).$$

The rate constants are given by Frankenhaeuser and Huxley (1964), relative to the resting potential, which we set to $-60\,\text{mV}$. The activation and inactivation variables, m and h, are further shifted to more positive potentials by $5\,\text{mV}$ and $15\,\text{mV}$, respectively. The kinetics of both m and h are slowed down by a factor of 2. Although some evidence for a secondary inactivation exists, it did not lead to any observable effect in our model. $\bar{g}_{Na} = 2\,\mu\text{S}$. This implies a density of about $40\,\text{mScm}^2$. $E_{Na} = 50\,\text{mV}$. The midpoint for m_∞ is $-20.7\,\text{mV}$, for m_∞^2, $-10.8\,\text{mV}$, and for h_∞, $-37.6\,\text{mV}$.

Activation variable:

$$\frac{dm}{dt} = \frac{m_\infty - m}{\tau_m}$$

$$\tau_m = \frac{2}{\alpha_m + \beta_m}$$

$$m_\infty = \frac{\alpha_m}{\alpha_m + \beta_m}.$$

The forward and backward rate constants are given by

$$\alpha_m = \frac{0.36(V + 33)}{1.0 - e^{-(V+33)/3}} \quad \text{and} \quad \beta_m = \frac{-0.4(V + 42)}{1.0 - e^{+(V+42)/20}}.$$

Inactivation variable:

$$\frac{dh}{dt} = \frac{h_\infty - h}{\tau_h}$$

$$\tau_h = \frac{2}{\alpha_h + \beta_h}$$

$$h_\infty = \frac{\alpha_h}{\alpha_h + \beta_h}.$$

The forward and backward rate constants are given by

$$\alpha_h = \frac{-0.1(V + 55)}{1 - e^{(V+55)/6}} \quad \text{and} \quad \beta_h = \frac{4.5}{1 + e^{-V/10}}.$$

Fast Calcium Current

$$I_{Ca} = \bar{g}_{Ca}mh(V - E_{Ca}),$$

where $\bar{g}_{Ca} = 0.116\,\mu S$.

We felt it necessary to include a threshold for activation of this current at $-32\,mV$. In other words, $m_\infty = 0$ if $V < -32\,mV$. Inactivation does not depend on the membrane potential but on $[Ca^{2+}]_i$. The reversal potential E_{Ca} is variable (natural log assumed) with

$$E_{Ca} = 12.5 \cdot \log \frac{[Ca^{2+}]_o}{[Ca^{2+}]_i},$$

where $[Ca^{2+}]_o$, the fixed extracellular concentration of Ca^{2+}, is equal to $4\,mM$, and $[Ca^{2+}]_i$ is the concentration of Ca^{2+} in the shell just below the membrane (see section 4.6). Initially, we have $E_{Ca} = 141.2\,mV$. The midpoint for m_∞ is $3\,mV$ and for h_∞ is $0.01\,mM$.

Activation variable:

$$\frac{dm}{dt} = \frac{m_\infty - m}{\tau_m}$$

$$\tau_m = \frac{7.8}{e^{+(V+6)/16} + e^{-(V+6)/16}}$$

$$m_\infty = \frac{1}{1 + e^{-(V-3)/8}}.$$

Inactivation variable:

$$h = \frac{K}{K + [Ca^{2+}]_i},$$

where $K = 0.01\,mM$.

Transient, Outward Potassium Current

$$I_A = \bar{g}_A mh(V - E_K),$$

where $\bar{g}_A = 0.120\,\mu S$, and

$$E_K = 25.0 \cdot \log \frac{[K^+]_o}{[K^+]_i},$$

where $[K^+]_o$ is the variable extracellular and $[K^+]_i$ is the constant intracellular potassium concentration, equal to $140\,mM$. The midpoint for m_∞ is $-42\,mV$ and for h_∞, $-110\,mV$.

Activation variable:

$$\frac{dm}{dt} = \frac{m_\infty - m}{\tau_m}$$

$$\tau_m = 1.38$$

$$m_\infty = \frac{1}{1 + e^{-(V+42)/13}} \, .$$

Inactivation variable:

$$\frac{dh}{dt} = \frac{h_\infty - h}{\tau_h}$$

$$\tau_h = 50 \quad \text{if} \quad V < -80 \, \text{mV; else 150}$$

$$h_\infty = \frac{1}{1 + e^{+(V+110)/18}} \, .$$

Two of our currents, I_A and I_K, have time constants that are modeled using either a constant value or step functions. These parameters were modeled in this fashion because experimental data in these cases was sketchy; constant value functions lay within the variance of the data.

Noninactivating Muscarinic Potassium Current

$$I_M = \bar{g}_M m (V - E_K),$$

where $\bar{g}_M = 0.084 \, \mu S$. The midpoint for m_∞ is $-35 \, \text{mV}$.
    Activation variable:

$$\frac{dm}{dt} = \frac{m_\infty - m}{\tau_m}$$

$$\tau_m = \frac{1{,}000}{3.3(e^{+(V+35)/40} + e^{-(V+35)/20})}$$

$$m_\infty = \frac{1}{1 + e^{-(V+35)/10}}$$

Delayed, Rectifying Potassium Current

$$I_K = \bar{g}_K m^2 h (V - E_K),$$

where $\bar{g}_K = 1.17 \, \mu S$, and

$$E_K = 25 \cdot \log \frac{[K^+]_o}{[K^+]_i} \, .$$

The midpoint for m_∞ is $-12.1 \, \text{mV}$; for m_∞^2, $-1.6 \, \text{mV}$; and for h_∞, $-25 \, \text{mV}$.
    Activation variable:

$$\frac{dm}{dt} = \frac{m_\infty - m}{\tau_m}$$

$$\tau_m = \frac{1}{\alpha_m(V) + \beta_m(V)}$$

$$m_\infty = \frac{\alpha(V - 20)}{\alpha_m(V - 20) + \beta_m(V - 20)}.$$

The forward and backward rate constants are given by

$$\alpha_m(V) = \frac{-0.0047(V + 12)}{e^{-(V+12)/12} - 1} \quad \text{and} \quad \beta_m(V) = e^{-(V+147)/30}.$$

Inactivation variable:

$$\frac{dh}{dt} = \frac{h_\infty - h}{\tau_h}$$

$$\tau_h = 6{,}000 \quad \text{if} \quad V < -25\,\text{mV; else } 50$$

$$h_\infty = \frac{1}{1 + e^{+(V+25)/4}}.$$

Noninactivating Calcium-Dependent Potassium Current

$$I_C = \bar{g}_C m(V - E_K),$$

where $\bar{g}_c = 1.2\,\mu\text{S}$.
Calcium-dependent activation variable:

$$\frac{dm}{dt} = \frac{m_\infty - m}{\tau_m}$$

$$\tau_m = \frac{1}{f(V, \text{Ca}) + b(V)}$$

$$m_\infty = \frac{f(V, \text{Ca})}{f(V, \text{Ca}) + b(V)}$$

The forward and backward rated constants are given by

$$f(V, \text{Ca}) = 250[\text{Ca}^{2+}]_i e^{+V/24} \quad \text{and} \quad b(V) = 0.1 e^{-V/24}.$$

Voltage-Independent, Calcium-Dependent Potassium Current

$$I_{AHP} = \bar{g}_{AHP} m^2(V - E_K),$$

where $\bar{g}_{AHP} = 0.054\,\mu\text{S}$. The midpoint for m_∞^2 is 220 nM.
Calcium-dependent activation variable:

$$\frac{dm}{dt} = \frac{m_\infty - m}{\tau_m}$$

$$\tau_m = \frac{1{,}000}{f(\text{Ca}) + b}$$

$$m_\infty = \frac{f(\text{Ca})}{f(\text{Ca}) + b}.$$

The forward and backward rate constants are given by

$$f(\text{Ca}) = 1.25 \cdot 10^8 [\text{Ca}^{2+}]_n^2 \quad \text{and} \quad b = 2.5.$$

Passive Components

$$I_{leak} = \bar{g}_{leak}(V - E_{leak}),$$

where $\bar{g}_{leak} = 0.02\,\mu\text{S}$ (50 MΩ) and $E_{leak} = -10\,\text{mV}$. The experimentally measured total membrane cell capacity is $C_N = 0.150\,\text{nF}$. The input resistance of our standard cell can be measured by injecting very small de- or hyperpolarizing currents into the soma and measuring the resulting stationary de- or hyperpolarization. In our case, 0.05 nA of injected current changes the membrane potential by approximately 0.554 mV, corresponding to an input resiance of about 11.1 MΩ. The passive values used correspond to an unusual high specific capacity of about $3.0\,\mu\text{F}\,\text{cm}^{-2}$ and a specific membrane leak resistance of about $2,500\,\Omega\,\text{cm}^2$.

Fast, Nicotinic Synaptic Input

$$I_{syn} = g_{sym}(t)(V - E_{syn}),$$

where

$$g_{syn}(t) = \text{const} \cdot t e^{-t/t_{peak}}.$$

In order to match experimental data, we assumed $E_{syn} = -10\,\text{mV}$ and $t_{peak} = 2.5\,\text{msec}$ (Kuba and Nishi 1979). The peak conductance change, g_{peak}, achieved at $t = t_{peak}$, varied between 20 and 350 nS. For our standard cell, the minimal peak conductance change necessary to elicit an action potential, $g_{peak} = \text{const} \cdot t_{peak} \cdot e^{-1}$, is 26.75 nS.

5 Modeling Active Dendritic Processes in Pyramidal Neurons

Zachary F. Mainen and Terrence J. Sejnowski

5.1 Introduction

The role of active ion channels in dendritic function is among the most interesting and complex aspects of information processing in single neurons (reviewed in Mel 1994; Segev, Rinzel, and Shepherd 1995; Yuste and Tank 1996; Johnston et al. 1996; Koch 1997, Borg-Graham, 1997). While the behavior of isolated channels or the passive electrical properties of dendrites can be studied in isolation, the interaction of multiple nonlinear ionic currents within a geometrically complex structure is described by equations that cannot be solved analytically and often resist intuition. Detailed computer models thus provide a crucially needed framework within which hypotheses about active dendritic mechanisms can be expressed and tested. Realistic neuronal models help determine whether known biophysical properties can account for experimental observations and provide insight into computational functions of these mechanisms.

The chief obstacle in constructing such models is obtaining constraints for their parameters. Until recently, not enough experimental data were available on the physiological properties of cortical neurons to be able to create accurate models. In early models of hippocampal and neocortical neurons (e.g., Traub and Llinás 1979; Shepherd et al. 1985; Bernander et al. 1991; Lytton and Sejnowski 1991), the kinetic properties of the channels were mixed and matched from cortical and noncortical neurons, including motoneurons in the spinal cord, sympathetic ganglion cells, and even the squid giant axon. Still scantier data were available regarding the spatial distribution of channels present in dendrites, axons, and synaptic terminals. Fortunately, the application of dendritic patch recordings, Ca^{2+} imaging, and immunocytochemistry and other molecular techniques is now yielding an abundance of precise data on the properties and localization of ion channels in the dendritic membrane. Furthermore, dendritic recordings and imaging of Ca^{2+}- or voltage-sensitive dyes provide windows into dendritic behavior not available with traditional somatic recordings. Thus the time is ripe for detailed models of active dendritic computation.

The basics of compartmental models are presented in chapter 3, this volume, and numerical methods for solving them in chapter 14. In the present chapter, we show how compartmental simulations can be used to model neurons with active dendritic ion channels; our focus is chiefly on modeling pyramidal neurons such as those of the neocortex and hippocampus, but much of the material can be applied more widely. In section 5.2, we present definitions of channel types, their densities, and their localization, and we discuss the steps involved in combining experimental data into a model of an active, spatially extended neuron. In section 5.3, we present applications, concentrating on models that exemplify the close interactions possible between simulations and physiology. Finally, in section 5.4, we discuss techniques for simplifying and analyzing complex models.

5.2 Passive Cable Models

Compartmental modeling (Rall 1964; Segev, Rinzel, and Shepherd 1994 and chapter 2, this volume) provides a general framework within which chemical and electrical signaling can be described at the level of single neurons. The strategy of this technique is to approximate the partial differential cable equations using both spatial and temporal discretization (see chapter 2, this volume). The advantage of this strategy over analytical techniques is that arbitrary geometries and ionic currents can be included and examined. The disadvantages are that simulations of complex dendritic geometries can be highly computation-intensive and that the parameters to be measured or estimated are legion (see section 5.2.6 on exploring parameters). Two high-quality public domain compartmental simulation environments are available: NEURON (Hines and Carnevale 1997; and chapter 3, this volume) and GENESIS (Bower and Beeman 1995; and chapter 12, this volume). Both provide efficient techniques for numerical solution of the cable equations as well as powerful languages and convenient graphic interfaces for programming and controlling the simulations. (For an introduction to NEURON, used for some of the simulations presented in this chapter, see the appendix to chapter 3, this volume.)

The first task in developing a model is to determine the structure of the neuron and the behavior of its ion channels (see chapter 3, this volume, for a general discussion of the passive properties of neurons and the influence of the various parameters on the cable properties of branched structures). Section 5.2 will focus on how the neuronal morphology is specified and on recent estimates for the properties and densities of voltage-dependent ion channels in cortical neurons, a subject that is rapidly changing as more data become available.

5.2.1 Passive Electrical Structure

Geometry Whereas in a single-compartment model, all channel currents combine linearly to produce a total membrane current, in a spatially extended neuron, the electrotonic structure of the neuron defines a much more complex spatiotemporal interplay between ion channels. The specification of the linear cable properties can be considered the first step in defining an active model and here entails translating a neuroanatomical description into a set of discrete connected compartments. In NEURON, these are cylinders with specified lengths, "L," and diameters, "diam."

Because the choice of compartment size ("segment" size in NEURON) will affect the accuracy of a compartmental simulation (Hines and Carnevale 1997), care must be taken to choose a sufficiently fine discretization to avoid numerical errors. In simulations with active currents that can be much faster or more localized than the passive currents, there is no absolute rule for an adequate spatial discretization. A compartment size no larger than $0.05\,\lambda$ has been suggested (Cooley and Dodge 1966; De Schutter and Bower 1994a). As in temporal discretization, "dt," a good strategy is to compare the results at a given maximum compartment length with the those at a finer discretization (e.g., doubling the number of compartments). As the number of compartments increases, the quantitative results from the simulations should converge, indicating that the compartment size is sufficiently small.

Although most models begin with a reconstructed neuron in the form of a computer file, it is worth enumerating the factors one should consider in evaluating such digitized anatomical data. Although care in reconstruction is obviously most important, albeit somewhat difficult to evaluate from the finished product, there are a number of other important factors that go into accurately representing a dendritic arbor from a dye-filled neuron. These factors can have a considerable effect on the ultimate electrical structure of the modeled neuron. Furthermore, variation in techniques may lead to difficulties in comparison of structures of neurons reconstructed in different laboratories. (See also chapter 3 for a corresponding discussion.)

• *Completeness.* Some methods, such as Golgi stains, may not completely penetrate fine processes, giving an incomplete fill. Methods involving intracellular injection of small molecules (e.g., lucifer yellow, biocytin) are generally preferable because they result in more complete fills.

• *Shrinkage.* Before a neuron can be reconstructed, the neural tissue in which it is embedded must generally be fixed, a process whereby proteins are chemically crossed-linked to immobilize them. Fixation results in varying amounts of tissue shrinkage depending on the exact method applied and a correction for this shrinkage must be determined or estimated. Some reconstructions will be corrected, while others will not. Shrinkages of 10%–20% are typical (Major et al. 1994; Mainen et al. 1996).

• *Wiggle.* Some fixation procedures, particularly those required for electron microscope (EM) processing, produce tissue distortion resulting in significant dendritic "wiggle." Failure to account for this tortuosity by sampling too few points during digital reconstruction will result in an underestimation of the dendritic length. In some cases, a correction factor may be applied, the value of which will depend on the exact reconstruction technique (Major et al. 1994).

• *Diameter estimation.* Estimation of small branch diameters can be problematic when these approach the resolution of the microscope. Systematic overestimation of small branch diameters is a strong possibility for ordinary light microscopy (Mainen et al. 1996). Although confocal microscopy offers better resolution of small processes, confocal reconstruction systems are still uncommon.

• *Spine membrane.* The dendrites of pyramidal neurons are studded with dendritic spines that are typically not included in dendritic reconstructions. A simple method to account for these spines is to increase the membrane surface area to compensate for the additional spine membrane area, which can be as much as 50% (see Stratford et al. 1989; Rapp, Yarom, and Segev 1992; and Major et al. 1994). Measurements of spine densities for pyramidal neurons of several types are available (neocortex: Larkman 1991; CA1: Harris, Jensen, and Tsao 1992). Although EM measurements of spine dimensions are also available (neocortex: Peters and Kaiserman-Abramof 1970; CA1: Harris, Jensen, and Tsao 1992), these numbers may not apply to cells of other areas or different ages.

• *Translation.* The data produced by digital reconstruction systems can usually be translated directly into a form suitable for incorporation into a simulation environment. The program NTSCable translates Eutectics, Nevin, and several other format files into NEURON code. Care must be taken with such automated translation programs because errors in reconstruction may be introduced by the translation. For example, there may be missing links between branches and trunks of dendrites. Representation of the soma is particularly problematic and often requires hand correction.

Passive Properties Along with the geometry, the passive membrane parameters complete a description of the cable properties of the neuron. These parameters are the membrane capacitance, C_m ("cm" in NEURON), the membrane resistivity, R_m ("1/g_pas" in NEURON), and the cytoplasmic or axial resistivity, R_i ("Ra" in NEURON). Although direct measurement of these parameters is difficult, experimental measurements combined with compartmental models provide indirect estimates (see chapter 2, this volume). Recent studies (Stratford et al. 1989; Spruston, Jaffe, and Johnston 1994; Major et al. 1994; Spruston and Stuart 1996, see also chapter 3, this volume) based on tight-seal whole-cell recordings (which are considered more accurate due to a smaller somatic "shunt") have generally arrived at estimates in the following ranges:

$R_m = 20\text{--}100\,\mathrm{k\Omega\,cm}^2$

$C_m = 0.5\text{--}1.5\,\mathrm{\mu F\,cm}^{-2}$

$R_i = 100\text{--}300\,\Omega\,\mathrm{cm}$

In perhaps the most direct measurement to date, a study of neocortical pyramidal cells using double simultaneous whole-cell recordings from soma and apical dendrite and subsequent reconstruction and compartmental modeling (Spruston and Stuart 1996) found $R_i \approx 150\,\Omega\,\mathrm{cm}$.

The passive membrane properties are often taken to be uniform (e.g., Spruston and Johnston 1992; Major et al. 1994; Mainen et al. 1996). Although there is little or no direct support, the possibility that the passive parameters are nonuniform across the cell has been considered in several modeling studies (e.g., Fleshman, Segev, and Burke 1988; Rall et al. 1992; Rapp, Segev, and Yarom 1994; Stratford et al. 1989 and chapter 3, this volume). Because the leak conductance is thought to result from the one or more K^+ or mixed cation channels, possibly the ORK1 channel (Goldstein et al. 1996) that are active (and linear) near the resting potential (Theander, Fahraeus, and Grampp 1996), a nonuniform distribution of these channels could result in non-uniform R_m (Spruston and Stuart 1996). The case for nonuniformity of C_m or R_i is less clear. It is also worth noting that nonuniformity of spine density (Larkman 1991) can be considered to contribute to an effective nonuniformity of both C_m and R_m once the additional spine membrane area is added.

5.2.2 Active Channels

Chapter 4 describes active channel properties from voltage clamp data (also see Johnston and Wu 1995; Hille 1992). We focus here on issues particularly relevant to constraining models with spatially distributed active channels: estimating channel densities and localization of channel types.

Current through an ion channel can be described by an equation of the form

$$I(V_m, t) = \bar{g}p_o(V_m, t)(V_m - E), \tag{5.1}$$

where I is the total current, $\bar{g}$ the maximum conductance, p_o a dynamic state variable representing the probability of channel opening or fraction of open channels (ranging from 0 to 1), V_m the membrane potential, and E the reversal potential of the channel in question. This equation assumes a linear or ohmic current-voltage relation. For most voltage-gated channels except those permeable primarily to Ca^{2+}, the ohmic approximation is reasonable. For Ca^{2+} channels, a more precise description of the driving force is offered by the Goldman-Hodgkin-Katz equation (see chapter 6, this volume; Hille 1992).

The equations for channel activation, p_o, are generally based on the gate activation, m, and inactivation, h, formalism of Hodgkin and Huxley (1952; see chapter 4, this volume), although a more general description using kinetic equations is often used by biophysicists (see Destexhe, Mainen, and Sejnowski 1994). The same kinetic formalism can be used to describe ligand-gated ion channels (see chapter 1, this volume).

5.2.3   Temperature Dependence

Because many physiological studies are performed at room temperature ($22°-25°$ C) rather than at physiological temperature ($37°-40°$ C), it is often necessary to compensate for the impact of temperature on model parameters, in particular, channel kinetics and conductances. The usual strategy employed is to scale the rate constants by a temperature coefficient, Q_{10} (fractional rate increase per $10°$ C temperature increase). However, the kinetics of different channels are not necessarily equivalent in their temperature dependence, and even the activation and inactivation rates of a given channel may depend differently on temperature. For example, in a study of the temperature dependence of Na^+ currents (Schwarz and Eikhof 1987), the steady-state parameters were found to be insensitive to temperature (in accord with the usual assumption), while the activation and inactivation rates had Q_{10} values of 2.2 and 2.9, respectively. Temperature also may affect the conductance of ions through a channel and hence $\bar{g}$. For example, a Q_{10} of 1.4 was reported for the conductance of one type of calcium channel (Acerbo and Nobile 1994). Despite the significance of these findings for the construction of accurate kinetic models, voltage clamp experiments at physiological temperature and the necessary data on temperature dependence are still both scarce.

5.2.4   Density Estimation

A serious problem in models that include a variety of ion channels spread non-uniformly across the neuron is the huge number of parameters available to describe the channel densities. In the majority of detailed compartmental modeling studies (e.g., Lytton and Sejnowski 1991; Traub et al. 1991; Rhodes and Gray 1994; Jaeger, De Schutter, and Bower 1997), the channel densities have been considered as free parameters that are altered systematically (or haphazardly) until the desired physiological behavior is produced. Because the fitting of a highly complex model to experimental data is severely underconstrained, the need for independent estimates of channel density and localization is clearly critical. Although this information was in the past essentially absent, through recent physiological and anatomical studies, many of these vitally needed parameters are now becoming available. Due to the importance of the topic, we will consider in some detail the process of incorporating channel density data into neural models.

While most compartmental models express channel density in terms of a maximal conductance, $\bar{g}$, this parameter cannot be measured experimentally, but rather must be calculated. Generally speaking, data on conductance densities are provided by two classes of experimental technique: anatomical and physiological, both of which have their advantages and limitations.

Anatomical Density Estimation   Using techniques of molecular biology such as immunocytochemistry, anatomical techniques offer the possibility of superb specificity and resolution of subcellular channel localization. To resolve the distribution of ion channels, the channel must be bound by a probe molecule such as a specific toxin or, more commonly, a specific antibody. The primary probe is detected by attaching a secondary probe that is visible either fluorescently (typically a secondary antibody conjugated to a fluorophore) or by electron microscopy (typically a gold particle).

Given estimates of channel density, if the single-channel conductance is also known, then $\bar{g}$ ($pS/\mu m^2$) can simple be calculated from

$$\bar{g} = \gamma\rho, \tag{5.2}$$

where γ is the single-channel conductance (in pS) and ρ is the channel density (in channels/μm^2).

Although molecular techniques make it possible to measure precisely and quantitatively the distribution of various channels, they have a number of limitations. First, most ion channels have several subunits, each with a variety of subtypes that can be recognized differentially by immunocytochemical probes. The properties of a given type of channel may vary widely depending on the precise subunit composition, yet in many cases the properties of these possible channel subtypes are not known. Second, most ion channels are subject to biochemical modulation, and therefore the true functional channel density will reflect not only the anatomical density but also the functional state of these channels. These limitations reinforce the value of physiological techniques.

Whole-Cell Recording   Whole-cell and sharp-electrode voltage clamp recordings sample channel activity from both local and distant cell regions with a weighting that depends on the electrotonic structure of the cell and the frequency of the currents in question (White, Sekar, and Kay 1995; Zador, Agmon-Snir, and Segev 1995). Thus estimating channel density in spatially complex neurons by whole-cell methods is at best a tricky proposition. Such estimates are typically only useful in cells lacking dendritic arbors, or those treated by enzymes to remove the dendrites (i.e., acutely dissociated cell cultures).

On the other hand, whole-cell and intracellular recordings can be used to qualitatively assay regional differences in channel densities by comparing currents in somatic and dendritic recordings (e.g., Andreasen and Lambert 1995) or by applying channel-blocking drugs in a local fashion to test for the presence of channels in particular region of the neuron (e.g., Huguenard, Hamill, and Prince 1989; Schwindt and Crill 1995; Lipowsky, Gillessen, and Alzheimer 1996; Colbert and Johnston 1996). The spatial resolution of these methods is clearly limited because (1) currents are measured over a range of electrotonic distances from the recording site; (2) electrotonically remote active channels cannot be voltage-clamped (White, Sekar, and Kay 1995); and (3) confirmation of the region of drug application is difficult. Nevertheless, local application of blocking drugs can provide invaluable qualitative tests of hypotheses regarding the function of channels in a compartment (Lipowsky, Gillessen, and Alzheimer 1996; Colbert and Johnston 1996).

Maximal conductance, $\bar{g}$, can be calculated from an isolated, voltage-clamped current if the driving force and fraction of open channels are known, using

$$\bar{g} = \frac{I}{p_o(V - E)A}, \tag{5.3}$$

where I is the maximal current amplitude, p_o the fraction of channels open at the maximal observed current, V the clamp potential, E the reversal potential of the channel, and A the area of membrane sampled. Note that if I is measured in pA, V in mV, and A in μm^2 then $\bar{g}$ will be measured in $nS/\mu m^2$. Although it is commonly assumed that $p_o = 1$ (all channels open during the maximal observed current), for many channels, $p_o < 1$ due to channel inactivation. For example, in some models, peak open probability for the Na^+ channel is substantially less than one (Aldrich and Stevens 1987). This will lead to an underestimate of $\bar{g}$, which can be corrected by estimating the true p_o from a kinetic model of the channel in question. Note that the estimation of the area sample (A) may be the most difficult parameter in this equation to determine.

Single-Channel Recording   Using patch clamp recordings in the outside-out or cell-attached configuration (Sakmann and Neher 1995b), it is possible to sample isolated single-channel currents from any location on a neuron that can be patched. This method, although more difficult, avoids many of the problems inherent in whole-cell voltage clamp experiments by confining the membrane examined to a small patch drawn into the patch pipette. Thus both excellent voltage clamp and high spatial resolution are achieved. With the advent of visually guided patch techniques (reviewed in Stuart, Dodt, and Sakmann 1993), the repertoire of targets now includes larger dendritic processes (reviewed in Stuart and Spruston 1995) and proximal portions of the axon (Stuart and Sakmann 1994; Hausser et al. 1995; Colbert and Johnston 1996) as well as the soma.

Channel densities can be estimated directly from peak currents observed in patch recordings by eq. 5.3, or where single-channel currents can be observed, from

$$\rho = \frac{I}{p_o i A},$$ \hfill (5.4)

where I is the peak current observed, i the single-channel current amplitude at the same holding potential, and A the estimated patch area. As described above, since $p_o \leq 1$, this is a lower bound on the actual number of channels and should be corrected using the actual p_o. In cases where single-channel currents cannot be resolved, fluctuation analysis (Sigworth and Zhou 1992) can be used to estimate the number of channels and single-channel conductance, providing $\bar{g}$ by eq. 5.2.

There are two caveats to keep in mind when converting currents observed in patches to a $\bar{g}$ parameter. First, patch areas are relatively difficult to estimate and most often measured indirectly. Area estimates may be fairly sensitive to errors in measurement of the pipette diameter and the amount of membrane drawn into the pipette. In one of the few systematic studies (Sakmann and Neher 1995a), membrane area in patches obtained with typical (2–3 MΩ) pipettes ranged from 5 μm^2 to 20 μm^2. Extrapolation to smaller pipettes used in dendritic or axonal patches is difficult because of the high variance and lack of measurements of higher resistance pipettes. For example, in measurements of dendritic Na$^+$ channel density with similar patch clamp techniques, Stuart and Sakmann (1994) estimated a 1.5 μm^2 patch area, while Magee and Johnston (1995a) estimated 3 μm^2.

And second, in outside-out patches, channel activity may be increased or decreased relative to normal conditions due to perturbation of the cytoplasmic environment. For example, Na$^+$ channels are regulated by protein kinase C, cAMP-dependent protein kinase, and phosphoprotein phosphotases (Murphy et al. 1993). Basal levels of cAMP-dependent kinase have been shown to produce significant functional inhibition of Na$^+$ currents in intact cells (Li et al. 1992). The absence of endogenous kinase and phosphotase activity in the outside-out patch configuration might thus be expected to result in higher Na$^+$ channel activity in outside-out patches compared to the intact cell.

Imaging Optical imaging of membrane potential or intracellular ion concentrations can also provide useful data on channel densities. The most successful method so far has been Ca^{2+} imaging. Because resting intracellular Ca^{2+} concentration is typically less than $100\,nM$, increases in Ca^{2+} concentration provide an excellent signal of voltage-dependent Ca^{2+} channel activity. Comparing the Ca^{2+} signal and time course of Ca^{2+} rises at different dendritic locations, it has been possible to localize the site of Ca^{2+} entry and thereby pinpoint the locations of ion channels selective for Ca^{2+} (see below). Recent advances, such as two-photon laser scanning microscopy (Denk et al. 1994), have opened up new avenues including the ability to observe Ca^{2+} entry in the dendrites of cortical neurons in vivo (Svoboda et al. 1997). However, although Ca^{2+} enters through several varieties of voltage-dependent calcium channel (see below), it also enters through the NMDA-type glutamate receptor (see chapter 1, this volume) and can also be released from intracellular stores (reviewed in Pozzan et al. 1994). Thus the interpretation of Ca^{2+} imaging data can be tricky (some of the issues involved are discussed in more detail in chapter 6, this volume).

Na^+ Imaging Na^+-sensitive dyes such as Na^+-green are available and have been used to localize Na^+ channels (e.g., Jaffe et al. 1992; Tsubokawa and Ross 1996; and see below). Because internal Na^+ concentration is fairly high, the signal-to-noise of these dyes is low. Nonetheless, it has been possible to show, for example, that the axon hillock region of Purkinje cells in the cerebellum are a "hot spot" for Na^+ entry, suggesting a higher density of Na^+ channels there than in the soma and dendritic regions (Lasser-Ross and Ross 1992).

Membrane Potential Imaging Voltage-sensitive dyes, used for some time to measure events in small processes of cultured neurons (Grinvald, Ross, and Farber 1981), have recently been used to examine passive properties (Fromherz and Muller 1994) and spike initiation (Zečević 1996). Newly developed dyes (Kogan et al. 1995; Antić and Zečević 1995; Gonzalez and Tsien 1995) promise better signal-to-noise and hence better resolution.

5.2.5 Channel Types

This section briefly reviews the chief players in active dendritic processing, the voltage-gated ion channels, with particular attention to their subcellular localization in pyramidal neurons (table 5.1). We generally combine data from hippocampal and neocortical pyramidal neurons with data from other cell types that may be particularly applicable. Let us start with some general comments on these data (axonal currents are considered separately in section 5.2.6).

Table 5.1
Table of currents discussed in this chapter

Current	Channel	γ (pS)	Activation	τ_{inact} (ms)
I_{Na}	Na^+(Na)	15–20	$\uparrow = V_\theta$	1
I_{Na_p}	Na^+(Na)	15–20	$\uparrow < V_\theta$	—
I_T	Ca^{2+}(LVA)	7–10	$\uparrow \approx V_\theta$	50
I_{Ca-NR}	Ca^{2+}(HVAm)	14–18	$\uparrow > V_\theta$	100
I_{Ca-L}	Ca^{2+}(HVAl)	25–30	$\uparrow > V_\theta$	—
I_A	K^+(Kv)	5–10	$\uparrow \approx V_\theta$	5–25
I_{Kd}	K^+(Kv)	5–10	$\uparrow > V_\theta$	—
I_C	K^+(BK)	?100	$\uparrow Ca^{2+}$(L)	—
I_M	K^+(eag?)	small	$\uparrow < V_\theta$	—
sI_{AHP}	K^+(?)	?	$\uparrow Ca^{2+}$(R)	—
I_{AHP}	K^+(SK)	5–20	$\uparrow Ca^{2+}$(N)	—
I_H	K^+/Na^+(Kir?)	?	$\downarrow < V_\theta$	—
I_{IR}	K^+/Na^+(Kir)	?	$\downarrow < V_\theta$	—

Where it is known, the channel underlying the observed currents is given (? indicates that the channel is still unknown or speculative). The single-channel conductance (γ) is useful for converting between channel densities and conductance densities. The entries in the "Activation" column describe whether the channel is activated ($\uparrow$) or inactivated ($\downarrow$) by Ca^{2+} or depolarization. The parenthetical letters refer to the subtype of Ca^{2+} channel believed to be associated with different Ca^{2+}-activated K^+ currents. The voltage range of activation relative to action potential threshold (V_θ) is also given. The rightmost column gives the approximate time constant of inactivation (if present). References are given in the text.

General Observations

• A wide variety of voltage-dependent channels are present in dendritic membranes, and include all major families of sodium, potassium, and calcium channels.

• Some channel subtypes are confined to dendritic, somatic, or axonal compartments (e.g., Westenbroek, Merrick, and Catterall 1989; Hell et al. 1993; Sheng et al. 1992); this may be primarily for differential modulation because functional properties of the different subtypes are often similar.

• Some channel types, notably, certain Ca^{2+} and Ca^{2+}-dependent K^+ subtypes (Sah 1995), may coassociate, forming functionally specific units.

• Some voltage-gated channels show microscale dendritic clustering, including exclusion or enrichment in dendritic spines (e.g., Ahlijanian, and Catterall Westenbroek, 1990; Turner et al. 1994); the electrophsiological impact of this clustering is not well known.

• Above the microscale, changes in channel density appear to be relatively gradual through the dendrites and soma, while possibly more abrupt in the axon.

• Voltage-gated channel densities in dendrites estimated by patch clamp recordings are generally within a fairly narrow range (<10 channels/μm^2; see figure 5.1), although density estimates by various molecular methods for axonal Na^+ channels and synaptic receptors can be extremely high ($>1,000$ channels/μm^2).

Sodium Channels   Electrophysiological and modeling studies have differentiated between a fast or transient Na^+ current, I_{Na}, and a persistent Na^+ current, I_{Na_p} (reviewed in Crill 1996). The transient current mediates the fast action potential, while the persistent current activates below threshold, may boost synaptic currents in dendrites (Stuart and Sakmann 1995; Schwindt and Crill 1995; Lipowsky, Gillessen, and Alzheimer 1996), and contribute to bursting (Franceschetti et al. 1995) and subthreshold oscillations (Gutfreund, Yarom, and Segev 1995) in neocortical neurons.

KINETICS   Single-channel recordings indicate that the fast and persistent Na^+ currents are mediated by the same type of Na^+ channel, entering either a rapidly or a slowly inactivating mode (Kirsch and Brown 1989; Alzheimer, Schwindt, and Crill 1993; Brown, Schwindt, and Crill 1996; Magee and Johnston 1995a). Because complex gating is not readily incorporated into the Hodgkin-Huxley framework, all models to date have treated I_{Na} and I_{Na_p} as two distinct currents. A full Markov model of the Na^+ channel (e.g., Vandenberg and Bezanilla 1991; Destexhe, Mainen, and Sejnowski 1994) would be desirable. I_{Na} kinetics can be difficult to determine because the currents are large and fast and therefore hard to voltage-clamp without introducing artifacts (White, Sekar, and Kay 1995). I_{Na} kinetics described by Huguenard and colleagues (Huguenard, Hamill, and Prince 1988; Hamill, Huguenard, and Prince 1991; Mainen et al. 1995) in dissociated neocortical pyramidal cells are very similar to those observed in rat brain Na^+ channels expressed in oocytes (Stühmer et al. 1987), and those measured in rat and human neocortex (Cummins, Xia, and Haddad 1994). The steepness of the activation curve (9 mV/e-fold) is about half as steep as that used in an I_{Na} model introduced by Traub and colleagues (1991, 1994) and used in a number of other recent models. The kinetics of I_{Na_p} were described by French et al. (1990) in hippocampal neurons, and their data has formed the basis for the current used in most recent models (e.g., De Schutter and Bower 1994a; Gutfreund, Yarom, and Segev 1995; Lipowsky, Gillessen, and Alzheimer 1996). The model includes an activation variable only.

DISTRIBUTION   Assuming that I_{Na} and I_{Na_p} derive from the same underlying channel, the distributions of their currents should be the same, although the magnitude of I_{Na_p} is approximately 1% of the transient Na^+ current (Crill 1996). However, it is possible

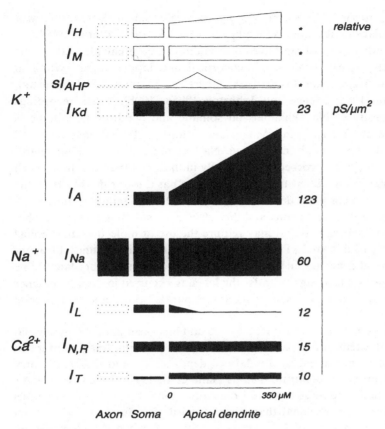

Figure 5.1
Schematic diagram of conductance densities ($\bar{g}$) in pyramidal cells estimated by direct, cell-attached patch recordings (*shaded*: $I_{Kd}, I_A, I_{Na}, I_{Ca}$) or inferred from combined modeling and electrophysiology studies (*white boxes*: I_H, I_M, sI_{AHP}). *Dotted lines*: not measured. Conductance densities are those reported by the authors or calculated from reported channel densities, using eq. 5.2. The apical dendritic distance scale is approximately correct, but the somatic and axonal distances are not to scale. Numbers on the right indicate the maximum average peak conductance density for each channel. I_H, I_M from Hutcheon et al. 1996; sI_{AHP} from Sah and Bekkers 1996; I_{Kd}, I_A from Hoffman Magee, and Johnston 1996; Hoffman et al. 1997; I_{Na} from Stuart and Sakmann 1994; Magee and Johnston 1995a; Colbert and Johnston 1996; $I_L, I_{N,R}$, from Magee and Johnston 1995a.

that the ratio of I_{Na} to I_{Na_p} differs across subtypes of Na^+ channel, which show a nonuniform subcellular distribution (Westenbroek, Merrick, and Catterall 1989).

Single-channel dendritic recordings have allowed direct measurements of dendritic Na^+ channels on the apical dendrite of neocortical and hippocampal pyramidal neurons (Huguenard, Hamill, and Prince 1989; Stuart and Sakmann 1994; Spruston, Jonas, and Sakmann 1995; Magee and Johnston 1995a, 199b). These recordings indicate that the density of Na^+ channels on somatic and dendritic membrane is similar, in the range of 30–60 pS/μm². Magee and Johnston (1995a) have provided evidence that the developmental increase in Na^+ channel density (Huguenard, Hamill, and Prince 1988) may proceed more rapidly in the soma than dendrites, such that in juvenile animals (<4 weeks) the apical dendrite has a lower density than the soma. Although these recordings definitively establish the presence of functional dendritic Na^+ channels, their uniformity and their density on small-diameter branches and spines are not yet determined and may require the use of molecular anatomical techniques. One study of this kind (Turner et al. 1994) found Na^+ channels throughout the apical and basal dendrites, in pyramidal cells of the electrosensory lateral line lobe of the weakly electric fish. Significantly, the labeling occurred in discrete patches rather than uniformly and was absent from the dendritic spines and subsynaptic membrane.

A possible difference between neocortical layer-5 and hippocampal CA1 pyramidal neurons is the spatial extent of Na^+ channels in the apical dendrite. Imaging of intracellular Na^+ ions in hippocampal pyramidal cell dendrites showed that Na^+ entry was confined to the proximal dendritic regions (Jaffe et al. 1992). Likewise, in CA1 neurons Ca^{2+} elevations produced by antidromically propagating action potentials are substantially greater in proximal than distal dendrites (Jaffe et al. 1992), even though a more uniform pattern of Ca^{2+} entry can be seen when K^+ channels are blocked (Jaffe et al. 1992). In contrast, Ca^{2+} elevations in layer-5 neurons are high throughout the dendritic arbor (Schiller, Helmchen, and Sakmann 1995), suggesting that antidromically propagating spikes can fully invade the dendrites in slice preparations, although the extent of the invasion may be regulated in vivo (Svoboda et al. 1997). These observations suggest that while Na^+ channel density in distal dendrites may be lower than in more proximal regions in CA1 pyramidal cells, this gradient may not be as large in neocortical pyramidal cells, although differences in experimental methods and animal age may also contribute to the differences in these findings.

Calcium Channels Voltage-dependent Ca^{2+} channels (VDCCs) appear to be present throughout the dendrites of pyramidal cells. Ca^{2+} entering through these VDCCs can contribute to a wide variety of biochemical cascades triggered by Ca^{2+}, including neurotransmitter release and synaptic plasticity. Ca^{2+} entry through VDCCs activates Ca^{2+}-dependent K^+ channels (see below), which leads to hyperpolarization that tends to limit cell firing. Under some conditions, Ca^{2+} channels participate in regenerative bursting or plateau potentials (Wong, Prince, and Basraum 1979; Kim and Connors 1993; Yuste et al. 1994; Hirsch, Alonso, and Reid 1995).

SUBTYPES There are two main classes of VDCCs; low-voltage- and high-voltage-activated (LVA and HVA). The LVA class corresponds to I_T (T-current) which is activated in the subthreshold voltage range. Possible functions suggested for I_T include generation of low-threshold spikes that lead to burst firing, promotion of intrinsic oscillatory behavior, boosting of calcium entry for hyperpolarized cells, and synaptic potentiation (reviewed in Huguenard 1996). The HVA class includes L-, N-, P-, Q-, and R-type currents (Tsien et al. 1988; Randall and Tsien 1995). While the different HVA Ca^{2+} channels vary in their distribution, pharmacological sensitivity, modulation, and inactivation properties, all are activated in similar superthreshold voltage ranges and may produce currents of essentially identical kinetics during physiological activity (Brown, Schwindt, and Crill 1993). As a consequence, in most models of pyramidal neurons, a single channel type (often simple called I_{Ca}) has been used to represent all classes of HVA channel (e.g., Traub et al. 1991, 1994; Reuveni et al. 1993; Warman, Durand, and Yuen 1994; Rhodes and Gray 1994; Mainen and Sejnowski 1996), although Ca^{2+} imaging experiments suggest that N- (slowly inactivating) and L-type (noninactivating) currents can be distinguished in more detailed models (Jaffe and Brown 1994; Migliore, Alicata, and Ayala 1995).

DISTRIBUTION The range of data on dendritic VDCCs in hippocampal and neocortical pyramidal neurons is growing rapidly. Ca^{2+} imaging studies have shown that VDCCs are located throughout the dendritic arbor (Regehr, Connor, and Tank 1989; Miyakawa et al. 1992; Jaffe et al. 1992; Schiller, Helmchen, and Sakmann 1995) including dendritic spines (Jaffe, Fisher, and Brown 1994; Segal 1995; Denk et al. 1996), as well as in the axon initial segment (Schiller, Helmchen, and Sakmann 1995) and, of course, presynaptic terminals. Localized calcium influx produced by subthreshold synaptic events (Markram and Sakmann 1994; Magee et al. 1995) occurs through LVA channels that can be activated by such stimuli (Magee and Johnston 1995b). In contrast, HVA channels are activated by backpropagating Na^+ action potentials (Schiller, Helmchen, and Sakmann 1995; Spruston, Jonas, and Sakmann 1995a; Markram, Helm, and Sakmann 1995; Helmchen, Imoto, and Sakmann 1996; Svoboda et al. 1997; Magee and Johnston 1997; Markram et al. 1997), dendritic Ca^{2+} bursting (Yuste et al. 1994) or by repetitive trains of synaptic stimuli (Miyakawa et al. 1992).

Pharmacological dissection of the contribution of various VDCCs to dendritic Ca^{2+} influx suggests that in CA1 neurons, I_T (LVA Ca^{2+} channels) are preferentially located in more distal dendrites while HVA Ca^{2+} channels are more concentrated in the soma and proximal dendrites (Christie et al. 1995). I_T is also concentrated in the distal dendrites of thalamic neurons (Destexhe et al. 1996). Single-channel patch recordings in apical dendrites of pyramidal cells support these findings (Magee and Johnston 1995a). In CA1 neurons the overall combined density of dendritic Ca^{2+} channels is about 50%–75% that of voltage-gated Na^+ channels (Magee and Johnston 1995a).

Immunocytochemical methods yield findings generally consistent with the physiological data, suggesting that VDCCs are clustered rather than uniformly distributed in the dendrites (Jones, Kunze, and Angelides 1989), with L-type channels localized to the base of major dendrites as well as the soma (Westenbroek, Ahlijanian, and Catterall 1990). Similar methods show N-type channels are present in the soma, dendrites, and a subset of dendritic spines (Mills et al. 1994). Further dissection of the subcellular localization of various VDCC subunits (Hell et al. 1993; Westenbroek et al. 1995; Yokoyama et al. 1995; Sakurai et al. 1996) is providing a basis for an even finer-grained analysis of the subcellular distribution of VDCCs and other channels. Models that take subcellular localization into account could help in exploring the functional consequences of VDCC clusters.

Potassium Channels K^+ channels are a large and diverse group (see reviews by Storm 1990; Christie 1995; Sah 1996). Functionally, the K^+ currents can be divided into three primary groups according to function: (1) spike repolarization, I_A, I_{Kd}, I_C; (2) spike frequency adaptation, I_M, I_{AHP}, sI_{AHP}; and (3) anomalous rectification, I_H, I_{IR}. While several other types of K^+ current have been described, including Na^+-dependent K^+ currents (Schwindt, Spain, and Crill 1989) and several very slow voltage-gated currents such as I_D (Storm 1988), these have not yet been incorporated into models.

FAST SPIKE REPOLARIZATION   In pyramidal neurons, action potentials are repolarized by both voltage- and Ca^{2+}-dependent K^+ currents (Storm 1987). The former are members of the large and diverse Kv family of voltage-gated K^+ channels (Christie 1995), and include a class of inactivating currents, I_A, as well as noninactivating or delayed-rectifier currents, I_{Kd}. In addition to these voltage-gated currents, I_C, which is activated by both voltage and Ca^{2+}, also contributes significantly to spike repolarization (Lancaster and Nicoll 1987; Storm 1987). I_C is mediated by the large-conductance (BK) class of K^+ channel (Christie 1995).

Models for I_A are given by Banks, Haberly, and Jackson (1996, based on recordings from pyriform cortical neurons) and Hoffman et al. (1997, based on recordings in hippocampal CA1 neurons). A model for I_{Kd} is given by Mainen et al. (1996), based on data from neocortical neurons described in Hamill, Huguenard, and Prince (1991). Although the calcium and voltage dependence of I_C have been characterized in nonneuronal cells (Barrett, Magleby, and Pallotta 1982), kinetic descriptions from neocortical or hippocampal pyramidal neurons are not yet available. Consequently, models of I_C in these neurons are still based on data culled from diverse preparations and can be considered somewhat less than canonical. A model of I_C based on studies in muscle cells by Moczydlowski and Latorre (1983) is included in NEURON; another, based on data from bullfrog sympathetic ganglia, is given in chapter 4. Models of I_C in pyramidal cells based on modifications of these and other data are given by Traub et al. (1991); Lytton and Sejnowski (1991); De Schutter and Bower (1994a); and Warman, Durand, and Yuen (1994).

Owing to the relatively slow repolarization of dendritic action potentials (e.g., Wong, Prince, and Basraum 1979; Turner et al. 1991; Stuart and Sakmann 1994), modeling studies have assumed that the density of fast K^+ currents is higher in the soma and proximal dendrites (Mainen et al. 1995; Rapp, Yarom, and Segev 1996; Traub et al. 1994). There is however, no direct physiological or molecular evidence for this assumption, and some recent evidence argues for higher densities of dendritic K^+ channels farther from the soma (Hoffman, Magee, and Johnston 1996; Hoffman et al. 1997).

Different subtypes of Kv channels show highly specific patterns of cell type specific expression and subcellular localization (Sheng et al. 1992, 1994; Wang et al. 1994; Maletic-Savatic, Lenn, and Trimmer 1995; Weiser et al. 1995). These complex and diverse patterns clearly provide a rich substrate for possible differential regulation, a subject which is just starting to be unraveled. To the extent that dendritic K^+ channels are important for the transformation of synaptic currents into spike firing patterns, it should be expected that even among various subclasses of pyramidal cells, variability in K^+ channel expression may lead to heterogeneity in cellular integration properties. In the hippocampus, I_{Kd}-mediating subtypes (Kv1.5, Kv2.1, and Kv2.2) are expressed in proximal dendrites, while I_A-mediating subtypes (Kv1.4 and Kv4.2) are present in the distal dendrites of a subpopulation of neurons (Maletic-Savatic, Lenn, and Trimmer 1995). Another I_A subtype (Kv1.2) is also specifically expressed in the dendrites of neocortical and hippocampal pyramidal cells (Sheng et al. 1994).

Channels with properties corresponding to I_A, I_{Kd}, and I_C have been described in dendritic patches from CA1 pyramidal neurons (Hoffman, Magee, and Johnston

1996; Hoffman et al. 1997). The channel densities measured by this technique show a pattern of K^+ channel segregation consistent with the anatomical data: relatively constant I_{Kd} and I_A increasing in the dendrites with distance from the soma (Hoffman et al. 1997; discussed further in section 5.3).

SPIKE FREQUENCY ADAPTATION   Like spike repolarization, spike frequency adaptation is mediated by both voltage- and Ca^{2+}-dependent K^+ channels (Madison and Nicoll 1984). These channels are essential to determining the relative sensitivity of a neuron to transient versus sustained inputs and limiting the response to large inputs, enabling a wide dynamic range of synaptic currents to be mapped to physiological firing frequencies (Mainen 1996; Tang, Bartels, and Sejnowski 1997). Electrophysiologically, the currents from these channels can also be seen as afterhyperpolarizations (AHPs) following a spike train (Madison and Nicoll 1984; Schwindt et al. 1988; Storm 1990) or sometimes a single spike or subthreshold event (e.g., Stuart and Sakmann 1995; Lipowsky, Gillessen, and Alzheimer 1996). Whereas the fast K^+ currents I_A, I_{Kd} and I_C contribute to what is known as the fast AHP, the much slower K^+ currents give rise to the medium AHP (I_M and I_{AHP}) or the slow AHP (sI_{AHP}; Schwindt et al. 1988; Storm 1989; Sah 1996).

   I_M is a slow, muscarine-sensitive, voltage-dependent K^+ current (Adams, Brown, and Constanti 1982) present in neocortical and hippocampal pyramidal neurons (Halliwell 1986; Schwindt et al. 1988; Storm 1989). I_M activates near threshold and does not inactivate (Adams, Brown, and Constanti 1982) and is one of several currents that contribute to the mAHP (Storm 1989). In addition to its role in modulating firing sensitivity and adaptation, I_M is partially activated at the resting membrane potential and, combined with I_{Na_p}, can give rise to subthreshold oscillations in cortical pyramidal neurons (Alonso and Klink 1993; Gutfreund, Yarom, and Segev 1995). The kinetics of I_M ($\tau \approx 30{-}50$ msec) are intermediate between the fast K^+ currents described above and the Ca^{2+}-dependent K^+ currents (I_{AHP} and sI_{AHP}). The channels underlying I_M are not yet firmly established, but may belong to a family of proteins (*eag*) related to the Kv family (Christie 1995). A model of an I_M current based on data from neocortical neurons is given by Gutfreund, Yarom, and Segev (1995).

   There at least two types of slow Ca^{2+}-dependent K^+ currents that contribute to spike frequency adaptation: I_{AHP} (or mI_{AHP}) and sI_{AHP} (Madison and Nicoll 1984; Lancaster and Adams 1986; Schwindt et al. 1988; Schwindt, Spain, and Crill 1992; Sah 1996). These two types of currents, which have often been confused, can be distinguished by their time course and pharmacological profiles. The faster I_{AHP} (1–5 msec rise, 100–200 msec decay) is believed to correspond to the SK class of K^+

channel (Sah 1996), while the channel underlying the slower sI_{AHP} (>100 msec rise, >1 sec decay) is not known at present, but may be a subtype of SK channel (Sah 1996). Because the biophysical mechanisms underlying these currents are poorly understood, the existing models of I_{AHP}/sI_{AHP} are still quite speculative and are based on a mixture of data from different neuronal types (examples are found in Traub et al. 1991; Warman, Durand, and Yuen 1994).

There is evidence that Ca^{2+} ions rather than channel kinetics determine the time courses of these currents, as well as I_C (Lancaster and Zucker 1994; Sah 1993). It is not precisely known how different K^+ channel types would access Ca^{2+} signals with the necessary differences in time course, but the molecular coupling of the Ca^{2+}-dependent K^+ channels and the Ca^{2+} channels that are the source of their activation signal is thought to play a crucial role. In rat sympathetic neurons, it has been shown that Ca^{2+} entry via L-type channels selectively activates BK K^+ channels (producing the action potential–repolarizing I_C), while Ca^{2+} entry via N-type channels selectively activates SK K^+ channels (producing I_{AHP}), and Ca^{2+} entry via R-type Ca^{2+} channels activates Ca^{2+} release from intracellular stores (producing sI_{AHP}; Davies, Ireland, and McLachlan 1996). A similar story might hold in pyramidal neurons. Conventional compartmental models have generally simulated one or more pools of intracellular Ca^{2+} that directly gate the K^+ channel (e.g., Warman, Durand, and Yuen 1994; Migliore, Alicata, and Ayala 1995). Ca^{2+} handling is treated in detail in chapter 6, this volume. An interesting avenue to explore would be models in which specific K^+ channel types are coupled to specific Ca^{2+} channel types and Ca^{2+} stores.

Relatively little is known about the density or distribution of slow voltage-dependent K^+ currents in pyramidal neurons, though a number studies have implicated a dendritic localization of slow K^+ currents. First, insofar as I_M is responsible for subthreshold oscillations, dendritic recordings indicate that it must be present in the apical dendrites in order to reproduce the observed resonance properties of neocortical neurons (Hutcheon et al. 1996). Dendritic recordings from CA1 neurons have also suggested the presence of a slow dendritic Ca^{2+}-dependent K^+ current (Andreasen and Lambert 1995). In an interesting combined modeling and electrophysiological study, Sah and Bekkers (1996) argued that sI_{AHP} must be localized to the proximal apical dendrite (within $\approx 200\,\mu m$) in order to reproduce the interaction of the current with inhibitory postsynaptic potentials (IPSPs) and the observed offset of the current under voltage clamp. Whether their findings reflect localization of the K^+ channels or of the Ca^{2+} signals activating these channels has not been determined.

INWARD RECTIFICATION   The final class of K^+ currents (which includes mixed cation currents), are tonically active at subthreshold membrane potentials, are activated by *hyperpolarization* rather than depolarization, and do not inactivate. The slow mixed-cation (Na^+/K^+) current I_H (also sometimes known as I_Q) underlies slow oscillatory behavior in several cell types and has been shown to be present in neocortical pyramidal neurons and to contribute to subthreshold membrane resonance (Spain, Schwindt, and Crill 1990; Perkins and Wong 1995; Hutcheon, Miura, and Puil 1996a, 1996b). The anomalous rectifying K^+ current, I_{IR} has similar properties to I_H, but with much faster kinetics (Constanti and Galvan 1983; Sutor and Hablitz 1993).

The inwardly rectifying currents belong to a relatively large class of K^+ channels, known logically as the "inward rectifier family" (Kir; reviewed in Doupnik, Davidson, and Lester 1995). Not much is known about the subcellular distribution of these channels. Based on dendritic recordings and modeling of subthreshold oscillations in neocortical pyramidal neurons, Hutcheon, Miura, and Puil (1996a) argued for the presence of I_H in the dendrites (as well as the soma). Because the inward rectifiers are tonically active at resting membrane potentials, a nonuniform distribution of these channels would result in an effectively nonuniform membrane resistance. The possibility of dendritic membrane enriched in I_H or I_{IR} could complicate substantially the interpretation of passive membrane models. Based on a study combining dual somatic/dendritic recordings and compartmental modeling, Spruston and Stuart (1996) have suggested that I_H may indeed be concentrated in the apical dendrite.

5.2.6   Axonal Structure and Function

In a passive compartmental model, the axon contributes very little to dendritic or somatic behavior because its fine caliber and electrical isolation from the remainder of the cell produce little passive load (Rall et al. 1992). In models with active properties, however, the axon (or at least its proximal segments) may contribute substantially to the behavior of the neuron due to the contribution of voltage-gated Na^+ channels that make the axon the site of action potential initiation (Coombs, Curtis, and Eccles 1957a; Stuart and Sakmann 1994; Spruston, 1995; Colbert and Johnston 1996). Although the majority of published compartmental models omit the axon, several recent models of pyramidal cells have incorporated axonal anatomy as an essential component (e.g., Traub et al. 1994; Mainen et al. 1995; Rapp, Yarom, and Segev 1996).

Anatomy   In pyramidal cells, the axon arises from the soma or in some cases from a basal dendrite. The transitional region where the axon meets the soma is known as the "axon hillock." The *initial segment* of the axon is an ultrastructurally specialized region that generally extends to the first myelinated segment and is the target of about 20–50 axoaxonic inhibitory synapses (Peters, Proskauer, and Kaiserman-Abramof 1968; Jones and Powell 1969; Fariñas and DeFelipe 1991) made by a special class of GABA-ergic inhibitory interneurons called "chandelier cells" (Somogyi, Freund, and Cowey 1982).

In pyramidal neurons of the neocortex and hippocampus, the length of the initial segment ranges from about 20 µm to 50 µm (Sloper and Powell 1978; Somogyi, Freund, and Cowey 1982; Fariñas and DeFelipe 1991; Colbert and Johnston 1996) with an average diameter in the range of 1–2.5 µm (Westrum 1970; Fariñas and DeFelipe 1991). There is generally a 2- to 4-fold taper from the hillock to the distal end (Fariñas and DeFelipe 1991).

In myelinated axons, the myelin sheath begins at the end of the initial segment and is interrupted regularly by the nodes of Ranvier. In the terminal arbors of cat cortical axons, an internodal length of around 100 µm is typical (Waxman and Melker 1971; Deschênes and Landry 1980a), but systematic studies of internodal lengths of proximal axonal arbors are not available. The myelinated segments are thicker than the initial segment or nodes of Ranvier (Palay et al. 1968), with diameters in the range of 0.5–2 µm (Haug 1968). It is also important to note that myelination is only partially developed in the juvenile rats used in many electrophysiological studies.

Sodium Channels   The propagation of nerve impulses in myelinated axons depends critically on localization of Na^+ channels to the nodes of Ranvier (Black, Kocsis, and Waxman 1990). Similarly, localization of Na^+ channels to the axon initial segment (Angelides et al. 1988; Kobayashi et al. 1992) has been proposed to contribute to the role of this structure as the site of action potential initiation (Coombs, Curtis, and Eccles 1957a; Dodge and Cooley 1973; Mainen et al. 1995; Rapp, Yarom, and Segev 1996). A primary distinguishing feature of both the initial segment and the nodes of Ranvier is the presence of an electron-dense undercoating (Peters, Proskaucr, and Kaiserman-Abramof 1968), which has long been thought to be related to electrical conduction (Peters, Proskauer, and Kaisermann-Abramof 1968; Palay et al. 1968), presumably reflecting to an elevated density of Na^+ channels. The existence of structural barriers to diffusion of Na^+ channels between the axon hillock and soma (Srinivasan et al. 1988; Kobayashi et al. 1992) could provide the molecular basis for the trapping of channels in the initial segment. Conventional estimates of nodal Na^+ channel density are 1,000–2,000 channels/µm², compared with a 30-fold lower density in internodal regions (Black, Kocsis, and Waxman

1990; Waxman and Ritchie 1993). But is there a similar difference in channel density between soma and initial segment?

Measurements with fluorescent toxin–binding studies (Angelides et al. 1988) have shown up to 30-fold higher Na^+ channel density in the initial segment compared to the soma in cultured spinal cord neurons, consistent with the analogy to node and internode, although lower differences (<10-fold) were found in cortical neurons (Angelides et al. 1988) and retinal ganglion cells (Wollner and Catterall 1986). Moreover, using direct patch clamp recordings from the initial segments of subicular pyramidal cells, Colbert and Johnston (1996) found *no difference* between somatic and initial segment densities. Because the Na^+ channels of the initial segment may be clustered (Angelides et al. 1988; Turner et al. 1994), it is possible that sampling problems hampered the patch clamp estimates. On the other hand, Colbert and Johnston (1996) also found no evidence for a substantially lower threshold at the initial segment compared to the soma, throwing considerable doubt on the applicability of the classical model to action potential initiation in pyramidal cells (see also below).

Other Properties   Because of their small diameters, central axons are very difficult to measure electrophysiologically. There is consequently very little such data on axonal specializations of voltage-dependent channels or other electrical properties. As for dendrites, all major channel types are likely to be found in axonal membranes, albeit perhaps different subtypes at different densities. The presence of a variety of Ca^{2+} channels in axon terminals responsible for neurotransmitter release is well documented (reviewed in Reuter 1996). Various members of the Kv family of K^+ channels (corresponding to I_A and I_{Kd}) have been localized to axons in immunocytochemical studies.

Myelinated axon segments generally have very low capacitance (Black, Kocsis, and Waxman 1990; Hille 1992), for example, $0.04\,\mu F/cm^2$ (Graham and Redman 1994). While there may be very little leak current or other channels associated with myelinated axonal segments, the resistance of the nodes is believed in some cases to be substantially lower than even that of somatodendritic membrane (Blight 1985; Black, Kocsis, and Waxman 1990), for example, $50\,\Omega\,cm^2$ (Graham and Redman 1994). This lower resistance could help to repolarize the membrane following an action potential in the absence of a delayed rectifier current, although various K^+ channels are known to be present in axons (Sheng et al. 1992, 1994; Wang et al. 1994; Maletic-Savatic, Lenn, and Trimmer 1995; Weiser et al. 1995). In addition, several recent modeling studies have used lower axonal than dendritic axial resistivity, for example, 70–$100\,\Omega\,cm$ versus 200–$300\,\Omega\,cm$ (Traub et al. 1994; Rapp, Yarom, and

Segev 1996; Migliore 1996), although there is little experimental evidence to support a disparity.

Propagation   Compared to dendritic processing, the subject of computation in the axons of pyramidal neurons has received relatively little attention (see reviews in Waxman 1975; Wall 1995). Three main classes of computation have been examined: (1) history-dependent spatiotemporal filtering of impulses (Chung, Raymond, and Lettvin 1970; Deschênes and Landry 1980b; Lüscher and Shiner 1990); (2) temporal delay processing (Manor, Koch, and Segev 1991); and (3) presynaptic inhibition of impulse conduction (Segev 1990; Graham and Redman 1994). These studies have been based on relatively simple models of action potential propagation (i.e., based on classical Hodgkin-Huxley Na^+ and K^+ currents), although evidence suggests that most of the channels contributing to the complexity of dendritic behavior are also present in axons. The potential impact of non-Hodgkin-Huxley channels on action potential conduction in axonal arbors (Lüscher et al. 1994b, 1994a) certainly bears further examination in compartmental models.

5.2.7   Exploring Parameters

From the data reviewed above, it is apparent that the practice of treating dendritic channel densities as free, unconstrained parameters is rapidly becoming untenable. It is nevertheless true that any model of a spatially extended neuron with active conductances will retain some degree of flexibility in assigning channel densities. Heterogeneity among cell subtypes and over developmental ages as well as variability across individual cells means that the idea of a canonical channel distribution will at best be a rough sketch. "Tuning" channel densities to fit a set of electrophysiological data will therefore be necessary. Indeed, this is considered to be the most arduous task in constructing a compartmental model and raises an interesting theoretical issue as to how each neuron determines and regulates these densities. One intriguing possibility is that local information in the time-varying membrane potentials and ion concentrations may control the local densities of particular channel types through up- and down-regulation as well as other biophysical mechanisms (Bell 1992; Siegel, Marder, and Abbot 1994 and chapter 10, this volume). The immediate concern of most modelers, however, is to find some way to constrain the parameters by matching simulations to experimental recordings.

In most studies, channel densities (and other parameters) are tuned by hand; that is, by trial and error, starting with plausible values for the parameters and changing them in some systematic way (e.g., Lytton and Sejnowski 1991; Traub et al. 1991, 1994; Rhodes and Gray 1994; Migliore, Alicata, and Ayala 1995; Mainen and

Sejnowski 1996). Although, in some cases, individual parameters may be directly related to specific electrophysiological variables, the correspondence is seldom simple: most behaviors are the net result of the interaction of multiple currents with the electrotonic structure of the neuron (Mainen and Sejnowski 1996). There is very little explicit description in the modeling literature about how the process of parameter tuning is carried out. In the best cases, a particular final set of channel densities is loosely justified in terms of direct measurements and their effects on net electrophysiolgical behavior (e.g., Traub and Llinás 1979, Traub 1982; Traub et al. 1985, 1991; Quadroni and Knöpfel 1994). A promising approach in this regard is the use of a combination of in vitro and in vivo recordings from the same cell type: constraints can be added progressively, starting with in vitro recordings from dissociated neurons without dendrites, and proceeding to recordings from a slice preparation in which the dendrites are present but there is minimal synaptic activity, and finally to in vivo recordings from neurons that reflect the full complexity of a dynamic, nonstationary environment (Destexhe et al. 1996).

A number of attempts to systematize the process of parameter tuning have been described (e.g., Foster, Ungar, and Schwaber 1993; Bhalla and Bower 1993; Eichler-West and Wilcox 1995; Baldi, Vanier, and Bower 1996). The number of combinations of parameters that must be searched goes up exponentially with the number of parameters, so that in even the simplest one-compartment model with a few dozen parameters, an exhaustive search over all possible combination is simply not feasible. While there are ways to find optimal combinations of parameters in high-dimensional spaces, they suffer from both local minimum and uniqueness problems. A set of parameters may be locally optimal in the sense that making small changes to the parameters increases the error of the fit (Bhalla and Bower 1993), but there may be a better overall set of parameters in a different part of the parameter space that has not been tested. An approach based on genetic algorithms offers a way to make large jumps in the values of some combinations of parameters (Eichler-West and Wilcox 1995). The problem with uniqueness is that there may be many combinations of parameter values that fit the limited data equally well. Without a sufficiently rich set of data to constrain all the parameters in the model, it is impossible to have any confidence in the interpretation of the model.

The primary difficulty of systematic approaches based on optimization has been the time required to compute a single "evaluation function" (i.e., a simulation run) —typically seconds. Increases in computer performance are making these approaches more practical. In particular, the fastest supercomputers are multiple instruction, multiple data (MIMD) machines that have thousands of microprocessors. Because each processor can run the same simulation program with a different set of parameters, taking full advantage of the computational power in a data-parallel way, these machines are ideal for exploring parameter spaces (see chapter 12, this volume).

A few general points are worth mentioning about confronting a complex model with thousands of parameters. First, there is a wide choice for the evaluation function, ranging from timing the occurrences of action potentials in response to current injection to matching statistical measures such as current-frequency curves (Foster, Ungar, and Schwaber 1993). Second, experimental data from a variety of conditions are needed to constrain most models, e.g., including the responses of neocortical neurons to fluctuating current injection, which is closer to in vivo conditions, as well as more conventional step current pulses (Mainen and Sejnowski 1995; Tang, Bartels, and Sejnowski 1997). Third, the problem of searching the space can be reduced to some extent by identifying parameters that covary; that is, the result may depend only on the ratios of some parameters, or on some other functional combination. A Bayesian framework offers a systematic way to take such dependencies into account (Baldi, Vanier, and Bower 1996). The most highly sensitive parameters in reproducing a particular result may be the most critical ones to constrain experimentally, and this may be one of the most important insights gained from the model.

Finally, if the goal of a model is to make a new discovery, in addition to summarizing existing data, the search for anomalies and failures of the model to fit aspects of the data may be more important than finding a perfect fit. When a model fails, the assumptions that went into constructing the model must be critically assessed, which can lead to new insights.

5.3 Applications

This section presents a few selected applications of compartmental models that have explored active dendritic function. Several examples have been chosen to illustrate how a detailed model helped to guide or illuminate electrophysiological studies along three lines of investigation: (1) synaptic integration in dendrites; (2) spike initiation and dendritic propagation; and (3) generation of firing patterns.

5.3.1 Synaptic Integration

Historically, dendrites have been seen as impeding current flow from synapses to the soma (Rinzel and Rall 1974). As a number of modeling studies have shown, synaptic inputs to distal dendritic locations suffer considerable attenuation in passive dendritic arbors of reconstructed neurons (Spruston et al. 1993; Zador, Agmon-Snir, and Segev 1995; Major et al. 1994; Mainen et al. 1996). A major role for excitable dendritic currents has been seen in boosting distal synaptic input to enhance its propagation to the soma (Perkel and Perkel 1985; Shepherd et al. 1985; Pongracz 1985; Segev and Rall 1988; Jaslove 1992; Wathey et al. 1992).

The problem of synaptic attenuation and the possible role of active currents was addressed by Connors and colleagues (Cauller and Connors 1992; Amitai et al. 1993; Cauller and Connors 1994). Although it was found electrophysiologically that stimulation of layer-1 input to the distal tuft of layer-5 pyramidal cells could produce a surprisingly strong somatic excitatory postsynaptic potential (EPSP), a model neuron with a passive dendritic tree and massive layer-1 input could not reproduce a somatic EPSP as large as those observed experimentally (figure 5.2). Two problems contributed to weakening the effects of distal input on the soma:

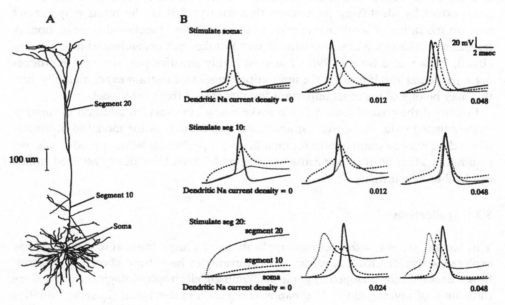

Figure 5.2
Simulations of soma-dendritic Na$^+$ spiking in a layer-5 pyramidal cell. (A) Camera lucida drawing of the modeled cell. Labels designate the locations of the three sites from which voltage charges are illustrated in panel B. (B) Effects of dendritic Na$^+$ channels and stimulus site on dendritic spiking; superimposed voltage responses from the soma (solid line), the trunk of the apical dendrite (segment 10; dashed line), and the end of apical trunk (segment 20; dotted line) while simulating with a step depolarizing pulse of current (intensity adjusted in each case to 1.5 times somatic spike threshold). Current was applied either at the soma (top row), to segment 10 (middle row), or to segment 20 (bottom row). Active Na$^+$ currents in the apical dendrites were assumed to be either absent (left column), at a relatively low density (middle column), or at a higher density (right column). Note that when the apical dendrites were passive (bottom left), it was not possible to bring the soma to spike threshold by stimulating segment 20, even when the local dendritic potential was positive.

1. The relatively high impedance of the distal branches leads to saturation of the synaptic current as the local membrane potential quickly depolarizes the neuron to near the synaptic reversal potential.

2. The cable properties (particularly the large axial resistance) of the dendritic arbor produce a large voltage drop between the distal site and the soma.

This anomaly between the model and the experimental results led to the hypothesis that low densities of Na^+ channels in the apical dendrite could boost layer-1 input enough to fire the cell (Cauller and Connors 1992; Amitai et al. 1993; Cauller and Connors 1994). This circumvents problem 2 by a counteracting the voltage drop along the apical dendrite. Bernander, Koch, and Douglas (1994) expanded on this idea by tackling problem 1 in addition to problem 2. By adding a depolarization-activated outward current to the apical dendrite, their model compensated for saturation of synaptic current, helping to counteract the local depolarization produced by large inputs. They derived the voltage-dependence of a K^+ current necessary to accomplish exact linearization and showed that a biophysically reasonable K^+ current would be roughly suitable. Thus, in principle, a combination of Na^+ boosting and K^+ linearization could serve to compensate for the effects of the passive cable properties on synaptic input.

Recently, several physiological studies have directly tested the actual contribution of Na^+ currents to synaptic potentials (Stuart and Sakmann 1995; Schwindt and Crill 1995; Lipowsky, Gillessen, and Alzheimer 1996). Studying CA1 neurons, Lipowsky, Gillessen, and Alzheimer (1996) demonstrated that the amplitude of distal synaptic EPSPs, measured at the soma, was reduced by tetrodotoxin (TTX) locally applied to the apical dendrite (and to a much lesser extent by TTX applied to the axon or soma). Interestingly, the shape of the EPSP was not affected by TTX. To ensure that TTX was not acting presynaptically (TTX blocks presynaptic action potentials as well as postsynaptic Na^+ channels), they used a local field potential recording of the synaptic current (which was not affected by TTX) and postsynaptic hyperpolarization (which reduced the observed boosting). Examined in a compartmental model, these observations were consistent with physiological densities of I_{Na} in the main apical dendrite. Moreover, a dendritically located low-voltage-activated K^+ current was also needed to reproduce the data: specifically, to account for the lack of significant shape change of the boosted EPSPs.

In a study of layer-5 pyramidal cells, Stuart and Spruston (1995) also demonstrated the ability of a persistent Na^+ current to boost subthreshold synaptic currents, although they arrived at somewhat different conclusions about the location of the Na^+ channels contributing to the synaptic boost. Their technique was to use a dendritic patch clamp electrode to inject current into the dendrite to mimic a synaptic current. This allowed them to use TTX to block I_{Na_p}. Interestingly, using local TTX application, they found that axosomatic Na^+ channels had a much greater effect than dendritic Na^+ channels in boosting the subthreshold current injection. Furthermore, dual axonic and somatic recordings showed that the site of greatest amplification was in fact the axon rather than the soma, consistent with suggestions that the axon initial segment contains a high density of Na^+ channels (Mainen et al. 1995; see also section 5.3.2). Schwindt and Crill (1995) also showed a contribution of I_{Na_p} to subthreshold amplification in layer-5 cells by examining the effect of TTX on iontophoretically applied pulses of glutamate.

One interpretation of the differences between these studies is a significantly different distribution of Na^+ channels between cortical layer-5 pyramidal cell and hippocampal CA1 pyramidal cells (Lipowsky, Gillessen, and Alzheimer 1996). The neocortical pyramidal cells may have a relatively higher axonal density of Na^+ channels.

Given the complexity and variety of the voltage-dependent Na^+, Ca^{2+}, and K^+ channels in dendrites, the possibility arises that nonlinear synaptic integration more complex than amplification could occur. Even in the passive case, synaptic conductance changes could themselves cause current shunting and nonlinear interactions between nearby synapses (Rall 1964; Wang and Zhang 1996). Relative timing of a few milliseconds between neighboring excitatory and inhibitory synapses could significantly affect the current that reaches the spike-initiating region. (For a detailed model of the effects of voltage-dependent dendritic currents on synaptic integration in cerebellar Purkinje cells, see chapter 6, this volume.)

Before the properties of active dendritic conductances were firmly established, the theoretical possibility of performing logical operations (AND, OR, XOR) between synaptic inputs was explored with simulations (Shepherd and Brayton 1987; Rall and Segev 1987; Zador, Claiborne, and Brown 1992; Fromherz and Gaede 1993). A strictly logical function would be difficult to arrange, however, and low-order polynomial functions offer a more likely mathematical approximation to synaptic integration (Mel 1993). Sums of polynomial functions computed in different dendritic branches could be used to approximate a wide range of nonlinear functions, including the properties of complex cells in visual cortex (Mel, Ruderman, and Niebur 1996), which could be learned through long-term potentiation at excitatory synapses through activation of NMDA receptors (Mel 1992). This literature is necessarily more speculative and, thus far, less tied to physiological data (see Mel 1994 for a review). As recordings from dendrites become better refined, it should be possible to arrive at much better approximations to the types of spatial and temporal nonlinearities that neocortical neurons could compute. The results of these experiments may have profound implications for theories of function of the neocortex.

5.3.2 Spike Initiation

The initiation of an all-or-none action potential is the point at which a neural signal is transformed from analog to pulse-coded information. The site at which this transformation occurs is critical to the nature of signal processing carried out by a neuron. A number of modeling studies have examined the possibility of dendritic spike initiation (e.g., Shepherd et al. 1985; Softky and Koch 1993; Softky 1994). This work has been based less on physiological data than on the appeal of the richer computational properties offered by nonlinear processing in dendrites. For example, using simulations, Shepherd et al. (1985) showed that the presence of Hodgkin-Huxley conductances in dendritic spines could give rise to nonlinear interactions between neighboring synaptic inputs, as well as saltatory dendritic conduction of action potentials. Similarly, Softky (1994) modeled a mechanism for submillisecond synaptic coincidence detection based on brief dendritic spikes carried by fast Na^+ and K^+ currents. The relevance of speculative proposals such as these depends critically on resolving the actual locus of spike initiation.

In the classical description of spike initiation derived from the motoneuron, initiation normally occurs in proximal segments of the axon (in the region of the axon hillock or initial segment); when orthodromic stimulation is increased, the site of initiation may move into the dendrites (Coombs, Curtis, and Eccles 1957b; Fatt 1957; Fuortes, Frank, and Becker 1957). In the hippocampus and neocortex, the possibly greater excitability of pyramidal cell dendrites could tend to favor dendritic spike initiation (Spencer and Kandel 1961).

Both orthodromic and antidromic dendritic spike propagation in the hippocampus were described originally using current source density measurements (Richardson, Turner, and Miller 1987; Turner et al. 1991; Turner, Meyers, and Barker 1993). Dual dendritic/somatic recordings confirmed that the axon is a preferential site for spike initiation in neocortical and hippocampal pyramidal cells (Stuart and Sakmann 1994; Spruston, Jonas, and Sakmann 1995; Colbert and Johnston 1996), but that dendritic spike initiation can occur in mature animals during strong synaptic stimulation (Turner et al. 1991; Regehr et al. 1993; Stuart and Sakmann 1996).

When spikes initiate first in the axon, the action potential backpropagates into the dendritic tree (Turner et al. 1991; Stuart and Sakmann 1994). This antidromically propagating action potential could signal the firing time of the neuron throughout the dendritic arbor, leading, for example, to Hebbian plasticity (Markram et al. 1997; Magee and Johnston 1997). The degree of invasion of the backpropagating action potential is not fixed (Spruston, Jonas, and Sakmann 1995; Svoboda et al. 1997) but can be regulated through Na^+ channel inactivation by previous spikes (modeled by Migliore 1996), K^+ channel activation, excitatory (Magee and Johnston 1997; Hoffman et al. 1997) or inhibitory (Buzsaki et al. 1996; Tsubokawa and Ross 1996) synaptic potentials, and, potentially, neuromodulators such as acetylcholine, norepinephrine, and serotonin.

Two recent modeling studies of spike initiation have attempted to account for the above experimental results using known anatomical and physiological properties of pyramidal cells (Mainen et al. 1995; Rapp, Yarom, and Segev 1996). Both studies used reconstructed cortical neurons and just two voltage-dependent currents, I_{Na} and I_{Kd}, assuming that the contributions from the other currents would not be significant during on the short time scale of spike initiation. The conclusions of the two studies were similar (figure 5.3):

1. The passive electrical load biases the neuron toward spike propagation in the antidromic direction. This is analogous to the greater ease with which a voltage signal is passed outward from the soma than inward toward the soma, (see chapter 2, this volume) although geometrical considerations alone are insufficient to account for a strong bias for axonal initiation.

2. The presence of a larger source of Na^+ current—either a very high density (Mainen et al. 1995) or a moderate density with altered kinetics (Rapp, Yarom, and Segev 1996)—in the axon initial segment can account for preferential axonal initiation (but compare with Colbert and Johnston 1996, discussed earlier).

3. Although density measurements for the dendritic and somatic Na^+ channels are similar (Stuart and Sakmann 1994), the experimentally observed decrement of the backpropagating spike can be reproduced because this density is low. The axonal Na^+ source serves to increase the amplitude of the somatic action potential.

4. A developmental increase in Na^+ density (Huguenard, Hamill, and Prince 1988) can account for the increased tendency toward dendritic initiation in older animals (Stuart and Sakmann 1996).

A recent physiological study (Hoffman et al. 1997) has shown that dendritic K^+ channels may also have a major role in the locus of initiation and control of dendritic action potential. An enrichment of an I_A-like current in the dendritic arbor (Maletic-Savatic, Lenn, and Trimmer 1995) can limit the size of transient events such as EPSPs and spikes, thereby shunting dendritic spikes. By activating during the rising phase of the action potential, this current could also reduce the amplitude of a backpropropagating spike, allowing for a relatively higher dendritic Na^+ current

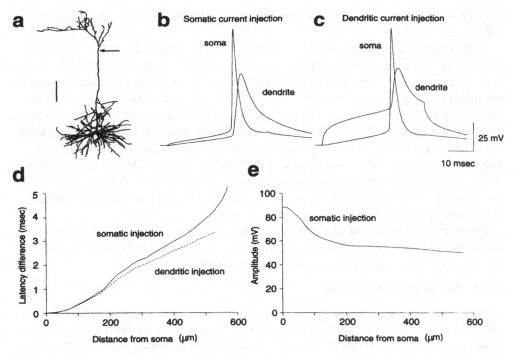

Figure 5.3
Site of action potential initiation in a model of a neocortical pyramidal neuron (compare to Stuart and Sakmann 1994, figure 1). (a) Digitally reconstructed layer-5 pyramidal neuron (courtesy of D. K. Smetters and S. Nelson, unpublished). Arrow indicates dendritic recording/stimulation site in panels b–c. Scale bar is 100 μm. (b) Simulation of action potentials evoked by a current step injected at the soma. Voltage traces from the soma and apical dendrite are shown. (c) Similar to panel b, but current injection is made at the dendritic site. (d) Latency difference between peak somatic and peak dendritic potential at different distances from the soma. Action potentials were elicited by somatic (solid line) or dendritic (dashed line) current injection. Latencies were measured using time-to-peak amplitude. (e) Action potential amplitude plotted as function of distance from the soma under the same conditions as in panel b following somatic injection. This figure is based on Mainen et al. 1995. NEURON code, including ".mod" files describing the active currents and ".hoc" code describing the morphologies and simulation setup, used to generate this figure is available; see "Internet Resources."

density, even while maintaining a decremental antidromic invasion (Hoffman et al. 1997).

In contrast to the many models that explore the consequences of Na^+ and Ca^{2+} currents in dendrites, models that explore the functional roles of dendritic K^+ currents have been few (e.g., Wilson 1995; Hoffman et al. 1997), in part because patch recordings and anatomical studies of K^+ currents are not as far advanced (Softky and Koch 1993; Bernander, Koch, and Douglas 1994; Wilson 1995; Andreasen and Lambert 1995). Both Rapp, Yarom, and Segev (1996) and Mainen et al. (1995) used a low density of dendritic K^+ channels to reproduce the relatively slow repolarization of the dendritic spike and the lack of AHP in the dendrites (Stuart and Sakmann 1994). However an I_A that inactivates rapidly enough may exert its influence primarily on the upstroke of a dendritic spike and become inactivated without contributing to a fast repolarization or AHP (Hoffman et al. 1997).

Given the importance of spike initiation for cortical signaling—all the information that flows into, out of, and between cortical areas is coded by spike trains—the axon hillock and initial segment deserve much more attention.

5.3.3 Intrinsic Firing Patterns

Different types of neurons produce different intrinsic rhythmic firing patterns when stimulated with a simple depolarizing current pulse in vitro in the absence of synaptic activity. For pyramidal neurons, these intrinsic patterns are typically either bursting (stereotyped clusters of two or more spikes firing at rates of up to 1,000 Hz) or adapting (firing at rapidly or gradually slowing rates; McCormick et al. 1985). The impression of these intrinsic properties can be seen in the characteristic firing modes of different types of neurons in vivo (e.g., complex spikes fired by hippocamal pyramidal cells, which relect their intrinsic bursting properties). Thus the temporal pattern of spikes emitted by a neuron in vivo reflects both the pattern of synaptic and modulatory input the neuron receives and the sculpting of this input by the dendritic, somatic, and axonal conductances that generate the spike train (Llinás 1988).

Modeling (and experimental) studies have begun to explore three important issues in the relationship between intrinsic firing patterns and neural signaling:

1. How are intrinsic firing patterns determined by the interplay of intrinsic conductances and neural geometry (see below)?

2. How do intrinsic currents interact with synaptic currents (e.g., Reyes and Fetz 1993; De Schutter and Bower 1994b, 1994c; Jaeger, De Shutter, and Bower 1997; Mainen and Sejnowski 1995; Tang, Bartels, and Sejnowski 1997)?

3. How do different temporal spike patterns interact with the filtering characteristics of synaptic transmission (e.g., Markram and Tsodyks 1996; Tsodyks and Markram 1997; Abbott et al. 1997; Lisman 1997)?

While all three issues are crucial to understanding the propagation of a neural signal, with respect to the modeling literature, the first is by far the best developed.

Models of bursting and repetitive firing in pyramidal neurons were pioneered by Traub and colleagues (Traub and Llinás 1979; Traub 1979, 1982; Traub et al. 1991, 1994). The original Traub model (Traub and Llinás 1979) laid out basic mechanisms by which slow dendritic Ca^{2+} and K^+ channels, partially coupled with somatic Na^+ channels, gave rise to rhythmic bursting in hippocampal pyramidal neurons. This model also documented the ability of dendritic Na^+ "hot spots" on fine dendrites to produce the fast prepotentials described in these neurons (Spencer and Kandel 1961). A revision of this model (Traub 1982) was constructed to account for data showing bursts generated locally in the dendrites (Wong, Prince, and Basraum 1979); this required the addition of dendritic inactivating K^+ conductances (I_A), a prediction that appears to have been borne out by the recent data (Hoffman et al. 1997).

The elaboration of the bursting model in Traub et al. (1994), which included an axon and more complex dendrites, combined synaptic and intrinsic voltage-dependent conductances. Versions of the Traub model have served as the starting point for other models aimed at exploring the influence of intrinsic properties of neurons on the interactions between neurons in area CA3 of the hippocampus. The model CA3 pyramidal neuron was also modified to serve as a CA1 pyramidal neuron by increasing I_{Kd} and decreasing dendritic I_{Ca} and I_C. After these alterations, tonic depolarization of the soma leads to adapting repetitive firing, whereas stimulation of the distal dendrites leads to bursting. A related model of bursting in neocortical neurons emphasized the importance of dendritic I_{Na} in propagating the somatic spike into the dendrites to trigger I_{Ca} (Rhodes and Gray 1994). Bursting in this model depended critically on the amount of I_{AHP} activation, and hence on the level of intracellular Ca^{2+}.

In these models of bursting, the Ca^{2+} currents in the dendrites produce the prolonged depolarization that initiates the fast Na^+ spikes, but there is increasing evidence that Na^+ currents themselves can produce bursts in some neurons (Turner et al. 1994; Franceschetti et al. 1995; Azouz, Jensen, and Yaari 1996). Because Na^+ currents are quite brief, the longer time scale of the burst must arise somehow from the geometry of the neuron and the interaction between different conductances in different compartments. Using reconstructed cortical neurons with different dendritic structures but a fixed distribution of ion channels, Mainen and Sejnowski (1996) have shown that the entire range of intrinsic firing patterns, including nonadapting, adapting, and bursting types, can be reproduced in a set of neurons that differ only in their geometry (figure 5.4). In their study, reconstructed layer-5 pyramidal cells with large dendritic arbors produced repetitive bursting to current injection, while more compact layer 2/3 pyramidal cells produced regular spiking behavior. These results demonstrated that the electrotonic structure of a neuron shapes the dynamic inter-actions between nonuniformly distributed ion channels, and may thereby shape the pattern of repetitive firing. The wide anatomical variety of neocortical dendrites (Peters and Jones 1984), supported the idea of a continuous spectrum of neocortical firing patterns (McCormick et al. 1985; Connors and Gutnick 1990), rather than discrete categories.

Mainen and Sejnowski (1996) suggested a causal relationship for the observed correlations between dendritic structure and firing properties (Connors and Gutnick 1990; Chagnac-Amitai, Luhmann, and Prince 1990; Mason and Larkman 1990; Franceschetti et al. 1995; Yang, Seamans, and Gorelova 1996) and emphasized the importance of active dendritic conductances in neuronal function. Quadroni and Knöpfel (1994) have also demonstrated in simulations that the number of dendrites may affect the firing patterns of medial vestibular neurons. Heterogeneity of den-dritic structure can thus parsimoniously explain some aspects of the heterogeneous firing properties of neurons in terms of their anatomical diversity, but heterogeneity in the distribution of channel may also be important. Indeed, a modeling study by Migliore, Alicata, and Ayala (1995) demonstrated that the effects of small differences in morphology can be overridden by tuning the relative densities of intrinsic currents such as sI_{AHP}.

Most of these models are based on data from cortical slices that lack the sponta-neous background firing activity and tonic neuromodulation that occurs in vivo. Models that take these conditions into account (Bernander et al. 1991; Rapp, Yarom, and Segev 1992; Tang, Bartels, and Sejnowski 1997) may reveal other properties of neurons that are important for their participation in perceptual and cognitive states.

5.4 Analysis

This chapter has focused on highly detailed models of pyramidal cells derived from anatomical and physiological data. The resulting models of active dendritic processes are complex, yet, however exhaustively their behavior may be scrutinized, new tools for analysis may be needed to achieve a deeper understanding of the phenomena they display. The development of these methods is still nascent, but several useful avenues are worth mentioning.

5.4.1 Reduced Models

If the complex behavior of a realistic model can be captured in a much simplified version of the model, understanding of the model can be enormously improved. Collapsing the number of compartments in a model is a good starting point for simplification. For passive electrical structures, several straightforward methods are discussed in chapter 3, this volume. With active models, reducing both the number of active conductances and the number of compartments may be useful (e.g., Lytton and Sejnowski 1991; chapter 10, this volume).

A single-compartment model will be sufficient when the electrotonic structure of the neuron is not relevant to its behavior, but otherwise, a minimal model consists of two compartments. Pinsky and Rinzel (1994) developed a simplification of the model of Traub et al. (1991) with just two compartments, identified as a soma and a dendrite. The electrical geometry was reduced to two parameters: the ratio of soma to dendrite area, ρ; and the coupling resistance between then, κ. Despite this simplicity, the model captured essential aspects of the generation of bursting in the Traub model not found in a single-compartment model (Pinsky and Rinzel 1994). The reduced number of parameters allows the model to be used efficiently in network simulations and aids in understanding the role played by electrical structure in the behavior of the model. (See more in chapter 10, this volume.)

Mainen and Sejnowski (1996) also used a two-compartment model similar to that of Pinsky and Rinzel (1994) to elucidate the effects of electrical geometry on the firing patterns of neocortical neurons. The full range of regular spiking responses, adaptation, afterdepolarizations, and repetitive bursting observed in recordings and in models of reconstructed pyramidal cells and inhibitory neurons could be reproduced in the two-compartment model. This reduced model shed light on the mechanisms responsible for the effects of geometry on the spike firing pattern observed in more detailed models of reconstructed neurons.

5.4.2 Current-Voltage Curves

One of the more informative analyses for understanding how a model neuron will respond to inputs is the current-voltage relationship (I-V curve). Because data from experimental recordings are often presented in this way, the I-V curve of the model can be compared directly with measurements. The steady-state, or static I-V curve, $I_\infty^{static}(V_m)$, is obtained by voltage clamping the soma to V_m and determining the asymptotic current. The slope of this curve defines the steady-state input conductance of the neuron as a function of membrane potential. The momentary, or instantaneous, I-V curve, $I_0(V_m)$, is obtained by changing the membrane potential

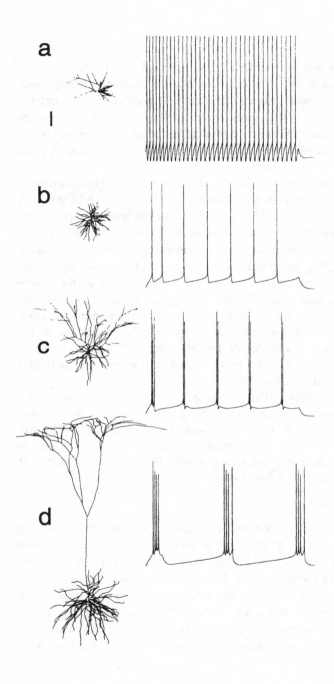

rapidly from the resting level to a new value, V_m, more rapidly than all the conductances (except for I_{Na}, which has an activation time of less than 100 μsec).

Koch, Bernander, and Douglas (1995) have analyzed the threshold of a model cortical pyramidal cell using the I-V relationships (figure 5.5). Near the spiking threshold, there is a local maximum in the $I_\infty^{static}(V_m)$, which corresponds to the current threshold for sustained inputs. The voltage threshold, which applies to rapid synaptic currents or current injection, occurs at a zero-crossing of $I_0(V_m)$, which is more depolarized than $I_\infty^{static}(V_m)$. Koch, Bernander, and Douglas (1995) define a third, dynamic I-V relationship, while the cell is spiking. The relationship between current inputs in the dendrites and spiking in the soma can also be studied using similar techniques (Jaeger, De Schutter, and Bower 1997).

5.4.3 Phase Plane Analysis

Because the previous histories of the ionic currents are also important in determining the response of a neuron to an input, the I-V curves defined above only give a rough idea of how a cell will respond to a more complex time-varying input. Hysteresis occurs already at the start of a simulation because the states of the activation and inactivation variables of all the ionic currents affect the subsequent dynamics. Phase plane analysis can be used to visualize and analyze the complex dynamics exhibited by neurons during simulations.

The "phase" in phase plane analysis refers to variables such as the membrane potential and current that dynamically change during a simulation but it also includes other variables such as the activation and inactivation variables for the ionic currents and ion concentrations. In the phase plane of current against membrane potential, the neuron follows a trajectory on a two-dimensional graph (see chapter 7, this volume). The current through specific channels or the internal Ca^{2+} concentration can also serve as axes in a phase plane. For example, Lytton and Sejnowski

Figure 5.4
Distinct firing patterns in model neurons with identical channel distributions but different dendritic morphology. Digital reconstructions of dendritic arbors of neurons from rat somatosensory cortex (panel a) and cat visual cortex (panels b–d). (a) Layer-3 aspiny stellate. (b) Layer-4 spiny stellate. (c) Layer-3 pyramid. (d) Layer-5 pyramid. Somatic current injection evoked characteristic firing patterns. Panel a shows only the branch lengths and connectivity, while panels b–d show a two-dimensional projection of the three-dimensional reconstruction. Scale bars: 250 μm (anatomy), 100 msec, 25 mV. Dendritic reconstructions were provided by J. Anderson, K. Martin, R. Douglas, L. Cauller, and B. Connors. Active conductances included four active currents: I_{Na} from Mainen et al. 1995; I_{Kd} from Mainen et al. 1995; I_M from Gutfreund, Yarom, and Segev 1995; I_{Ca} from Reuveni et al. 1993; and sI_{AHP} from Reuveni et al. 1993. This figure is based on Mainen and Sejnowski 1996. NEURON code, including ".mod" files describing the active currents and ".hoc" code describing the morphologies and simulation setup, used to generate this figure is available; see "Internet Resources."

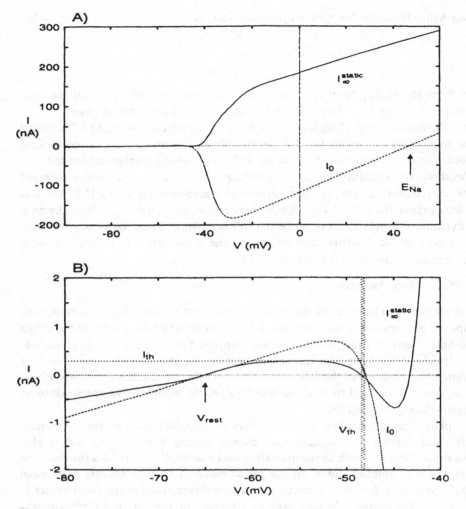

Figure 5.5
Current-voltage relationship for a model cell (Koch, Bernaabe and Douglas, 1995). The somatic membrane potential V_m was voltage-clamped and the clamp current '$I_\infty^{static}(V_m)$', recorded once steady state was reached. The instantaneous current-voltage curve '$I_0(V_m)$', assumes that the membrane potential is instantaneously displaced from V_{rest} to its new value at V_m. All somatic membrane conductances retain the values they had at V_{rest} with the sole exception of the fast sodium activation process—due to its very fast time constant (50 μsec) we assume that it reaches its steady-state value at V_m. (A) Full range. Note the very large amplitudes of I_0 (due to I_{Na} activation) and of $I_\infty^{static}(V_m)$ (due to I_{Dr} activation). The instantaneous current I_0 crosses over close to the reversal potential for I_{Na}. (B) Detail of panel A in the vicinity of the resting potential and spike threshold. Both curves reserves at V_{rest}. The slope of $I_\infty^{static}(V_m)$ corresponds to the inverse of the input resistance at rest. The right zero-crossing of I_0 occurs at $V_m = -48$ mV and that of $I_\infty^{static}(V_m)$ at -48.5 mV. The amplitude of $I_\infty^{static}(V_m)$ at the local peak around -54 mV represents the current threshold, I_{th}, for spike initiation, while the location of the middle zero-crossing of I_0 corresponds to the voltage threshold V_{th} for spike initiation (indicated by the thin gray area).

(1991) used phase plane analysis with these variables to explore the entrainment of cortical pyramidal neurons by inhibitory postsynaptic potentials. In some cases it is possible to gain a qualitative feel for the dynamics by plotting the null clines on the phase plane, which correspond to lines along which the derivatives of variables are zero (Murray 1989).

Phase plane analysis can reveal more about the mechanisms underlying dynamics through the application of bifurcation theory. As one parameter, such as input current or a conductance, is changed slowly, the phase plane trajectory for a repetitively firing neuron may qualitatively shift, for example, from a regular spiking mode to a bursting mode (see chapter 7, this volume; Butera, Clark, and Byrne 1996). This sudden shift indicates that a bifurcation has occurred in the dynamics; that is, a discontinuous change in the behavior of the system. In the theory of dynamical systems, the types of bifurcations that can occur have been classified and analyzed. Although this approach is normally used on simplified models of neurons that can be characterized by a few differential equations, new automated software systems such as XPP (Bard Ermentrout; see chapter 7, this volume; ftp://ftp.math.pitt.edu/pub/bardware/tut/start.htm) and "DsTool" (John Guckenheimer; ftp://macomb.tn.cornell.edu/pub/dstool) make it feasible to analyze the bifurcations in more realistic models systems represented by dozens of differential equations.

Internet Resources

An increasing number of valuable resources are available on the Internet. At our web site, http://www.cnl.salk.edu/CNL/simulations/methods.html, we have compiled a directory that includes code used to generate several of the models illustrated here (figures 5.3 and 5.4), as well as links to simulation software (e.g., NEURON and GENESIS) and models. This directory will be periodically updated.

Acknowledgments

The preparation of this chapter was supported by Howard Hughes Medical Institute, National Institutes of Health, and the Office of Naval Research. We are grateful to Venkatesh Murthy and Brian Christie for comments on this chapter.

6 Calcium Dynamics in Large Neuronal Models

Erik De Schutter and Paul Smolen

6.1 Introduction

Calcium is an important intracellular signaling molecule with rapid effect on the kinetics of many processes. As a consequence, almost all biophysically realistic models of neurons have to account for Ca^{2+} dynamics in some way, whether to model transmitter release or synaptic plasticity at individual synapses or to simulate the activation of K^+ channels in a complete cell. While most neuronal models have only considered Ca^{2+} inflow through voltage- or ligand-gated channels, release from intracellular Ca^{2+} stores may be physiologically as important.

This chapter builds on the basic approach to modeling ionic currents, Ca^{2+} diffusion, buffers, and pumps introduced in chapter 4, this volume, and assumes familiarity with those concepts. We describe how to simulate Ca^{2+} concentrations, $[Ca^{2+}]$, Ca^{2+} release activated by Ca^{2+} itself or by inositol-1,4,5-triphosphate (IP_3), and several other Ca^{2+} processes in complex models of dendritic trees (figure 6.1). Whenever appropriate, we describe how we implemented the equations[1] in the GENESIS neural simulator (described in chapter 12, this volume; see also Bower and Beeman 1995).

We use biophysically realistic models of Ca^{2+} dynamics in cerebellar Purkinje cells to investigate the dendritic physiology of these cells (for a recent review of the biology of Ca^{2+} signaling in Purkinje cells, see Eilers, Plant, and Konnerth 1996). An intriguing characteristic of the Purkinje cell is its very active dendrite, capable of generating large Ca^{2+} spikes (Llinás and Sugimori 1980), combined with the tremendous synaptic convergence of over 150,000 excitatory parallel fiber synapses onto this dendrite (Harvey and Napper 1991). In an earlier model of a rat Purkinje cell, using Hodgkin and Huxley–like equations (1952), we focused on accurately reproducing the properties of the different channel types (De Schutter and Bower 1994a). To model the activation of one of these, the large-conductance (BK or maxi-K) Ca^{2+}-activated K^+ channel, researchers have to compute $[Ca^{2+}]$ (Latorre et al. 1989). We choose to use a simple exponentially decaying Ca^{2+} pool (eq. 6.1), which is usually considered sufficient (e.g., Traub et al. 1991; Buchholtz et al. 1992; McCormick and Huguenard 1992). A very important advantage of this approach was that only one parameter β needed to be defined for the entire model (eq. 6.1). In fact, when building a large active membrane model that includes Ca^{2+} dynamics, one encounters a feedback loop: the Ca^{2+}-activated K^+ channels hyperpolarize the membrane, leading to reduced Ca^{2+} influx. In other words, modifying the Ca^{2+} dynamics will alter Ca^{2+} influx, which is functionally equivalent to changing the maximum

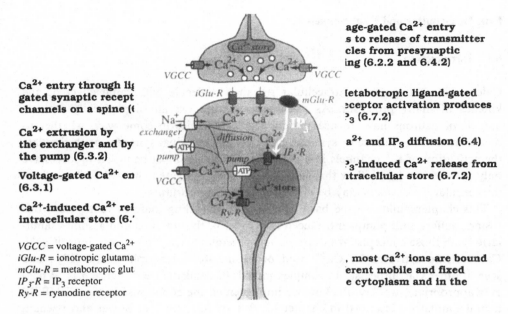

Ca²⁺ entry through li[
gated synaptic recept
channels on a spine ((

Ca²⁺ extrusion by
the exchanger and by
the pump (6.3.2)

Voltage-gated Ca²⁺ en
(6.3.1)

Ca²⁺-induced Ca²⁺ rel
intracellular store (6.'

VGCC = voltage-gated Ca²⁺
iGlu-R = ionotropic glutama
mGlu-R = metabotropic glut
IP₃-R = IP₃ receptor
Ry-R = ryanodine receptor

age-gated Ca²⁺ entry
s to release of transmitter
cles from presynaptic
ing (6.2.2 and 6.4.2)

letabotropic ligand-gated
eceptor activation produces
?₃ (6.7.2)

a²⁺ and IP₃ diffusion (6.4)

?₃-induced Ca²⁺ release from
itracellular store (6.7.2)

, most Ca²⁺ ions are bound
erent mobile and fixed
e cytoplasm and in the

Figure 6.1
Overview of Ca²⁺ processes in a presynaptic ending and a dendritic spine. The boldface text describes each process and points to the corresponding section in this chapter. Similar Ca²⁺ processes occur in the dendrite and soma.

conductance levels, $\bar{g}$, of the Ca²⁺ channels. Finding the appropriate $\bar{g}$ levels for the channels at different locations in the model was difficult enough without the additional complications of simulating detailed Ca²⁺ dynamics. But even if [Ca²⁺] is needed only to simulate the activation of K⁺ channels, the exponentially decaying pool model may not be sufficient. In fact, the slower activating small-conductance (SK or AHP) Ca²⁺-activated channel seems to sense different [Ca²⁺] from that sensed by the BK channel (Lancaster and Zucker 1994) and may even depend on Ca²⁺-activated Ca²⁺ release (Sah 1996). Multiple types of Ca²⁺-activated K⁺ channels are present in Purkinje cells (Gruol, Jacquin, and Yool 1991), but kinetic data on their Ca²⁺ dependence are lacking.

Our earlier version of the Purkinje cell model was quite successful in reproducing synaptic responses (De Schutter and Bower 1994b): it predicted that a small, localized parallel fiber input could cause a focal activation of dendritic Ca²⁺ channels (De Schutter and Bower 1994c), which was later confirmed experimentally (Eilers, Augustine, and Konnerth 1995). This dendritic Ca²⁺ channel activation amplifies parallel fiber–evoked excitatory postsynaptic potentials (EPSPs), making the somatic response of the Purkinje cell model insensitive to the location of its parallel fiber inputs. This is in direct contrast to the predictions from passive membrane modeling (see chapters 2 and 3, this volume). Even more interesting, the active dendrite amplifies subthreshold background synaptic inputs as well, resulting in an increased variability of the somatic response to synchronous parallel fiber input (De Schutter 1995). This turns out to be caused by the Ca^{2+}-activated K^+ channels and raises the question of whether other mechanisms influencing dendritic $[Ca^{2+}]$ could modify synaptic responses also.

It has been long known that Purkinje cell dendrites contain high densities of intracellular Ca^{2+} stores (Martone et al. 1993), making these cells a popular preparation for the study of Ca^{2+} release mechanisms (Berridge 1993). Calcium release from these stores can be activated both by synaptic stimulation of metabotropic glutamate receptors (Llano et al. 1991) and by Ca^{2+} itself (Llano, DiPolo, and Marty 1994; Kano et al. 1995). But the physiological role of these processes remains unclear, and positive evidence for Ca^{2+} release under normal in vivo conditions is still lacking. It is unlikely that this question will soon be resolved experimentally because the present recording techniques are not sensitive enough (see section 6.6.4, on the limitations of fluorescent Ca^{2+} indicators). Another problem experimentalists face is the lack of a fast "calcium clamp," similar to the voltage clamp procedure. As a consequence, the kinetics of many Ca^{2+} related procedures have been studied exclusively under steady-state conditions, and only a few gating studies of Ca^{2+}-activated K^+ channels are available (e.g., Moczydlowski and Latorre 1983; Dichiara and Reinhart 1995). The introduction of caged release of Ca^{2+} and of second messengers (Wang and Augustine 1995) has made possible more detailed kinetic studies (Györke and Fill 1993).

These experimental limitations make developing realistic models of Ca^{2+} dynamics in Purkinje cells both more important and more difficult. We and others have demonstrated that compartmental models of neurons incorporating Hodgkin and Huxely–like channels can be used to probe single-cell function in vivo (Bernander et al. 1991; De Schutter and Bower 1994b; see chapters 4 and 5, this volume). This is important because, in the case of the Purkinje cell, even simple experiments demonstrate that the firing properties in vivo are completely different from those in slice (Jaeger, De Schutter, and Bower 1997). Similarly, we expect our modeling to contribute to a better understanding of the role of intracellular Ca^{2+} release in vivo and of the importance of Ca^{2+} channels on spines (Denk, Sugimori, and Llinás 1995).

In this chapter we describe how we developed a more detailed model of the Ca^{2+} dynamics in the Purkinje cell, presenting some preliminary results to demonstrate the importance of simulating these mechanisms. We also consider other models of ionic concentrations. Indeed, we start by considering models that are not realistic at all.

6.2 Phenomenological Models of Calcium Dynamics

The first question that should always be asked is whether it is necessary to simulate Ca^{2+} dynamics with a complete biophysical model including Ca^{2+} diffusion, buffers, and pumps. If the only reason to simulate $[Ca^{2+}]$ is to couple two processes of interest to the modeler, it might be better to use a simple ad hoc model that computes an "effective $[Ca^{2+}]$." Such a "phenomenological" model will contain fewer parameters than a biophysical model and will therefore be much easier to constrain with experimental data. Especially if the relevant Ca^{2+} concentrations have never been measured, a biophysical model of $[Ca^{2+}]$ may bear little resemblance to the real system, however realistic the model may appear.

6.2.1 The Simple Pool Model of Calcium Concentration

The exponentially decaying Ca^{2+} pool (Traub and Llinás 1977) is the most frequently used model of $[Ca^{2+}]$ in neuronal simulations. It describes the change in $[Ca^{2+}]$ in a single compartment as

$$\frac{d[Ca^{2+}]}{dt} = -\frac{I_{Ca}}{2Fv} - \beta([Ca^{2+}] - [Ca^{2+}]_{min}). \tag{6.1}$$

The first term of this equation describes the change caused by Ca^{2+} inflow into a compartment with volume v (F is Faraday's constant; see eq. 4.15); the second is a decay term that causes $[Ca^{2+}]$ to relax exponentially with a time constant $1/\beta$ to the baseline concentration $[Ca^{2+}]_{min}$. Often referred to as a "diffusion rate constant" (McCormick and Huguenard 1992) or a "Ca^{2+} buffering constant" (LeMasson, Marder, and Abbott 1993), the constant β lumps together many different mechanisms causing a reduction in $[Ca^{2+}]$.

The implicit formulation of eq. 6.1 used in the GENESIS neural simulator is based on the trapezoidal rule and depends on the computation of I_{Ca} at a time offset by half a time step Δt from the time at which voltage is computed (see section 14.3.6):

$$[Ca^{2+}]_{t+\Delta t} = [Ca^{2+}]_{min} + \frac{([Ca^{2+}]_t - [Ca^{2+}]_{min})(1 - \beta\frac{\Delta t}{2})}{1 + \beta\frac{\Delta t}{2}} - \frac{\Delta t}{1 + \beta\frac{\Delta t}{2}}\frac{I_{Ca,t+\Delta t/2}}{2Fv}. \tag{6.2}$$

Values for β range from $0.02\,\text{msec}^{-1}$ (Traub and Llinás 1977) to $10\,\text{msec}^{-1}$ (De Schutter and Bower 1994a). A large β makes $[Ca^{2+}]$ follow changes in I_{Ca} closely with minimal accumulation of Ca^{2+}. An often used modification to eq. 6.1 is to restrict v to the volume of a submembrane shell (Traub et al. 1991; De Schutter and Bower 1994a).

Eq. 6.1 is useful for neuronal models where $[Ca^{2+}]$ is needed only to simulate the activation of the large conductance (BK) Ca^{2+}-activated K^+ channel (Latorre et al. 1989). But it can also be used in more complex models that include Ca^{2+}-regulated molecular processes. A nice example is the activity-dependent regulation of channel densities in a model by LeMasson, Marder, and Abbott (1993). The $[Ca^{2+}]$ was computed by eq. 6.1 and then used to dynamically change the densities ($\bar{g}$) of all the ionic channels represented in the model:

$$\tau \frac{d\bar{g}}{dt} = \frac{G_T}{1 + e^{\gamma([Ca^{2+}] - C_T)}} - \bar{g}. \tag{6.3}$$

In eq. 6.3, a rise of $[Ca^{2+}]$ above C_T will cause a slow increase in the maximum conductance $\bar{g}$ of K^+ channels ($\gamma < 0$) and a decrease in the conductance of Ca^{2+} and Na^+ channels ($\gamma > 0$). LeMasson, Marder, and Abbott showed that, depending on the target concentration C_T and the maximum conductance G_T, the conductance levels in single-compartment models change dynamically until the modeled cell becomes silent, regularly firing, or bursting. The same method was later successfully applied to a multicompartmental model of a pyramidal neuron (Siegel, Marder, and Abbott 1994). These results demonstrate how one can combine biophysically realistic models (Hodgkin and Huxley–like equations) with an extremely simple ad hoc model to simulate complex dynamic processes.

6.2.2 A Model of Synaptic Transmitter Release

If the exponentially decaying pool of eq. 6.1 is not sufficient to model the dynamics of the system, it might still be appropriate to use an ad hoc model, with its parameters directly fitted to the available physiological data. Such ad hoc models can replicate the desired behavior to a high degree of accuracy. This approach was used in a model of graded synaptic transmission between leech neurons (De Schutter, Angstadt, and Calabrese 1993). In this case, our goal was to study the role of graded synaptic inhibition in the generation of oscillatory network activity (Calabrese and De Schutter 1992). The actual mechanisms controlling transmitter release were not relevant to this goal, but the model needed to replicate the relation between presynaptic voltage (V_{pre}) and postsynaptic current (I_{syn}) accurately. Because voltage-gated Ca^{2+}inflow is responsible for spike-mediated synaptic transmission (Augustine, Charlton, and Smith 1985; Parnas, Parnas, and Hochner 1991; Sabatini and Regehr 1997), it seemed evident to postulate a similar mechanism for graded release.

Extensive experimental data were available, consisting of dual voltage clamps of coupled interneurons, which simultaneously measured the Ca^{2+} currents (I_{Ca}) in the presynaptic cell and the synaptic current (I_{syn}) in the postsynaptic cell (Angstadt and Calabrese 1991). We decided to build an ad hoc model relating these two variables:

$$\frac{d[P_{pre}]}{dt} = \max\left(-I_{Ca} - A(V_{pre}), 0\right) - B(V_{pre})[P_{pre}] \tag{6.4}$$

$$I_{syn} = \bar{g}[P_{pre}]^3(V_{post} - E_{syn}). \tag{6.5}$$

These equations relate an effective Ca^{2+} concentration $[P_{pre}]$ to the voltage-gated Ca^{2+} inflow I_{Ca} (eq. 6.4), with transmitter release and the postsynaptic conductance proportional to the third power of $[P_{pre}]$ (Augustine, Charlton, and Smith 1985; eq. 6.5). The Ca^{2+} currents were described by conventional Hodgkin and Huxley–like equations. A first version of the ad hoc model contained only the Ca^{2+} inflow I_{Ca} and the removal factor B (similar to β in eq. 6.1 with $[Ca^{2+}]_{min} = 0$), but such a model could not adequately fit the data. A transient I_{Ca} is activated at the beginning of each depolarizing voltage step, causing the initial Ca^{2+} inflow to be much larger than I_{syn}. Therefore, a parameter A that subtracts the part of the Ca^{2+} current ineffective in causing transmitter release was introduced in eq. 6.4. All that remained to be done was to find voltage-dependent equations for the parameters A and B by fitting the model to each of six voltage steps (De Schutter, Angstadt, and Calabrese 1993).

This simple model of computing an "effective Ca^{2+} concentration" $[P_{pre}]$ from the Ca^{2+} inflow was highly effective in reproducing the oscillatory firing behavior of two reciprocally coupled interneurons (Calabrese and De Schutter 1992; De Schutter, Angstadt, and Calabrese 1993). Subsequently, the model was further improved by making the dependence on $[P_{pre}]$ in eq. 6.5 saturating (Nadim et al. 1995) which allowed several model predictions to be confirmed experimentally (Olsen and Calabrese 1996).

This example demonstrates the advantages and disadvantages of such phenomenological models. Quite effective in the network simulations for which it was built, the model computed rapidly and was robust for large variations of its other parameters (Nadim et al. 1995). Yet it also required specific modifications to the simulator code before it could be used. Most general neural simulators (De Schutter 1992) require at least a recompilation and often also modifications of the source code before they can run an ad hoc model.

Another consequence of this approach is that the properties of the model will reflect the kind of data used to generate it. In this specific example, both parameters A

and B are voltage-dependent. This was an artifact caused by the use of voltage clamp data, where the membrane potential is of course accurately known. While there is some evidence for the involvement of voltage-dependent processes in transmitter vesicle docking mechanisms (Parnas, Parnas, and Hochner 1991), it should be emphasized that the voltage dependence of the parameters in eq. 6.4 has no biophysical meaning. In practice, however, the relevance of such models may be unclear unless it is made very plain which parts are biophysically realistic (the Hodgkin-Huxley equations) and which are not (e.g., eq. 6.4).

6.3 Rectifying Calcium Channels and Pumps

In this section we describe methods to model nonohmic currents and the electrogenic effect of pumps (the simulation of ohmic currents, i.e., currents with a linear dependence on voltage, is described in chapter 4, this volume). We also briefly describe the results obtained with the new Purkinje cell model (more detailed information on this model, the parameter values used, and how to obtain the GENESIS scripts to run it can be found in chapter appendix A).

6.3.1 Goldman-Hodgkin-Katz Equation

The standard model of ionic currents introduced by Hodgkin and Huxley (1952) is ohmic, that is, it assumes the instantaneous current-voltage relation is linear. This is not true if the external concentration of the permeant ion is very different from the internal one, causing current to pass more easily in one direction (rectification; Hille 1992). Calcium ions have a concentration ratio of about 50,000:1, which makes outward Ca^{2+} currents very small. The concentration-dependent rectification of ionic currents is usually described by the Goldman-Hodgkin-Katz constant field equation, commonly called the "GHK equation" (Goldman 1943; Hodgkin and Katz 1949a):

$$I_{Ca} = P_{Ca} z_{Ca}^2 \frac{VF^2}{RT} \frac{[Ca^{2+}]_i - [Ca^{2+}]_o \, e^{-z_{Ca} FV/RT}}{1 - e^{-z_{Ca} FV/RT}}, \tag{6.6}$$

with P_{Ca} as the channel permeability to Ca^{2+} ions, z_{Ca} the valency (here equal to $+2$), V the voltage and R, F, and T the gas constant, Faraday constant, and absolute temperature, respectively. The assumptions underlying this equation can be found in Jack, Noble, and Tsien 1975 and in Hille 1992. When the GHK equation is used, Ca^{2+} currents become quite nonlinear and small above 0 mV, but they will still reverse above $+120$ mV, that is, at the Nernst potential for Ca^{2+}. To obtain the reversal potential of between $+40$ mV and $+70$ mV that is observed experimentally, a second GHK equation must be included to model the permeability of the Ca^{2+} channel to K^+ ions (Hille 1992).

To use eq. 6.6 in standard compartmental models the voltage-dependent gating of I_{Ca} needs to be incorporated. Strictly speaking, the gating concept is incompatible with the GHK equation because the latter does not consider membrane pores at all (Hille 1992)! The permeability, P_{Ca}, is in fact a measure of how easily Ca^{2+} ions diffuse across the cell membrane (units m/sec) and is usually expressed relative to other permeabilities, for example, P_{Ca}/P_{Na} is the relative permeability of a Na^+ channel to Ca^{2+} ions. In practice, however, Hodgkin and Huxley–like equations can be used to compute m_{Ca} and h_{Ca} (see chapter 4, this volume) and, from these, the voltage-dependent membrane permeability to Ca^{2+}:

$$P_{Ca}(V) = \bar{g}' m_{Ca}^2 h_{Ca}. \tag{6.7}$$

Note that in this approximation $\bar{g}'$ has the dimensions of a permeability (m/sec) and should be about 10^7 times smaller than the corresponding maximum conductance $\bar{g}$ (in siemens; eq. 4.5) to obtain a similar amplitude I_{Ca}. Once P_{Ca} is computed, it is trivial to use eq. 6.6 to replace the ohmic equation for I_{Ca} in the voltage equation if a forward Euler method is used (eq. 14.46). But how should eq. 6.6 be incorporated into an implicit method (e.g., eq. 14.47)? One solution is to accept that the GHK equation makes the voltage equation nonlinear and use iterative solution methods (see chapter 14, this volume). We have implemented a faster, but potentially less accurate, method in the GENESIS simulator, which uses a local linearization of the GHK equation. In addition to eq. 6.6, its derivative over V, the slope conductance (Jack, Noble, and Tsien 1975), is also computed:

$$
\begin{aligned}
g'_{Ca} &= \frac{dI_{Ca}}{dV} \\
&= P_{Ca} z_{Ca}^2 \frac{F^2}{RT} \frac{[Ca^{2+}]_i - [Ca^{2+}]_o e^{-z_{Ca}FV/RT}}{1 - e^{-z_{Ca}FV/RT}} \\
&\quad - P_{Ca} z_{Ca}^3 \frac{F^3}{R^2 T^2} ([Ca^{2+}]_i - [Ca^{2+}]_o) \frac{V e^{-z_{Ca}FV/RT}}{(1 - e^{-z_{Ca}FV/RT})^2}.
\end{aligned}
\tag{6.8}
$$

Assuming that I_{Ca} is linear for V over the step Δt, the slope conductance g'_{Ca} can be used to compute a "slope reversal potential":

$$E'_{Ca} = \frac{g'_{Ca} V - I_{Ca}}{g'_{Ca}}. \tag{6.9}$$

As long as g'_{Ca} is positive, it can be used together with E'_{Ca} in eq. 14.47. This solution was perfectly stable and fast for the computation of the two Ca^{2+} currents in the Purkinje cell model. The local linearization approach of eqs. 6.8–6.9 works because the GHK current deviates most from linearity when it is small (Hille 1992, 343).

6.3.2 Calcium Pumps

Other types of nonohmic currents in the Purkinje cell model include membrane pumps. Usually the electrogenic component of such pumps is neglected (see, for example, chapter 4, this volume), but we will demonstrate that these pumps can carry a sizable current. As described in section 4.6.4, two major types of plasma membrane Ca^{2+}-pumping mechanisms have been identified. The Ca^{2+}-ATPase pump is a high-affinity, low-capacity pump causing an outward current. Its Ca^{2+} dependence can be approximated with a Michaelis and Menten function (1913; Garrahan and Rega 1990; Zador, Koch, and Brown 1990):

$$I_{Ca-ATP} = z_{Ca} F a_i V_{max} \frac{[Ca^{2+}]_i}{K_d + [Ca^{2+}]_i}, \tag{6.10}$$

where V_{max} is the maximal pump rate (units of $mol\,cm^{-2}\,msec^{-1}$, taking into account the surface density of the pump), K_d the dissociation constant, and a_i the outer membrane surface area of the compartment. Eq. 4.15 can be used to compute the decrease in $[Ca^{2+}]_i$ caused by the pump. Because eq. 6.10 has no voltage dependence, it can be considered constant during the step Δt in the voltage equation. Consequently, it can be divided by the membrane capacitance C_m and added as $(\Delta t/C_m)I_{Ca-ATP}$ to the right sides of eq. 14.46 or 14.47.

Na^+-Ca^{2+} Exchanger The second pump is the Na^+-Ca^{2+} exchanger, which has a lower affinity for Ca^{2+}, but a higher capacity to remove Ca^{2+}. It uses the transmembrane Na^+ gradient to move Ca^{2+} ions, with a stoichiometry of $3:1$. DiFrancesco and Noble (1985) have developed a model of the cardiac Na^+-Ca^{2+} exchanger, which has been applied to neuronal models (Gabbiani, Midtgaard, and Knöpfel 1994):

$$I_{NaCa} = k_{NaCa} a_i \left([Ca^{2+}]_o [Na^+]_i^3 e^{\gamma FV/RT} - [Ca^{2+}]_i [Na^+]_o^3 e^{(\gamma-1)FV/RT} \right), \tag{6.11}$$

with k_{NaCa} (units of $\mu A\,mM^{-4}\,cm^{-2}$) as a factor controlling the maximum exchange current and γ as a partition parameter representing the fractional position within the membrane of the voltage-sensitive energy barrier (usually taken to be 0.38; Hille 1992). If $[Ca^{2+}]_i$ is sufficiently high, eq. 6.11 results in an inward current. Eq. 4.15

with a net "effective valency" z of -1 can be used to compute the change of $[Ca^{2+}]_i$. This current is, like the GHK current, voltage-dependent and nonohmic. To solve it implicitly, we have used a similar approach by computing a slope conductance g' and using eq. 6.9 to compute the "slope reversal potential." Unfortunately, the dependence of the Na^+-Ca^{2+} exchange current on voltage becomes less linear when I_{NaCa} increases due to a rise in $[Ca^{2+}]_i$; because it remains a small current (see figure 6.2), however, the inaccuracies introduced by the local linearization are small.

Purkinje Cell Model   The Ca^{2+}-ATPase pump was modeled using eq. 6.10 with a V_{max} of $9 \cdot 10^{-11}$ mol cm^{-2} msec^{-1} and a K_d of 1 µM. The Na^+-Ca^{2+} exchanger had a k_{NaCa} of $1.4 \cdot 10^{-3}$ µA mM^{-4} cm^{-2} (eq. 6.11). Na^+ concentrations were assumed to be constant at 10 mM inside and 125 mM outside (Aidley 1991).

Figure 6.2 compares the electrogenic currents to the voltage-gated currents during dendritic Ca^{2+} spikes. As expected from their stoichiometry, the pump caused an outward current and the exchanger an inward one. In between dendritic spikes, the high-affinity pump dominated, contributing significantly to the total outward current of the model. During the dendritic spike, the exchanger partially counteracted the pump current, but not completely. This is because the depolarization diminished the exchange current, without affecting the Ca^{2+}-ATPase pump. The relative contributions of both depended, however, on the exact maximum pump rates V_{max} and k_{NaCa} used, parameters for which unfortunately little data are available.

The electrogenic current of the pump and exchanger contributed significantly to the resting membrane potential (-68 mV in the model, with a resting $[Ca^{2+}]$ of 40 nM). At rest, the outward pump current (-0.81 pA in the compartment shown is figure 6.2) counteracted the small inward I_{Ca} currents (0.92 pA). At rest, the Na^+-Ca^{2+} exchanger was also outward (-0.27 pA), but its size depended critically on the resting $[Na^+]_i$. Outward exchanger currents have been described in the experimental literature (Reeves 1990).

Tabulated Equations   Because solving eq. 6.6 and eqs. 6.8–6.9 (or eq. 6.11) requires many computations, the GENESIS neural simulator uses precomputed tables whenever possible. If $[Ca^{2+}]_o$, $[Na^+]_i$, and $[Na^+]_o$ are constant, a two-dimensional table indexed by V and $[Ca^{2+}]_i$ can be precomputed to rapidly obtain the slope conductance and reversal potential.

It is always difficult to predict whether the use of precomputed tables will increase simulation speed. Two factors determine the speed of tabulated functions: memory access, which tends to be slower than floating point operations on modern computers, and interpolation. Interpolation may not be necessary for purely voltage-dependent functions (see chapter 14, this volume). But with Ca^{2+}-dependent functions,

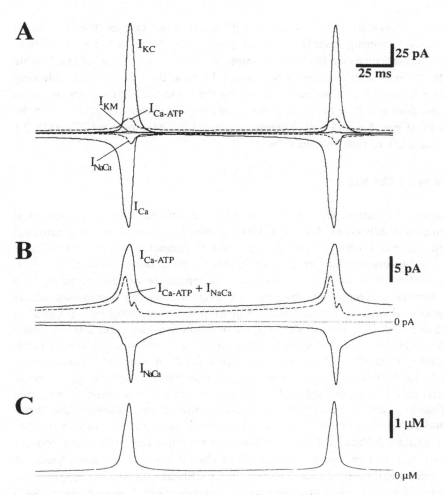

Figure 6.2
Voltage and Ca^{2+}-gated currents in a spiny dendritic compartment during two Ca^{2+} spikes in the Purkinje cell model. (A) Comparison of the electrogenic Ca^{2+}-ATPase pump and Na^{+}-Ca^{2+} exchanger currents (broken lines) with the Ca^{2+} and K^{+} currents (full lines). The persistent outward Ca^{2+}-ATPase pump current is the largest dendritic current in between the two spikes. (B) The two electrogenic currents and their sum (broken line) are shown at a larger scale. (C) $[Ca^{2+}]$ in the submembrane shell of the same spiny dendritic compartment.

it is difficult to make the table increment sufficiently small because the table must include a range covering several orders of magnitude. Also, in the case of two-dimensional tables, memory limitations simply do not allow the use of small table increments. Even if they are not faster, tables do have the advantage of allowing many different functions to be implemented by the same code. Moreover, if tables are used, one does not have to check continuously for singularities (e.g., $V = 0$ in the denominator of eqs. 6.6 and 6.8). Therefore, the implicit methods in GENESIS 2.1 make extensive use of interpolated tables.

6.4 Diffusion of Calcium

In this section, we extend the solution for buffered diffusion in a single spherical compartment (introduced in chapter 4, this volume) to diffusion in large neuronal models with several compartments having different geometries. A compartment is considered to be isopotential (see chapter 3, this volume), but because of the short space constant of diffusion (see section 6.6.5), it cannot be isoconcentration. In a complete biophysical representation, the coupling between compartments occurs both by potential and by concentration (potential has been described in detail in chapters 2 and 3, this volume, as the axial current flow between compartments; here we consider only diffusion). In general, diffusion of Ca^{2+} and other molecules needs to be treated in three dimensions (see also section 6.4.2). But, if Ca^{2+} fluxes are assumed to be uniform across the membrane of a cylindrical compartment, no longitudinal gradients will be created within the compartment. As a consequence, only radial diffusion needs to be considered within compartments, allowing the three-dimensional diffusion system to be reduced to a one-dimensional system that is much easier to compute. Although such a one-dimensional approach neglects the concentration gradients between compartments, which should cause longitudinal fluxes, in practice, concentration gradients between compartments (at similar depths) are much smaller than the radial gradients within compartments (compare figure 6.6D to figure 6.7A).

6.4.1 One-Dimensional Diffusion in Cylinders and Spheres

Fick's first law (1855) states that the diffusion flux $J_{Ca,D}$ is proportional and opposite to the concentration gradient:

$$J_{Ca,D} = -aD_{Ca}\frac{\partial[Ca^{2+}]}{\partial x}, \tag{6.12}$$

where the one-dimensional flux $J_{Ca,D}$ has the units of mol/sec, a is the area across which diffusion occurs, and D_{Ca} is the diffusion constant for Ca^{2+}. Discretization of eq. 6.12 leads to

$$J_{i \to j} = D_{Ca} \frac{a_{i,j}}{\delta_{i,j}} ([Ca^{2+}]_i - [Ca^{2+}]_j), \tag{6.13}$$

with $\delta_{i,j}$ as the distance between the points where $[Ca^{2+}]_i$ and $[Ca^{2+}]_j$ are measured. The change in $[Ca^{2+}]$ caused by the diffusion flux $J_{i \to j}$ will be determined by the volume v in which $J_{i \to j}$ is diluted. This leads to the explicit forward Euler formulation for the change in $[Ca^{2+}]_i$ due to one-dimensional diffusion between the shells i and $i + 1$:

$$[Ca^{2+}]_{i,t+\Delta t} - [Ca^{2+}]_{i,t} = \Delta t\, D_{Ca} C_{i,i+1} ([Ca^{2+}]_{i+1,t} - [Ca^{2+}]_{i,t}), \tag{6.14}$$

where the coupling constant $C_{i,i+1}$ is defined as

$$C_{i,i+1} = \frac{a_{i,i+1}}{v_i \delta_{i,i+1}}. \tag{6.15}$$

The coupling constant (units $1/m^2$) depends on the specific geometry of the shells and will usually be different for any pair of neighboring shells. The implicit Crank and Nicholson (1947) formulation of eq. 6.14 is

$$[Ca^{2+}]_{i,t+\Delta t} - [Ca^{2+}]_{i,t}$$

$$= \frac{\Delta t}{2} D_{Ca} C_{i,i+1} ([Ca^{2+}]_{i+1,t+\Delta t} - [Ca^{2+}]_{i,t+\Delta t} + [Ca^{2+}]_{i+1,t} - [Ca^{2+}]_{i,t}). \tag{6.16}$$

The Crank-Nicolson method is the preferred method for the solution of diffusion problems (Fletcher 1991; Press et al. 1992). Usually, a shell $i - 1$ will also be present. This gives rise to a second set of terms in eq. 6.14 and 6.16. For eq. 6.16, adding these terms and rewriting gives

$$-\frac{\Delta t}{2} D_{Ca} C_{i-1,i} [Ca^{2+}]_{i-1,t+\Delta t} + \left(1 + \frac{\Delta t}{2} D_{Ca}(C_{i-1,i} + C_{i,i+1})\right) [Ca^{2+}]_{i,t+\Delta t}$$

$$-\frac{\Delta t}{2} D_{Ca} C_{i,i+1} [Ca^{2+}]_{i+1,t+\Delta t}$$

$$= \frac{\Delta t}{2} D_{Ca} C_{i-1,i} [Ca^{2+}]_{i-1,t} + \left(1 - \frac{\Delta t}{2} D_{Ca}(C_{i-1,i} + C_{i,i+1})\right) [Ca^{2+}]_{i,t}$$

$$+ \frac{\Delta t}{2} D_{Ca} C_{i,i+1} [Ca^{2+}]_{i+1,t} + \frac{\Delta t}{2} \frac{J_{i,t+\Delta t/2}}{v_i}, \tag{6.17}$$

where we have added an unspecified flux J_i, which could be the transmembrane Ca^{2+} inflow into the volume v_i of shell i (see eq. 4.15) or the flux from an intracellular store (see section 6.7.3). The system of equations described by eq. 6.17 can be solved very efficiently because its corresponding matrix is tridiagonal with diagonal dominance (see section 14.3.4; Press et al. 1992). Although the Crank-Nicholson method is second-order accurate in both space and time, because the diffusion equation is parabolic, its accuracy depends completely on how exactly the boundary conditions are solved (Fletcher 1991). In most neuronal models, the most important boundary condition is the transmembrane flux J_i, which should be computed with the same Δt as in eq. 6.17.

Compartmental Models of Neurons Because electrical compartments usually represent cylinders, it is convenient to use similar geometries and cylindrical coordinates for the simulation of diffusion (see figure 6.3).

For radial diffusion into a cylinder the coupling constant (eq. 6.15) becomes

$$C_{i,i+1} = \frac{2(i+1)}{(2i+1)\Delta r^2}, \tag{6.18}$$

and for a sphere:

$$C_{i,i+1} = \frac{3(i+1)^2}{(3i^2+3i+1)\Delta r^2}, \tag{6.19}$$

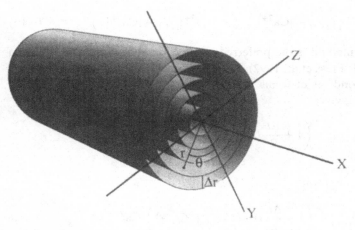

Figure 6.3
Comparison of Cartesian coordinates (x, y, z) and cylindrical ones (r, θ, x). To simulate radial one-dimensional diffusion, the cylindrical volume is discretized into a number of shells, each with a thickness Δr. While comparing with experimental data, $[Ca^{2+}]_{i,t}$ should be taken as the concentration in the center of shell i.

where Δr is the thickness of the shells (figure 6.3) and $i = 0$ is the central shell. The diameter of the electrical compartment should be $d = 2 \cdot n\Delta r$.

Equations 6.18–6.19 assume that all shells in a compartment have the same thickness Δr. It is not practical to keep the number of shells n constant in a multicompartmental model based on a reconstructed morphology. Because of the variability in compartmental diameters, this would require different values for Δr in each compartment. This is not a good solution because with each compartment having a different thickness Δr for the outer submembrane shell, the computed $[Ca^{2+}]$ will vary between compartments even if the activation of Ca^{2+} channels is identical. This not only complicates comparisons between $[Ca^{2+}]$ of different compartments but also leads to unphysiological differences in the activation of Ca^{2+}-activated K^+ channels.

It is better to use the same value for Δr throughout the model. This keeps the spatial resolution of the diffusion equations constant. Because the radius of any given compartment is usually not an integral multiple of Δr, one shell must have a different Δr and, for the reasons outlined in the previous paragraph, this cannot be the submembrane shell. The best choice is the central shell $i = 0$, and eq. 6.15 can be used to compute $C_{0,1}$, with $\delta_{0,1} = \Delta r_0 + \Delta r_1/2$. It is important to realize that eqs. 6.14 and 6.16 become unstable if the geometry is very asymmetric. For example, if Δr_i is much smaller than Δr_{i+1}, a small Δt will be needed for correct convergence. In practice, this means that Δr_0 should not be too small. In the GENESIS neural simulator, a thin central shell is created only if $\Delta r_0 > \Delta r/4$; otherwise, the central shell has a thickness of Δr plus the small remainder.

Carnevale and Rosenthal (1992) discuss the relation between Δr and the temporal accuracy of the discretized solution. In general, this accuracy will be poor in the submillisecond range for extremely fast changes in concentration, which fortunately are rare in biological simulations. Note that if $[Ca^{2+}]_{i,t}$ is used to compute the activation of Ca^{2+}-activated K^+ channels, a change of Δr throughout the model will always vary the fine details of the computed spiking pattern. In a typical neuronal model, one cannot expect the solution to converge for decreasing values of Δr, as it does for decreasing Δt.

Modeling Spines Calcium transients in spines have been modeled extensively to study the role of the Ca^{2+} influx through NMDA receptor channels (Mayer and Westbrook 1987) in the induction of synaptic plasticity (Artola and Singer 1993). As a rule, only one or a few spines are modeled in detail and coupled to a compartmental model of the dendritic tree (see chapter 3 for more details on modeling dendritic spines).

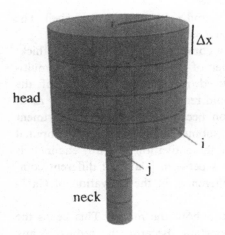

Figure 6.4
Diffusion is modeled in a spine by stacking short cylinders on top of each other. In this example, the spine head is represented by four cylinders with $\Delta x = 0.10\,\mu m$ and $r = 0.25\,\mu m$ and the neck by four cylinders with $\Delta x = 0.10\,\mu m$ and $r = 0.05\,\mu m$. One-dimensional diffusion is modeled along the X-axis.

Both the head and neck of the spine can be represented as a set of short cylinders stacked on top of each other (figure 6.4), with the diffusion along the axis of the cylinders. Eq. 6.14 or 6.16 can again be applied, with

$$C_{i,i+1} = \frac{1}{(\Delta x)^2} \quad \text{if } r_{i+1} \geq r_i \text{ and } \Delta x_i = \Delta x_{i+1} \tag{6.20}$$

between cylinders in the spine head or neck, and at the transition from head cylinder i to neck cylinder j, in the more general form

$$C_{i,j} = \frac{2r_j^2}{r_i^2 \Delta x_i (\Delta x_i + \Delta x_j)}. \tag{6.21}$$

Eq. 6.21 assumes a sharp transition between the spine head and the neck. In practice, eq. 6.21 works fine, although in several models the transition between head and neck has been modeled either as a large number of thin segments (Zador, Koch, and Brown 1990) or as a smooth function (Holmes and Levy 1990).

Examples of Spine Models   Koch and coworkers have implemented detailed models of Ca^{2+} transients in a spine coupled to simplified models of a hippocampal pyramidal neuron (Gamble and Koch 1987; Zador, Koch, and Brown 1990). They showed that the voltage-dependent Ca^{2+} entry through the NMDA receptor channel can be the factor that couples pre- and postsynaptic activity during Hebbian learning at synapses (Hebb 1949). Recently a phenomological model of Ca^{2+} stores was added to this model by Schieg et al. (1995). Holmes and Levy (1990) studied induction of long-term potentiation by simulating 100 spines on a detailed model of a dendate granule cell. GENESIS scripts for this model (De Schutter and Bower 1993) can be downloaded from http://bbf-www.uia.ac.be/CHAPTER/spine.html.

6.4.2 Multidimensional Diffusion

Calcium influx into presynaptic terminals causes localized increases in $[Ca^{2+}]$ to hundreds of μM in regions just below the channel pores, called "microdomains" (Llinás, Sugimori, and Silver 1992). Many models have simulated the $[Ca^{2+}]$ in these domains to better understand the relation between Ca^{2+} entry and transmitter release (Parnas, Hovav, and Parnas 1989; Yamada and Zucker 1992; Winslow, Duffy, and Charlton 1994). Such models require the simulation of three-dimensional diffusion of Ca^{2+}. The terminal is discretized into many cubic boxes, and diffusion is modeled as the summation of fluxes along each axis. For example, the diffusion along the X-axis can be approximated as

$$\frac{\partial^2 [Ca^{2+}]_{x,y,z,t}}{\partial x^2} \approx \frac{1}{\Delta x^2} ([Ca^{2+}]_{x-\Delta x,y,z,t} - 2[Ca^{2+}]_{x,y,z,t} + [Ca^{2+}]_{x+\Delta x,y,z,t}). \tag{6.22}$$

Applying similar equations along the Y- and Z-axes, one arrives at

$$[Ca^{2+}]_{x,y,z,t+\Delta t} - [Ca^{2+}]_{x,y,z,t}$$

$$= \Delta t D_{Ca} \left(\frac{\partial^2 [Ca^{2+}]_{x,y,z,t}}{\partial x^2} + \frac{\partial^2 [Ca^{2+}]_{x,y,z,t}}{\partial y^2} + \frac{\partial^2 [Ca^{2+}]_{x,y,z,t}}{\partial z^2} \right). \tag{6.23}$$

Eq. 6.23 is solved explicitly or using standard PDE solvers (see chapter 14, this volume). Boundary conditions are an important problem in multidimensional diffusion because the simulated volume is often assumed to be part of a much larger volume without diffusional constraints. The standard solution is to model the complete volume where $[Ca^{2+}]$ will be perturbed in detail and to add at the periphery (progressively) larger boxes until one reaches zones where $[Ca^{2+}]$ remains at rest. Small time steps are necessary (about 0.1 μsec) and even with adaptive box sizes, one easily ends up with millions of boxes (Yamada and Zucker 1992). Such models obviously require very long computation times.

Alternating Direction Implicit Method   An elegant method to solve this problem is the alternating direction implicit (ADI) method (Press et al. 1992; Fletcher 1991), which we will describe for the Crank-Nicholson formulation of two-dimensional diffusion in a cylinder. The cylinder is discretized into many annuli, which are shells divided into short segments along the X-axis. Diffusion is described in a cylindrical coordinate system $(r, \theta, x$; see figure 6.3) and the concentration function is considered cylindrically symmetric (i.e., independent of θ). Each time step is divided into two steps of size $\Delta t/2$ and in each substep a different independent variable is treated implicitly:

$$[Ca^{2+}]_{i,j,t+\Delta t/2} - [Ca^{2+}]_{i,j,t} = \frac{\Delta t}{4} D_{Ca}\big(C_{i,i+1}([Ca^{2+}]_{i+1,j,t+\Delta t/2} - [Ca^{2+}]_{i,j,t+\Delta t/2})$$

$$+ C_{j,j+1}([Ca^{2+}]_{i,j+1,t} - [Ca^{2+}]_{i,j,t})) \qquad (6.24)$$

$$[Ca^{2+}]_{i,j,t+\Delta t} - [Ca^{2+}]_{i,j,t+\Delta t/2} = \frac{\Delta t}{4} D_{Ca}\big(C_{i,i+1}([Ca^{2+}]_{i+1,j,t+\Delta t/2} - [Ca^{2+}]_{i,j,t+\Delta t/2})$$

$$+ C_{j,j+1}([Ca^{2+}]_{i,j+1,t+\Delta t} - [Ca^{2+}]_{i,j,t+\Delta t})), \qquad (6.25)$$

where first diffusion along the r-coordinate is solved implicitly (i variable in eq. 6.24) and then over the x-coordinate (j variable in eq. 6.25). Eqs. 6.24 and 6.25 are written like eq. 6.16, that is, for diffusion to one side from i to $i + 1$ and from j to $j + 1$ only, but it should be obvious how to convert them to the form of eq. 6.17, which includes diffusion to both sides. Again, the two matrices corresponding to the systems of coupled equations of 6.24–6.25 are tridiagonal with diagonal dominance and can be solved very efficiently. In two dimensions, the ADI scheme for diffusion is unconditionally stable for the full time step and second-order accurate in both space and time, provided the appropriate boundary conditions are used (Fletcher 1991; see also Holmes 1995 for using the two-dimensional ADI method with cylindrical coordinates in a model of glutamate diffusion). The ADI scheme can also be used to model three-dimensional diffusion with substeps of $\Delta t/3$, but it is only conditionally stable (Fletcher 1991).

Cylindrical coordinates allow modelers to faithfully represent the geometry of the submembrane region, usually the most important one in neuronal models of diffusion. Unfortunately, modeling three-dimensional diffusion in cylindrical coordinates is awkward because the volume elements become extremely small close to the center. To simulate three-dimensional diffusion in a complex geometry like a spine, a finite-element method might be indicated. These can be implemented using standard mathematical packages (e.g., Aharon, Parnas, and Parnas 1994), but are again very computation-intensive.

Domain Model   Repeating the message from section 6.2, it may not be necessary to model Ca^{2+} diffusion in three dimensions if the high concentrations inside the Ca^{2+} microdomains (Chad and Eckert 1984; Llinás, Sugimori, and Silver 1992) are needed only to inactivate Ca^{2+} channels or to activate K^+ channels or transmitter release. A highly simplified model sets the domain Ca^{2+} concentration directly proportional to the current through the Ca^{2+} channel (Sherman, Keizer, and Rinzel 1990):

$$[Ca^{2+}]_{d,i} = -\frac{\gamma}{a_i} I_{Ca,i},$$ (6.26)

where a_i normalizes the current for membrane surface and γ converts from units of current to concentration and incorporates any additional effects of diffusion and buffering. Although this model has obvious limitations and becomes inaccurate when the membrane potential approaches the reversal potential, it is very fast.

6.5   Electrodiffusion Models

6.5.1   Description

In section 6.4.1, simple models of $[Ca^{2+}]$ in a dendritic spine (Zador, Koch, and Brown 1990) were described. It was implicitly assumed that the voltage transients and the ionic concentrations in these models can be computed separately and interact only through the transmitter-gated ionic influx. But even relatively small ionic fluxes cause large changes in ionic concentration in the limited volume of a spine head (Koch and Zador 1993) and change the ionic equilibrium potential. A first improvement is to use the Nernst equation (eq. 4.16) or, even better, the constant field equation (eq. 6.6; Holmes and Levy 1990) to compute the synaptic current.

Qian and Sejnowski (1989) have argued, however, that this is not sufficient, proposing instead that concentrations in spines be described by an electrodiffusion model based on the Nernst-Planck equation (Nernst 1888; Planck 1890; Hille 1992). If one again assumes only diffusion along the axis of the compartment cylinder, the Nernst-Planck equation for Ca^{2+} can be reduced to

$$\frac{\partial [Ca^{2+}]}{\partial t} = D_{Ca}\frac{\partial^2 [Ca^{2+}]}{\partial x^2} + D_{Ca}\frac{z_{Ca}F}{RT}\frac{\partial}{\partial x}\left([Ca^{2+}]\frac{\partial V}{\partial x}\right) - \frac{1}{v}J_{Ca}.$$ (6.27)

Eq. 6.27 states that $[Ca^{2+}]$ can change due to pure diffusion (first term), the potential gradient (second term), and the transmembrane flux J_{Ca} (computed with the GHK equation, i.e., eq. 6.6). An additional equation is needed to compute the effect of changes in ionic concentration on the membrane potential, and Qian and Sejnowski

(1989) suggest using the total charge taken over the concentration of every ion inside a cylindrical compartment:

$$V(x, t) = V_{rest} + \frac{r}{2C_m} F \sum_{ions} z_{ion}([ion](x, t) - [ion]_{rest}),$$
(6.28)

where r is the radius and C_m the capacitance. Eq. 6.27 can be converted to a finite-difference equation and solved together with eq. 6.28 using the forward Euler method, but the electrodiffusion system is quite computation intensive.

To circumvent this problem, the same authors have suggested a simple modification of the standard compartmental model (see chapter 3, this volume) that approximates the electrodiffusion model. Besides computing changes in concentration caused by transmembrane fluxes and using the GHK equation (eq. 6.6) to compute ionic currents, the axial current is replaced by several axial fluxes caused by the electrochemical gradients. Effectively, the axial current (compare to eq. 14.25) is decomposed into a series of parallel currents, one for each ionic species that is modeled:

$$C_m \frac{V_{i,t+\Delta t} - V_{i,t}}{\Delta t} = \sum_j \left(\frac{a_{i,j}}{2(\Delta x)^2} \sum_{ions} \frac{E_{i,j,ion} + V_{i,t} - V_{j,t}}{R_{i,ion}} \right) - \bar{g} V_{i,t} - \sum_{ions} I_{ion},$$
(6.29)

where $a_{i,j}$ is the cross-sectional area coupling compartments i and j, $E_{i,j,ion}$ the electrochemical driving force for each ion (computed as the Nernst potential between adjoining compartments), and $R_{i,ion}$ the coupling resistance for each ionic species, which needs to be computed at every time step. Thus, for Ca^{2+}:

$$R_{i,Ca} = \frac{RT}{D_{Ca} z_{Ca} F} \frac{1}{z_{Ca} F [Ca^{2+}]_i}.$$
(6.30)

Finally, the changes in concentration due to the ion specific axial currents need to be added to those caused by the membrane currents I_{ion}. Eqs. 6.29–6.30 give a reasonable approximation of eq. 6.27, except during fast changes in transmembrane current (see Qian and Sejnowski 1989, which also describes how to compute electrodiffusion at branches).

6.5.2   Applicability and Examples

Qian and Sejnowski (1989) suggest that the electrodiffusion equation (eq. 6.27), or its compartmental approximation (eq. 6.29), should be used whenever one wants to model electrical events in a structure with a diameter smaller than 1 μm, as, for example, silent inhibition onto a spine. Cable modeling suggests that when a spine is contacted by both a Cl^- inhibitory synapse (reversal potential close to rest) and by an excitatory synapse, the inhibitory synapse can block excitatory input by shunting the EPSP without producing a measurable inhibitory postsynaptic potential (IPSP; Koch, Poggio, and Torre 1982). This concept does not work in the electrodiffusion model because the inflow of Cl^- ions reduces the inhibitory reversal potential (Qian and Sejnowski 1990). Because the different results in the electrodiffusion model can be explained by the use of the Nernst equation (eq. 4.16), however, it remains unclear if the computation of the axial electrochemical flux (eq. 6.29) qualitatively changes the conclusion.

Moreover, the increased biophysical fidelity of the electrodiffusion model forces one to consider which charge carriers are responsible for the axial current. Qian and Sejnowski (1990) make the simple assumption that axial current is carried by the same ions as the transmembrane current, namely, Na^+, K^+, and Cl^-. But is this correct? Many other ions and small molecules carry charge along the dendritic axis. Taking into account their mobility in water and their intraneuronal concentrations, the most important carriers are expected to be K^+ (R_i of $97\,\Omega$ cm at $20°$ C), Mg^{2+} (R_i of $304\,\Omega$ cm), and phosphates (R_i of $327\,\Omega$ cm) (Milazzo 1963; Guyton 1986; Hille 1992). These R_i values assume that the ions are not buffered in the cytoplasm, which is unlikely for Mg^{2+} (Zhou and Neher 1993). All other ions have cytoplasmic resistivities of more than $2,000\,\Omega$ cm at rest. In fact, because these resistivities operate in parallel, neglecting all ions except for K^+, Mg^{2+}, and phosphates changes the cytoplasmic resistivity at rest only from $55\,\Omega$ cm to $60\,\Omega$ cm! Obviously these values vary as the ionic concentrations change due to transmembrane fluxes, but the $[Na^+]$ has to rise more than fivefold or the $[Cl^-]$ tenfold to reduce its R_i below $300\,\Omega$ cm.

These simple calculations suggest that electrodiffusion models are not necessary to model spines or small dendrites. It is more important to use the GHK equation and to consider that most ligand-gated channels are permeable to multiple ions; for example, Na^+, K^+, and Ca^{2+} ions permeate through the NMDA receptor channel (Mayer and Westbrook 1987) and Cl^- and HCO_3^- through the $GABA_A$ receptor channel (Staley, Soldo, and Proctor 1995). Electrodiffusion theory has been successfully applied, however, in axonal models to study the effects of injury (van Egeraat and Wikswo 1993).

6.6 Buffer Capacity and Buffer Diffusion

Until now, we have only considered free diffusion. Most ions, in particular divalent ones such as Ca^{2+} and Mg^{2+}, bind to cytoplasmic buffers (Thayer and Miller 1990; Neher and Augustine 1992; Zhou and Neher 1993). To elaborate the second-order buffering scheme introduced in chapter 4, this volume:

$$Ca^{2+} + B \underset{b}{\overset{f}{\rightleftharpoons}} CaB. \tag{6.31}$$

It should be noted that eq. 6.31 is only an approximation because most Ca^{2+}-binding proteins have multiple binding sites with different f and b rates (Linse, Helmersson, and Forsen 1991) and require more complex equations to be modeled accurately. In practice, however, experimental data for the binding rates are often not available.

6.6.1   Buffer Capacity

An important parameter for models of Ca^{2+} buffering is the buffer capacity, the fractional amount of bound Ca^{2+} per free Ca^{2+}:

$$\kappa = \frac{d[CaB]_i}{d[Ca^{2+}]_i}. \tag{6.32}$$

The buffer capacity can be estimated using specific Ca^{2+}-sensitive dye imaging procedures (Neher and Augustine 1992; Zhou and Neher 1993); it ranges from about 45 (98% of Ca^{2+} entering the cell is bound to the buffer) in chromaffin cells (Zhou and Neher 1993) to more than 4,000 (99.97% of Ca^{2+} entering the cell is bound to the buffer) in Purkinje cells (Llano, DiPolo, and Marty 1994). If endogenous buffers have a low affinity (high dissociation constant $K_d = b/f$), which seems to be the case (Neher and Augustine 1992), the total buffer concentration $[B]_T$ can be estimated from κ:

$$\kappa \approx \frac{[B]_T}{K_d} \quad \text{if } [Ca^{2+}]_i \ll K_d. \tag{6.33}$$

6.6.2   Buffer Diffusion

Eq. 6.33 raises the issues of what the intracellular buffers and their K_d are and whether the buffers are mobile. Zhou and Neher (1993) estimated that about 25% of the buffer capacity in adrenal chromaffin cells is represented by slowly mobile buffers (D_B of about $1 \cdot 10^{-7}\ cm^2\ sec^{-1}$), postulating that inorganic anions and small metabolites should act as highly mobile buffers (D_B of $2 \cdot 10^{-6}\ cm^2\ sec^{-1}$). They estimated the highly mobile buffer capacity to be less than 15%. More important, most indicator dyes used in Ca^{2+} imaging experiments also act as highly mobile buffers. The effects of the indicator fura-2 on Ca^{2+} diffusion have been modeled extensively using explicit forward Euler methods (Sala and Hernandez-Cruz 1990; Blumenfeld, Zablow, and Sabatini 1992; see also section 6.6.5).

To study the effects of diffusible buffers, eqs. 6.16 and 6.31 need to be combined. The implicit Crank-Nicholson equation for buffer diffusion is

$$-\frac{\Delta t}{2} D_B C_{i-1,i}[B]_{i-1,t+\Delta t} + \left(1 + \frac{\Delta t}{2} D_B(C_{i-1,i} + C_{i,i+1}) + \frac{\Delta t}{2}(b + f[Ca^{2+}]_{i,t})\right)[B]_{i,t+\Delta t}$$

$$+\frac{\Delta t}{2} f[B]_{i,t}[Ca^{2+}]_{i,t+\Delta t} - \frac{\Delta t}{2} D_B C_{i,i+1}[B]_{i+1,t+\Delta t}$$

$$=\frac{\Delta t}{2} D_B C_{i-1,i}[B]_{i-1,t} + \left(1 - \frac{\Delta t}{2} D_B(C_{i-1,i} + C_{i,i+1}) - \frac{\Delta t}{2} b\right)[B]_{i,t}$$

$$+\frac{\Delta t}{2} D_B C_{i,i+1}[B]_{i+1,t} + \Delta t\, b[B]_{T,i}, \tag{6.34}$$

where f and b are, respectively, the forward and backward rates of the buffer binding reaction (eq. 6.31) and D_B is the diffusion constant of the buffer. Similarly, for buffered Ca^{2+}-diffusion:

$$-\frac{\Delta t}{2} D_{Ca} C_{i-1,i}[Ca^{2+}]_{i-1,t+\Delta t} + \frac{\Delta t}{2}(b + f[Ca^{2+}]_{i,t})[B]_{i,t+\Delta t}$$

$$+\left(1 + \frac{\Delta t}{2} D_{Ca}(C_{i-1,i} + C_{i,i+1}) + \frac{\Delta t}{2} f[B]_{i,t}\right)[Ca^{2+}]_{i,t+\Delta t} - \frac{\Delta t}{2} D_{Ca} C_{i,i+1}[Ca^{2+}]_{i+1,t+\Delta t}$$

$$=\frac{\Delta t}{2} D_{Ca} C_{i-1,i}[Ca^{2+}]_{i-1,t} + \left(1 - \frac{\Delta t}{2} D_{Ca}(C_{i-1,i} + C_{i,i+1})\right)[Ca^{2+}]_{i,t}$$

$$+\frac{\Delta t}{2} D_{Ca} C_{i,i+1}[Ca^{2+}]_{i+1,t} - \frac{\Delta t}{2} b[B]_{i,t} + \Delta t b[B]_{T,i} + \frac{\Delta t}{2} \frac{J_{i,t+\Delta t/2}}{v_i}. \tag{6.35}$$

Eq. 6.34 assumes that $[B]_{T,i}$ is constant, in other words, that D_B is identical for the free and bound forms of the buffer. Taking into account the relative sizes of Ca^{2+} and most buffer molecules, this is a reasonable assumption. Eqs. 6.34 and 6.35 should be solved together, resulting in a diagonally banded matrix with three bands for the Ca^{2+} diffusion and two bands extra for each buffer modeled. The most efficient ordering of the matrix is by shells, mixing $[Ca^{2+}]$ and $[B]$ so that the first row computes the buffer equations for the innermost shell. Because such a matrix is more complex to solve than the tridiagonal matrix of eq. 6.17, introducing buffers into a model will have an impact on computation speed.

6.6.3 Purkinje Cell Model

Radial diffusion of Ca^{2+} was modeled using concentric shells with a Δr of $0.2\,\mu m$, resulting in a total of 7,471 shells for the 1,604 compartments in the model. Although simulations were usually run with a Δt of $10\,\mu sec$, to obtain an increased accuracy, a Δt of $5\,\mu sec$ was used for the figures in this chapter.

We used a D_{Ca} of $2 \cdot 10^{-6}\,cm^2\,sec^{-1}$. This value is three times slower than D_{Ca} in water (see chapter 4, this volume) and is based on measurements of Ca^{2+} diffusion rates in cytoplasm (Albritton, Meyer, and Stryer 1992). In general, diffusion constants listed in standard textbooks (e.g., Hille 1992) apply to very dilute solutions, while cytoplasm is estimated to have twice the viscosity of water (Albritton, Meyer, and Stryer 1992).

A very high buffer capacity has been estimated for Purkinje cells (Llano, DiPolo, and Marty 1994; Fierro and Llano 1996). We have put the nonmobile buffer capacity at 2,080 by including $4\,mM$ of a buffer with a K_d of $1.9\,\mu M$. The relative slow binding rates ($f = 1.3 \cdot 10^6\,M^{-1}\,sec^{-1}$) indicate that this buffer modeled Ca^{2+} uptake by both endogenous buffers and internal stores. Additionally, we simulated fura-2, represented as $75\,\mu M$ of a mobile buffer ($D_{fura} = 2 \cdot 10^{-6}\,cm^2\,sec^{-1}$) with a K_d of $0.2\,\mu M$ ($f = 4 \cdot 10^8\,M^{-1}\,sec^{-1}$). Buffer concentrations were identical in all shells. This is different from many other models where the submembrane shell had a higher buffer content (see, for example, chapter 4, this volume). While there is some evidence for higher submembrane buffer concentrations in cell bodies (Naraghi et al. 1995), this seems less likely to be the case for tiny dendritic branches.

Results   Figures 6.5 and 6.6 show the Ca^{2+} dynamics of the Purkinje cell model during a $1.5\,nA$ somatic current injection. While the somatic firing pattern looked very similar to that of the earlier Purkinje cell model (De Schutter and Bower 1994a), the dendritic spiking pattern had improved considerably. In particular, dendritic spikes were sharper and had a larger amplitude. The steady state $[Ca^{2+}]$ in between spikes rose to $200\,nM$, which was closer to reported changes in $[Ca^{2+}]$ during current injection (Lev-Ram et al. 1992) and higher than in the earlier model that used eq. 6.1 ($[Ca^{2+}]$ of $100\,nM$).

The $[Ca^{2+}]$ profiles showed a significant radial gradient in all compartments, which can be explained by the effect of the buffers on Ca^{2+} diffusion (see section 6.6.5). This was most obvious in the smooth dendrite (figure 6.7A), where the submembrane shells sensed fast changes in Ca^{2+} inflow during somatic spikes, while the central core $[Ca^{2+}]$ reflected highly attenuated dendritic spikes only. The gradient was less outspoken in the spiny dendrite shown in figure 6.5C, where the amount of free nonmobile buffer decreased progressively during long periods of bursting. This

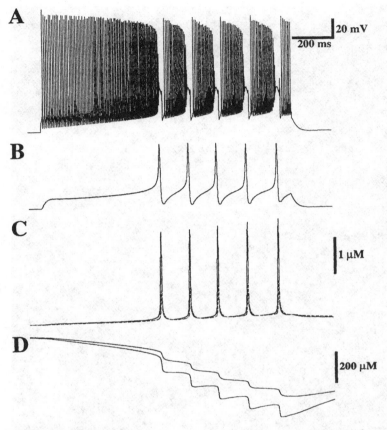

Figure 6.5
Response of the Purkinje cell model to a 1.2 sec long 1.5 nA current injection in the soma. (A) Membrane potential in the soma shows that the model produces initially fast somatic Na^+ spikes only. Later, the dendrite starts spiking, too. (B) Membrane potential in a spiny dendrite demonstrates the initial plateau phase followed by dendritic Ca^{2+} spikes. (C) $[Ca^{2+}]$ in the submembrane (full line) and core shells (broken line) of the same spiny dendritic compartment, which has a diameter of 1.3 µm. (D) Free fixed buffer concentration in the same shells. During the current injection [B] decreased from 3.9 mM to 3.4 mM.

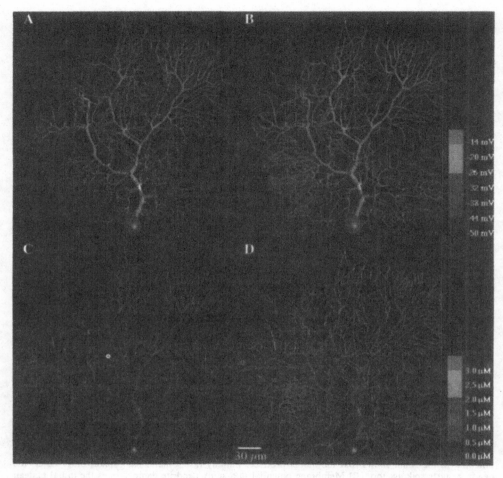

Figure 6.6
Membrane potential (photos A–B) and [Ca^{2+}] in the submembrane shell (photos C–D) during a dendritic spike in the Purkinje cell model. Photos B and D were taken 5 msec later than photos A and C. In this example the dendritic spike initiated in the upper right dendrite, but this was not always the case in the model. Note that the increase in [Ca^{2+}] was delayed compared to the depolarization. The lower [Ca^{2+}] in the thick branches (the smooth dendrite) compared to the thinner branches (the spiny dendrite) was caused by the surface-to-volume ratio effect (see section 6.6.5) as the Ca^{2+} channel density was identical in all dendritic compartments. Morphology for the Purkinje cell model was reconstructed by M. Rapp (Rapp et al. 1994).

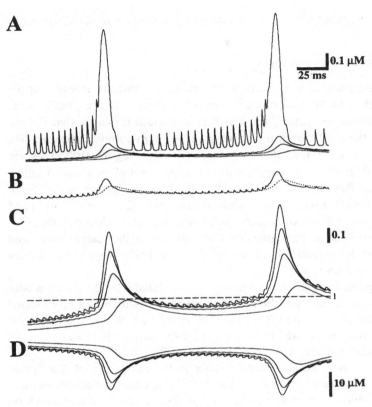

Figure 6.7
Simulation of fura-2 signals during the first two Ca^{2+} spikes of figure 6.5. (A) Calcium concentrations in a smooth dendritic compartment. The $[Ca^{2+}]$ in the submembrane shell, in shells $0.5\,\mu m$ and $1.0\,\mu m$ below the membrane and in the core shell are shown. (B) Spatial average of $[Ca^{2+}]$ (full line) and the estimated $[Ca^{2+}]$ (broken line) derived from the fura-2 signals (eq. 6.38) in the same compartment. (C) F_1/F_2 ratios in the same shells as shown in panel A. (D) Free fura-2 concentrations in the same shells as in panel A. The free fura-2 decreased from about $55\,\mu M$ to about $35\,\mu M$ in the submembrane shell.

caused a slow rise of the steady state $[Ca^{2+}]$, leading by activation of K^+ channels to a slower dendritic spiking.

6.6.4 Modeling Calcium Indicator Dyes

Whenever a biophysical model is built, it is important to constrain it with experimental data if available. In the case of Ca^{2+} dynamics, these data are usually measurements with fluorescent indicator dyes. It is very important to realize that the use of such dyes distorts the Ca^{2+} signal in two ways. First, high-affinity indicators like fura-2 have binding properties that affect the measured signal significantly: they are easy to saturate and their slow backward reaction rate does not allow them to follow rapid $[Ca^{2+}]$ changes. Regehr and Atluri (1995) compare the properties of high-affinity dyes such as indo-1, fura-2, fluo-3, and calcium green-2 (K_d in the 0.1–1 μM range) with those of low-affinity dyes such as furaptra and BTC. Second, these indicators act as mobile buffers, changing the Ca^{2+} dynamics themselves (Sala and Hernandez-Cruz 1990; Blumenfeld, Zablow, and Sabatini 1992; Wagner and Keizer 1994; Gabso, Neher, and Spira 1997).

Therefore, it is impossible to directly compare the simulated $[Ca^{2+}]$ transients with measured indicator signals. Instead, the indicator response itself should be modeled so that the experimentally estimated $[Ca^{2+}]$ can be computed. We will describe the simulation of fura-2 indicators, which consists of three parts; it is trivial to apply similar methods to other indicators.

First, fura-2 must be included as a mobile buffer in the simulation of $[Ca^{2+}]$ (see section 6.6.2), which requires an estimate of the dye's $[B]_T$, often impossible to measure experimentally, and of its D_B, f, and b. The last three factors depend on the ionic environment of the dye (Grynkiewicz, Poenie, and Tsien 1985) and values found in the literature vary widely. For example, D_B values range from $4 \cdot 10^{-7}\,cm^2\,sec^{-1}$ to $2 \cdot 10^{-6}\,cm^2\,sec^{-1}$, f values from $0.25 \cdot 10^8\,M^{-1}\,sec^{-1}$ to $6.0 \cdot 10^8\,M^{-1}\,sec^{-1}$, and what is more important for distortions, the backward rate constant b values from $17\,sec^{-1}$ to $380\,sec^{-1}$ (Timmermann and Ashley 1986; Kao and Tsien 1988; Blumenfeld, Zablow, and Sabatini 1992; Hollingworth et al. 1992; Zhou and Neher 1993).

Next, the fluorescence emitted by bound and unbound fura-2 in response to excitation at 340 nm, F_1, or at 380 nm, F_2 (Grynkiewicz, Poenie, and Tsien 1985), must be computed in every shell i:

$$F_{j,i} = S_{b,j}[CaFura]_i + S_{f,j}[Fura]_i \quad j = 1, 2. \tag{6.36}$$

The S factors are measured experimentally using calibration solutions. $S_{f,j}$ and $S_{b,j}$

are the fluorescence measured as $[Ca^{2+}]_i$ approaches zero (F_1) and full saturation (F_2) of fura-2, respectively. Typical values are $S_{b1} = 1.0\,\text{mM}^{-1}$, $S_{f1} = 0.455\,\text{mM}^{-1}$, $S_{b2} = 0.051\,\text{mM}^{-1}$, and $S_{f2} = 1.006\,\text{mM}^{-1}$ (Blumenfeld, Zablow, and Sabatini 1992).

Finally, the limitations of the recording setup must be compensated for. Unless a confocal laser microscope or dual photon microscope (Denk and Svoboda 1997) is used, the measured excitation will be a spatial summation of different fluorescence levels throughout the radial axis of the cylinder (in the case of a dendrite). This means that the volume-weighted average should be computed over all shells i of the fluorescence levels $F_{j,i}$:

$$F_j = \frac{\sum_i v_i F_{j,i}}{\sum_i v_i} \quad j = 1, 2. \tag{6.37}$$

The total fluorescence levels F_1 and F_2 or their ratio can be compared directly to the measurements. Often the data are presented as an estimated $[Ca^{2+}]$ (Grynkiewicz, Poenie, and Tsien 1985), which should then be computed also:

$$[Ca^{2+}]_{est} = K_{d,fura} \frac{S_{f2}}{S_{b2}} \frac{F_1/F_2 - S_{f1}/S_{f2}}{S_{b1}/S_{b2} - F_1/F_2}. \tag{6.38}$$

Many additional refinements to this fura-2 model are possible. For example, one can explicitly model the spatial blur and the temporal filtering of the recording system (Blumenfeld, Zablow, and Sabatini 1992) or the effect of background fluorescence and of Ca^{2+}-insensitive fura-2 (Zhou and Neher 1993).

Purkinje Cell Model   Figure 6.7 shows a simulation of the fura-2 signal (using eqs. 6.36–6.38) in the smooth dendrite. As predicted, the fura-2 signal (figure 6.7C) gave a filtered version of the $[Ca^{2+}]$. This is most obvious in the signal from the outer shell, where the somatic spikes were damped and the rise and decay phase of the dendritic spikes were slowed down significantly. Note that fura-2 did not saturate during the simulation (figure 6.7D). The spatially averaged fura-2 signal (figure 6.7B) was only a poor measure of the rich $[Ca^{2+}]$ dynamics in the smooth dendrite as it approximated most the $[Ca^{2+}]$ 1.0 µm submembrane. The approximation was better for a spiny dendritic compartment because of the smaller $[Ca^{2+}]$ gradients and the absence of fast $[Ca^{2+}]$ changes caused by the passively propagated somatic spikes (figure 6.5C).

6.6.5   Predictions from Linearized Calcium Theory

Several groups have developed simplified equations for buffered diffusion (Wagner and Keizer 1994; Zador and Koch 1994). We will briefly discuss the properties of the linearized Ca^{2+} theory (Zador and Koch 1994), but its derivation is beyond the scope of this chapter.

If the $[Ca^{2+}]$ is sufficiently small to neglect any buffer saturation ($[Ca^{2+}] \ll K_d$) and if the buffering reaction can be considered to be at equilibrium with respect to the diffusional processes, one can describe buffered diffusion as:

$$\frac{r}{2}(1 + \kappa)\frac{\partial [Ca^{2+}](x,t)}{\partial t} = \frac{r}{2}(D_{Ca} + \kappa D_B)\frac{\partial^2 [Ca^{2+}](x,t)}{\partial x^2} - P_m[Ca^{2+}](x,t)$$

$$+ K_\infty P_m I_{Ca}(x,t), \tag{6.39}$$

where r is the radius of the cylinder, κ is defined in eq. 6.33, and P_m is the pump rate (units of m/sec). The last term converts the Ca^{2+} current into concentration with K_∞ as a proportionality constant. Although the usefulness of eq. 6.39 for the solution of $[Ca^{2+}]$ transients is limited (Zador and Koch 1994), it allows one to gain an intuitive feeling for axial diffusion in a cylinder. Indeed, eq. 6.39 is identical in form to the equation for propagation of voltage along a one-dimensional fiber (see chapter 2, this volume):

$$C_m \frac{\partial V(x,t)}{\partial t} = \frac{r}{2R_i}\frac{\partial^2 V(x,t)}{\partial x^2} - \frac{1}{R_m}V(x,t) + \frac{R_\infty}{R_m}I_{Ca}(x,t). \tag{6.40}$$

By substituting the proper parameters, one can therefore define space and time constants for the Ca^{2+} reaction-diffusion system:

$$\lambda_{Ca} = \sqrt{\frac{r(D_{Ca} + \kappa D_B)}{2P_m}} \tag{6.41}$$

$$\tau_{Ca} = \frac{r(1 + \kappa)}{2P_m} \tag{6.42}$$

Comparison of eqs. 6.41 and 6.42 with the corresponding electrical λ and τ (see chapter 2, this volume) produces useful insights into the properties of buffered diffusion. First, both the space and time constant depend on r, while the electrical time constant is independent of r. The effect of r on the dynamics of diffusion (eq. 6.42) is often described by experimentalists as the "surface-to-volume ratio effect," which in effect states that the equilibration speed scales with $2/r$ for a cylinder and with $3/r$ for a sphere. Second, the space constant for Ca^{2+} and other second messengers is in general 1,000 times smaller than the electrical space constant (Kasai and Petersen 1994). Changes in $[Ca^{2+}]$ tend therefore to stay much more localized within the dendritic tree than electrical transients, which has important consequences for Ca^{2+} signaling. The difference in λ also explains why diffusion shells should be much smaller than the spatial discretization needed for solving the nonlinear cable equation. For example, in the Purkinje cell model the shells have a thickness of $0.2\,\mu m$; the mean length for electrical compartments is $7.5\,\mu m$. The space constant decreases with higher pump rates (the pumps are equivalent to membrane conductance in the voltage equation), while high diffusion constants have the opposite effect.

Finally, buffers can change both the capacity of the system and the effective diffusion rate. The capacity of the system is $(r/2)(1 + [B]_T/K_d)$ (eq. 6.39). Without buffers, the capacity is determined by the surface-to-volume ratio. Buffers increase the capacity of the system by an amount proportional to their total concentration (eq. 6.33) and to their affinity $(1/K_d)$. The effect of buffers on diffusion can be modeled as a change in the diffusion constant for Ca^{2+}. Neglecting the last two terms of eq. 6.39, and dividing both sides by the capacity, one can define an apparent diffusion coefficient (Wagner and Keizer 1994; Zador and Koch 1994):

$$D_{app} \approx \frac{1}{1+\kappa} D_{Ca} + D_B \quad \text{if } [Ca^{2+}]_i \ll K_d \text{ and } \kappa \gg 1. \tag{6.43}$$

The cytoplasmic D_{app} caused by the endogenous buffer capacity (κ) of 45 or more (Neher and Augustine 1992) is therefore expected to be more than an order of magnitude smaller than D_{Ca} in solution. Indeed, Albritton, Meyer, and Stryer (1992) found that D_{app} was only $1.3 \cdot 10^{-7}\,cm^2\,sec^{-1}$ for buffered Ca^{2+} diffusion, compared to $2.2 \cdot 10^{-6}\,cm^2\,sec^{-1}$ for free diffusion in cytoplasm. Diffusible buffers will increase D_{app} and λ_{Ca} because they transport Ca^{2+}. This is a consequence of the bound buffer generating a second concentration gradient besides the $[Ca^{2+}]$ gradient (Sala and Hernandez-Cruz 1990). The bound buffer will diffuse toward regions of low $[CaB]$, which of course have also a low $[Ca^{2+}]$, and this increases the apparent diffusion rate by D_B (eq. 6.43). Because D_B is not scaled by $1/(1 + \kappa)$, it will have a big effect on D_{app}, despite D_B being smaller than D_{Ca}.

Wagner and Keizer (1994) have shown that the effects on D_{app} are actually more complex, especially for high-affinity buffers like fura-2. If enough mobile buffer is present to prevent immediate saturation, it will first bind Ca^{2+} without releasing it and will have a capacitative effect only. Later, when enough Ca^{2+} is bound, the mobile buffer will start to release Ca^{2+} and the diffusive effect will become apparent: D_{app} will increase over time.

This last point demonstrates the importance of buffer saturation, something linearized Ca^{2+} theory cannot predict. A systematic modeling study was done by Nowycky and Pinter (1993), who found that the submembrane transients during Ca^{2+} influx were shaped much more by the forward rate factor f than by K_d.

Moreover, if fixed [*CaB*] could be measured, this would give a much better representation of the spatial [Ca^{2+}] gradient than diffusible [*CaB*] (e.g., fura-2). Finally, during fast changes in [Ca^{2+}], other Ca^{2+} binding proteins that have fast binding rates (e.g., calmodulin; Linse, Helmersson, and Forse 1991) will compete with the indicator dye and cause it to bind less Ca^{2+}. This may lead to an underestimate of the Ca^{2+} influx in experiments where this influx is measured using very high concentrations of fura-2 (Tempia et al. 1996).

6.7 Uptake and Release from Calcium Stores

Calcium release from intracellular stores plays a central role in the generation of Ca^{2+} oscillations and Ca^{2+} waves (Berridge 1993). Ca^{2+} oscillations are cyclic changes in the cytoplasmic [Ca^{2+}] caused by repetitive periods of release of Ca^{2+} from stores, followed each time by reuptake. Cytoplasmic Ca^{2+} waves are the spatial transmission of similar processes. Because of their ubiquitous nature, these processes have generated tremendous interest from both experimentalists and modelers, although frequently outside the context of the nervous system. The models differ in the relative roles attributed to different release mechanisms in maintaining oscillations (Goldbeter, Dupont, and Berridge 1990; De Young and Keizer 1992) and to Ca^{2+} versus IP_3 diffusion in generating waves (Safri and Keizer 1995; Sneyd et al. 1995), details beyond the scope of this chapter. It is important to realize, however, that these phenomena are much slower than most neuronal signals, with time scales of seconds and beyond.

Two separate mechanisms cause release from intracellular stores: Ca^{2+}-induced Ca^{2+} release (CICR) and IP_3-induced Ca^{2+} release (Berridge 1993). CICR is mediated by a receptor that binds the muscle-paralyzing alkaloid ryanodine and that is activated by caffeine (Coronado et al. 1994). IP_3 is a second messenger created by the hydrolysis of lipid precursors, stimulated, in turn, by the activation of G-protein–linked receptors such as the metabotropic glutamate receptor (Schoepp and Conn 1993). Calcium uptake into the stores is mostly by a Ca^{2+}-ATPase pump (Lytton et al. 1992). Recent measurements suggest that free [Ca^{2+}] in the stores is in the $100\,\mu M$ (Hofer and Machen 1993) to $5\,mM$ range (Kendall, Dormer, and Campbell 1992). Stores contain large amounts of low-affinity buffers such as calsequestrin (Takei et al. 1992) and calretinin.

In Purkinje cells, the Ca^{2+} stores are part of the endoplasmic reticulum (ER). Because the ryanodine and IP_3 receptors have differential distributions, it has been suggested that the ER is subcompartmentalized into separate pools (Takei et al.

1992). Anatomical studies suggest, however, that the ER is one contiguous structure throughout the whole cell (Martone et al. 1993; Terasaki et al. 1994).

6.7.1 Calcium Uptake and CICR

Goldbeter, Dupont, and Berridge (1990) were first to describe a model of CICR-mediated $[Ca^{2+}]$ oscillations still used extensively (Sneyd, Charles, and Sanderson 1994). Although such models give reasonable approximations of slow changes in $[Ca^{2+}]$, they have two notable limitations in the context of simulating neuronal Ca^{2+} transients. First, both the Ca^{2+} uptake flux J_U and the release flux J_{CICR} are described phenomenologically by Michaelis and Menten (1913) functions (e.g., eq. 6.45); in other words, the binding of Ca^{2+} to pumps and receptors is assumed fast enough to be at equilibrium. While this assumption of steady-state kinetics is a sensible simplification at time scales of seconds, experiments using caged release of Ca^{2+} have measured a time constant for activation of CICR of 1.1 msec (Györke and Fill 1993). Second, because Goldbeter, Dupont, and Berridge assume that CICR ends because of depletion of the pool, their model works only if the store concentration $[Ca^{2+}]_s$ is in the low μM range, which is unlikely (Hofer and Machen 1993; Kendall, Dormer, and Campbell 1992). We have assumed release to have a threshold and a lower affinity (Györke and Fill 1993) than uptake, so that uptake will compensate release once the cytoplasmic $[Ca^{2+}]_i$ increases sufficiently, and we have neglected slow inactivation of release (Györke and Fill 1993). As a first step to more realistic kinetics for the Ca^{2+} uptake and CICR processes, we let the fluxes relax to the steady-state Michaelis-Menten function with a fixed time constant:

$$\frac{dJ_k([Ca^{2+}], t)}{dt} = \frac{J_{k,\infty}([Ca^{2+}]) - J_k([Ca^{2+}], t)}{\tau_k},$$

(6.44)

with $k = U, CICR$;

$$J_{U\infty} = V_U \frac{[Ca^{2+}]_i^2}{K_U^2 + [Ca^{2+}]_i^2}$$

(6.45)

$$J_{CICR_x} = V_{CICR} \frac{[Ca^{2+}]_i}{K_{CICR} + [Ca^{2+}]_i} ([Ca^{2+}]_s - [Ca^{2+}]_i)$$

(6.46)

$$J_{CICR_x} = 0.0 \quad \text{for } [Ca^{2+}]_i \le K_T,$$

(6.47)

where V_U and V_{CICR} are the maximum rates of uptake and release, respectively. (The parameters to eqs. 6.44–6.46 can be found in chapter appendix B.) Eq. 6.45 describes the steady-state kinetics of many different types of Ca^{2+}-ATPase pumps, which are all activated cooperatively by Ca^{2+} with a Hill coefficient of 2 (Lytton et al. 1992). A limitation of eq. 6.45 is that it does not depend on $[Ca^{2+}]_s$, while empty stores have a higher rate of uptake (Missiaen et al. 1990).

6.7.2 IP₃-induced Calcium Release

The IP₃ receptor seems to have more complex dynamics than the ryanodine receptor. It has a bell-shaped steady-state curve for dependence on $[Ca^{2+}]$, with a sharp peak around $0.2\,\mu M$ (Bezprozvanny, Watras, and Ehrlich 1991). De Young and Keizer (1992) have proposed a model for IP₃ receptor gating that includes IP₃ binding steps and Ca^{2+} activation and inactivation steps, resulting in eight possible states. This model was later reduced by Li and Rinzel (1994) to a Hodgkin and Huxley–like set of equations, with an activation gate m and an inactivation gate h, which can be incorporated easily into neuronal models. We have again adapted these to include a time constant for the combined IP₃ and Ca^{2+} activation:

$$J_{IP_3} = V_{IP_3} m^3 h^3 ([Ca^{2+}]_s - [Ca^{2+}]_i) \tag{6.48}$$

$$m_\infty = \frac{[IP_3]_i}{[IP_3]_i + d_{IP_3}} \frac{[Ca^{2+}]_i}{[Ca^{2+}]_i + d_{act}} \tag{6.49}$$

$$\tau_m = \frac{1}{b_{IP_3} + a_{IP_3}[Ca^{2+}]_i} \tag{6.50}$$

$$h_\infty = \frac{Q([IP_3])}{Q([IP_3]) + [Ca^{2+}]_i} \tag{6.51}$$

$$\tau_h = \frac{1}{a_{inh}(Q([IP_3]) + [Ca^{2+}]_i)} \tag{6.52}$$

$$Q = d_{inh} \frac{[IP_3]_i + d_{IP_3}}{[IP_3]_i + d_{dis}}, \tag{6.53}$$

where V_{IP_3} is the maximum rate of IP₃-induced release. (The parameters to eqs. 6.48–6.52 and a brief description of the different variables are summarized in chapter appendix B.) A similar set of equations can be found in Sneyd et al. 1995.

IP₃ Concentration Most models have assumed that [IP₃] increases are pulsatile and that degradation follows linear (De Young and Keizer 1992) or saturable kinetics (Sneyd et al. 1995). In neuronal models where IP₃ is generated by activation of the metabotropic glutamate receptor (Llano et al. 1991), it seems most appropriate to model the generation of IP_3 with an alpha function:

$$\frac{d[IP_3]_i}{dt} = \gamma t e^{-t/t_{peak}} - \beta([IP_3]_i - [IP_3]_{min}), \tag{6.54}$$

where t_{peak} is the time to peak, γ determines the maximum amount of IP_3 production, and β is the removal rate. More complex models have also included diffusion of IP_3 and the positive feedback of $[Ca^{2+}]$ onto IP_3 production (De Young and Keizer 1992).

6.7.3 The Complete Model of Release from Stores

Combining eqs. 6.44–6.54 gives a set of equations describing the change of $[Ca^{2+}]$ in the cytoplasm:

$$\frac{\partial[Ca^{2+}]_i}{\partial t} = D_{Ca}\frac{\partial^2[Ca^{2+}]_i}{\partial x^2} + (b[CaB]_i - f[Ca^{2+}]_i[B]_i)$$

$$+ \frac{J_{CICR} + J_{IP_3} - J_U + V_{leak}([Ca^{2+}]_s - [Ca^{2+}]_i)}{v_i} \tag{6.55}$$

The first and second terms of eq. 6.55 represent the diffusion and buffering term from eq. 6.35. The last term describes all the store-related fluxes and a leak flux, with a constant rate V_{leak}, which is important to compensate the Ca^{2+} uptake by J_U at rest. An equation similar to eq. 6.55, but without the diffusion term and with the fluxes reversed, describes the change of $[Ca^{2+}]_s$. During the implicit solution of the reaction-diffusion system the last term is evaluated at $t + \Delta t/2$ (like the Hodgkin-Huxley equations; see section 14.3.6).

Eq. 6.55 implicitly assumes that the Ca^{2+} fluxes do not change the electrical gradient across the ER membrane. The sarcoplasmic reticulum, which is a specialized ER found in muscle, has a membrane potential of about $+20\,mV$ compared to the cytoplasm (Stephenson, Wendt, and Forrest 1981). Jafri and Gillo (1994) have made a model where eqs. 6.44–6.46 are used to compute a $\bar{g}$ that, combined with the Nernst potential (eq. 4.16) across the ER membrane, gives a Ca^{2+} current. This model produced correct ER membrane potentials only if the movement of counterions like K^+ into the ER was included also.

Purkinje Cell Model The Purkinje cell model presented thus far did not contain Ca^{2+} stores. Figure 6.8 presents some preliminary results of a model where a Ca^{2+} store was included in every shell. Based on an electron microscopic reconstruction of

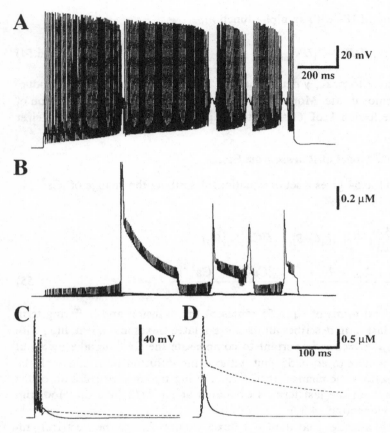

Figure 6.8
Ca^{2+}-induced Ca^{2+} release in the Purkinje cell model. (A) Membrane potential in the soma during a 1.5 nA somatic current injection. (B) Ca^{2+} concentrations in the same shells of a smooth dendritic compartment as in figure 6.7 A. (C) Comparison of somatic membrane potentials during a complex spike in model without (full line) and with Ca^{2+} stores (broken line). The subtle differences in spiking during the initial burst are functionally not significant, but the subsequent plateau depolarization in the Ca^{2+} store model is. (D) Fura-2 estimated [Ca^{2+}] in a spiny dendrite during the same complex spikes.

the ER in Purkinje cells (Martone et al. 1993), the stores were assumed to occupy 20% of the volume of each shell. This store volume was converted into store surface using the assumption that the ER could be represented as a long tube with a diameter of 0.050 μm (Palay and Chan-Palay 1974).

In practice, we found that beyond the limitations imposed by the use of Michaelis-Menten functions in eqs. 6.44–6.46, the CICR model was also very sensitive to the values of its parameters, most of which are no better than educated guesses (see chapter appendix B). In particular, CICR produced reasonable results only if calsequestrin was assumed to have extremely slow backward binding rates (b of 1 to $10\,\mathrm{sec}^{-1}$). With faster rates, CICR dumped the complete contents of the stores fast enough to raise the cytoplasmic $[Ca^{2+}]$ beyond 20 μM. We used also higher threshold values ($K_T = 200\,\mathrm{nM}$) than reported for Purkinje cells (Kano et al. 1995) because the experimental values are distorted by the spatial averaging of the fura-2 signal (figure 6.7B). In fact, the apparent $[Ca^{2+}]$ threshold for CICR that can be estimated from the computed fura-2 signal in a spiny dendrite of the model (80 nM) is very close to the experimental values (Kano et al. 1995).

We have tuned the parameters of the CICR model so that CICR is activated during somatic current injection without causing noticeable changes to the Purkinje cell firing pattern (figure 6.8A). Compared to the Purkinje cell model without Ca^{2+} stores (figure 6.5A), the firing pattern looks similar and the subtle differences are within the normal range. This corresponds to the experimental observation that firing patterns look normal in cells where subsequent addition of low concentrations of caffeine evokes large Ca^{2+} signals due to CICR. Nevertheless, CICR caused complex changes to the cytoplasmic Ca^{2+} levels during the dendritic spikes (figure 6.8B). Each dendritic spike evoked CICR, causing prolonged increases of the sub-membrane $[Ca^{2+}]$. Note that the first dendritic spike was initiated sooner due to the CICR itself. The CICR remained localized to the submembrane region and did not cause a Ca^{2+} wave traveling toward the center of the compartment. This can be explained by the relative high threshold for CICR intitiation (K_T).

Using the same parameters, CICR had a profound effect on the shape of the complex spike (figure 6.8C). The complex spike is a distributed synaptic response evoked by climbing fiber stimulation that activates Ca^{2+} channels everywhere in the dendritic tree of the Purkinje cell (Miyakawa et al. 1992a). In the presence of Ca^{2+} stores, the increase in $[Ca^{2+}]$ due to Ca^{2+} infow was markedly enhanced by CICR (figure 6.8D). This activated the Na^+-Ca^{2+} exchanger, causing the prolonged depolarization in the model with CICR. Depolarizing plateaus evoked by complex spikes have been reported in the literature (Ekerot and Oscarsson 1981).

6.8 Conclusions

This chapter has given an overview of up-to-date techniques to model biophysically realistic Ca^{2+} dynamics in a compartmental model of a dendritic tree. Many of these techniques can easily be applied to the simulation of other ionic species or of second messengers.

The model we have presented is a first step toward understanding the role of Ca^{2+} release in Purkinje cell physiology. Over the coming years, we expect the model to become more complex. We have neglected, for example, diffusion of IP_3 and have modeled radial diffusion of Ca^{2+} only. Although, because of buffering, Ca^{2+} has a very low D_{app} and presumably also slight longitudinal effects, this may not be true for Ca^{2+} release mechanisms. Because IP_3 is not buffered, it is expected to diffuse much further than Ca^{2+} (Kasai and Petersen 1994; but see also Wang and Augustine 1995), and it has been hypothesized that CICR could transmit Ca^{2+} gradients down a dendrite (Sah 1996). We have also neglected the morphology of the ER and other organelles in the cytoplasm, which can obstruct diffusion (Kargacin 1994). Nor can we expect release mechanisms to be uniformly distributed (Martone et al. 1993).

Finally, as regards correctly modeling $[Ca^{2+}]$ in spines, a quick calculation shows that a 25 nM concentration corresponds to exactly one ion in the volume of a 0.5 µm diameter sphere, which is about the size of a spine head! This raises doubts about the use of differential equations to describe $[Ca^{2+}]$ in spines. We believe that a Monte Carlo method, which Bartol et al. (1991) have used to study transmitter diffusion, might be the best technique to study $[Ca^{2+}]$ diffusion in three dimensions (Bormann and De Schutter 1996).

Acknowledgments

This research is supported by National Institute of Mental Health grant 1-R01-MH52903, by the National Fund for Scientific Research (Belgium) and by European Science Foundation grant 156. The authors thank Guy Bormann for his help in the conversion to LATEX, and Christof Koch, Reinoud Maex, and Alex Protopapas for their comments on earlier versions of this chapter.

Note

1. For clarity we will use the same convention for the sign of membrane currents as used in chapter 4, this volume, which is opposite to the convention used in GENESIS.

Appendix A: Purkinje Cell Model Description

The equations and parameters specific to the simulation of $[Ca^{2+}]$ dynamics are presented in this chapter and in chapter appendix B. For the sake of brevity, we will not list all the parameters for the passive properties of the model and for the voltage-gated channels. The complete Purkinje cell model can be obtained at http://bbf-www.uia.ac.be/CHAPTER/Purkinje.html.

The current model simulates the same morphology, reconstructed by M. Rapp (Rapp, Segev, and Yarom 1994), and utilized in our earlier one (De Schutter and Bower 1994a) except for the addition of an axon hillock four compartments long, making the total number of compartments 1,604. The membrane capacitance was changed to $1\,\mu F\,cm^{-2}$, the standard value used in most models (Jack, Noble, and Tsien 1975).

All the compartments in the model are active. Channel kinetics are simulated using Hodgkin and Huxley–like equations and a set of nine channel types similar to those used before. The soma has fast and persistent Na^+ channels (NaF and NaP), T-type and P-type Ca^{2+} channels (CaT and CaP), a delayed rectifier (Kdr), an A-current (KA), noninactivating K^+ channels (KM), and an anomalous rectifier (Kh). The dendritic membrane includes CaT and CaP channels, a Ca^{2+}-activated K^+ channel (KC), and a KM channel. Additionally, a transitional zone called the "main dendrite" also contains Kdr and KA channels. The axon hillock has NaF and Kdr channels in a slightly higher density than the soma. The total number of channels and pumps in the model without stores is 9,842.

The Hodgkin and Huxley–like equations for the CaP and KA channels were updated, based on newer data from Purkinje cells. Because the conductance of the KC channel in the earlier model did not have a realistic dependence on $[Ca^{2+}]$ (De Schutter and Bower 1994a), the equation for KC was replaced by the kinetic description of a rat muscle BK channel (Moczydlowski and Latorre 1983). These equations were based on measurements of channels incorporated in artifical lipid bilayers, a procedure which is known to affect the Ca^{2+} affinity of the channel (Kapicka et al. 1994). We therefore increased the affinity in the model by a factor of 33 (e.g., Gabbiani, Mitgaard, and Knöpfel 1994), bringing it closer to the values for maximal KC activation measured in whole cells (Prakriya, Solaro, and Lingle 1996).

Appendix B: Parameters for Calcium Stores

Ca^{2+} uptake parameters (eq. 6.45):

$$V_U = 4 \cdot 10^{-9}\,\mu M\,cm^{-2}\,msec^{-1}$$

$$K_U = 1.0\,\mu M$$

$$\tau_U = 1.0\,msec.$$

Ca^{2+}-induced Ca^{2+} release parameters (eq. 6.46):

$$V_{CICR} = 3 \cdot 10^{-8}\,cm^{-2}\,msec^{-1} \qquad \tau_{CICR} = 1.2\,msec$$

$$K_{CICR} = 0.3\,\mu M \qquad K_T = 0.2\,\mu M$$

IP$_3$-induced Ca^{2+} release parameters (eqs. 6.48–6.53):

$$V_{IP_3} = 1.0 \cdot 10^{-8}\,cm^{-2}\,msec^{-1} \qquad b_{IP_3} = 4.1 \cdot 10^{-3}\,msec^{-1}$$

$$a_{inh} = 2.0 \cdot 10^{-4}\,\mu M\,msec^{-1} \qquad a_{IP_3} = 0.42\,\mu M^{-1}\,msec^{-1}$$

$$d_{inh} = 1.05\,\mu M \qquad d_{IP_3} = 0.13\,\mu M$$

$$d_{act} = 8.2 \cdot 10^{-2}\,\mu M \qquad d_{dis} = 0.94\,\mu M.$$

Parameters a and b are respectively, forward and backward binding rate constants for IP_3 receptor binding (a_{IP_3} and b_{IP_3}) and inhibitive Ca^{2+} binding to the receptor (a_{inh}). Similarly, dissociation constants (b/a) are defined for IP_3 binding to the uninhibited (d_{IP_3}) and Ca^{2+}-inhibited receptor (d_{dis}), and for Ca^{2+} activation (d_{act}) and inhibition (d_{inh}) of the receptor.
Initial Ca^{2+} concentrations:

$[Ca^{2+}]_{i,rest} = 40\,nM$

$[Ca^{2+}]_{s,rest} = 200\,\mu M$.

Buffer in store (calsequestrin) parameters:

$K_d = 1\,mM$

$f_s = 10.0\,M^{-1}\,msec^{-1}$

$b_s = 0.01\,msec^{-1}$

$[B]_{T,s} = 100\,mM$.

7 Analysis of Neural Excitability and Oscillations

John Rinzel and Bard Ermentrout

7.1 Introduction

Qualitative features of excitable or oscillatory dynamics are shared by broad classes of neuronal models. Expressed in models for single-cell behavior as well as for ensemble activity, these features include excitability and threshold behavior; beating and bursting oscillations and phase locking; and bistability and hystersis. Our goal here is to illustrate, by exploiting a specific model of excitable membrane, some of the concepts and techniques that can be used to understand, predict, and interpret these dynamic phenomena biophysically. Our mathematical methods include numerical integration of the model equations, graphical or geometric representation of the dynamics (phase plane analysis), and analytic formulae for characterizing thresholds and stability conditions. The concepts are from the qualitative theory of nonlinear differential equations and nonlinear oscillations, and from perturbation and bifurcation theory. In this brief chapter, we will not consider the spatiotemporal aspects of distributed systems. Thus our methods apply directly only to a membrane patch, to a spatially uniform, equipotential cell, or to a network with each cell type perfectly synchronized.

Even seemingly simple models that exhibit one or two of the different dynamic behaviors, such as generation of individual or repetitive action potentials, may display a great variety of response characteristics when a broad range of parameters is considered. This means that a given cell or ensemble may behave in many different modes, for example, as a generator of single pulses, as a bursting pacemaker, as a bistable "plateauing" cell, or as a beating oscillator, depending upon the physiological conditions (neuromodulator or ionic concentrations) or stimulus presentations (applied currents or synaptic inputs). The nonlinear nature of the models provides the substrate for this broad repertoire; in contrast, linear models may be characterized by exponential or oscillatory time courses over their entire parameter ranges. It is important when studying a nonlinear model that stimulus-response properties be considered over ranges of the biophsical parameters.

In this chapter, we show that a simple, but biophysically reasonable, two-current excitable membrane model is sufficiently robust to exhibit such behavioral richness, as parameters are systematically varied. By adjusting channel densities, activation dynamics, and stimulus intensities, we find that the cell model can exhibit quite different threshold characteristics for spike generation (finite or infinite latency, with or without intermediate amplitude responses) and for onset of repetitive firing (finite or zero minimum frequency). The cell shows various types of bistable behavior: two different rest states, in one case, and a rest state with a coexistent oscillatory response around a depolarized level, in another. The latter situation can provide a mechanism for rhythmic bursting when additional slower processes (e.g., slow channel kinetics, or a channel affected by slow ion accumulation) respond differently at the two potential levels. Because the spike-generating dynamics significantly influence the burst's waveform, there can be several different types of bursting depending on the nature of the fast dynamics; for example, parabolic bursting does not depend on bistability in the spike-generating processes. Finally, by considering the phase-resetting behavior for a self-oscillatory cell, we show that the response to a single brief, arbitrarily timed, perturbing stimulus can often be used to predict phase-locking responses to periodic stimulation, and to predict the synchronization properties of weakly coupled cells.

The underlying qualitative structure for these behaviors will be revealed with graphical phase plane analysis, complemented by a few analytic formulas. The concepts we will cover include steady states, trajectories, limit cycles, stability, domains of attraction, and bifurcation of solutions. Phase plane characteristics and system dynamics will be interpreted biophysically in terms of activation curves, current-voltage relations, and the like. A user-friendly program, XPP (developed by G. B. Ermentrout) for X-windows computers allows modelers to interactively generate, explore, and visualize most of the behaviors described here in the same spirit as an experimental "setup." (XPP's numerical procedures are summarized in chapter appendix B.) The concepts apply to higher-order systems, for which appropriate projections of phase space, motivated by differences in time scales for certain variables, can lead to similar insights.

7.2 Models for Excitable Cells and Networks

Most models for excitable membrane retain the general Hodgkin-Huxley (HH) format (Hodgkin and Huxley 1952), and can be written in the form

$$C\frac{dV}{dt} + I_{ion}(V, W_1, \ldots, W_n) = I(t) \tag{7.1}$$

$$\frac{dW_i}{dt} = \phi\frac{[W_{i,\infty}(V) - W_i]}{\tau_i(V)}, \tag{7.2}$$

where V denotes membrane potential (say, deviation from a reference, or "rest" level), C is membrane capacity, and I_{ion} is the sum of V- and t-dependent currents through the various ionic channel types; $I(t)$ is the applied current. The $W_i(t)$ variables describe the fraction of channels of a given type that are in various conducting states (e.g., open or closed) at time t. The first-order kinetics for W_i typically involve V dependence in the time constant τ_i; ϕ is a temperature-like time scale factor that may depend on i. If the current, I_j, for channel type j may be suitably modeled as ohmic, then it might be expressed as

$$I_j = \bar{g}_j \sigma_j(V, W_1, \ldots, W_n)(V - V_j), \tag{7.3}$$

where $\bar{g}_j$ is the total conductance with all j-type channels open (product of single-channel conductance with the total number of j channels), σ_j is the fraction of j channels that are open (it may depend on several of the W_i variables), and V_j is the reversal potential (usually Nernstian) for this ion species. For some channel types the current-voltage relation may be more appropriately represented by the Goldman-Hodgkin-Katz equation, or by a barrier kinetics scheme (Hille 1992), and the gating kinetics might involve a multistate Markov description. In the classical HH model (Hodgkin and Huxley 1952) for squid giant axon, there are three variables W_i, denoted as m, h, and n, to describe the fractions $m^3 h$ and n^4 of open Na^+ channels and K^+ channels, respectively.

For some purposes, it is important that the current balance equation (eq. 7.1) contain terms to account for ionic pump currents. These currents, as well as some channel conductances, may depend upon time-varying second messengers or ionic concentrations, for example, in diffusionally restricted intracellular or extracellular volumes. For such considerations, additional variables and transport or kinetic balance equations would be included in the model, and these will carry along their own time scales. Indeed, some models that include the dynamics of intracellular free calcium handling have assumed time constants that are orders of magnitude greater than channel kinetics and thereby set the time scale for phenomena such as bursting oscillations (see, for example, Chay and Keizer 1983). We also note that the form of eq. 7.2 is not unique; in a phenomenological model of Rall (see Goldstein and Rall 1974), the corresponding equations are nonlinear in the W_i.

Some models for excitability contain many variables and represent numerous channel types, especially models designed to account for rather detailed aspects of spike shape and dependence on many different pharmacological agents. On the other hand, if qualitative or semiquantitative characteristics of spike generation and input-output relations are adepuate, say in network simulations, then a reduced model having just a few variables may suffice. Such reductions can sometimes be obtained when time scale differences allow relatively fast variables to be instantaneously relaxed to pseudo–steady-state values; thus, if τ_j is small relative to other time constants, then one might set $W_j = W_{j,\infty}(V)$ in eq. 7.2. Likewise, functionally related variables with similar time scales might be lumped together. In this spirit, FitzHugh (1960) considered reductions of the HH model (see also Rinzel 1985; Kepler, Abbott, and Marder 1992) and then introduced (FitzHugh 1961) and idealized, analytically tractable two-variable model (see also Nagumo, Arimoto, and Yoshizawa 1962) widely studied as a qualitative prototype for excitable systems in many biological and chemical contexts. A FitzHugh-Nagumo/Hodgkin-Huxley hybrid was formulated and studied by Morris and Lecar (1981), in the context of electrical activity of the barnacle muscle fiber. The model incorporates a V-gated Ca^{2+} channel and a V-gated, delayed-rectifier K^+ channel; neither current inactivates. A simple version of this model is represented by the equations

$$C \frac{dV}{dt} = -I_{ion}(V, w) + I \tag{7.4}$$

$$\frac{dw}{dt} = \phi \frac{[w_\infty(V) - w]}{\tau_w(V)}, \tag{7.5}$$

where

$$I_{ion}(V, w) = \bar{g}_{Ca} m_\infty(V)(V - V_{Ca}) + \bar{g}_K w(V - V_K) + \bar{g}_L(V - V_L). \tag{7.6}$$

In eqs. 7.4–7.6, w is the fraction of K^+ channels open, and the Ca^{2+} channels respond to V so rapidly that we assume instantaneous activation. One might introduce dimensionless variables, as in FitzHugh 1969 or Rinzel and Ermentrout 1989, in order (1) to reduce the number of free parameters and identify equivalent groups of parameters, and (2) identify and group "fast" and "slow" processes together. However, in the interest of clarity, we will keep all equations in their original form. In eq. 7.5, τ_w has been scaled so its maximum is now one, and ϕ equals the temperature factor divided by the prescaled maximum ($1\sqrt{\lambda_w}$ in Morris and Lecar 1981). (The V-dependent functions, m_∞, w_∞, and τ_w, and the reference parameter sets are given in appendix A). All the computations and figures in this chapter are based on eqs. 7.4–7.6, and extensions of them for generating bursting behaviors.

Even network models in certain approximations can reduce to a few variables. One example is the Wilson-Cowan model (1972; for another, see chapter 11, this volume):

$$\mu_e \frac{d\mathscr{E}}{dt} = -\mathscr{E} + S(\alpha_{ee}\mathscr{E} - \alpha_{ie}\mathscr{I} - \theta_e) \tag{7.7}$$

$$\mu_i \frac{d\mathscr{I}}{dt} = -\mathscr{I} + S(\alpha_{ei}\mathscr{E} - \alpha_{ii}\mathscr{I} - \theta_i), \tag{7.8}$$

where $\mathscr{E}$ and $\mathscr{I}$ represent the respective firing rates of a population of excitatory and inhibitory interneurons. The parameters μ_e, μ_i are the membrane time constants; θ_e, θ_i are the firing thresholds; α_{ee}, α_{ie}, α_{ei}, α_{ii} are the "synaptic weights"; and $S(\cdot)$ is a nonlinear saturating function similar in form to $m_\infty(V)$.

7.3   Understanding Dynamics via Phase Plane Analysis

While an experimenter typically can measure membrane potential, it is usually impossible to monitor other dynamic variables, such as ionic currents, during non-clamped activity. For a theoretical model, we must explicitly compute the time courses of all dependent variables; we can then compare the time courses of the different dynamic variables and identify their contributions and temporal relationships. A valuable way to view the response of multiple variables and their relationship to physiological functions at the same time is by phase plane profiles, that is, curves of one dependent variable against another. Moreover, such plots allow us also to geometrically represent and interpret aspects of the model (e.g., activation curves) along with the response trajectories. At a glance, we can see whether the model has one or multiple steady states, which stimuli might invoke switching between states, and where these steady states lie in relation to activation and current-voltage (I-V) characteristics. While the phase plane view provides a full description for two-variable models, judicious two-dimensional projections from phase spaces of higher-order systems can yield some of these same insights.

   Phase plane analysis was used effectively by FitzHugh (1960, 1961, 1969) to understand various aspects of the HH equations and the two-variable FitzHugh-Nagumo model. (FitzHugh 1969 also defines some basic mathematical terminology of nonlinear dynamics and supplements our presentation; for additional mathematical introduction, see also Edelstein-Keshet 1988 and Strogatz 1994.)

7.3.1   The Geometry of Excitability

We begin by considering the Morris-Lecar model (1981), in the case that there is a unique rest state and a thresholdlike behavior for action potential generation. Figure 7.1A shows the V responses to brief current pulses of different amplitudes. The peak V is graded, but the variation occurs over a very narrow range of stimuli; in this case, as in the standard HH model, the threshold phenomenon is not discrete, but rather, steeply graded. In figure 7.1B, these same responses are represented in the V-w plane. The solution path in the space of dependent variables is called a "trajectory," and direction of motion along a trajectory is often indicated by an

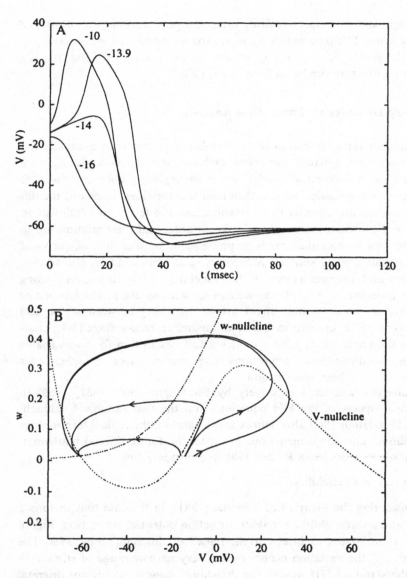

Figure 7.1
Response of the Morris-Lecar excitable system, eqs. 7.4–7.6, to a brief current pulse. For these parameters (see appendix A), the system has a unique stable rest state, $\bar{V} = -61\,mV$, $\bar{w} = .015$. The line $w = \bar{w}$ is shown lightly dashed. Four different stimuli lead to an instantaneous displacement of V from $\bar{V}$ to V_0 (values of V_0 are shown alongside the curves in panel A). Panel A shows the time course of the voltage. Notice that intermediate responses are possible with some stimuli: the threshold is graded; firing occurs with finite latency. Panel B shows trajectories in the V-w phase plane; nullclines are shown dashed and intersect only once. The effect of a stimulus is to displace the initial condition horizontally from rest.

arrowhead. In figure 7.1B, the flow is generally counterclockwise. All the trajectories shown here ultimately lead to the rest point: $V = \bar{V}, w = \bar{w} = w_\infty(\bar{V})$. The rest state is said to be "globally attracting." Each trajectory has a unique initial point, a horizontal displacement from the rest point corresponding to instantaneous depolarization by a brief current pulse. A trajectory's slope conveys the relative speed of w to V; thus a shallow slope means V is changing faster (see next paragraph). The trajectory of an action potential shows the following features: an upstroke with rapid increase in V (trajectory is moving rightward with little vertical component) and then the transient depolarized plateau with the delayed major increase in w, corresponding to the slower opening of K^+ channels. When w is large enough, the abrupt downstroke in V occurs—the trajectory moves leftward, nearly horizontal, as V tends toward V_K. Finally, as w decreases (the potassium channels close), the state point returns to rest with a slow recovery from hyperpolarization.

In the phase plane, the slope of a trajectory at a given point is dw/dV, which is simply the ratio of dw/dt to dV/dt, and these quantities are evaluated from the right-hand sides of the differential equations (eqs. 7.4–7.5). (The program XPP has a command to plot short vectors that indicate the flow pattern generated by the equations. This allows a global view of the flow without having to compute the trajectories. The program also computes nullclines, defined next.) Thus a trajectory must be vertical or horizontal where $dV/dt = 0$ or $dw/dt = 0$, respectively. The conditions

$$0 = -\bar{g}_{Ca}m_\infty(V)(V - V_{Ca}) - \bar{g}_K w(V - V_K) - \bar{g}_L(V - V_L) + I \tag{7.9}$$

$$0 = \phi \frac{[w_\infty(V) - w]}{\tau_w(V)} \tag{7.10}$$

define curves, the V and w nullclines, which are shown dashed in figure 7.1B. This provides a geometrical realization for where V and w can reach their maximum and minimum values along a trajectory in the V-w plane (notice how the trajectories cross the nullclines either vertically or horizontally in figure 7.1B). The w nullcline is simply the w activation curve, $w = w_\infty(V)$. The V nullcline, from eq. 7.9, corresponds to V and w values at which the instantaneous ionic current plus applied current is zero; below the V nullcline, V is increasing and above it, V is decreasing. The cubic-like shape seen here reflects the N-shaped *instantaneous I-V relation*, $I_{ion}(V, w)$ versus V with w fixed (eq. 7.6), typical of excitable membrane models in which the V-gated channels carrying inward current activate rapidly. From another viewpoint, motivated by the slower time scale of w, suppose we fix w, say, at a moderate value. Then the three points on the V nullcline at this w correspond to three pseudo–steady states; at the low-V state, small outward and inward currents cancel while at the high-V state, both currents are larger but are again in balance. These states are transiently visited during the plateau phase and the return-to-rest phase of an action potential. Notice how the trajectory is near the right and left branches of the V nullcline during these phases.

If ϕ were smaller still, then the phase plane trajectories (except when near the V nullcline) would be nearly horizontal (because dw/dV would be small); the action potential trajectory during the plateau and recovery phases would essentially cling to, and move slowly along, either the right or left branch of the V nullcline. The downstroke would occur at the knee of the V nullcline. The time course would be more like that of a cardiac action potential. Also, in the case of smaller ϕ, the threshold phenomenon would be extremely steep; the middle branch of the V null-cline would act as an approximate separatrix between sub- and superthreshold initial conditions. In contrast, for larger ϕ, the response amplitude is more graded. This theoretical conclusion led Cole, Guttman, and Bezanilla (1970) to demonstrate experimentally that, at higher temperatures, the action potential for squid axon does not behave in an all-or-none manner.

We note that phase plane methodology applies to autonomous systems, whose equations have no explicit time dependence and whose nullclines and flow field therefore do not change with time. (This would not be the case if, for example, I were periodic in t; periodic stimuli will be covered later.) The phase plane method extends, however, to cases where a step change in a parameter occurs. At the time a parameter's value jumps, the nullclines would change instantaneously, but not the present location of V and w. FitzHugh (1961) uses this trick to interpret anodal break excitation, and Somers and Kopell (1993) have used this to analyze the behavior of coupled Morris-Lecar oscillators when ϕ is very small.

7.3.2 Oscillations Emerging with Nonzero Frequency

In the phase plane treatment, the rest state of the model is realized as the intersection of the two nullclines; such steady-state solutions are also referred to as singular or equilbrium points. From the geometrical viewpoint, one sees how different parameter values could easily lead to multiple singular points—by changing the shapes and positions of the nullclines. In figure 7.1, the unique singular point is attracting. Technically, we say it is asymptotically stable, that is, for any nearby initial point the solution tends to the singular point as $t \to \infty$. In general, the local stability of a singular point can be determined by a simple algebraic criterion (Edelstein-Keshet 1988; Strogatz 1994). The procedure is to linearize the differential equations, evaluate the partial derivatives at the singular point (this matrix of partial derivatives is called the Jacobian), and to determine whether the exponential solutions to this constant coefficient system have any growing modes. If so, then the singular point is unstable; if all modes decay, then it is stable. For eqs. 7.4–7.6, the linearized equations that describe the behavior of small disturbances, $V \approx \bar{V} + x$, $w \approx \bar{w} + y$, from the singular point are

$$\frac{dx}{dt} = ax + by \tag{7.11}$$

$$\frac{dy}{dt} = cx + dy, \tag{7.12}$$

where

$$a = -\frac{\partial I_{ion}(V, w)}{\partial V} \tag{7.13}$$

$$b = -\frac{\partial I_{ion}(V, w)}{\partial w} \tag{7.14}$$

$$c = \frac{\phi}{\tau_w} \frac{dw_\infty}{dV} \tag{7.15}$$

$$d = -\frac{\phi}{\tau_w}. \tag{7.16}$$

Solutions are of the form $\exp(\lambda_1 t)$, $\exp(\lambda_2 t)$, where $\lambda_{1,2}$ are the eigenvalues of the Jacobian matrix in eqs. 7.11–7.12; they are roots of the quadratic

$$\lambda^2 - (a + d)\lambda + (ad - bc) = 0. \tag{7.17}$$

For the parameters of figure 7.1, the two eigenvalues are both real and negative.

As parameters are varied, the singular point may lose stability. In our example, the rest state could then no longer be maintained and the behavior of the system would change—it may fire repetitively or tend to a different steady state (if a stable one exists). Let us consider the effect of a steady applied current and ask how repetitive firing arises in this model. We will apply linear stability theory to find values of I for which the steady state is unstable. First, we note that for eqs. 7.4–7.6, and for nerve membrane models of the general form of eqs. 7.1–7.2, a steady-state solution $\bar{V}$ for a given I must satisfy $I = I_{ss}(\bar{V})$, where $I_{ss}(V)$ is the steady-state I-V relation of the model given by

$$I_{ss}(V) = I_{ion}(V, w_\infty(V)). \tag{7.18}$$

If I_{ss} is N-shaped, there will be three steady states for some range of I. If however, I_{ss} is monotonic increasing with V, as in the case of figure 7.1, then there is a unique $\bar{V}$ for each I; moreover, $(\bar{V}, \bar{w})$ cannot lose stability by having a single real eigenvalue pass through zero. Destabilization can only occur by a complex conjugate pair of eigenvalues crossing the axis $Re\,\lambda = 0$ as I is varied through a critical value I_1. At such a transition, a periodic solution to eqs. 7.4–7.6 is born—and we have the onset of repetitive activity. This solution, for I close to I_1, is of small amplitude and frequency proportional to $Im\lambda$. Emergence of a periodic solution in this way is called a Hopf bifurcation (Edelstein-Keshet 1988; Strogatz 1994).

From eqs. 7.11–7.12, or eq. 7.17, we know that $\lambda_1 + \lambda_2 = a + d$. Thus loss of stability occurs for the I whose corresponding $\bar{V}$ satisfies

$$\frac{\partial I_{ion}(V, w)}{\partial v} + \frac{\phi}{\tau_w} = 0. \tag{7.19}$$

The first term here is the slope of the instantaneous I-V relation and the second is the rate of the recovery process; this condition also applies approximately to the HH model (Rinzel 1978). From eq. 7.19 we conclude that loss of stability occurs: (1) only if the *instantaneous I-V relation* has negative slope at $\bar{V}$; (2) when the destabilizing growth rate of V from this negative resistance just balances the recovery rate; and (3) only if recovery is sufficiently slow, i.e. if ϕ is small (low "temperature"). In figure 7.2A, $\bar{V}$ is plotted versus I (this is the *steady-state I-V relation*, but shown as V against I) and the region of instability is shown dashed.

Figure 7.2A also shows the maximum and minimum values of V for the oscillatory response. Just as a singular point can be unstable, so, too, can a periodic solution (Strogatz 1994); unstable periodics are indicated by open circles. Here we see that the small amplitude periodic solution born at $I = I_1 = 93.85\,\mu A/cm^2$ from the loss in stability of $\bar{V}$ is itself unstable; it would not be directly observable. (In the phase plane, but not generally for higher-order systems, an unstable periodic orbit can be determined by integrating backward in time.) Note that solutions along this branch depend continuously on parameters and they gain stability at the turning point or knee at $I = I_v = 88.3\,\mu A/cm^2$. A stable periodic solution is called a "limit cycle." The upper branch (solid) corresponds to the limit cycle of observed repetitive firing. The frequency increases with I over most of this branch (figure 7.2B). At sufficiently large I, repetitive firing ceases (depolarization block) as $\bar{V}$ regains stability at $I = I_2 = 212\,\mu A/cm^2$. This figure is referred to as a "bifurcation diagram"; it depicts steady-state and periodic solutions, and their stability, as functions of a parameter

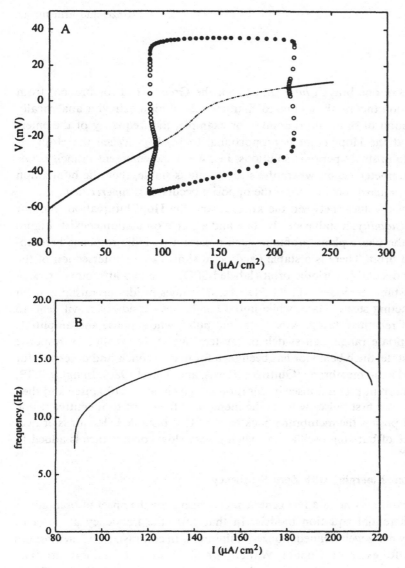

Figure 7.2
Repetitive firing in the Morris-Lecar model for steady current. Bifurcation diagram in panel A shows the steady-state voltage $\bar{V}$ versus I (thin lines; stable are solid, unstable are dashed) and the maximum and minimum voltage for periodic solutions shown as filled (stable) and unfilled (unstable) circles. The unstable branch of periodic solutions meets the branch of steady-state oscillations at $I = I_1 = 94 \, \mu\text{A/cm}^2$ and $I = I_2 = 212 \, \mu\text{A/cm}^2$ (Hopf bifurcation points). The unstable branch of periodic solutions coalesces with the stable branch of periodic solutions at $I = I_v = 88 \, \mu\text{A/cm}^2$. A similar coalescence occurs near $I = 215 \, \mu\text{A/cm}^2$. For these parameters, the steady-state I-V curve is monotonic. Furthermore, panel B shows that the frequency (plotted in Hz, and only for the stable limit cycles) as a function of current is always bounded away from zero. Parameters are as figure 7.1.

and it shows where one branch *bifurcates* (from the Greek word for branch) from another. Bifurcation theory allows one to characterize solution behavior analytically in the neighborhood of bifurcation points; for example, the frequency of the emergent oscillation at the Hopf point is proportional to $|Im\lambda_{1,2}|$. When the Hopf bifurcation leads to unstable periodic solutions, i.e., when the emergent branch bends back into the parameter region where the steady state is stable, then the bifurcation is *subcritical* (i.e., a hard oscillation); if the opposite occurs, it is *supercritical*.

For a range of I values (between the knee, I_v and the Hopf bifurcation, I_1), our model exhibits *bistability*: a stable steady state and a stable oscillation coexist. Figure 7.3A illustrates the phase plane profile in such a case; a periodic response here appears as a closed orbit. There is a stable fixed point shown as the intersection of the two nullclines and a stable periodic orbit (labeled SPO). The two attractors are separated by an unstable periodic orbit (UPO). Initial values inside the unstable orbit tend to the attracting steady state, while initial conditions outside of it will lead to the limit cycle of repetitive firing. A brief current pulse, whose phase and amplitude are in an appropriate range, can switch the system out of the oscillatory response back to the rest state. Such behavior has been seen for many models and observed, for example, in squid axon membrane (Guttman, Lewis, and Rinzel 1980). In figure 7.3B, two $30\,\mu A/cm^2$ current pulses 5 msec in duration are given, at $t = 100$ msec and then at $t = 470$ msec. The first pulse switches the membrane from rest to repetitive firing, while the second pushes the membrane back to rest. This bistable behavior is critical for the occurence of bursting oscillations when a very slow conductance is added to the model.

7.3.3   Oscillations Emerging with Zero Frequency

The Hopf bifurcation is one of a few generic mechanisms for the onset of oscillations in nonlinear differential equation models. In that case, the frequency at onset of repetitive activity has a well-defined, nonzero minimum. In contrast, some membranes and models (see, for example, Connor, Walter, and McKown 1977) exhibit zero (i.e., arbitrarily low) frequency as they enter the oscillatory regime of behavior; Rall's model (Goldstein and Rall 1974) also behaves this way. A basic feature in such systems is that I_{ss} versus V is N-shaped rather than monotonic, as in the previous section. For eqs. 7.4–7.6, this occurs if the V dependence of K^+ activation is translated rightward (see appendix A, and note value of V_3), so that the inward component of I_{ss} dominates over an intermediate V range. Thus, for some values of I, below the repetitive firing range, there are three singular points in the phase plane and the system is excitable. We discuss this case first. In figure 7.4B, we see the nullclines

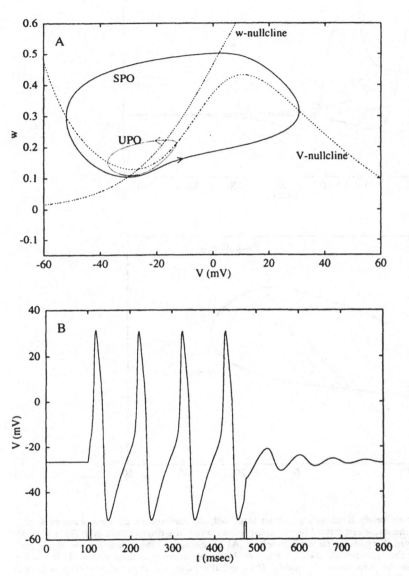

Figure 7.3
Bistability for steady current near the threshold for repetitive firing for the Morris-Lecar model with parameters as in figure 7.1 and $I = 90\,\mu A/cm^2$. In this region, where I is between the first Hopf bifurcation point, I_1, and the "knee," I_v, there are two stable states (cf figure 7.2): a rest state (the intersection of the nullclines) and a stable oscillation (SPO) separated by an unstable periodic solution (UPO). This is shown in panel A. Panel B demonstrate switching from rest to oscillation and then back to rest for two brief appropriately timed depolarizing current pulses.

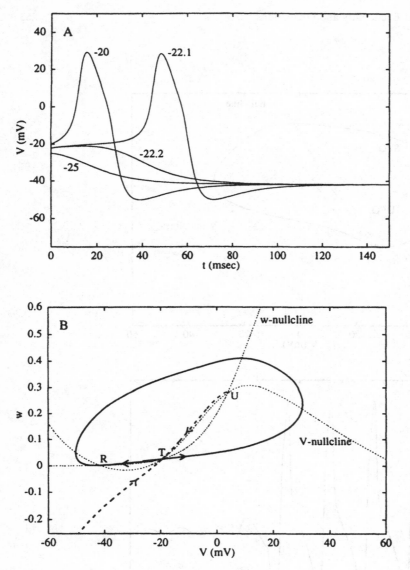

Figure 7.4
Excitability with three steady states and a distinct threshold; the response of the membrane to a brief current pulse from the stable rest state. Four different stimuli result in a displacement of V from $\bar{V}$ to V_0 (values of V_0 are given alongside the curves in panel A). (A) Time course of the voltage for $I = 30\,\mu A/cm^2$. (B) Phase plane for the dynamics illustrated in panel A. Nullclines intersect at three places: (1) R a stable rest state, (2) T, a saddle point threshold, and (3) U an unstable node. The thick solid line shows the unstable manifold for the saddle point; here, unstable refers to movement in opposing directions away from T (indicated by arrowheads). The manifold's two branches lead to the stable rest state and form a smooth loop in phase space. The heavy dashed line shows the stable manifold for the saddle point (arrowheads pointing toward T). Any initial conditions to the left of this manifold decay to rest. Initial conditions to the right lead to an action potential before returning to rest. Parameters are as in figure 7.1, except $\bar{g}_{Ca} = 4\,mS/cm^2$, $V_3 = 12\,mV$, $V_4 = 17.4\,mV$, $\phi = 1/15$.

intersecting three times. As determined by linear stability theory, the singular points are the stable rest state (**R**), and unstable saddle point threshold (**T**), and an unstable spiral (**U**). The system is excitable, with the lower state being a globally attracting rest state: initial conditions near R lead to a prompt decay to rest, while larger stimuli lead to an action potential—a long trajectory about the phase plane. The phase plane portrait moreover reveals that this case of excitability indeed has a distinct threshold which is due to the presence of the saddle point, **T**. To understand this, we note that associated with the saddle are a unique pair of incoming trajectories (bold dashed lines) corresponding to the negative eigenvalue of the Jacobian matrix; together, these represent the *stable manifold*. Corresponding to the positive eigenvalue are a pair of trajectories (bold lines) that enter the saddle as $t \to -\infty$; these are the *unstable manifold*. (XPP has a command that generates these manifolds.) The stable manifold defines a separatrix curve in the phase plane that sharply distinguishes sub- from superthreshold initial conditions. For initial conditions near the threshold separatrix, there is a long latency before a firing or decaying subthreshold response (see figure 7.4A). This is because the trajectory starts close to (but not exactly on) the stable manifold and thus the solution comes very near the saddle singular point (where it moves very slowly) before taking off. If w is started at rest, w_R, then there is a unique value of $V = V_T$ (between -22.1 and $-22.2\,\text{mV}$ in the present example) called the "voltage threshold," where the stable manifold intersects the line $w = w_R$.

The action potential trajectory follows along the unstable manifold (bold lines), which passes around the unstable spiral and eventually tends to the rest point. Such a trajectory joining two singular points is called a "heteroclinic orbit." The other branch of the unstable manifold is also a heteroclinic orbit from the saddle to the rest point. This heteroclinic pair forces any trajectory that begins outside it to remain outside it—thus preserving the amplitude of the action potential. In this case we do not find graded responses for any brief current pulses from the rest state.

This case also provides a counterexample to the common misconception that if there are three steady states, then the "outer" two are stable, while the "middle" one is unstable. In fact, in some parameter regimes this model has three singular points, none of which is stable.

Next, we tune up I and ask when repetitive firing occurs. Because I_{ss} is N-shaped, we know that the lower and middle values of $\bar{V}$ move toward each other as I increases, and there is a critical value I_1 where they meet. In the phase plane, this means that the rest point and the saddle coalesce and then disappear; this is called a "saddle node bifurcation." Moreover, the heteroclinic pair become a single closed loop, a limit cycle, which for I just above I_1 has very long period (figure 7.5). Thus,

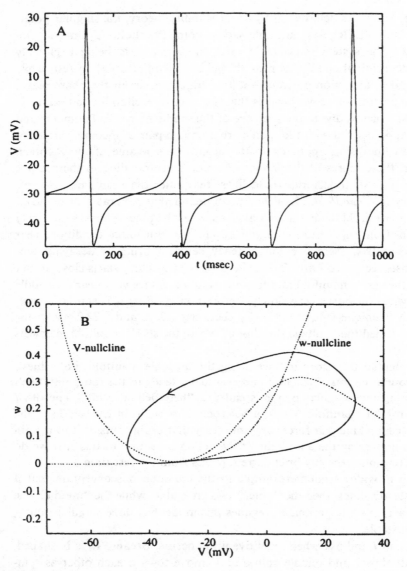

Figure 7.5
Onset of repetitive firing with arbitrarily low frequency for a constant current, $I = 40.76\,\mu A/cm^2$ shows an oscillation with a period of about 220 msec. Panel A shows the voltage time course and panel B shows the phase plane. Note the "narrow channel" between the two nullclines near $-30\,mV$, which accounts for most of the oscillation period (see Rinzel and Ermentrout 1989). Parameters are as in figure 7.4.

in this parameter regime, the transition to repetitive firing is marked by arbitrarily low frequency (figure 7.6B). For I near the critical current, the frequency is proportional to $\sqrt{I - I_1}$ (Strogatz 1994). When $I = I_1$, the limit cycle has infinite period; it is called a "saddle node loop" or SNIC (saddle node on an invariant circle). Generally, an infinite period limit cycle is called a "homoclinic orbit," one that begins and ends at a singular point. The saddle node loop is one type of homoclinic orbit; we will encounter another type in the next section. This type of zero-frequency onset is generic and occurs over a range of parameters. Changing another parameter will typically lead to a smooth change in I_1. We emphasize that this mechanism allows arbitrarily low firing rates without relying on channel gating kinetics, which are necessarily slow. Such low rates have been associated with the inactivating potassium A-type current (Connor, Walter, and McKown 1977), although the underlying mathematical structure of the saddle node loop does not, of course, require an A-current (Rush and Rinzel 1995). We have found the fast spike dynamics in several recent models (e.g., Traub et al. 1991) for cortical pyramidal cells to have this same zero-frequency onset of repetitive firing (unpublished observations by the authors). The value I_1 is determined by evaluating I_{ss} at the value of V for which $\partial I_{ss}/\partial v = 0$, and this latter condition is equivalent to having the determinant $ad - bc$ of the Jacobian matrix equal zero.

The global picture of repetitive firing is shown in the bifurcation diagram of figure 7.6A, with frequency versus I in figure 7.6B. The branch of steady states (unstable shown dashed) form the S-shaped curve, and the oscillatory solutions are represented by the forked curve whose open end begins at $I = I_1$. As I increases beyond I_1 the peak-to-peak amplitude on the stable (repetitive firing) branch decreases and the frequency increases. The family of periodic solutions terminates at $I = I_2$ via a subcritical Hopf bifurcation. Except for I in a small interval of this upper range, this system is monostable. Annihilation of repetitive firing, as in figure 7.3, cannot be carried out for I near I_1 in this case (although at the high-current end where there is bistability, annihilation can occur).

7.3.4 More Bistability

It is important to realize that the solution behavior we have described in our bifurcation diagrams depends on other parameters in the model. The temperature parameter ϕ is particularly convenient, with useful interpretative value for additional parametric tuning: it plays no role in I_{ss} and thus does not affect the values along the S-shaped curve of steady states in figure 7.6, or the corresponding curve in figure 7.2. The *stability* of a steady state does, however, depend on ϕ. As is seen from eq. 7.19,

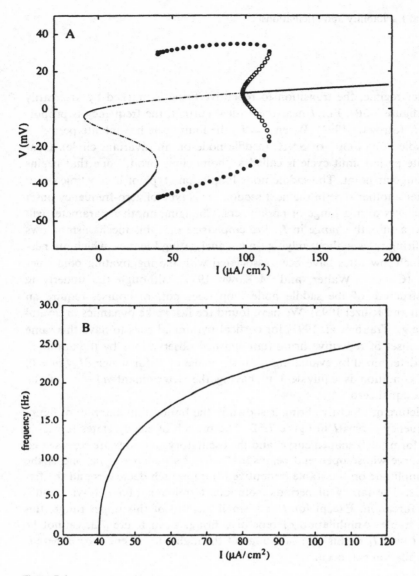

Figure 7.6
Multiple steady states and periodic orbits for a steady current when the I_{ss}–V relation is N-shaped. (A) Bifurcation diagram (line types as in figure 7.2A; parameters are as in figures 7.4–7.5). In spite of the coexistent states, the system is monostable for I between $I_1 = 40$, the turning point of the steady states, and $I_2 = 98$ where there is a Hopf bifurcation. Onset of repetitive firing at zero frequency occurs at $I = I_1$ where two fixed points coalesce. This corresponds to figure 7.4B when the unstable manifolds of the saddle point form a closed loop. The branch of periodic orbits has a turning point at $I = 116$ before terminating at the Hopf bifurcation point, $I = I_2$. All current values in $\mu A/cm^2$. (B) Frequency (in Hz) of stable branch of periodic orbits.

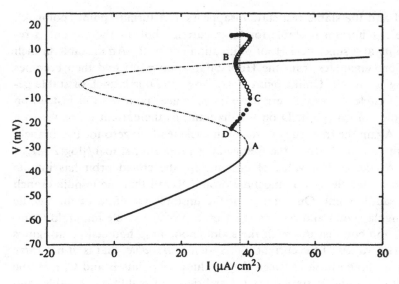

Figure 7.7
Bifurcation diagram (as in figure 7.6 but for $\phi = 0.23$). Point A shows where the two lower steady states coalesce, point B shows the Hopf bifurcation for the upper steady state, point C shows the coalescence of the stable and unstable periodic branches, and point D shows where the branch of stable oscillatory solutions terminates on the branch of saddle points (not on the knee, as in figure 7.6) at a saddle loop homoclinic. For currents between points B and A, there are three stable states: (1) a low-voltage rest state, (2) a high-voltage rest state, and (3) an oscillatory state. Note that the steady-state branch is identical to that of figure 7.6; ϕ only affects the stability of the steady states and the behavior of the periodic orbits. Vertical line at $I = 37.5\,\mu\text{A/cm}^2$ shows a current for which there are three stable states (cf. figure 7.8).

when ϕ is large, oscillatory destablization is precluded; Hopf bifurcation from a steady state only occurs when the time scale of w is slow compared to that of V. Thus, for large ϕ, both the upper and lower branches of the S-curve are stable; the middle branch is of course unstable. This system is bistable. In this large-ϕ limit, the kinetics of the K^+ system are so fast (essentially instantaneous, with $w = w_\infty(V)$) that the model reduces to one dynamic variable, V. Then stability is determined only by the slope of I_{ss}, with the two "outer" states being stable and the "middle" unstable. This simple example also shows that sometimes a model can be conveniently reduced to a lower dimension when there are significant time scale differences between variables.

For intermediate values of ϕ, the dynamics of both V and w influence stability, and the upper branch is unstable for a certain range of I. Figure 7.7 shows a bifurcation diagram analogous to that in figure 7.6A, in which the branch of steady states is S-shaped and the stable rest state disappears at a turning point (point A). The high voltage equilibrium is stable for large currents but, as the current is reduced, loses stability at a subcritical Hopf bifurcation (point B). An unstable branch of periodic solutions emanates from the Hopf bifurcation point and then becomes stable at a turning point (C). Unlike figure 7.6A, however, this branch of stable periodic orbits (solid circles) does not terminate on the knee (point A) but instead on the unstable middle branch (point D on the diagram) as the current decreases to a critical value, I_D. Again the frequency of the limit cycle tends to zero for this branch, but not as the square root. Rather, the frequency is proportional to $1/|\log(I - I_D)|$ (Strogatz 1994). At the critical value of current, I_D, the closed orbit has infinite period; it is called a "saddle loop homoclinic orbit." Recall that the middle branch of solutions is a saddle point. One branch of the unstable manifold of this saddle point exits the singular point and returns via a branch of the stable manifold (compare figure 7.8A) and contrast this with the saddle node loop homoclinic in figures 7.4–7.6). For certain values of the current, this system is *tristable*, that is, it has three stable states. If I is chosen to lie between the I values for points B and C, then the lower branch still exists and is stable, the upper branch of equilibria is stable, and there is a stable periodic orbit. Figure 7.8A shows the phase plane for this case. The stable manifold for the saddle point (bold dashed trajectory) acts to separate the stable periodic orbit (SPO) from the lower rest state. The small unstable periodic orbit (UPO) separates the upper rest state from the stable periodic solution. As in figure 7.3B, we can use brief current pulses to switch between states. Figure 7.8B shows the effect of three 5 msec current pulses switching from the periodic orbit to the lower rest state, back to the periodic orbit, and then to the upper rest state. (Note that perturbations from the upper rest state decay very slowly.) The HH model, adjusted for higher than normal external potassium, exhibits similar multistable behavior (Rinzel 1985).

This example of coexistence between a depolarized limit cycle and a lower resting state is important because it also forms the basis for a general class of bursting phenomena.

7.4 Bursting and Adaptation: Spiking Dynamics with Slow Modulation

Many neurons exhibit much more complicated firing patterns than the simple repetitive firing we have described here. *Bursting*, the clustering of spikes followed by relative quiescence, is a common mode of firing in neurons and other excitable cells (see Wang and Rinzel 1995 for a brief review). Bursting cannot happen in two-variable

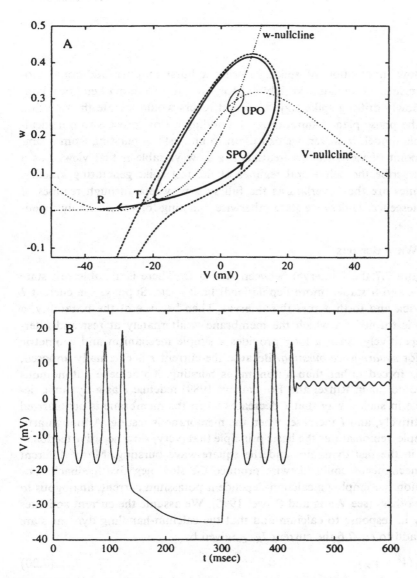

Figure 7.8

Multistability for a current between points B and A in figure 7.7 ($I = 37.5 \,\mu\text{A/cm}^2$; other parameters are as in figure 7.7). Panel A depicts the V-w phase plane. The nullclines intersect at three places representing steady states: (1) a lower stable rest state (R), (2) an unstable saddle point (T), and (3) an upper stable rest state (unlabeled). The left branch of the unstable manifold of the saddle point (bold line) connects to the lower steady state. The right branch wraps around the stable periodic orbit (SPO). The branches of the stable manifold of the saddle point (bold dashed line) form a separatrix between the lower stable rest state and the stable periodic orbit. The unstable periodic orbit (UPO) separates the stable upper steady state from the stable periodic orbit. Panel B shows the effects of three successive depolarizing current pulses. Starting on the stable oscillation, the membrane is switched to the lower stable steady state. Another brief pulse pushes it back to the stable oscillation and a third pulse switches it to the upper steady state. No single brief current pulse can switch it from the lower steady state directly to the upper steady state, although the opposite transition is possible.

models. The slow modulation of spiking during a burst requires additional biophysical mechanisms and dynamic variables. Moreover, just from mathematical considerations, a slowly drifting spike trajectory that recurs would violate the rule that
trajectories in the phase plane cannot cross. By adding a slow process to our idealized two-variable model, however, we can use it to understand bursting from a simple geometric point of view. In this treatment, a slow variable is first viewed as a
parameter to describe the behavioral regimes of the fast spike-generating kinetics;
the slow dynamics are then overlaid as the full system sweeps through regimes of
spiking and quiescence. Unless we state otherwise, bursting for us will imply repetitive bursting.

7.4.1 Square-Wave Bursters

Consider in figure 7.7 the I interval between A and D. There is a stable rest state
around $-35\,\mathrm{mV}$ and a stable (more depolarized) limit cycle. Suppose the current I
slowly varies back and forth across this interval. Then because of the bistability, a
hysteresis loop is formed, in which the membrane is alternately at rest and alternately firing repetitively. Such a loop provides a simple mechanism and geometric
interpretation for *square-wave bursting*. Because the current I is externally imposed,
however, this is forced rather than autonomous bursting. To achieve autonomous
bursting, one could (as in Rinzel and Ermentrout 1989) redefine I as a dynamic dependent variable in such a way that I decreases when the membrane is depolarized
and firing repetitively, and I increases when the membrane is resting. Although artificial, this example demonstrates the basic principle that (very) slow negative feedback
and hysteresis in the fast dynamics underlie square-wave bursting. Many different
ionic current mechanisms could likewise produce the slow negative feedback. For
further illustration, we employ a calcium-dependent potassium current, analogous to
that studied by others (see Wang and Rinzel 1995). We assume the current activates
instantaneously in response to calcium and that the calcium-handling dynamics are
slow. Thus we add to eq. 7.6 the current I_{K-Ca} given by

$$I_{K-Ca} = g_{K-Ca}z(V - V_K), \tag{7.20}$$

where g_{K-Ca} is the maximal conductance for this current and z is the gating variable
with a Hill-like dependence on Ca (the near-membrane calcium concentration scaled
by its dissociation constant for activating the gate, K_D):

$$z = \frac{Ca^p}{Ca^p + 1}. \tag{7.21}$$

(For simplicity, we set the Hill exponent $p = 1$, although this is not required.) The balance equation for Ca is

$$\frac{dCa}{dt} = \varepsilon(-\mu I_{Ca} - Ca), \qquad (7.22)$$

where the parameter μ is for converting current into a concentration flux and involves the ratio of the cell's surface area to the calcium compartment's volume. The parameter ε is a product of the calcium removal rate and the ratio of free to total calcium in the cell. Because calcium is highly buffered, ε is small and thus the calcium dynamics are slow. This is a greatly simplified model; one could have, for example, more complicated calcium handling, including diffusion of calcium in the cytoplasm, nonlinear removal of calcium by pumps/exchangers, perhaps even release of calcium from intracellular pools. If the conductance g_{K-Ca} of this outward current is large, the membrane is hyperpolarized; if it is small, then the membrane can fire. Thus, when a bifurcation curve is drawn as a function of this conductance, it is reversed from that of figure 7.7, which plots the behavior as a function of an *inward* current. When the membrane is firing, intracellular calcium slowly accumulates, turning on this outward conductance and thereby terminating the firing. Figure 7.9A shows a bursting solution to the three-variable model, eqs. 7.4–7.6 coupled with the slow calcium dynamics, eq. 7.22. Projecting the solution onto the z-V plane, where z is defined in eq. 7.21, shows how the burst's trajectory slowly tracks the attracting branches of the fast subsystem (figure 7.9B). Rapid transitions occur when the branches terminate at bifurcation points and turning points. We note that any number of alternate mechanisms could provide the slow negative feedback for bursting including a slow gating kinetics for z with fast calcium handling, or slow inactivation of I_{Ca}, driven by V or Ca.

7.4.2 Chaos and Poincaré Maps

We emphasize that even our minimal three-variable model exhibits the complex dynamics of bursting oscillations. Moreover, because of its simplicity and the geometric viewpoint we offer, the role of each variable is clear; V and w are for fast spike generation with bistability, and Ca provides the slow modulation. Finally, the model is sufficiently robust that in certain parameter ranges, it appears to exhibit chaotic behavior. Increasing the K_D for the calcium-dependent potassium conductance, equivalent to decreasing μ, can switch the membrane into a repetitively firing regime. The transition between the bursting and repetitive regimes is very complicated. For example, when $\mu = 1/59$, the burst pattern has period 4, that is, every fourth burst is the same. When $\mu = 1/60$, behavior is aperiodic (time course not shown); its

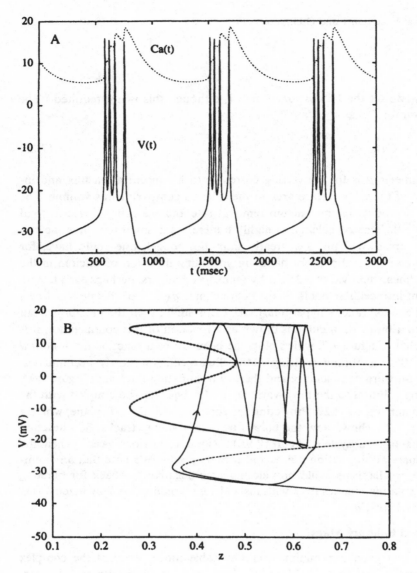

Figure 7.9
Bursting solution to eqs. 7.4–7.6 coupled with the calcium-dependent potassium current, eqs. 7.20–7.22. Parameters are as in figure 7.7, with $I = 45\,\mu A/cm^2$, $\varepsilon = 0.005$, $\mu = 0.2$, $g_{K-Ca} = 0.25\,mS/cm^2$. Panel A shows the voltage trace (use mV for ordinate scale) and the calcium concentration (for plotting clarity, the dimensionless Ca values have been multiplied by ten; ordinate scale is unitless in this case). The burst's active phase ends when calcium rises too high and the membrane hyperpolarizes. During the silent phase calcium is removed and after the calcium-dependent potassium current diminishes enough the membrane depolarizes to initiate the next burst. Panel B shows the projection of the bursting solution on the z-V plane along with the bifurcation diagram with $z = Ca/(1 + Ca)$ as a parameter. The trajectory alternately tracks the stable periodic solution (SPO in figure 7.8A) and the lower steady state. Panel C shows that for a slightly different value, $\mu = 0.01667$, the solution is chaotic; data points plot the value of calcium at successive times as the voltage decreases through 0 mV. The solid diagonal line is the identity function.

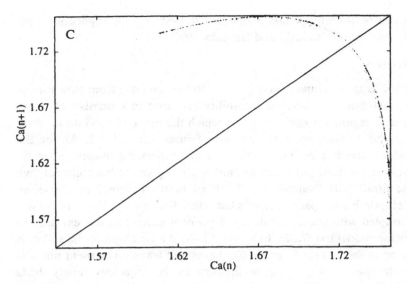

Figure 7.9 (continued)

dynamics can be described as follows. Each time that V passes a given value (here when V decreases through $0\,\mathrm{mV}$), we record the concentration of calcium, as well as the value of w. For this particular model, the recorded values of w are all about 0.35. The value of calcium, however, varies between 1.56 and 1.73. The solution is approximately represented by the time series of values for the calcium, $Ca_1, Ca_2, \ldots$ We can generate the one-variable dynamic rule whose solutions approximate these time series as follows. With initial conditions $V = 0$ and $w = 0.35$, we specify a value for calcium, and then integrate the full differential equations until V crosses 0, again getting the next value of calcium. Thus we have a *map* taking a value of calcium, Ca, to a new value of calcium, $F(Ca)$. This map is called a "Poincaré map." The entire dynamics of our burster are captured by this simple map. For $\mu = 1/60$, this map is shown in figure 7.9C. From the figure, it is evident that there is an intersection of the line $y = x$ and $y = F(x)$. That means that there is a single concentration of calcium, Ca^*, to which the trajectory returns after one cycle. This corresponds to a periodic solution to the model equations. If $|F'(Ca^*)| > 1$ (as is the case here), the periodic solution is unstable. This type of map is characteristic of dynamics that have *chaotic behavior*, that is, the successive values of calcium appear to be random and aperiodic. By reducing the three-dimensional differential equation to a simple one-dimensional iteration, we can understand the essence of the transition from constant repetitive firing to chaos as we vary a parameter, say μ. (More details on one-dimensional maps and chaos can be found in Glass and Mackey 1988; for an application to a neuronal bursting system, see Hayashi and Ishizuka 1992.)

7.4.3 Elliptic Bursters

Bursting that differs from the square-wave pattern above can arise from slow modulation of bistable fast dynamics because bistability can arise in a number of ways. Consider a parameter regime for eqs. 7.4–7.6 in which the onset of oscillations is via a subcritical Hopf bifurcation, such as shown in figures 7.2 and 7.3. As for the square-wave burster, there is a regime where the spike-generating dynamics are bistable; a limit cycle and a fixed point coexist, although, unlike the bistability shown in figure 7.7, the limit cycle "surrounds" the fixed point. Figure 7.10 shows an example of an "elliptic burst" pattern generated when the fast dynamics of figures 7.2 and 7.3 are coupled with the slow calcium-dependent potassium current used in the previous bursting model (eq. 7.22). In figure 7.10A, the envelope of the spikes is "elliptical" in shape as the amplitude gradually waxes and wanes. The silent phase is characterized by damping and growing oscillations as the trajectory slowly drifts through the Hopf bifurcation of the fast subsystem. This type of activity pattern has been seen in sleep spindles, and a cellular model related to it involves the same mathematical mechanism (Destexhe, McCormick, and Sejnowski 1993; see also Wang and Rinzel 1995, and Rush and Rinzel 1995). As with a square-wave burster, this type of bursting can also have complex dynamics such as quasi-periodic behavior and chaos.

7.4.4 Parabolic Bursting: Two Slow Processes

Bursting can arise even without bistability in the spike-generating dynamics. Minimal models for the most widely known endogenous cellular burster, the *Aplysia* R-15 neuron, operate in a regime where the fast dynamics are monostable (Rinzel and Lee 1987). Suppose the spiking dynamics are as in figures 7.4–7.6, where the onset of repetitive firing is through a saddle-node-loop bifurcation and there is no bistability. (Ignore the bistable behavior at high currents. We are interested in the low-current regime only, where the rest state is more negative than $-30\,mV$.) The mechanisms for bursting that depend on *one* slow variable cannot produce bursting in this parameter regime because there is no longer a hysteresis loop. A model with a single slow variable interacting with these fast dynamics will, in response to a steady input, slowly approach a maintained state of repetitive firing or rest. The slow transient phase for a depolarizing input could show increasing or decreasing activity depending on whether the slow variable provides positive or negative feedback. Figure 7.11A illustrates that $I_{K\text{-}Ca}$ with slow Ca dynamics provides a mechanism for adaptation in repetitive firing behavior.

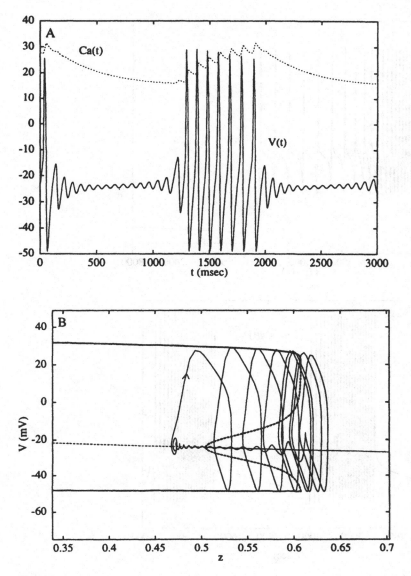

Figure 7.10
Elliptic burster formed when the Morris-Lecar model, equations 7.4–7.6 in the parameter regime of figure 7.2, is coupled to the calcium-dependent potassium current, equations 7.20–7.22. Parameters are as in figure 7.2, with $I = 120\,\mu A/cm^2$, $\mu = 0.3$, $\varepsilon = 0.002$, $g_{K\text{-}Ca} = 0.75\,mS/cm^2$. Panel A shows the time courses of voltage and calcium (ordinate scales as in figure 7.9A). As in figure 7.9, when the calcium is high and the calcium-dependent potassium channel is activated, the membrane tends toward rest; when calcium is low enough, it is oscillatory. Panel B shows the projection of the burst on the z-V plane as in figure 7.9B. During the active and silent phases, the burst trajectory slowly tracks attractors of the fast subsystem. Actually during the later phase of the silent period, the trajectory drifts well into the unstable regime of the fast subsystem's rest state (left of the Hopf point, $z < 0.5$), and this feature is explainable.

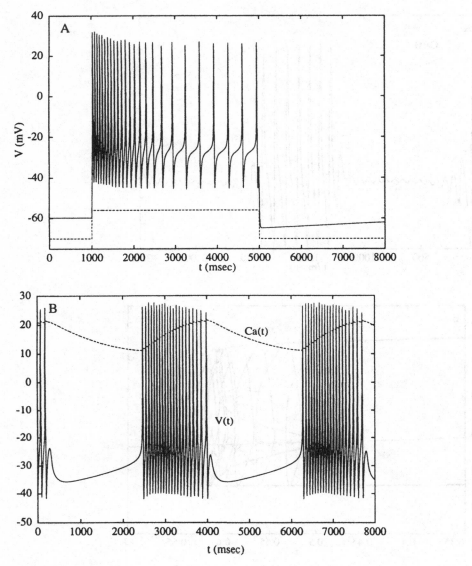

Figure 7.11
Modulation of the Morris-Lecar model, equations 7.4–7.6 in the regime of figure 7.4, by slower processes. Panel A shows how coupling with the calcium-dependent potassium current, eqs. 7.20–7.22, results in adaptation to a long current pulse. Parameters are as in figure 7.4, with $g_{K\text{-}Ca} = 1\,\text{mS/cm}^2$, $\mu = 0.025$, $\varepsilon = 0.0005$. The current pulse is $70\,\mu\text{A/cm}^2$. The membrane initially fires repetitively at 17 Hz and eventually slows to 3 Hz, more than a fivefold decrease. Panel B shows that a parabolic burster is formed by adding an additional slow inward current governed by eq. 7.23 with $I = 65\,\mu\text{A/cm}^2$, $g_{Ca,s} = 1\,\text{mS/cm}^2$, $\tau_s = 0.05\,\text{msec}$. Other parameters are as in panel A. This plot shows the membrane potential and the dimensionless calcium concentration as functions of time (ordinate scales as in figure 7.9A). For plotting convenience, Ca has been multiplied by ten. Panel C shows the projection of the burst onto the z-s plane. The dashed line is the curve of saddle-node-loop bifurcations of the fast dynamics, viewing s and z as parameters. Above this line, the membrane is oscillatory; below it, there is only a stable rest state.

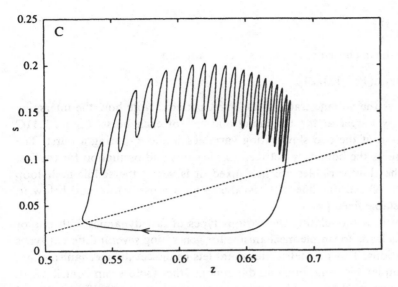

Figure 7.11 (continued)

To obtain the slow oscillation that underlies parabolic bursting, we need yet another slow variable so that there are opposing influences of slow positive (auto-catalytic) and slow negative feedback. Suppose, therefore, that we add a slow *inward* current to the model, which means there are two slow variables. As the inward current slowly activates, it causes the membrane to fire repetitively; this, however, turns on the slow outward current, which then shuts the membrane down. If the threshold for the slow inward current is low enough, it can start up once again and the process repeats. Thus a combination of a slow outward current and slow inward current can produce slow oscillations that move the fast dynamics into and out of the repetitively firing regime. The generality of this mechanism for parabolic bursting (also realiz-able with an inward current that slowly activates and then slowly inactivates, as in Rinzel and Lee 1987) has been described by a number of authors (e.g., Baer, Rinzel, and Carrillo 1995).

To illustrate with the Morris-Lecar model (that includes I_{K-Ca} as above), we need only add a slow autocatalytic process. With considerable freedom of choice, we add an additional slowly activating calcium current:

$$I_{Ca,s} = g_{Ca,s}s(V - V_{Ca}),$$

where

$$\tau_s \frac{ds}{dt} = \varepsilon(s_\infty(V) - s).$$ (7.23)

For simplicity, we have chosen $\tau_s = 0.05$ as a constant and

$$s_\infty(V) = 0.5[1 + \tanh(V - 12)/24].$$

Figure 7.11B shows the voltage trace of the burst pattern. Note how the interspike interval is relatively longer at the beginning and end of each burst. Figure 7.11C shows the projection of the two slow gating variables, s and z, during a burst. The dashed line represents the boundary between fixed points and oscillation for the fast dynamics when the slow variables are held fixed; it is where the saddle-node-loop bifurcation occurs. Above this line, the fast dynamics are oscillatory and below it, there is a unique stable fixed point.

We have shown how modulating the various types of fast dynamics with one or two slow processes leads to simple mechanisms for generating several different types of bursting oscillations. This geometric viewpoint lets us dissect the mechanisms that underlie some complex neuronal bursting dynamics. Other factors can contribute to burst rhythmogenesis including cable properties and spatially nonuniform channel densities, and nonlinear regenerative factors in the calcium handling system (cf. Wang and Rinzel 1995).

7.5 Phase-Resetting and Phase-Locking of Oscillators

We now turn our attention to a brief description of periodically forced and coupled neural oscillators. The behaviors generally involve issues that are very difficult to analyze and we will only touch on them briefly. Before treating a specific example, it is useful to discuss certain important aspects of oscillators. We say that a periodic solution to an autonomous (time does not explicitly appear in the right-hand side) differential equation is (*orbitally*) "asymptotically stable" if perturbations from the oscillation return to the oscillation as $t \to \infty$. The difference between asymptotic stability of an oscillation and that of a steady-state solution is that, for the oscillation, the time course may exhibit a shift. That is, we do not expect the solution of the perturbed oscillation to be the same as the unperturbed; rather, there will be a shift (see figure 7.12A) due to the time translation invariance of the periodic solution. Indeed, in phase space, the periodic trajectory is unchanged by translation in time. The shift that accompanies the perturbation of the limit cycle can be exploited in order to understand the behavior of the oscillator under external forcing. Suppose that an oscillator has a period, say T. We may let $t = 0$ correspond to the time of

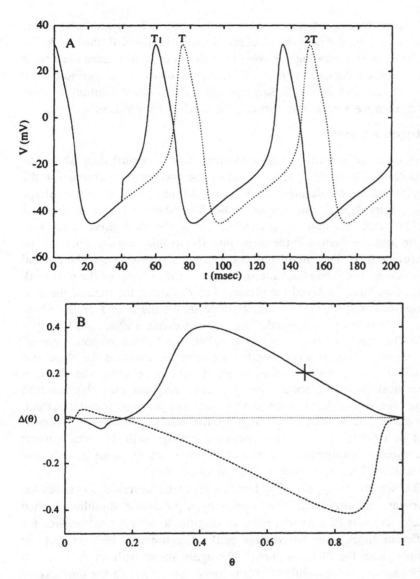

Figure 7.12
Phase-resetting of a Morris-Lecar oscillator. (A) A brief depolarizing stimulus can shorten the onset of the next spike and thus advance the phase. (B) Phase response curve (PRC) for the Morris-Lecar equations with parameters as in figures 7.4–7.6 and an applied current $I = 50\,\mu A/cm^2$. The stimulus is a 0.5 msec pulse with amplitude of $\pm 480\,\mu A/cm^2$ delivered at time $t = 40$ msec. The solid line shows the PRC for a depolarizing stimulus and the dashed for a hyperpolarizing pulse. The cross on the depolarizing PRC corresponds to the experiment in figure 7.13.

peak value of one of the oscillating variables, so that at $t = T$ we are back to the peak. Given that we are on the periodic solution, if some t is specified, then we know precisely the state of each oscillating variable. This allows us to introduce the notion of *phase* of the periodic solution. Let $\theta = t/T$ define the phase of the periodic solution so that $\theta = 0, 1, 2, \ldots$ all define the same point on the periodic solution. For example, if $\theta = 8.5$, then we are halfway through the oscillator's ninth cycle.

7.5.1 Phase Response Curves

With the notion of phase defined, we now examine how a perturbation shifts the phase of the oscillator. In figure 7.12A, we show the voltage time course for the Morris-Lecar system in the oscillating regime. At a fixed time, say t, after the voltage peak, we apply a brief depolarizing current pulse. This shifts the time of the next peak (figure 7.12A) and this shift remains for all time (the solid curve is the perturbed oscillation and the dashed is the unperturbed—in this case the time for the next peak is shortened). If the time of the next peak is shortened from the natural time, we say that the stimulus has "advanced the phase"; if the time of the next peak is lengthened, that we have "delayed the phase." Let T_1 denote the time of the next peak. The phase shift is $(T - T_1)/T$, and T_1 depends on the time t or the phase $\theta = t/T$ at which the stimulus is applied. Thus we can define a phase shift $\Delta(\theta) \equiv (T - T_1(\theta))/T$. The graph of this function is called the "phase response curve" (PRC) for the oscillator. If $\Delta(\theta)$ is positive, the perturbation advances the phase and the peak will occur sooner. On the other hand, if $\Delta(\theta)$ is negative, the phase is delayed and the next peak will occur later. We can easily compute this function numerically, and the same idea can be used to analyze an experimental system. Moreover, this curve can be used as a rough approximation of how the oscillator will be affected by repeated perturbation (periodic forcing) with the same current pulse. (More complete descriptions and numerous examples of phase models and PRCs can be found in Glass and Mackey 1988; Winfree 1980.)

In figure 7.12B, we show a typical PRC for the Morris-Lecar model computed for both a depolarizing stimulus (solid line) and a hyperpolarizing stimulus (dashed line). The stimulus consists of a current pulse of magnitude $480\,\mu\text{A}/\text{cm}^2$ applied for $0.5\,\text{msec}$ at different times after the voltage peak. The time of the next spike is determined, which yields the PRC, as above. The figure agrees with our intuition; if the depolarizing stimulus comes while $V(t)$ is increasing (i.e., during the upstroke or slow depolarization of recovery), the peak will occur earlier and we will see a phase advance. If the stimulus occurs while $v(t)$ is decreasing (i.e., during the downstroke), there will be a delay. The opposite occurs for hyperpolarizing stimuli. The curves show that it is difficult to delay the onset of an action potential with a depolarizing stimulus or advance it with a hyperpolarizing one. For different sets of parameters, these curves may change. As we have seen in the previous section, it is sometimes possible to completely stop the oscillation if a stimulus is given at the right time. In this case, the PRC is no longer defined; nearby phases can then have arbitrarily long latencies before firing.

We now show how this function can be used to analyze a periodically forced oscillator. Suppose that every P time units a current pulse is applied to the cell. Let θ_n denote the phase right before the time of the nth stimulus. This stimulus will either advance or delay the onset of the next peak depending on the phase at which the stimulus occurs. In any case, the new phase after time P and just before the next stimulus will be $\theta_n + \Delta(\theta_n) + P/T$. To understand this, first consider the case where there is no stimulus: after time P the oscillator will advance P/T in phase, but because the stimulus advances or delays the phase by an amount $\Delta(\theta_n)$, this amount is just added to the unperturbed phase, resulting in an equation for the new phase just before the next stimulus:

$$\theta_{n+1} = \theta_n + \Delta(\theta_n) + P/T. \tag{7.24}$$

This difference equation can be solved numerically. Here we consider the natural question of whether the periodic stimulus can entrain the voltage oscillation. That is, we ask whether there is a periodic solution to this forced neural oscillation. In general, a periodic solution is one for which there are M voltage spikes for N stimuli, where M and N are positive integers. When such a solution exists, we have what is known as "$M:N$ phase-locking."

Finding $M:1$ phase-locked solutions is quite easy. We require the oscillator to undergo M oscillations per stimulus period. In terms of eq. 7.24, this means we seek a solution that satisfies

$$\theta + M = \theta + \Delta(\theta) + P/T \tag{7.25}$$

for some value of θ. If such a solution exists and is stable (to be defined below), then, starting near θ, we can iterate eq. 7.24 and end up back at θ. This θ is the locking phase just before the next stimulus and because it does not change from stimulus to stimulus, the resulting solution must be periodic. Obviously, a necessary condition for a solution to eq. 7.25 is that $M - P/T$ lie between the maximum and minimum of $\Delta(\theta)$, that is, we must solve

$$M - P/T = \Delta\theta. \tag{7.26}$$

Having solved eq. 7.26, we need to determine the stability of the solution. For equations of the form of eq. 7.24, a necessary and sufficient condition for θ to be a stable solution is that $-2 < \Delta'(\theta) < 0$. Because $\Delta(\theta)$ is periodic and continuous, there will in general be two solutions to eq. 7.26 (see figure 7.12B). But because only one of them will occur where $\Delta(\theta)$ has a negative slope, there will be a unique stable solution. We must also worry about whether the negative slope is too steep (i.e., more negative than -2); for small stimuli, this will never be the case—stability is assured. When $\Delta'(\theta) < -2$ (instability), very complex behavior can occur such as chaos (see, for example, Glass and Mackey 1988). The case of $M : N$ phase-locking where $N > 1$ is more difficult to explain and will not be considered here. It is clear that if the stimulus is weak, the magnitude of $\Delta(\theta)$ will also be small so that $M - P/T$ must be small in order to achieve $M : 1$ locking. On the other hand, if the stimulus is too strong, then we must be concerned with the stability of the locked solution. We note that, in a sense, eq. 7.24 is only valid for stimuli that are weak compared to the strength of attraction of the limit cycle; for stronger stimuli, it will take the solution more than a single oscillation to return to points close to the original cycle. The PRC in figure 7.12B shows that, when the stimulus is depolarizing, it is easier to advance the Morris-Lecar oscillator and thus force it at a higher frequency ($0 < P/T < 1$) than it is to force the oscillator at a lower frequency ($P/T > 1$). For hyperpolarizing stimuli, we can more easily drive the oscillator at frequencies lower than the natural frequency. (The counterresults are possible, but only for small ranges of parameters; see also Perkel et al. 1964)

To illustrate these concepts, we have periodically stimulated the Morris-Lecar model (natural period of 95 msec) with the same brief depolarizing current pulse repeated every 76 msec. Figure 7.13 shows that the oscillation is quickly entrained to the new higher frequency. Equation 7.26 allows us to predict the time after the voltage peak that the stimulus will occur for 1:1 phase-locking. From the PRC we can see that $\Delta(\theta) = 1 - 76/95 = 0.2$ corresponds to two values of θ, one stable (cross in figure 7.12B) $\theta = 0.702$ and the other unstable. Thus the locking time after the voltage peak, that is, when the stimulus occurs, is predicted from the PRC to be $t = T \cdot \theta = 67$ msec. This is exactly the shift observed in figure 7.13.

The technique illustrated here is useful for analyzing the behavior of a single oscillator when forced with a short pulsatile stimulus. For more continuous types of forcing, such as an applied sinusoidal current, other techniques must be used. One such technique is the *method of averaging*, applicable when the forcing is weak. Periodic forcing is a special case of coupling, which we will now describe.

7.5.2   Averaging and Weak Coupling

Although the general behavior of coupled neural oscillators is very difficult to analyze, limiting cases can be treated (Kopell 1988). We will describe one method, the

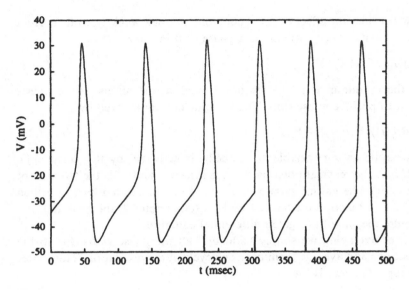

Figure 7.13
Phase-locking (1:1) of the Morris-Lecar model to a series of four current pulses with interpulse period of 76 msec. Intrinsic period of the membrane oscillator is 95 msec. Parameters are as in figure 7.12B. After phase-locking is achieved, the stimulus is seen to occur about 67 msec after the action potential's peak, just as predicted by the PRC.

method of averaging, used successfully to study the dynamics of two or more neural oscillators that are *weakly coupled* (e.g., Hansel, Mato, and Meunier 1995; Ermentrout and Kopell 1991). In this limit, the coupling is sufficiently weak that each oscillator's trajectory remains close to its intrinsic limit cycle. The primary effect of the coupling is to perturb the relative phase between the oscillators, much as we described above. Because the perturbation per cycle is small (with weak coupling), however, the net effect occurs only over many cycles, and the per cycle effect is seen as averaged. For illustration, we summarize the use of averaging to describe the phase-locking properties of two identical Morris-Lecar oscillators when coupled with identical mutually excitatory synapses. Detailed derivations of the equations can be found in the above-mentioned papers.

We assume that motion of each oscillator along its limit cycle can be rewritten in terms of a phase variable. Thus an oscillator's membrane potential is periodic with period T and follows the function $V(\theta_j)$, where θ_j is the phase of the jth oscillator, $j = 1, 2$, and V is the voltage component of the limit cycle trajectory. In the absence of coupling, the dynamics are given simply as $\theta_j = t + C_j$, where C_j is an arbitrary phase shift. Now consider the effect of small coupling. A brief, weak synaptic current I_{syn} to cell i from activity in cell j will cause a phase shift in cell i:

$$\Delta\theta_i = -V^*(\theta_i(t))I_{syn}(\theta_i(t), \theta_j(t)), \tag{7.27}$$

where $V^*(t)$ is the infinitesimal phase response function, the minus sign converts excitatory current to positive phase shift. The synaptic current is given by

$$I_{syn}(\theta_i, \theta_j) = g_c\alpha(\theta_j(t))(V(\theta_i(t)) - V_{syn}), \tag{7.28}$$

where the postsynaptic gating variable $\alpha(t)$ is cell i is activated by the presynaptic voltage $V(\theta_j)$, V_{syn} is the reversal potential for the synapse, and g_c is the strength of the synaptic coupling. The gating variable $\alpha(t)$ could be represented by a so-called (event-triggered) alpha function introduced by Rall (cf. chapter 2, this volume). Alternatively, it could obey a voltage-gated differential equation.

In the method of averaging we simply "add up" all the phase shifts due to the synaptic perturbations and average them over one cycle of the oscillation. Thus, after averaging, the coupled system is found to satisfy

$$\frac{d\theta_1}{dt} = 1 + g_cH(\theta_2 - \theta_1) + O(g_c^2) \tag{7.29}$$

$$\frac{d\theta_2}{dt} = 1 + g_cH(\theta_1 - \theta_2) + O(g_c^2), \tag{7.30}$$

where H is a T-periodic "averaged" interaction function, given by

$$H(\phi) = \frac{1}{T}\int_0^T V^*(t)\alpha(t + \phi)(V_{syn} - V(t))\,dt. \tag{7.31}$$

The key to these models is the computation of H (see Ermentrout and Kopell 1991; Kopell 1988).

In figure 7.14A, we show the function $V^*(t)$ along with the synaptic gating variable $\alpha(t)$ over one cycle for exactly the same parameters as in figure 7.12B. Here $\alpha(t) = 0.04\,te^{-t/5}$ is an alpha-function with a 5 msec time constant. Note the similarity (except for scale) of the excitatory PRC and the infinitesimal PRC, $V^*(t)$. As with the PRC, $V^*(t)$ is mainly positive, showing that the predominant effect of depolarizing perturbations is to advance the phase or, equivalently, to speed up the oscillator. In only a very small interval of time can the phase be delayed, and this is a general property of membranes that become oscillatory through a saddle node bifurcation (Ermentrout 1996).

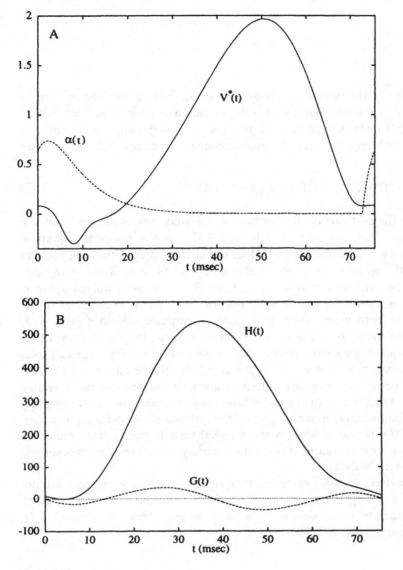

Figure 7.14
The method of averaging for two weakly coupled identical Morris-Lecar oscillators. Parameters for the oscillators are as in figures 7.4–7.6 (and figure 7.12A) and an applied current $I = 50\,\mu A/cm^2$. (A) Solid line shows the infinitesimal PRC, $V^*(t)$ and the dashed line shows the time course of the excitatory synaptic conductance (for plotting convenience, here multiplied by ten), modeled as an alpha function with a 5 msec time constant and peak of about $0.075\,mS/cm^2$. The alpha function "turns on" when V crosses 20 mV. (B) Interaction function $H(t)$ and its odd part $G(t)$ for the synaptic dynamics shown in panel A and a synaptic reversal potential of 0 mV. Zeros of the function $G(t)$ correspond to phase-locked solutions to the weakly coupled system; stable solutions have positive slopes and unstable have negative slopes.

Figure 7.14B shows the function $H(t)$ defined in eq. 7.31 for that figure's alpha function and for $V_{syn} = 0\,\text{mV}$. We can use this function along with eqs. 7.29–7.30 to determine the stable phase-locked patterns for this coupled system. Let $\Theta = \theta_2 - \theta_1$ denote the phase difference between the two oscillators. From eqs. 7.29–7.30 we see that Θ satisfies

$$\frac{d\Theta}{dt} = g_c(H(-\Theta) - H(\Theta)) + O(g_c^2) \equiv -2g_c G(\Theta) + O(g_c^2). \tag{7.32}$$

Here $G(\Theta)$ is just the odd part of the function H. Because the coupling is weak, the higher-order terms, $O(g_c^2)$ are ignored. Equation 7.32 is just a first-order equation. Phase-locked states are those for which Θ does not change, that is, they are roots of the function $G(\Theta)$ and they are stable fixed points if $G'(\Theta) > 0$. Because any odd periodic function has at least two zeros, $\Theta = 0$ and $\Theta = T/2$, there will always exist phase-locked states, although, these may not be stable. Synchronous solutions ($\Theta = 0$) imply that both membranes fire together. Antiphase solutions ($\Theta = T/2$) are exactly one-half cycle apart. Figure 7.14B shows the function $G(\Theta)$, from which we see there are four distinct fixed points: the *synchronous* (precisely in-phase) solution; the *antiphase* solution; and a pair of phase-shifted solutions at $\Theta \approx \pm 15\,\text{msec}$. Both the synchronous and antiphase solutions are unstable but the phase-shifted solution is stable. Thus, if two of these oscillators are coupled with weak excitatory coupling and the parameters chosen as above, they will phase-lock with a phase shift of about 20% of the period. Although the classical view is that mutual excitation leads to perfect synchrony, computations with a variety of neuronal models suggest that this is not generally the case.

This type of analysis is easily extended to systems where the oscillators are not exactly identical, coupling is not symmetric, and there are many more oscillators. The behavior of such phase models and the forms of the interaction functions, H, are the topics of current research.

7.6 Summary

We have introduced and used some of the basic concepts of the qualititative theory of differential equations to describe the dynamic repertoire of a representative model of excitability. We believe that a geometrical treatment, as in the phase plane, gives one an opportunity to see more clearly and to appreciate the underlying qualitative structure of models. One can see which initial conditions, for example, those resulting from a brief perturbing stimulus, will lie in the domain of attraction of any particular stable steady state or limit cycle. This is especially helpful for the design of experiments to switch a multistable system from one mode to another. Analytic methods are also important—for determining and interpreting the stability of solutions (e.g., eq. 7.19 for the Hopf bifurcation) and for approximating aspects of the solution behavior (e.g., eq. 7.25 for phase-locking). Another useful conceptual device is the bifurcation diagram by which we have provided compact descriptions of the system attractors. Although in several of our illustrations, the bifurcation parameter was I, and the steady-state I-V relation appeared explicitly in the diagram, channel density, synaptic weight (as in the Wilson-Cowan network model), or any other parameter can be used.

We have shown how a minimal but biophsically reasonable membrane model can be massaged to exhibit robustly a variety of physiologically identifiable firing behaviors. For the simplest two-variable Morris-Lecar model, we illustrated some qualitative differences in threshold behavior. When the steady-state current-voltage relation is monotonic, action potential size may be graded, although generally quite steeply with stimulus strength, and latency for firing is finite; when it is N-shaped, there is a true (saddle point) threshold for action potentials, latency may be arbitrarily long, and intermediate-sized responses are not possible. Correspondingly, for a steady stimulus, the monotonic case leads to onset of oscillations with a well-defined, nonzero frequency (Hopf bifurcation), and with possibly small amplitude (supercritical). In contrast, in the N-shaped case repetitive firing first appears with zero frequency (homoclinic bifurcation). These features are consistent with some of those used by Hodgkin (1948) to distinguish axons with different repetitive firing properties, class II and class I, respectively. Additionally, we have provided a geometric interpretation of some common forms of bursting neurons. Many bursters can be dissected into fast dynamics coupled to one or more slow processes that move the fast dynamics between resting and oscillatory states. Coupled and forced oscillators can often be reduced to maps or to continuous low-dimensional systems of phase equations, especially when the interactions are weak.

With regard to implementation of models, there are sophisticated software packages and subroutines available nowadays to help make theoretical experimentation and analysis a real-time endeavor; the "tooling-up" time is greatly reduced. Programs like XPP incorporate a mix of numerical integration and analytic formulation (linear stability analysis, bifurcation analysis, averaging—carried out numerically) with graphical representation all in an interactive framework. (The numerical methods employed by XPP are described in chapter appendix B.) To set up and get the Morris-Lecar model running should take less than fifteen minutes. Although we have used XPP here for the two-variable model, it can also deal with higher-order systems (like the bursting models of section 7.4). Stability of steady states can be computed, and time courses plotted interactively. The generalization of nullclines to surfaces is not available computationally, but two-variable projections of trajectories from the higher-order phase space can be insightful (e.g., figure 7.9). A widely distributed subroutine we have also found valuable for dissecting nonlinear systems in AUTO (Doedel 1981), which automatically generates bifurcation diagrams (as in figures 7.2, 7.6, 7.7; see chapter appendix B). The main components of AUTO are included in the package XPP, thus making AUTO an interactive program. We used XPP-AUTO for the fast/slow analysis of the bursting models in section 7.4. For the evaluation and algebraic manipulation of analytic prescriptions (e.g., lengthy perturbation and bifurcation formulas), many modelers have used symbol manipulation programs like Mathematica and MAPLE with success (see Rand and Armbruster 1987). As regards numerical packages, we advise that one be generally familiar with the methods being employed, and with their limitations. It is not so uncommon to pose a problem that seems to just miss the criteria for suitablity of a given technique—and one should be careful to recognize the symptoms of breakdown of the particular method being used.

Finally, we emphasize the value of using idealized, but biophysically reasonable, models in order to capture the essence of system behavior. If models are more detailed than necessary, identification of critical elements is often obscured by too many possibilities. On the other hand, if justified by adequate biophysical data, more detailed models are valuable for quantitative comparison with experiments. The modeler should be mindful and appreciative of these two different approaches: which one is chosen depends on the types of questions being asked and how much is known about the underlying physiology.

Acknowledgment

Bard Ermentrout was partially supported by National Science Foundation grant DMS 96–728. Much of John Rinzel's contribution to this chapter was completed while he was with the Mathematical Research Branch, NIDDK at the National Institutes of Health.

Appendix A: Morris-Lecar Equations

The differential equations and V-dependent functions are

$$C\frac{dV}{dt} = -\bar{g}_{Ca}m_\infty(V)(V - V_{Ca}) - \bar{g}_K w(V - V_K) - \bar{g}_L(V - V_L) + I \tag{7.33}$$

$$\frac{dw}{dt} = \phi\frac{[w_\infty(V) - w]}{\tau_w(V)}, \tag{7.34}$$

where

$$m_\infty(V) = 0.5 * [1 + \tanh\{(V - V_1)/V_2\}], \tag{7.35}$$

$$w_\infty(V) = 0.5 * [1 + \tanh\{(V - V_3)/V_4\}], \tag{7.36}$$

and

$$\tau_w(V) = 1/\cosh\{(V - V_3)/(2 * V_4)\}. \tag{7.37}$$

For Figures 7.1–7.3, we use the parameters $V_1 = -1.2$, $V_2 = 18$, $V_3 = 2$, $V_4 = 30$, $\bar{g}_{Ca} = 4.4$, $\bar{g}_K = 8.0$, $\bar{g}_L = 2$, $V_K = -84$, $V_L = -60$, $V_{Ca} = 120$, $C = 20\,\mu\text{F/cm}^2$, and $\phi = 0.04$. (All conductances are in mS/cm^2 and voltages in mV.) These same parameters are used for figures 7.4–7.6, with the following exceptions: $V_3 = 12$, $V_4 = 17.4$, $\bar{g}_{Ca} = 4.0$, and $\phi = 1/15$. In figures 7.7–7.8, the parameters are as in figures 7.4–7.6 but $\phi = 0.23$. The current, I (in $\mu\text{A/cm}^2$), is generally the only free parameter.

Appendix B: Numerical Methods

Most of the figures shown in this chapter were produced by numerically solving the Morris-Lecar equations. We have used a program XPP, written by Bard Ermentrout, which uses a variety of numerical integration methods to solve the equations on any computer that runs X-windows. It is available via anonymous ftp from ftp.math.pitt.edu/pub/bardware, and there is an extensive tutorial geared toward neurobiology available on the World Wide Web at http://www.pitt.edu/~phase. For the all but the bursting simulations, we have used a fourth-order Runge-Kutta algorithm. The bursting simulations employed a variable-time-step Gear algorithm (Press et al. 1986).

For the Morris-Lecar model, the nullclines can be found explicitly by solving each of the equations for w as a function of v, although this is generally not easy and thus calls for numerical techniques. All of the phase plane pictures were found by numerically computing the nullclines. This is done by breaking the phase plane into many small boxes, evaluating the functions on each point, and then using a linear interpolation to find the zero contours.

Singular points are found using Newton's method with a numerically computed Jacobian. Once a steady state is found, the Jacobian is computed and the QR algorithm is used to find the eigenvalues. These determine the stability of the singular point.

For certain steady states in the Morris-Lecar model, we want to find special trajectories called the "unstable" and "stable manifolds." This is done by computing an eigenvector for a particular eigenvalue (the eigenvectors are tangent to these manifolds) by inverse iteration. Once the eigenvector is known, the equations are integrated either forward or backward in time with initial conditions that are on the eigenvector and slightly off of the singular point.

The qualitative behavior of higher-dimensional systems as a parameter is varied can be understood and described compactly by determining the bifurcation diagrams. AUTO (Doedel 1981) was used in this chapter (through its interface with XPP) to trace, essentially automatically, the bifurcation curves as any parameter is varied. This program is able to find all steady states and periodic solutions regardless of their stability. The characteristics of stability, eigenvalues for steady states and Floquet exponents for periodic solutions, are computed along with the frequencies of periodic solutions. Two-parameter bifurcation diagrams (similar to figure 7.11C) indicating where steady states and periodic solutions exist and where they gain or lose stability can also be computed by AUTO.

The computation of the "infinitesimal PRC" is done automatically as part of the XPP package. Essentially, it solves an allied linear equation until a particular periodic orbit is found. The integral required for averaging is automatically computed.

A general and practical reference to many of the above numerical methods, which also leads to more literature, is Press et al. 1986.

8 Design and Fabrication of Analog VLSI Neurons

Rodney Douglas and Misha Mahowald

8.1 Introduction

There is a growing interest in the design and fabrication of artificial neural systems whose architecture and design principles are derived from biological nervous systems (Mead 1989, 1990; Douglas, Mahowald, and Mead 1995). These artificial systems are usually composed of analog electronic circuits fabricated in the complementary metal oxide semiconductor (CMOS) medium using very large-scale integration (VLSI) technology. They are predominantly analog circuits, which express directly the relevant physical processes of the neural systems they emulate. One interesting line of research in this field is the development of analog VLSI (aVLSI) neurons that emulate the electrophysiological behavior of real neurons. Such neurons could provide a basis for the construction of large neural networks that operate in real-time (Mahowald and Douglas 1991; Elias 1993; Murray and Tarassenko 1994). The aim of this chapter is to introduce the aVLSI approach by describing the principles of operation, design, and fabrication of a single simple silicon neuron. This chapter will help researchers new to this field to evaluate the benefits and costs of using aVLSI as a medium for modeling biologically realistic neurons.

Electronic neurons that emulate real neurons with various degrees of accuracy have been built in the past (Hoppensteadt 1986; Keener 1983). Although these neurons could be wired together to form small networks, because the neurons were usually constructed of discrete components, the complexity of the individual neurons and the size of their networks were very limited. Now, the development of VLSI technology has made it possible to envisage very large networks of realistic CMOS neurons operating in real time, and interacting directly with the world via sensors and effectors.

VLSI designers have taken a wide range of approaches to the design of neurons for artificial neural networks (Ramacher and Ruckert 1991; Murray and Tarassenko 1994). While many of these designs use pulse-based encoding, similar to the action potential output encoding of real neurons (Murray, Hamilton, and Tarassenko 1989), in most of these cases, it is the connectivity between neurons that is the focus of effort. The responses of the individual neurons are simplified to a fixed input-output relations that conform to the models used in artificial neural network research. Less effort is devoted to a study of the complex biophysical mechanisms that underlie neuronal discharge, and what their significance might be.

In this chapter, we describe how to construct more realistic silicon neurons by combining modular circuits that emulate the various biophysical properties of neurons relevant to their electrophysiological behavior (Mahowald and Douglas 1991). These neurons are based on the Hodgkin-Huxley formalism (1952) for channel kinetics (see chapter 4, this volume). The input-output relationship of the silicon neuron results from the concurrent dynamical activity of its coupled circuit modules, just as the input-output relationship of the biological cell arises from the biophysical interaction of its primitive elements.

8.2 Mapping Neurons into aVLSI

The strategy for mapping neurons into aVLSI circuits is similar to the compartmental modeling methods used in digital simulations of neurons (Traub and Miles 1991; see chapter 3, this volume). The continuous neuron is divided into compartments that represent segments of dendrite, soma, axon, and so on (figure 8.1). Each compartment is considered to be isopotential and spatially uniform in its properties. The model neuron is composed of convenient-sized cylindrical compartments that approximate the electrotonic properties of a real neuron, and the compartments are connected to each other as a tree that represents the neuron's morphology according to standard approximations (Rall 1977; Douglas and Martin 1993; chapter 3, this volume; see figure 8.1a). The morphology of the cell can be approximated by any number of compartments to varying degrees of accuracy. The resolution of the segmentation is a compromise between the questions that must be addressed by the model, the resources required by each compartment and error tolerance (Douglas and Martin 1993; Traub and Miles 1991, chapter 3, this volume).

In numerical simulations, the behavior of the compartments is governed by sets of ordinary differential equations that express the properties of membrane conductances, current flow, and so on. In the silicon neurons, the compartments are populated by modular subcircuits, each of which emulates the physics of a particular ionic conductance rather than its mathematical model. The performance of these modules can be adjusted by setting the voltage parameters, just as a numerical simulation can be controlled by the values of its parameters.

The foundation of each compartment is the passive, linear behavior due to the axial conductance offered by the intracellular fluid, the conductance of the cell membrane, and the membrane capacitance (Rall 1977). The axial conductance, G_a, establishes the electrical coupling between adjacent compartments. We implement this conductance using circuit GA (Douglas and Mahowald 1995),[1] which is an Hres circuit whose value can be varied over many orders of magnitude by a control voltage (Mead 1989). Hres has a limited linear response range (about 100 mV), outside

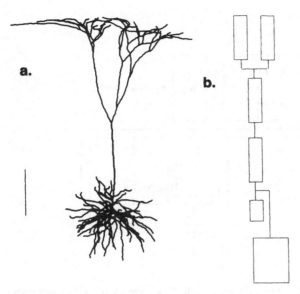

Figure 8.1
Mapping neurons in CMOS aVLSI circuits. (a) Biophysical characteristics and morphology of neurons are obtained from intracellular recordings and single-cell labeling, followed by three-dimensional recon-struction. This example shows a layer 5 pyramidal neuron in cat visual cortex reconstructed in three dimensions. Scale bar is 250 μm. (b) To construct a silicon neuron, the detailed pyramidal data must be simplified into a compartmental model. The degree of simplification is a compromise that depends on the problem being addressed. In this prototype, the pyramidal cell has been reduced to seven compartments (rectangles) that represent (bottom to top) the basal dendrites, soma, trunk of the apical dendrite (two compartments), and the branched apical tuft.

of which the current through the resistor saturates, thus limiting the amount of current that can flow into the soma of the cell. It is important to consider this effect when designing the neuron morphology. The membrane conductance, G_l, accounts for non-specific ion leakage across the cylinder membrane. The ion currents that flow across this average conductance drive the membrane voltage toward a potential, E_l, which is a weighted average of the reversal potentials of the various ions that leak across G_l. The leakage conductance circuit, GLEAK, is implemented by a wide-input-range transconductance amplifier (Mead 1989; Douglas and Mahowald 1995), which has a central linear range and saturating behavior. The conductance in the linear range can be varied over orders of magnitude by a control voltage. The capacitance of the cell membrane is emulated by the intrinsic capacitances of the CMOS material.

A switched-capacitor approach to emulating the passive linear biophysics of neu-ronal dendritic compartments has been successfully used by Elias (1993). Switched

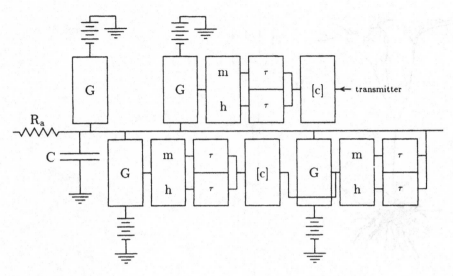

Figure 8.2
Example compartment comprising an axial resistor, *Ra*, a capacitor, *C*, a passive leak conductance, (isolated G at top left), and three types of modulated conductance, one voltage-sensitive (bottom right G), one ligand- (transmitter-) sensitive (top G), and one that is sensitive to ion concentration (bottom left G). The lower concentration, [c], element is shown connected to a voltage-sensitive conductance because the concentration, [c], of the ion is affected by the voltage-regulated flow of the ion into the cell. As in the Hodgkin-Huxley formalism, *m* stands for an activation process and *h* stands for an inactivation process; τ stands for a first-order temporal filter.

capacitors have the advantage of complete linearity and the effective membrane conductance and axial resistances can be varied by orders of magnitude. The disadvantage of switched-capacitor circuits is that clock signals must be generated to control the switching rate and thus the effective resistance values.

Passive linear models of dendrites are attractive because they are mathematically tractable, although there is substantial experimental evidence that, beside the action potential mechanisms of the soma, many kinds of neuron also have a variety of active conductances in their dendritic membranes (McCormick 1990; Stuart and Sakmann 1994). A representative compartment is shown in figure 8.2 that incorporates both active and passive conductances.

8.3   Active Channels

The building block of the CMOS neuronal circuits is the transistor, an active, three-terminal device. Current flows from the source terminal through the semiconductor channel into the drain terminal.[2] The channel current is controlled by the voltage on the gate terminal. In CMOS technology the transistors are of two types; N and P. In a P-type transistor (denoted by a circle on its gate), positive current flows from a source of positive potential into the relatively negative drain, while in the N-type transistor, positive current flows from the drain through the channel into the more negative source. The channel current of these transistors is a function of the voltage difference between the source and the gate. Beneath a voltage of about 0.8 V, called the "threshold," the function is exponential; above 0.8 V, it becomes a power function. In conventional digital and analog CMOS circuits, the transistors operate in the suprathreshold regime, where the behavior of components is much more uniform. By contrast, silicon neurons operate largely in the subthreshold regime, where they achieve the slow time behavior characteristic of biological neurons and can exploit the exponential device characteristics and low power consumption.

In the subthreshold regime, the same Boltzmann physics that governs populations of channels in the neuron's membrane dominates the flow of charge through the transistor channel. The transistor gate voltage controls the height of the energy barrier over which the charge carriers with Boltzamann-distributed energies must pass in order to flow across the channel. Current through the transistor cannot change more steeply than a factor of e for every 25 mV voltage change on the gate, and typically changes a factor of e for every 40 mV. The situation is slightly different in biological membranes, where the gating charges of the channel proteins rather than the ions themselves obey a Boltzmann distribution. Thus, if n gating charges are moved through the membrane per channel opening, the dependence of the number of open channels on membrane voltage will be n times steeper than the dependence of current through the transistor on the transistor gate voltage. Because the amount of current flowing across the nerve membrane is proportional to the number of open channels, the current through a population of active channels changes by a factor of e every $25/n$ mV, where n is the gating charge of the channel. In order to use the physics of the transistor to represent neuronal channel activation, the voltage range of the silicon neuron is scaled to be n (≈ 10) times larger than the voltage range of a real neuron. By scaling the voltage range, the degree of activation of the channel population (or conductance) as a fraction of the neuron's operating range is conserved.

The conductance of a population of voltage-dependent channels is modeled by using a differential pair circuit, which is a pair of transistors having a common source. This circuit is shown in figure 8.3a, where a bias transistor is interposed between the power (or ground) rail and a differential pair of transistors. The gate voltage of the bias transistor will set the constant current that must be the sum of

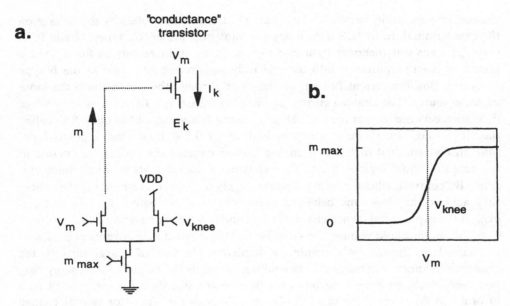

Figure 8.3
Example of a neuromorphic CMOS aVLSI circuit for potassium current. (a) Basic circuit that emulates transmembrane ion currents in the silicon neuron (Mahowald and Douglas 1991). A differential pair of transistors have their sources are linked to a single bias transistor (bottom). The voltage, m_{max}, applied to the gate of the bias transistor, sets the bias current, which is the sum of the currents flowing through the two limbs of the differential pair. The relative values of the voltages, V_m and V_{50}, applied to the gates of the differential pair determine how the current will be shared between the two limbs. (b) Relationship between V_m and the output current, m, in the left limb. The current, m, is the activation variable that controls the potassium (in this example) current, I_k, that flows through the "conductance" transistor interposed between the ionic reversal potential, E_k, and the membrane potential.

the currents flowing through the limbs of the differential pair. This bias current sets the maximum current that can flow through the population of neuron channels that the circuit emulates. The bias current is shared between the two limbs according to the relative gate voltages of the differential pair. The current flowing through the left-hand limb, for example, is described by

$$I_1 = I_b \frac{e^{\kappa V_m}}{e^{\kappa V_m} + e^{\kappa V_{50}}}.$$

This function is sigmoidal, with half activation at $V_m = V_{50}$, when half the bias current flows through each limb. When V_m is less than V_{50}, the bias current flows predominantly through the right limb; when V_m is greater than V_{50}, through the left. The coefficient, κ, is an efficiency factor. This simple three-transistor circuit is the basis of the all the activation and inactivation circuits that make up the ion conductance modules of the silicon neurons.

The dynamics of conductance activation and inactivation are approximated by first-order low-pass filters composed of a transconductance amplifier and a capacitor (figure 8.6, labeled τ). The transconductance amplifier supplies a current onto the capacitor that is proportional to the hyperbolic tangent of the voltage difference between its two input terminals. The voltage applied to the bias transistor of the transconductance amplifier sets the constant of proportionality, and can be used to control the time constant of the circuit over orders of magnitude.

In real neurons, the ion current that flows through the membrane depends on the conductance for that ion and the driving potential, which is the difference between the reversal potential of the ion and the intracellular potential. The same relationship holds in silicon neurons, although the silicon conductance is less linear than the real membrane conductance. Fortunately, the errors that arise from this nonlinearity are small because the membrane potential of the neuron hovers close to the threshold for action potential generation, and thus is nearly constant (figure 8.3a); detailed descriptions of the analog circuits can be found in Mead 1989; Douglas and Mahowald 1995.

8.4   The Action Potential

The most fundamental active neuronal phenomenon that the circuit modules must emulate is the generation of action potentials. The current that flows during the action potential can be decomposed into two components: the sodium current and the potassium current (Hodgkin and Huxley 1952). The action potential is triggered by a depolarization (increase) of the membrane voltage caused by an external current source. As the membrane voltage increases, the sodium current is activated and flows into the cell, further increasing the potential on the membrane capacitance. Eventually, the sodium current disappears, due to the delayed inactivation of the sodium channels. The potassium current is also activated by the membrane depolarization, although with a slower time constant. The potassium current flowing out of the cell discharges the membrane capacitance and abates when the membrane voltage falls below the level for its activation. The repolarization of the membrane allows the sodium channel to deinactivate, so that it is ready to generate another action potential.

When the action potential cycle of conductance change is completed, the cell either returns to rest or begins to depolarize again if the external current is still present. At high spike rates, the frequency of action potential generation depends on the magnitude of the external current relative to the potassium current as a function of time. When the input current exceeds the potassium current, the membrane depolarizes and another action potential begins. Ultimately, the occurrence of action potentials is limited by the requirement that the membrane hyperpolarize long enough for the sodium channel to deinactivate. If the input current is large enough to permanently depolarize the membrane so that deinactivation cannot occur, the action potential generation mechanism fails.

The action potential in the silicon neuron is generated the same way as in the biological neuron. A block diagram of a simple silicon neuron with membrane capacitor, leakage conductance, voltage-sensitive sodium conductance, and voltage-sensitive potassium conductance is shown in figure 8.4. The detailed activation/inactivation circuits are shown in figures 8.5 and 8.6. The kinetics of opening and closing of the sodium and potassium channels are controlled by the low-pass filters feeding the activation/inactivation circuits. A circuit structure called a "current mirror" (figure 8.5) is used to link the activation signal from the differential pair circuits to the gate of the conductance transistor, G. The mirror permits the output signal of a N-type circuit to control properly the P-type conductance transistor, in which the positive transmembrane current must flow from the sodium potential toward the membrane potential on the membrane capacitance. The current mirror controlled by the inactivation circuit subtracts current from the mirror that controls the conductance transistor and expresses the inactivation of the neuronal channels.

A simulation of the performance of these circuits is illustrated in figure 8.7. The membrane voltage, and delayed membrane voltages controlling all of the activation/inactivation differential pairs, and the resulting currents are all depicted as a function of time. The kinetics and scaled magnitudes of the currents giving rise to the action potential in the biological neuron are replicated by the concurrent dynamical interaction of the circuit modules.

A number of modules have been developed in addition to the action potential modules (Douglas and Mahowald 1995): the persistent sodium conductance, various calcium conductance, calcium-dependent potassium conductance, potassium A-conductance, nonspecific leak conductance, exogenous (electrode) current source, excitatory synapse, potassium-mediated inhibitory synapse, and chloride-mediated (silent) inhibitory synapse. The output of a neuron chip that includes these modules is shown in figure 8.8. While any desired combination of modules can be inserted into any of the compartments of the silicon neuron, all the circuit modules necessary to provide the required range of behavior of the neuron must of course be inserted at the time the chip is fabricated. Modules can be turned off by setting their conductance at maximal activation equal to zero, thereby effectively removing them

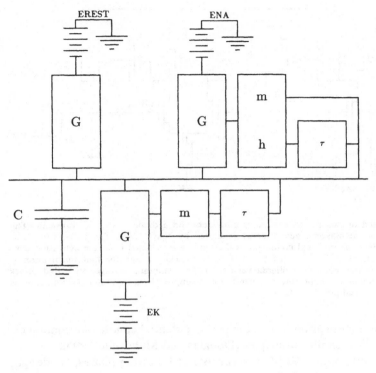

Figure 8.4
Simple silicon neuron able to generate action potentials. It comprises a capacitor, C, a leakage conductance (isolated G top left), a sodium conductance (top G) and a potassium conductance (bottom G). The sodium conductance has an activation module, m, and an inactivation module, h, that is driven through a temporal filter, τ. The potassium conductance has only an activation module, m, that is driven by a temporal filter, τ.

from the total neuronal circuit. Unfortunately, no new modules can be added after fabrication. If additional properties are required, another silicon neuron with different morphology or different types of channels can be fabricated using variations of the basic circuit modules.

8.5 Design and fabrication

The CMOS circuits are created by an iterative process of design, fabrication, and experiment. In the case of the silicon neuron, our strategy was to build a library of modules that could be used in a number of different contexts. In this section, we will

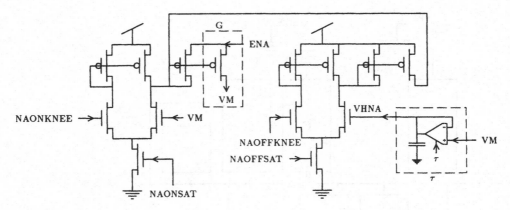

Figure 8.5
Sodium circuit is composed of two transconductance amplifiers and a diode connected transistor. The conductance of the module at maximal activation is generated by NAONSAT. The voltage for half-activation is NAONKNEE. The maximal conductance that will be subtracted from the activation conductance to produce inactivation is generated by NAOFFSAT. The voltage for half inactivation is NAOFFKNEE. VHNA is the temporally filtered version of the membrane voltage, VM, that drives sodium inactivation. The sodium current onto the membrane is supplied by a transistor, G, that sources current from the sodium reversal potential, ENA.

describe the design and fabrication of just the action potential conductance modules. The other modules follow similar principles (Douglas and Mahowald 1995).

The development cycle of an aVLSI chip consists of following phases; (1) design; (2) layout; (3) verification; (4) fabrication; and (5) testing (figure 8.9). Typically, designers execute each of these phases except the fabrication, which is done by a commercial silicon foundry. The foundry fabricates the chip according to a list of instructions contained in an ASCII file with a standard format, called "Caltech Intermediate Form" (CIF). Because the fabrication is automatic, what is assembled on the chip will depend entirely on what the designer has specified.

The circuits can fabricated on silicon chips of various standard sizes. Our silicon neuron was fabricated through the MOSIS service, on one of their "tinychips." MOSIS collects silicon designs from a number of sources and combines them into wafer-sized instruction sets to be fabricated by one of several professional silicon foundries. The MOSIS tinychip provides a silicon area of 2.3 × 2.3 mm, in a package with forty contact pins, at a cost of approximately 680 dollars for four pieces. This is the most economical prototype chip, and it provides ample silicon area for the needs of the novice designer.[3]

The design phase is usually the longest. During this phase the concept of the computation must be transformed into a legal and functionally correct aVLSI circuit. In

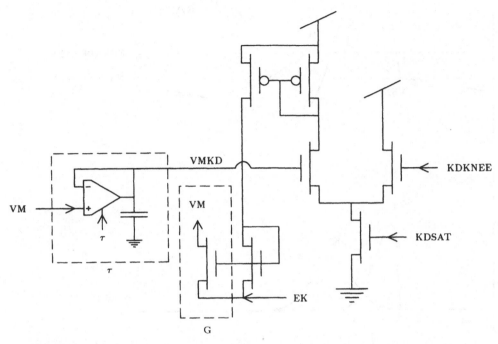

Figure 8.6
Potassium activation circuit has only one differential pair because this channel does not inactivate. The maximal conductance at full activation is generated by KDSAT. The voltage at half activation is KDKNEE. The membrane voltage, VM, is filtered by a temporal filter, τ, to yield the activation voltage, VMKD, which is compared to the half-activation voltage to determine the state of activation of the circuit. The potassium current flows onto the membrane voltage from the potasium reversal potential EK, through a transistor, G.

the design phase, the correspondence between elements of the analog circuit and those of the neural system is established and the variable parameters identified. The transformation involves recognizing certain functional elements in the process for which there are known electronic solutions. This is analogous to solving a particular differential equation by recognizing that it is a special case of a general form. As a result of the aVSLI research of the last decade, there is now a library of subcircuits whose properties are well understood. These subcircuits, or their modifications, will usually account for more than 90% of a simple circuit. Designers must combine these subcircuits to meet their ends, in the way that words are crafted into sentences. Figures 8.5 and 8.6 show how the action potential sodium and potassium circuits are specified in schematic form.

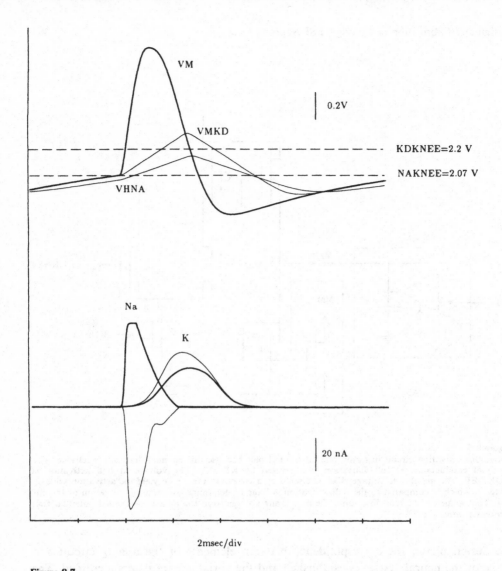

Figure 8.7
Action potential is generated by the dynamics of two channel modules that emulate the sodium channel and the delayed-rectifier potassium channel. The membrane voltage, VM, is plotted in thick line. The low-pass-filtered versions of the membrane voltage that control sodium inactivation. VHNA, and potassium activation, VMKD, are plotted in thin line. The threshold level for sodium activation and inactivation were set to the same voltage, indicated by NAKNEE. The threshold for potassium activation is indicated by KDKNEE. The lower plot shows the conductances (thick line) of the sodium and potassium channels during the spike, as well as the resulting currents (thin line) that flow onto the membrane capacitance. The notch in the sodium current relative to the sodium conductance is due to the diminished driving potential across the sodium conductance as the membrane voltage approaches the sodium reversal potential. These plots were obtained by circuit simulation in AnaLOG (see section 8.5), since not all of these variables were instrumented on fabricated chips.

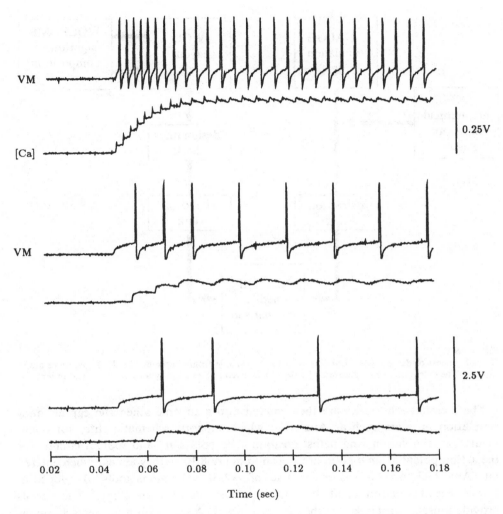

Figure 8.8
Real-time response of a silicon neuron emulating the response of a cortical pyramidal neuron to three different levels of a step of intrasomatic current injection. Only a somatic compartment and a compartment modeling a dendritic load were emulated. Each pair of response traces consists of the somatic membrane potential, V_m (2.5 V scale bar), and a voltage that is proportional to the intrasomatic free calcium concentration, $[Ca]$ (0.25 V scale bar). Notice the adaptation of discharge.

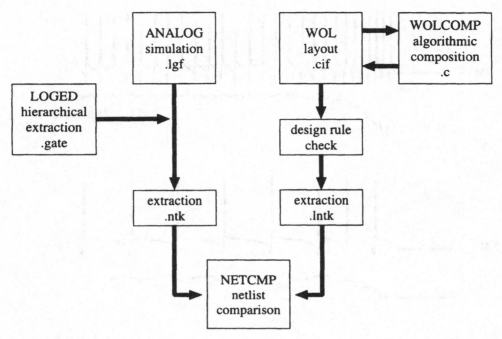

Figure 8.9
Overall process of designing a VLSI chip with tools available from Chipmunk Tools. Tool names are in capitals. The extension of files generated by the tool is given as ".ext;" programs are explained in text.

These circuit schematics are then entered into a suitable schematic capture-and-simulation program such as AnaLOG, which supports schematic entry for documentation, simulation, and netlist creation. The potassium and sodium circuits for the action potential simulation are shown in figure 8.10 as they appear when entered into AnaLOG. AnaLOG is one of a set of aVLSI "Chipmunk tools" developed in Carver Mead's laboratory at the California Institute of Technology.[4] These tools provide a useful starter set for the novice designer. AnaLOG is a particularly popular piece of software that provides accurate simulation of CMOS gates operating in their subthreshold regime. The circuit schematics are entered by a convenient computer-aided design (CAD) interface. The schematics can be previewed on-screen, and output to encapsulated Postscript or HPGL output files. The simulations are used for verifying the proposed operation of the circuits.

Although simulations and mathematical analyses of the proposed circuit subunits are useful during the design stage, they are nevertheless limited. Provided the overall

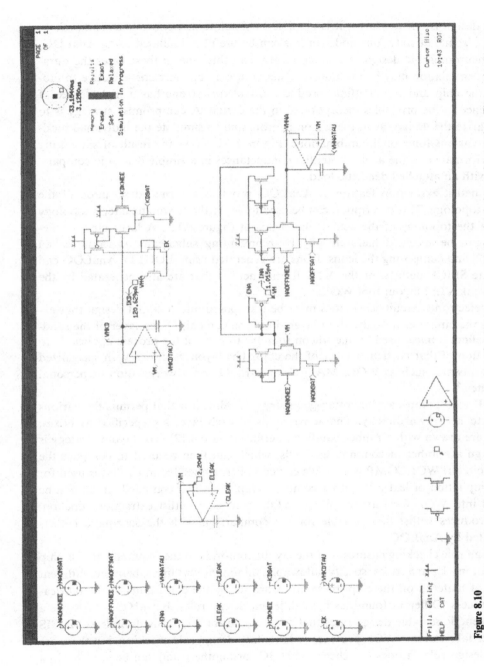

Figure 8.10
Example X-window from AnaLOG, illustrating the overall view of a simple neuron ready for simulation and extraction. The passive leak conductance and the potentiometers that set the control voltages for the neuron are shown on the left, the delayed-rectifier potassium circuit at the top of the page, and the sodium circuit at the bottom of the page. A subset of the library of components used to construct circuits is located at the bottom of the window.

circuit design is not too large, it is possible to simulate its performance comprehensively. Circuits of sixty-four nodes or less can be usefully simulated using AnaLOG. Most neuromorphic designs are much larger than this, and in these cases the durations of simulation may be prohibitive. Finally, it may be more cost-effective to fabricate the chip and test the final product, provided that one has a high degree of confidence in the principles incorporated in the design. A compromise strategy is to modularize the design, as in the silicon neuron, and to simulate the individual modules in various functional combinations. Figure 8.11 shows the result of simulating the performance of the action potential conductances in a simple dendritic compartment with an attached dendritic load.

The netlist extraction feature of AnaLOG provides a formal description of the circuit topology. This description can be used to verify the schematic circuit topology against the topology of the actual silicon layout (figure 8.12). A large circuit schematic can be specified hierarchically by representing subcircuits as icons (called "gates") and composing the icons. Icons are generated using LOGED. AnaLOG can generate SPICE netlists, or the NTK format netlists that are also generated by the Chipmunk VLSI layout tool WOL.

The electronic circuit schematics must be transposed into a layout design that expresses the circuit as a sandwich of layers in the silicon chip. Each layer of the sandwich defines a mask used by the silicon foundry to control the process applicable to fabrication of that particular layer of the chip. The layout is drawn with specialized CAD software, such as WOL, MAGIC, or L-EDIT, on a workstation or personal computer.[5]

WOL incorporates a Manhattan-geometry leaf cell editor that permits the various layers to be drawn directly. The active areas of each layer are specified as boxes, which are drawn with a rubber-banding interface (figure 8.12). The layout strategy is to design a number of common leaf cells, which can then be used to compose the larger circuit. WOLCOMP is a simple cell compiler, embedded in C, that is used for the compilation of leaf cells into a complete chip. The final compiled circuit can be loaded into WOL for further editing. WOL includes a netlist extraction function, that produces netlist files suitable for net comparison with the schematic netlists generated by AnaLOG.

Design rule checking ensures that the layout conforms to the requirements for chip fabrication. Design rules specify allowable minimum distances between different pieces of material on the chip; these limits are set by the constraints of the fabrication process. Different foundries have different design rules, but MOSIS provides a set of generic scalable design rules that can be used for any of the foundries MOSIS uses for fabrication.[6] WOL provides rudimentary design rule checking, but there are some design rules it does not check. MAGIC (or another tool) can be used to do a

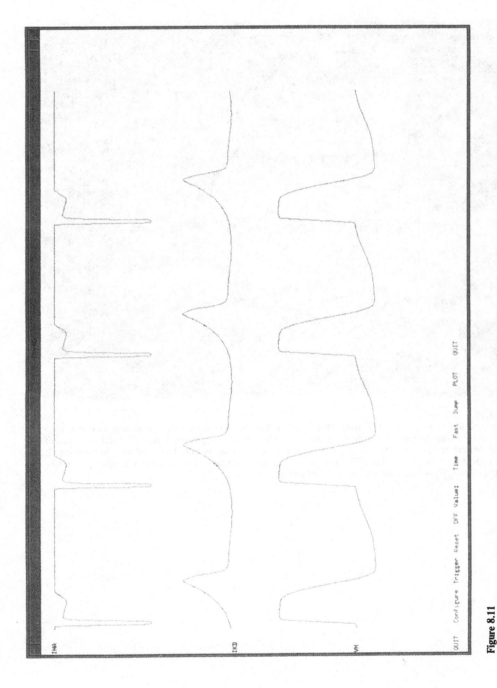

Figure 8.11
Example graphical output in an X-window of AnaLOG during simulation of the simple neuron, showing action potentials on the membrane voltage trace, VM (below); current through the sodium circuit, INA, onto the membrane (above); and current through the potassium circuit, IK, onto the membrane (middle).

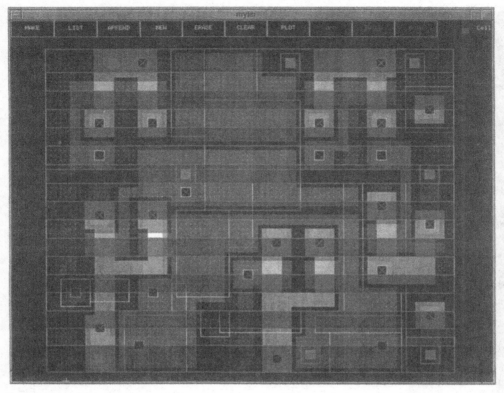

Figure 8.12
Layout represented in the WOL editor. This layout is for the delayed-rectifier potassium circuit shown schematically in figure 8.6. The different colors (not shown here) represent layers of different types of material. Where red polysilicon crosses green diffusion, there is a transistor. The conductance transistor is the very short one on the far right. The size of this layout fabricated on a 2μ process is $86x71\mu^2$. A tiny chip area of roughly $4\,mm^2$ can contain roughly 650 such circuits.

full-layout Design Rule Check (DRC). Tools exist to convert WOL CIF output to a form compatible with MAGIC.

The final layout instructions are sent by electronic mail to MOSIS, which returns the fabricated chip in about ten weeks.[7] Once the chip has been fabricated, its performance is explored using similar experimental methods to those used in a real neurophysiological preparation, except that many more variables can be observed. For example, the response of the analog circuits to stimulation is measured in real time, with an oscilloscope. Typically, the neuromorphic circuits will have a number of control parameters, inputs, and outputs, which are accessed via the pins of the chip package. The control parameters are usually voltages, which are applied to the pins by potentiometers. It is convenient to set up this ancilliary circuitry on a proto-typing grid, or on a prototype wire-wrap board.[8] It is convenient to assess the chip's performance using computer-assisted data logging, with instruments controlled via an IEEE-488 (GPIB) interface. Here again, the Chipmunk tools provide a useful package, VIEW. Alternatively, commercial packages such as MATLAB, or LABVIEW, can used.

Except for the variable parameters included in the design, the circuits cannot be altered after fabrication; thus errors in the specification of the neuron cannot be corrected as easily as in software simulations. Care must also be taken to plan experiments before the chip is fabricated so that instrumentation circuitry can be included to observe the state of interesting analog variables. The designs of circuits evolve with understanding gained by experiment. Often three to four revisions may need to be fabricated before the circuit is working as planned. It is therefore desirable to fabricate low cost tinychip prototypes for new circuit designs.

8.6 Conclusion

It is now possible to model interesting neuronal biophysical mechanisms in silicon. Although the CMOS transistor circuits described here are not an exact match for the equations used in digital simulation, they nevertheless emulate to a first approximation the behavior of biological neurons. The real-time emulation of neuronal electrophysiology is a first step to realizing artificial neural systems whose architecture and design principles are derived from biological nervous systems.

Acknowledgments

The preparation of this chapter and much of the research discussed in it were supported by grants to Rodney Douglas, Misha Mahowald, and Kevan Martin by the

Office of Naval Research, the United Kingdom Medical Research Council, and the
Swiss National Science Foundation. Fabrication facilities were provided by MOSIS.
We acknowledge the authors of the Chipmunk programs for the fine tools they have
placed in the public domain, and for the use of some of their documentation in this
chapter. We thank Brian Baker for electronic support and Philip Hafliger for pre-
paring the figures.

Notes

1. Subscripted notation will be used to denote physical properties, such as G_a, and uppercase to denote the
analogous circuit, such as GA.

2. The semiconductor "channel" is the path by which charge flows through a transistor; it is controlled by
the circuit performing a computation. Thus the meaning is slightly different from a biological membrane
"channel."

3. Prices for various chip types and sizes are available on the Internet at http://www.isi.edu/mosis/

4. AnaLOG is available from http://www.pcmp.caltech.edu/chipmunk/

5. WOL is a Chipmunk tool; MAGIC is available at http://www.research.digital.com/wrl/projects/magic/
magic.html; and L-EDIT is available from Tanner Research at http://www.tanner.com/

6. These design rules are available at http://www.isi.edu/mosis/

7. A complete layout for a tinychip with a small silicon neuron and associated schematics and netlist files
are available on the Internet at http://www.ini.unizh.ch/

8. Printed circuit boards suitable for testing the silicon neuron chip described in this chapter are available
from Brian Baker at baker@psych.ox.ac.uk

9 Principles of Spike Train Analysis

Fabrizio Gabbiani and Christof Koch

9.1 Introduction

Experiments in sensory neurophysiology often record action potential arrival times of nerve cells resulting from spontaneous or stimulus-evoked activity. When all action potentials are taken to be identical and only their localized times of occurrence are considered, one obtains a discrete series of time events, $\{t_1, \ldots t_n$, where $t_i =$ time of arrival of the ith spike$\}$, characterizing the spike train. It is this series of events that is transmitted down the axon to all of the cell's targets and that contains most, if not all, of the information the cell is conveying.

Most of this information is neglected when studying the *average rate*, the number of action potentials over some suitable interval usually lasting a fraction of a second or longer, as the relevant variable characterizing the neuronal response. Recently, the *temporal coding* of information in the patterns of spikes, both in the single cell as well as between multiple cells, has received renewed attention. The broad idea that spike timing, in particular across an ensemble of cells, plays an important role in encoding various aspects of the stimulus is supported by experiments in a variety of sensory systems such as locust olfaction, electric fish electrosensation, cat vision and olfaction, as well as monkey vision and audition (Chung, Raymond, and Lettvin 1970; Freeman 1975; Abeles 1990; Strehler and Lestienne 1986; Bialek et al. 1991; Eskandar, Richmond, and Optican 1992; Singer and Gray 1995; Decharms and Merzenich 1996; Laurent 1996; Wehr and Laurent 1996; Gabbiani et al. 1996; Lisman 1997).

The characteristics of the neuronal code are closely linked to the seemingly *stochastic* or *random* character of neuronal firing. Because little or no information can be encoded into a stream of completely regularly spaced action potentials, this raises the questions of how variable neuronal firing really is and what the relation is between variability and the neural code. It is the mathematical theory of stochastic point processes and the field of statistical signal processing that offer us the adequate tools for attacking these questions.

This chapter surveys a selection of such tools, starting with the classical interspike interval histograms commonly used in neurophysiological studies. The methods presented here are intended to shed additional light on two aspects of neuronal signal processing: (1) the integrative mechanisms underlying the activity of nerve cells; (2) the nature and reliability of stimulus encoding in neuronal spike trains.

To address these aspects and illustrate the methods presented here, we study the encoding of various signals in spike trains of certain simplified single-cell models, in particular integrate-and-fire neurons and Poisson spike train generators. This allows us to investigate in a controlled manner the effect of several biophysical parameters such as refractoriness or mean firing rate on the encoding of various signals. These models are described in detail in section 9.2. They can all be modeled using the MATLAB routines provided by us (see below and chapter appendix B).

Section 9.3 introduces the classical measure of variability associated with inter-spike interval distributions: the coefficient of variation, C_V. Its dependence on various biophysical and stimulus parameters is then investigated. In section 9.4, a different and complementary measure of variability of the neuronal response, the ratio of the variance to the mean spike count in a fixed time interval, F, is introduced. This measure plays an important role in determining the accuracy with which information can be conveyed in the mean spike count, as explained in section 9.5. Sections 9.6–9.7 are devoted to the analysis of information encoded in the timing of neuronal spiking. In section 9.6, the autocorrelation function and power spectrum of the time series of action potential events are defined. While the power spectrum is a measure of the frequency content of the spike train and can, under some assumptions, reflect to processing performed by the neuron on its input stimuli, it is also influenced by intrinsic properties of the neuron, like its refractory period or its tendency to fire regularly. The autocorrelation function, in turn, translates these properties in the time domain. Section 9.7 introduces a method that allows to directly assess the accuracy of the information transmitted by a neuron about a time-varying stimulus by estimating the stimulus from the spike train.

Increasingly fast computers and the availability of comprehensive software packages with practical graphical interfaces has made the analysis of neuronal data using the methods presented here more rapid and convenient. One of these packages, MATLAB, is well suited for such numerical work and was used to analyze our data. The corresponding programs (MATLAB M-files) can be freely accessed and downloaded from our web site (see chapter appendix B for a more detailed description as well as http://www.klab.caltech.edu/~gabbiani/signproc.html). All of the functions and spike generation models used in the following pages are defined within a simple and intuitive programming environment, based on the dynamical system simulation package of MATLAB called "Simulink." We also provide several tutorials that will allow the interested reader to directly generate and analyze the data from our models (as well as more elaborate variants, which are only briefly mentioned here) and to further explore topics not covered in this chapter. (For an early review and references on the subject of this chapter, see Schmitt 1970, chapters 51–58; see also Rieke et al. 1996.)

9.2 Models

We start by introducing several simplified models that will be used to illustrate the analysis methods explored in the following sections. We do not intend to perform biophysically detailed modeling of single neurons here (this subject is covered in chapters 3–6, this volume). The goal of this chapter is to incorporate some basic biophysical properties of real nerve cells, such as refractoriness, spike train variability or bursting, into idealized single-cell models, along with plausible processing schemes for input signals and to analyze the properties of the resulting spike trains. While none of the models described below can faithfully reproduce all the properties of a given neuronal spike train, each one of them has been shown in several instances to successfully capture at least some of them.

9.2.1 Perfect Integrate-and-Fire Neuron

We turn to a very simple, but quite powerful model of a spiking cell with a long and distinguished history, first investigated by Lapicque (1907, 1926). It is known as the "integrate-and-fire model" (Stein 1967a, 1967b; Knight 1972a; Tuckwell 1988) and assumes that the neuron integrates its inputs and generates a spike when a fixed voltage threshold is reached:

$$C_m \cdot \frac{dV_m}{dt} = I(t), \tag{9.1}$$

where $I(t)$ is the input current, integrated to yield the membrane voltage $V_m(t)$. In eq. 9.1, the resting membrane potential has been set to zero for convenience and the constant C_m represents the capacity of the model cell. With the help of an initial condition, such as $V_m(0) = 0$, eq. 9.1 specifies the evolution of the membrane potential in the subthreshold domain (figure 9.1).

A spike is generated each time that $V_m(t)$ reaches the threshold V_{th} and the membrane voltage is reset to zero immediately after a spike. Thus the successive times, t_i, of spike occurrence are determined recursively from the equation

$$\int_{t_i}^{t_{i+1}} I(t)\, dt = C_m V_{th}. \tag{9.2}$$

The response of such a model to a positive constant current step has the following characteristics: (1) the firing rate, f, is linearly related to the magnitude of the input current: $f(I) = I/C_m V_{th}$, in other words, the frequency-current or f-I curve is linear (see figure 9.2); (2) arbitrarily small input currents eventually lead to a spike, that is,

A

Perfect Integrate-and-Fire Unit

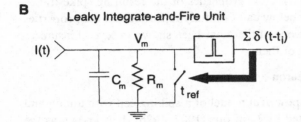

B

Leaky Integrate-and-Fire Unit

Figure 9.1
Two variants of integrate-and-fire "units." Common to both are passive integration within a single compartment for the subthreshold domain and a voltage threshold V_{th}. Whenever the membrane potential V_m reaches V_{th}, a pulse is generated and the circuit is short-circuited. For a duration t_{ref} following spike generation, any input $I(t)$ is shunted to ground (corresponding to an absolute refractory period). (A) Perfect or nonleaky integrate-and-fire model contains but a capacitance. (B) Leaky or forgetful integrate-and-fire unit accounts for the decay of the membrane potential by an additional component, a leak resistance R_m.

the model never "forgets" the occurrence of an input; and (3) the corresponding output spike train is perfectly regular.

Several simple modifications of this basic model lead to very different behaviors.

9.2.2 Refractory Period

In real neurons, the dynamic firing range is limited by the biophysical properties of the ionic membrane conductances responsible for action potential generation. In particular, neurons do not fire at arbitrarily high rates because sodium channels need to recover from inactivation between two action potentials. As a first approximation, this constraint can be implemented in the preceding model by assuming that after a spike the neuron is entirely inactive for a fixed period of time, t_{ref} (the absolute refractory period or dead time), before it resumes normal function. That is, for a fixed time after spike generation, all input current is shunted off. Such a refractory period limits the firing frequency to $f_{max} = 1/t_{ref}$ and thus introduces a nonlinear saturation in the f-I curve for large inputs:

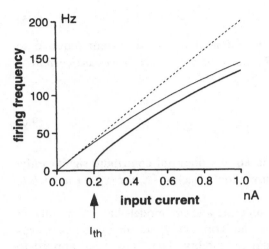

Figure 9.2
Graph of f-I curves for an integrate-and-fire model without and with refractory period (thin solid line and dashed line, respectively) and for a leaky integrate-and-fire model with refractory period (thick solid line). The f-I curve of the (leaky) integrate-and-fire neuron with refractory period saturates for high input currents at the inverse of the absolute refractory period (here 5 msec). The leaky integrate-and-fire model will not respond to currents less than I_{th} (arrow) because of its tendency to "forget" inputs, while for high currents its f-I curve becomes similar to the one of the perfect integrate-and-fire model. This and all following figures were generated using the MATLAB routines described in chapter appendix B and made available at our web site.

$$f(I) = \frac{I}{C_m V_{th} + t_{ref} \cdot I}$$ (9.3)

(see figure 9.2).

9.2.3 Leaky Integrate-and-Fire Neuron

The integrate-and-fire neuron considered above will sum linearly two subthreshold inputs irrespective of their temporal separation because it does not gradually forget the occurrence of events over time. A more realistic behavior is obtained by introducing a leak term in the dynamics of the subthreshold membrane voltage:

$$C_m \frac{dV_m}{dt} = I(t) - \frac{V_m}{R_m},$$ (9.4)

driving it toward its resting value, $V_m = 0$. The leak term is characterized by the resistance to current flowing out of the cell, R_m (figure 9.1).

In response to a constant current pulse I, this leaky integrate-and-fire model will relax exponentially toward a steady-state voltage $V_m = IR_m$:

$$V_m(t) = IR_m(1 - e^{-t/\tau_m}), \tag{9.5}$$

with time constant $\tau_m = R_m C_m$. Thus the minimal threshold current required to drive the cell to threshold is $I_{th} = V_{th}/R_m$ (also known as the "rheobase current"). The corresponding f-I curve is given by

$$f(I) = \begin{cases} 0 & \text{if } I \leq I_{th}, \\ \left[t_{ref} - \tau_m \log\left(1 - \frac{V_{th}}{IR_m}\right) \right]^{-1}, & I > I_{th}. \end{cases} \tag{9.6}$$

For large input currents, the leak term in eq. 9.4 does not contribute significantly; the f-I curve of eq. 9.3 is recovered (by using $\log(1 - x) \sim -x$, for $|x| \ll 1$ in eq. 9.6; see figure 9.2).

Due to the presence of the leak term, integrate-and-fire models have been difficult to fully characterize analytically (Poggio and Torre 1977) but have also been surprisingly successful in describing neuronal excitability. They have been applied to model the firing behavior of numerous cell types: neurons in the *Limulus* eye (Knight 1972b), α-motoneurons (Calvin and Stevens 1968), neurons in the visual system of the housefly (Gestri, Masterbroek, and Zaagman 1980), and cortical cells (Softky and Koch 1993; Troyer and Miller 1997), among others.

We will mostly consider the case of a perfect integrator model because it allows us to write down closed-form solutions for many variables of interest. However, the behavior of the leaky integrator will approach that of the perfect integrate-and-fire model if the average interspike interval is short compared to the time constant τ_m.

9.2.4 Poisson Spike Trains and Integrate-and-Fire Neurons with Random Threshold

While some neurons fire regularly in response to injected suprathreshold currents, many neurons show a considerable degree of variability in their sequence of action potentials, in contrast to (leaky) integrate-and-fire neurons. Irregular firing is particularly pronounced in the case of recordings carried out in vivo, rather than in brain slices or in cultured cells (Holt et al. 1996). We here consider a class of models able to produce irregular spike trains. The following description is phenomenological: possible causes for this variability will be considered more closely in section 9.3.

An irregular response to a constant current pulse can be obtained in a model that generates a spike at an average rate of $f = I/C_m V_{th}$, but in such a way that (1) every spike is generated randomly, (2) independently of other spikes and (3) with a uniform probability of occurrence in time. The resulting spike sequence is called "a Poisson spike train" and is highly variable because of the complete independence between the time of occurrence of neighboring spikes. Neuronal response variability is often compared to the variability of a Poisson spike train because of its simplicity. However, real spike trains usually have interspike intervals that are not independent from each other but that may depend on the preceding interspike intervals.

As a consequence of properties 1–3, the interspike interval distribution of a Poisson spike train is exponentially distributed with probability density

$$p(t) = (1/\bar{\imath})e^{-t/\bar{\imath}}, \tag{9.7}$$

where $\bar{\imath}$ is the mean interspike interval (figure 9.3A). The density function $p(t)$ is obtained experimentally by binning consecutive interspike intervals from spike trains, as in figure 9.3. In this guise it is called the "interspike interval" (ISI) histogram.

Because in an integrate-and-fire neuron the mean interspike interval is proportional to the voltage threshold, Poisson spike trains can be obtained from an integrate-and-fire neuron by reseting the threshold after each spike to a new random value according to the distribution $p(V) = (1/V_{th})e^{-V/V_{th}}$. The voltage V_{th} now denotes the mean value of the distribution $p(V)$. Similarly, by assuming that the random threshold is distributed according to a gamma distribution of order n,

$$p_n(V) = \frac{c_n V^{n-1}}{V_{th}^{n-1}} e^{-nV/V_{th}}, \tag{9.8}$$

with

$$c_n = \frac{n^n}{(n-1)!} \frac{1}{V_{th}}, \tag{9.9}$$

one obtains increasingly regular spike trains in response to a constant current injection as n increases. The case $n = 1$ corresponds to Poisson spike trains and in the limit $n \rightarrow \infty$, the usual integrate-and-fire neuron is recovered. The resulting interspike intervals are gamma distributed around their mean value (figure 9.3).

It could be argued that a random voltage threshold is not a very realistic physiological feature. After all, noise in the spiking mechanism is seldomly observed in real neurons (Calvin and Stevens 1968; Mainen and Sejnowski 1995), although, in the case of a perfect or nonleaky integrate-and-fire model, a random threshold can be shown to be equivalent to a random input current (Gestri, Masterbroek, and Zaagman 1980).

This point is most easily illustrated by considering an integrate-and-fire neuron that receives as input Poisson-distributed current pulses of size I_0 at an average frequency f_0 (as in figure 9.4). If n_{th} is the number of inputs needed to fire the cell (i.e., n_{th} is the smallest integer larger than $C_m V_{th}/I_0$; see eq. 9.1) then the average firing rate of the

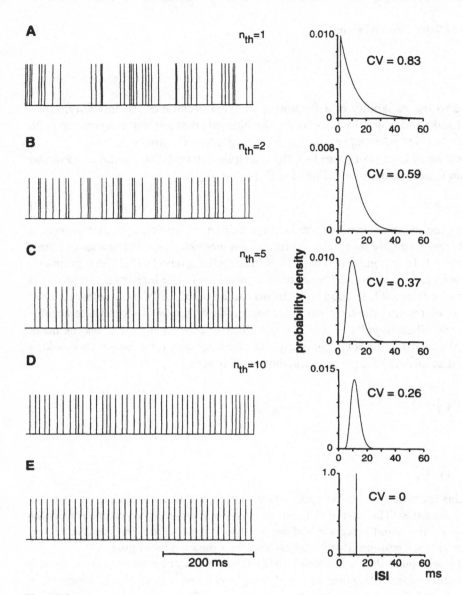

Figure 9.3
Sample spike trains and interspike interval (ISI) distributions from various models in response to a constant current input into a perfect integrator model. All models have an absolute refractory period of 2 msec and a mean firing rate of 83 Hz. (A) Poisson-distributed (i.e., exponential) random voltage threshold yields the most irregular spike train and an exponential ISI distribution. In the absence of a refractory period, C_V would be 1. (B–D) Gamma-distributed random thresholds of order 2, 5, and 10 yield increasingly regular ISI distributions, which are gamma-distributed of order 2, 5, and 10, respectively. (E) Integrate-and-fire model yields a perfectly regular spike train, corresponding to the limit $n \to \infty$. Spike trains with identical properties can be generated by a perfect integrator with fixed voltage threshold, Poisson-distributed synaptic input and, in panel A, $n_{th} = 1$ (i.e., each input triggers one output spike), in panels B–D, $n_{th} = 2, 5$, and 10 and, in panel E, a constant input current. The rate of the input Poisson process is adjusted to obtain the same mean firing rate in all cases.

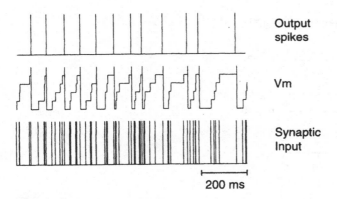

Figure 9.4
Perfect or nonleaky integrate-and-fire model averages out noise by summing its inputs until V_{th} is reached. While the Poisson synaptic input (lower trace) is highly irregular, the time to the next spike is averaged out in the membrane voltage (V_m, middle trace), yielding a more regular output spike train (top trace). In this example, $n_{th} = 5$ inputs are needed to reach threshold, thus yielding a spike train with gamma-distributed ISI distribution of order 5 (see figure 9.3C), whereas the synaptic input ISI distribution is exponential (see figure 9.3A).

model will be f_0/n_{th}. The distribution of spikes can be shown (Tuckwell 1988) to correspond to a gamma distribution of order n_{th}, identical to the interspike interval distribution considered in eq. 9.8 (figure 9.3; Tuckwell 1988).

Indeed, the statistical properties of the output spikes of both models are identical. That is, Poisson-distributed inputs into an integrator unit that requires n_{th} synaptic inputs to reach a fixed threshold V_{th} is equivalent to injecting a constant current $f_0 I_0$ into an integrator unit whose voltage threshold is distributed according to eq. 9.8 and where this constant input triggers the output spikes. Expressing the variability in terms of a random threshold distribution has mathematical and numerical advantages (see chapter appendix B). For example, the case of an *inhomogeneous Poisson process*, in which spikes are generated independently of each other with a time-varying rate $\lambda(t)$, is again equivalent to the case of injecting a deterministic current proportional to $\lambda(t)$ into the unit and having a random threshold of the form expressed in eq. 9.8.

9.3 Interspike Interval Distribution and Coefficient of Variation

The variability of a neuronal spike train is an important indicator of the type of processing a neuron performs on its synaptic inputs. The simplest measure of variability is the coefficient of variation of the interspike interval distribution, a dimensionless number defined as the standard deviation σ_t of the interspike interval

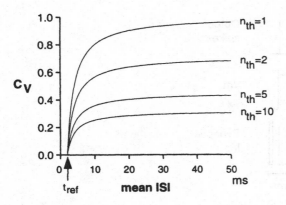

Figure 9.5
Coefficient of variation of an integrate-and-fire neuron with a 2 msec refractory period as a function of the mean ISI. The different curves denote the number of inputs n_{th} summed by the model to reach the voltage threshold. As the firing frequency increases toward the limit imposed by the refractory period t_{ref} (arrow), the spike trains becomes more regular ($C_V \to 0$ for mean ISI $\to 2$ msec). In other words, the refractory period exerts a regularizing effect on the spike train.

distribution normalized by the mean interspike interval $\bar{t}$:

$$C_V = \frac{\sigma_t}{\bar{t}}, \tag{9.10}$$

with

$$\bar{t} = \int_0^\infty t p(t)\, dt, \quad \text{and } \sigma_t^2 = \int_0^\infty (t - \bar{t})^2 p(t)\, dt, \tag{9.11}$$

where $p(t)$ is the probability density distribution of the interspike intervals. The coefficient of variation is equal to 1 for Poisson spike trains, since $\sigma_t = \bar{t}$, while for a gamma distribution of order n, $\sigma_t^2 = \bar{t}^2/n$ and $C_V = 1/\sqrt{n}$ (see eq. 9.8).

In other words, integrating over a large number of small inputs gives rise to very regular output spikes (figures 9.3–9.5). In the limit of an integrate-and-fire neuron under constant current input, $C_V \to 0$. Conversely, a neuron that is sensitive to a small number of random inputs is expected to generate very irregular spike trains. In real nerve cells, further potential sources of variability include the stochastic nature of synaptic transmission, nonlinear amplification of synaptic inputs by active dendritic conductances and network effects due to the interconnectivity of nerve cells (Softky and Koch 1993; Allan and Stevens 1994; Stuart and Sakmann 1994; van Vreeswijk and Sompolinsky 1996).

A refractory period lowers the C_V at high firing rates when it tends to force regularity in the interspike interval duration. In the ideal case of an absolute refractory period, the interspike interval probability density will simply be shifted to the right of the time axis, $p(t) \to p_{ref}(t) = p(t - t_{ref})$ and the new coefficient of variation is

$$C_{V_{ref}} = (1 - t_{ref}/\bar{t})C_V, \tag{9.12}$$

to that $C_{V_{ref}} \to 0$ as $\bar{t} \to t_{ref}$ (figures 9.3 and 9.5).

The time constant of integration of a leaky integrate-and-fire neuron will affect the coefficient of variation in a different way. If $n_{th} > 1$ coincident inputs are needed to fire the cell, a large τ_m will regularize the spike train by averaging the arrival of synaptic inputs over time, whereas a short τ_m will increase the sensitivity to coincident inputs and thus boost up variability.

In all of these examples, $C_V \leq 1$, with the upper bound given by a pure Poisson process, although in many instances interspike interval distributions of real neurons have C_V values greater than 1. This can be achieved in a Poisson neuron by assuming that the current (or the rate) driving the model is itself random in time. The resulting spike trains are termed *doubly stochastic Poisson* in the mathematical and engineering literature (Saleh 1978; Peřina 1985) because of the dual source of variability arising in the current and the spike generation mechanism. This is illustrated, for example, in a model that successfully describes several properties of retinal ganglion cell spike trains at low light levels (Saleh and Teich 1985). In this limit, the distribution of photons absorbed at the retina is expected to be Poisson. If each photon results in a slowly decaying input current to a ganglion cell that causes on average two output spikes per incoming photon (see figure 9.6A), then the interspike interval distribution of the model will have a C_V greater than 1 (figure 9.6B). The cause of this additional variability lies in the random number of spikes generated for each incoming Poisson pulse.

Other cell classes respond to inputs with a *burst* of spikes, that is, a small number of spikes separated by short interspike intervals. Several further special models and techniques have been developed to analyze the variability of such bursting cells (Bair et al. 1994; Franklin and Bair 1995; Holt et al. 1996).

9.4 Spike Count Distribution and Fano Factor

Although the C_V yields a useful measure of short-term variability, because this measure is obtained from the interspike interval distribution, it yields a complete characterization of variability only if the occurrence of a spike depends exclusively on the

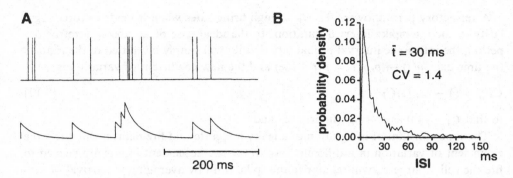

Figure 9.6
(A) Sample input current and spike train for the retinal ganglion cell model described in the main text, based on a doubly stochastic Poisson process. (B) Because of the added source of variability in the input current, the ISI distribution is more irregular than the one associated with a Poisson model (for which we would obtain $C_V = 1$).

time of the previous spike and not further on the past history of the spike train. This is the case for the Poisson- and gamma-distributed spike trains of figure 9.3; such spike trains are said to be generated by a *renewal process*. By definition, successive intervals between the spikes of a renewal process are independent (Cox 1962; Cox and Lewis 1966). Equivalently, the time of occurrence of a spike depends only on the previous one.

Information on variability beyond the first interspike interval can be gleaned from the distribution of spike counts measured over a time period of length T. To illustrate how the variability observed in the interspike intervals translates into variability of the spike count, we return to the examples of last section. For a Poisson spike train with mean firing rate $f = 1/\bar{t}$, the probability $p(n)$ of obtaining n spikes in the observation window T is

$$p(n) = \frac{(fT)^n e^{-fT}}{n!} \tag{9.13}$$

and is plotted in figure 9.7A.

For the model of retinal ganglion cell firing considered above, spike generation can be approximatively described as a cascade of two Poisson processes: the first one represents the absorption of photons at the retina and the second one the random generation of two spikes (on average) for each such photon.[1] The resulting spike count distribution (called a "Neyman type-A distribution"; see figure 9.7A; Teich 1981) is broader than a Poisson distribution of identical mean, consistent with the

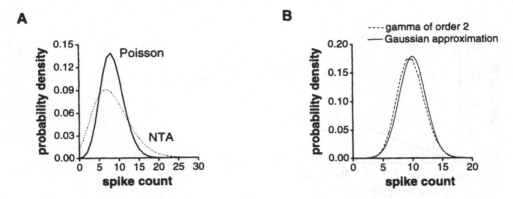

Figure 9.7
(A) Comparison of a Poisson (thick solid line) and Neyman type-A distribution (NTA, dotted line) of spike counts. The means of the two distributions are identical (8.35 spikes), but the variance of the NTA distribution is larger than the mean (the effective multiplication parameter k is equal to 1.45 in this example). (B) Spike count distribution (dashed line) obtained from a spike train with a gamma distributed ISI of order 2 (see figure 9.3B). The mean firing rate is $f = 50\,\text{Hz}$ and $T = 200\,\text{msec}$. The corresponding Gaussian approximation (solid line, see main text) is already very good, even though only 10 spikes are expected in this period.

higher variability observed in the interspike interval distribution ($C_V > 1$; figure 9.6B).

The variability in the spike count distribution is most conveniently characterized by the ratio of the variance, $V(T)$, to the mean, $N(T)$, of $p(n)$:

$$F(T) = \frac{V(T)}{N(T)} \quad \text{(in units of spk).} \tag{9.14}$$

This quantity is called the "index of dispersion" or "Fano factor." For a Poisson spike train, we obtain from eq. 9.13: $N(T) = fT$, $V(T) = fT$ and therefore $F(T) = 1$, independent of the duration T. For the Neyman type-A distribution, if we let f_{ph} denote the rate of incoming photons and k, the effective number of spikes per photon, then $N(T) = kf_{ph}T$, $V(T) = (k+1)f_{ph}T$ and therefore, $F(T) = 1 + k > 1$. Conversely, spike trains that are more regular than Poisson will have an index of dispersion smaller than 1. This is illustrated in figure 9.8 for a Poisson spike train with refractory period (Müller 1974) and for a gamma distribution of order 2 (Cox and Lewis 1966). In this latter case,

$$N(T) = \frac{T}{\bar{i}}, \quad V(T) = \frac{T}{2\bar{i}} + \frac{1}{8}(1 - e^{-4T/\bar{i}}), \tag{9.15}$$

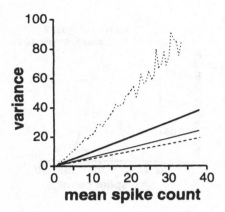

Figure 9.8
Variance as a function of mean spike count in several examples (the slope of these lines is the Fano factor of eq. 9.14). The curve with largest variance (dotted line) corresponds to the retinal ganglion cell model illustrated in figure 9.6 and was obtained by simulation. For a given mean spike count, the curve's variance is higher than the variance of a Poisson spike train (thick solid line), which has unit slope; that is, the variance increases as the mean number of spikes. Adding a 2 msec refractory period to the Poisson model (thin solid line) regularizes the spike count distribution, while the variance of a model with gamma-distributed ISI of order 2 (dashed line, see figure 9.3B) is only half of the mean spike count.

so that

$$F(T) = \frac{1}{2} + \frac{\bar{i}}{8T}(1 - e^{-4T/\bar{i}}).$$ (9.16)

While, for very small observation intervals, F converges to unity as in a standard Poisson process, for $T \to \infty$, F converges to $1/2$.

9.4.1 Relationship between Coefficient of Variation and Fano Factor

Two key results link the Fano factor to fundamental properties of the spike train. If the spike train can be described by a renewal process, the distribution of spike counts will be approximatively normally distributed for large counting times T, with mean $N(T) \cong T/\bar{i}$ and variance $V(T) \cong \sigma_i^2 T/\bar{i}^3$. This is illustrated in figure 9.7B for the gamma distribution of order 2. While a normal distribution for $p(n)$ is expected from the law of large numbers, the formulas for $N(T)$ and $V(T)$ depend explicitly on the renewal nature of the spike train. Thus, for large T, we obtain (Cox 1962)

$$F(T) \cong \frac{\sigma_i^2 T}{\bar{i}^3}\frac{\bar{i}}{T} = C_V^2.$$ (9.17)

The relation between $F(T)$ and C_V can be explicitly verified in the case of the gamma distribution of order 2 (from eq. 9.16 and using the previously obtained value, $C_V = 1/\sqrt{2}$). This result motivates the following algorithm to verify whether the variability observed in a spike train is solely due to variability in the interspike intervals: (1) compute $F(T)$ as a function of T for a given experimental spike train; and (2) randomly reshuffle the interspike intervals of the experimental spike train to obtain a renewal process and compute $F_{shuffled}(T)$. If, for large T, the Fano factor $F(T)$ is different from $F_{shuffled}(T)$, variability in the spike count cannot be accounted for by variability in the interspike intervals alone. Furthermore, $F_{shuffled}(T)^{1/2}$ provides an estimate of C_V, by eq. 9.17. This algorithm has been applied to sensory neurons and has consistently led to the conclusion that a substantial portion of spike train variability is not explained by interspike interval variability (for a review, see Teich, Turcott, and Siegel 1996).

9.4.2 Relationship between Fano Factor and the Autocorrelation Function

Another result allows for a more precise understanding of the origin of variability observed in the spike count. For a *stationary* spike train (Cox and Lewis 1966), the index of dispersion is related to the correlation in spike occurrence times by the following formula (Cox and Isham 1980; Teich 1989):

$$F(T) = 1 + \frac{2}{f} \int_0^T d\tau \left(1 - \frac{\tau}{T}\right) R_{xx}^+(\tau).$$ (9.18)

In this equation, f is the mean firing rate and $R_{xx}^+(\tau)$ the autocorrelation function of the spike train for τ positive, a measure of the statistical dependency between two spikes as a function of the time interval τ separating them ($R_{xx}^+(\tau)$ is identical to the usual autocorrelation function except for a δ-function at the origin, which is removed; it is defined and discussed in section 9.6). For a Poisson process, $R_{xx}^+(\tau) = 0$, and we recover $F(T) = 1$ from eq. 9.18. In the case of a gamma distribution of order 2, we recover eq. 9.16 by plugging the results of eqs. 9.31 and 9.32 (section 9.6) into eq. 9.18. It follows in particular from this formula that if the correlation between spikes is only slowly decaying over time, $R_{xx}^+(\tau) \sim \tau^{-\alpha}(0 < \alpha < 1)$, for large τ, then

$$F(T) \sim T^{1-\alpha},$$ (9.19)

for large T, or, equivalently,

$$V(T) \sim N(T)^{2-\alpha},$$ (9.20)

using $N(T) = fT$. In other words, long range correlations in spike occurrence times implies a power law increase of $V(T)$ as a function of $N(T)$.

To detect such power law behavior, it is convenient to plot $(N(T), V(T))$ pairs for different values of T in log-log coordinates (Usher et al. 1994).[2] For a Poisson process, this procedures yields a line with unit slope. A more variable process will be revealed by a slope that is larger than one. In the limit of a slope equal to two ($\alpha = 0$ in the above equation), the fluctuations are so high as to cancel any beneficial effect obtained by averaging for longer times. In practice, neurons seldom show such power relationships over very large ranges of T. For instance, as emphasized previously, a refractory period has the effect of reducing variability for values of $T \approx t_{ref}$. Cells in visual cortex typically cluster on a one of slope between 1 and 1.4 over the relevant range of firing frequencies (Vogels, Spileers, and Orban 1989; Snowden, Treue, and Andersen 1992; Softky and Koch 1993).

9.5 Signal Detection and Receiver Operating Characteristic Analysis

Spike count distributions can also provide useful insights on the encoding of stimulus information by neurons, in addition to shedding light on the issue of variability considered in the last section. Changes in the mean firing rate as a function of stimulus parameters are usually the most conspicuous feature of neurons responses.

One way of assessing the information conveyed in the mean spike count is to optimally discriminate two stimuli on the basis of differences between the firing rates measured in an interval of length T. This paradigm, based on the concept of an ideal observer, has been applied to a wide range of sensory neurons and experimental stimuli. In retinal ganglion cells, the presence or absence of a dim light flash can be inferred with good accuracy from the mean firing rate observed in a 200 msec time window (Barlow, Levick, and Yoon 1971). Further examples include the discrimination of stimulus orientation from the responses of orientation selective neurons in area V1 of the macaque monkey (Vogels and Orban 1990) or of the direction of motion from neurons in cortical area MT (Newsome, Britten, and Movshon 1989; Britten et al. 1992). Here the performance of individual neurons, as assessed using the *ideal observer paradigm* discussed below, was comparable to the performance of the trained animal on the corresponding psychophysical task. This places constraints on how information from single cells is integrated across pools of neurons to give rise to the behavior of the animal.

Let us imagine a classical *yes-no rating experiment* (Green and Swets 1966), in which either one of two stimuli is presented, called stimuli 0 and 1. On each trial and on the basis of an observation such as the mean spike count measured in an interval T, the subject has to decide which of stimuli 0 or 1 occurred. If the two stimuli result in different spike count distributions $p_0(n)$ and $p_1(n)$ being observed in an interval of duration T, an obvious strategy to determine the stimulus most likely to have caused a given spike count n_t is to compare the *likelihood ratio* $l(n) = p_1(n)/p_0(n)$ to a threshold criterion k and to choose stimulus 0 or 1 according to whether $l(n_t)$ is smaller or larger than threshold. The choice $k = 1$ corresponds to the inference[3]

$$p_1(n_t) < p_0(n_t) \rightarrow \text{stimulus } 0,$$

$$p_0(n_t) < p_1(n_t) \rightarrow \text{stimulus } 1.$$

The significance of values of k different from 1 will become clear as we proceed.

As a simple example, consider a Poisson neuron that fires at rates f_0 and f_1 ($f_0 < f_1$) in response to stimuli 0 and 1, respectively (Thibos, Levick, and Cohn 1979). From eq. 9.13

$$l(n) = \left(\frac{f_1}{f_0}\right)^n e^{-(f_1 - f_0)T}. \tag{9.21}$$

Two such Poisson spike count distributions and $l(n)$ are illustrated in figure 9.9A. The likelihood ratio of eq. 9.21 is a monotonic increasing function of n. In this case (the most common one), we can replace the criterion $l(n) \lessgtr k$ with the simpler rule

$$n < k' \rightarrow \text{stimulus } 0,$$

$$n > k' \rightarrow \text{stimulus } 1.$$

That is, if the observed spike count n is less than some threshold k', we infer that stimulus 0 was present; in the other case, we assume that stimulus 1 was present.

How good is this decision rule? Its performance can be precisely characterized by two quantities: (1) the *probability of false-alarm*, that is, the probability of concluding that stimulus 1 is present when in fact stimulus 0 occurred:

$$P_{FA} = \sum_{n \geq k'} p_0(n), \tag{9.22}$$

and (2) the *probability of correct detection*, that is, the probability of correctly concluding that stimulus 1 was present:

$$P_D = \sum_{n \geq k'} p_1(n). \tag{9.23}$$

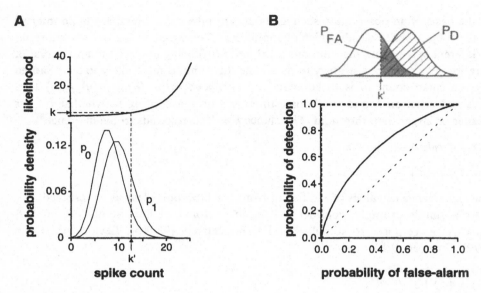

Figure 9.9
(A) Spike count distribution of a Poisson model with mean firing rates of 40 Hz and 50 Hz, respectively, corresponding to spike count densities p_0 (for stimulus 0) and p_1 (for stimulus 1; plotted for a $T = 200$ msec observation window). Likelihood ratio for these distributions shown on top. (B) ROC curve obtained by varying the threshold k' (see top illustration) from a very high value (in the limit of $k' \to \infty$, $P_D = P_{FA} = 0$) to a very low value (in the limit $k' \to -\infty$, $P_D = P_{FA} = 1$). For each value of the threshold k', the probability of false alarm P_{FA} (eq. 9.22; that is, believing that stimulus 1 was present while, in fact, stimulus 0 was present) is given by the integral of p_0 to the right of the threshold and is indicated by the gray surface (top illustration). The probability of detection P_D (eq. 9.23) of stimulus 1 corresponds to the integral of p_1 to the right of the threshold (hatched area). The ROC curve is a plot of this later area (P_D) as a function of P_{FA}. Dashed line below ROC curve: chance performance. On the opposite, the closer the ROC curve lies to the bold dashed lines, the better the performance.

It is clear from these equations that a fixed value of the threshold k' (or k) is equivalent to a fixed probability of false-alarm P_{FA} (or of correct detection P_D). Therefore, a plot of P_D as a function of P_{FA} completely characterizes the performance of the likelihood ratio test for all possible values of the threshold (see figure 9.9B). Such a plot is called the receiver operating characteristic of the likelihood ratio test or the ROC curve.[4] The diagonal line in figure 9.9B indicates chance performance ($P_{FA} = P_D$). The higher the ROC curve lies above the diagonal, the better the performance of the likelihood ratio test (the most favorable case being $P_D = 1$, independent of P_{FA}).

Remarkably, the likelihood ratio test is optimal: for a fixed probability of false-alarm P_{FA}, any alternative test used to decide between stimulus 0 and 1 from $p_0(n)$

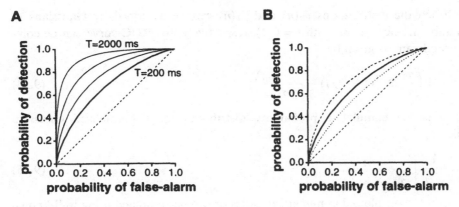

Figure 9.10
(A) ROC curves for the same model as in figure 9.9 and for increasing sampling times, $T = 200$ msec, $T = 500$ msec, $T = 1,000$ msec and $T = 2,000$ msec, respectively (only the two extreme curves are labeled). The performance of the ideal observer increases in parallel with the sampling time. In both panels A and B, the dashed straight line indicates chance level. (B) Middle curve (thick line) shows the discrimination performance of the ideal observer of two Poisson spike counts (same parameters as in figures 9.9B and 9.10A). The lower curve (dotted line) describes the performance of the ideal observer for spike counts distributed according to Neyman type-A (with same mean firing rates as in figure 9.9). The upper curve (dashed line) corresponds to the discrimination performance when the two spike counts are distributed according to gamma distributions of order 2 (see figure 9.7B).

and $p_1(n)$ will result in a smaller probability of detection P_D. In other words, any other test will yield an ROC curve below (or at best equal to) the ROC curve of the likelihood ratio test.[5] Note that because it remains unclear what type of decision rule nervous systems use, the optimal performance is the one obtained by an *ideal observer* who has complete access to the relevant probability distributions. Of course, the performance of the ideal observer will depend on properties of the spike trains and the interval chosen to measure the mean firing rate. In general, longer measuring intervals will lead to better performance by averaging out fluctuations, as illustrated for Poisson spike counts in figure 9.10A. Presently, the exact time interval over which neurons might average incoming information to perform a specific task is only weakly constrained. Similarly, spike trains that are more regular than Poisson ($C_V < 1$) will yield better discrimination performance, while spike trains with $C_V > 1$ will lead to worse performance (figure 9.10B).

As the measuring interval becomes large, the probability distribution of the spike count usually converges to a normal distribution by virtue of the law of large numbers (see section 9.4). In practice, the convergence can be quite fast, the Gaussian approximation being already accurate for spike counts as low as 10–20 (as in figure

9.7B). When the distributions $p_0(n)$ and $p_1(n)$ can be described by Gaussians of means and variances μ_i, σ_i (with $i = 0, 1$), respectively, the ROC curve can be computed exactly and is given by

$$P_D = 1 - \Phi\left(\frac{\sigma_0}{\sigma_1}\,\Phi^{-1}(1 - P_{FA}) - \frac{\mu_1 - \mu_0}{\sigma_1}\right), \tag{9.24}$$

where Φ is the cumulative probability distribution of a normalized Gaussian variable,

$$\Phi(x) = \frac{1}{\sqrt{2\pi}} \int_{-\infty}^{x} e^{-x^2/2}\,dx. \tag{9.25}$$

Values of $\Phi(x)$ are plotted in numerical tables or can be computed using well-known algorithms. Conversely, one can reexpress this equation in a different coordinate scale, $(\tilde{P}_{FA}, \tilde{P}_D)$, such that

$$P_{FA} = \Phi(\tilde{P}_{FA}), \quad P_D = \Phi(\tilde{P}_D). \tag{9.26}$$

This can be done using a simple command in MATLAB.

In this coordinate system, the ROC curve of eq. 9.24 corresponds to a straight line of slope $r = \sigma_0/\sigma_1$ and intercept $d' = (\mu_1 - \mu_0)/\sigma_1$ (Cohn, Green, and Tanner 1975). Changing coordinate scales is analogous to plotting exponential or power law functions on logarithmic paper, as illustrated in figure 9.11. In general, the larger the value of d', the easier the two distributions can be distinguished and the higher the performance.

When the standard deviations of the two spike count distributions are equal, $\sigma_1 = \sigma_0$, the ROC curve has unit slope and is completely characterized by the intercept d' commonly used in psychophysics (Green and Swets 1966). The value $d' = 1$ then corresponds to the two Gaussian distributions being separated by one standard deviation. However, usually for spike count distributions, the variance $V(T)$ is a function of the mean spike count $N(T)$, so that $\sigma_1 \neq \sigma_0$, and this special case is unlikely to occur.

9.6   Autocorrelation and Power Spectrum

While the mean spike count $N(T)$ is well suited to convey information about static components of a stimulus in a time interval of length T, stimulus parameters that vary over time during such an interval cannot be encoded by $N(T)$ alone. Modu-

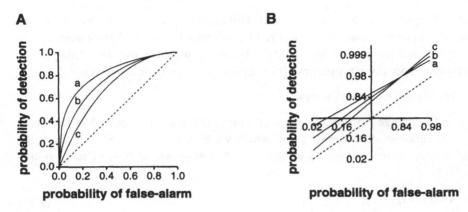

Figure 9.11
(A) Three ROC curves corresponding to the discrimination between two Gaussian distributions as the ratio of the two associated variances, $r = \sigma_0/\sigma_1$ and d' changes; d' is defined as the distance between the centers of the two Gaussians, normalized by σ_1. The parameters are: $r = 0.8$, $d' = 1.2$ for a, $r = 1$, $d' = 1$ for b and $r = 1.2$, $d' = 0.8$ for c. (B) On "normal" probability paper, corresponding to the change of coordinate of eq. 9.26, these curves are straight lines of slope r and intercept d' respectively (dashed line: chance level).

lation of the instantaneous firing rate around its mean value is an appropriate variable to encode such time-varying stimulus parameters.

Sections 9.6 and 9.7 survey a number of signal-processing techniques used to study stimulus encoding by means of instantaneous firing rate changes. In these techniques, the analysis of post stimulus time histograms (PSTHs) obtained from repeated presentations of a single stimulus is replaced by the analysis of average spike train properties in response to random stimulus ensembles. Such techniques represent a complementary approach to the more classical PSTH methods, shedding a different light on the encoding of time-varying stimuli in sensory neurons. By design, the techniques will work best if the neuronal system under study, whose input is the relevant stimulus parameter and whose output is the observed spike train, can be approximated by a linear, time-invariant (stationary) system. These assumptions are most likely to hold at early stages of sensory pathways (Wandell 1995; Rieke et al. 1996). Although further elaborations of these techniques can take into account non-linearities and changes in the stimulus or neuron response over time, as explained below, none of them is expected to capture the encoding of stimulus parameters when the precise pattern of spikes is of importance, as is likely to be the case in the olfactory system of insects, for instance (Laurent 1996; Wehr and Laurent 1996).

While the instantaneous firing rate might convey information on a time-varying stimulus, it will also reflect intrinsic properties of the neurons themselves. In the example of figure 9.3, fluctuations in instantaneous firing rate do not relate to the constant current input, but rather reflect different biophysical parameters (e.g., refractory period or passive time constant). We commence our investigation by characterizing how these properties affect the dynamics of neuronal firing.

9.6.1 The Autocorrelation Function

Second-order changes in the dynamics of neuronal firing are captured in the auto-correlation function of the spike train, which we now define. Let $x(t)$ be the spike train of a neuron, represented by a sequence of δ pulses at the time of spike occur-rences $\{t_k\}$,

$$x(t) = \sum_k \delta(t - t_k).$$ (9.27)

It helps to visualize $x(t)$ as the instantaneous firing frequency of the neuron in a particular trial or observation period (with units of spk/sec; see chapter appendix A). The mean firing frequency is defined as the average over such an ensemble of observations, $m = \langle x(t) \rangle$ and is assumed to be independent of t (i.e., we assume that the spike train is stationary). Furthermore, a single—albeit very long—spike train of the ensemble is often assumed to be representative of the response of the system, so that ensemble averages can be replaced by time averages over the single sample. This is known as the "ergodicity assumption." To clarify this point, we show that under the ergodicity assumption, the mean firing rate f of a single neuron in a single trial is equal to the mean firing rate m (in spk/sec) averaged over the ensemble. Figure 9.12 illustrates the same point graphically. If N is the number of spikes in a large interval T, then

$$m = \langle x(t) \rangle$$

$$= \frac{1}{T} \int_0^T x(t)\,dt, \quad \text{for large } T \text{ (by ergodicity)},$$

$$= \frac{N}{T},$$ (9.28)

where $N/T = f$ is the mean firing rate for the representative sample spike train. (Similarly, other statistical properties of the ensemble can be computed by time averaging, as explained in chapter appendix A.) The autocorrelation function is defined as the average joint probability density of a spike at time t and $t + \tau$, minus their mean values,

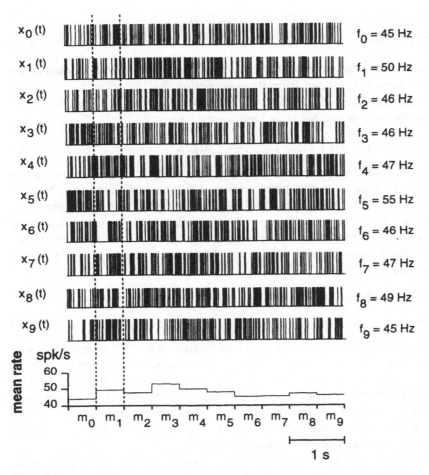

Figure 9.12
Traces labeled $x_0(t), \ldots, x_9(t)$ represent different spike trains of a Poisson neuron belonging to the same statistical ensemble which satisfies the assumptions of stationarity and ergodicity. They should be thought of as representing recordings from different nerve cells (assumed to be identical in their properties and response characteristics) or the response of a single cell to different realizations of a random stimulus. (Bottom) Mean firing rate m over 500 ms bins (m_0–m_9), obtained by averaging the firing rate of the ten samples (illustrated by two dashed lines for bin corresponding to m_1). Stationarity implies that m should be independent of the particular bin chosen: $m = m_0 = \cdots = m_9$ (i.e., a flat PSTH). Furthermore, m should be independent of the bin size (in the limit where the averaging is done over all spike trains of the ensemble). Ergodicity implies that the firing rate $f_0, \ldots, f_9$ for each single trace $x_0(t), \ldots, x_9(t)$ should be identical to m (in the limit where the recording time T is very long). Stationarity and ergodicity have analogous implications for higher order statistical functions, such as the autocorrelation.

$$R_{xx}(\tau) = \langle x(t)x(t+\tau) \rangle - m^2 \quad \text{(in units of (spk/sec}^2\text{)}$$

$$= \langle (x(t) - m)(x(t+\tau) - m) \rangle. \tag{9.29}$$

Again, by time invariance (stationarity), $R_{xx}(\tau)$ is assumed to be independent of the absolute time point t. It follows from this assumption that $R_{xx}(\tau) = R_{xx}(-\tau)$. Subtracting m^2 enforces the normalization $R_{xx}(\tau) \to 0$, for large τ, because we expect two spikes to be uncorrelated for large time separations:

$$\langle x(t)x(t+\tau) \rangle = \langle x(t) \rangle \langle x(t+\tau) \rangle = m^2 \quad \text{(for } \tau \text{ large)}. \tag{9.30}$$

For a Poisson process, $R_{xx}(\tau) = m\delta(\tau)$. The δ-function at the origin corresponds to the sure event of a spike at point t given a spike at point t, while for $\tau \neq 0$ the autocorrelation function $R_{xx}(\tau)$ vanishes identically, meaning that two spikes separated by an arbitrary time interval τ are completely uncorrelated. This extreme case of eq. 9.30 is, of course, a consequence of the complete independence between two events which defines the Poisson process (see section 9.2.4). An alternative way of writing the autocorrelation function is

$$R_{xx}(\tau) = R_{xx}^+(\tau) + m\delta(\tau)$$

$$= m(m_x(|\tau|) - m) + m\delta(\tau), \tag{9.31}$$

where $m_x(\tau), \tau > 0$ is to be interpreted as the probability density of observing a spike at time $t + \tau$ when a spike occurred at time t. (Note that $m_x(\tau)$ is the probability density of observing *any* spike at time τ following a spike, not only the first one; Cox and Lewis 1966.) Thus values of $m_x < m$ (or, equivalently, $R_{xx}^+(\tau) < 0$) correspond to a suppressed probability of spiking as compared to the mean m, while values of $m_x > m$ (or $R_{xx}^+(\tau) > 0$) correspond to an increased probability of spiking. We illustrate these two possibilities in the following examples.

The interspike interval distribution of a gamma process of order 2 has a reduced probability of firing for short intervals when compared to a Poisson process (see figures 9.3A and 9.3B). Thus one expects a reduced probability of firing $m_x(\tau)$ or, equivalently, a negative correlation for small values of τ. In fact, $m_x(\tau)$ can be shown (Cox and Lewis 1966) to relax exponentially to its mean value $m = f = 1/\bar{t}$, with a time constant $\bar{t}/4$:

$$m_x(\tau) = m(1 - e^{-4\tau/\bar{t}}), \quad \tau > 0. \tag{9.32}$$

The two functions $m_x(\tau)$ and $R_{xx}^+(\tau)$ are plotted in figure 9.13A. Quite generally, the

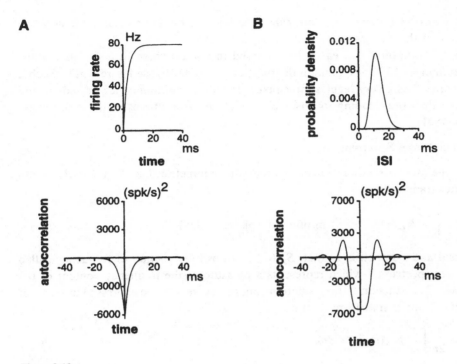

Figure 9.13
(A) Autocorrelation function R_{xx}^+ (bottom graph) of a renewal gamma process of order 2. The mean firing rate of the model is 80 Hz. The negative correlation for short values of τ is due to the relative refractoriness of the model following a spike. The corresponding firing probability density function m_x (see eq. 9.32) is plotted on top. Its value is zero immediately after a spike, recovering exponentially toward steady state (80 Hz) with a time constant of 3.125 msec. (B) Autocorrelation function of a renewal gamma process of order 10 ($m = 80$ Hz, bottom graph). The positive peaks in the autocorrelation at ± 12.5 msec reflect the regularity of the ISI distribution (top graph) and coincides with the peak in the ISI distribution. In both panels A and B, the δ-function of R_{xx} at the origin has been subtracted, see eq. 9.31.

refractory period immediately following a spike will manifest itself by a negative correlation at short times τ.

Positive correlations can easily be observed in regular spike trains. This is illustrated in figure 9.13B for a gamma distribution of order 10 (see figure 9.3D). Such a model neuron has a very regular interspike interval distribution concentrated around its mean value, thus leading to positive correlations at multiples of the mean interspike interval.

9.6.2 The Power Spectrum

Because the autocorrelation function is real and symmetric (i.e., $R_{xx}(\tau) = R_{xx}(-\tau)$), its Fourier transform

$$S_{xx}(\omega) = \int_{-\infty}^{+\infty} R_{xx}(\tau)e^{i\omega\tau}\,d\tau \quad \text{(in units of}(\text{spk/sec})^2/\text{Hz}), \tag{9.33}$$

is also real and symmetric. In fact, $S_{xx}(\omega)$ is a positive function of frequency called the "power spectrum," which represents a measure of the frequency content of the spike train. The autocorrelation function can, of course, also be expressed in terms of the inverse Fourier transform, that is,

$$R_{xx}(\tau) = \frac{1}{2\pi}\int_{-\infty}^{+\infty} S_{xx}(\omega)e^{-i\omega\tau}\,d\omega. \tag{9.34}$$

For a Poisson process, the Fourier transform of $R_{xx}(\tau)$ yields $S_{xx}(\omega) = m$, and thus all frequencies are equally represented. As is clear from eq. 9.31, the power spectrum will usually contain additional terms, causing a departure from a flat spectrum when the spike train differs from Poisson. In the case of a gamma-distributed process of order 2 (see figure 9.3B), we obtain

$$S_{xx}(\omega) = m\left(1 - \frac{8m^2}{16m^2 + \omega^2}\right). \tag{9.35}$$

Thus the reduced probability of firing at short times τ (see eq. 9.32) causes a dip in the power spectrum at low frequencies, as illustrated in figure 9.14A. This is the usual manifestation of refractoriness in the frequency content of the spike train (Bair et al. 1994; Franklin and Bair 1995).

For regular spike trains, the peaks in the autocorrelation at multiple intervals of the mean interspike interval translate into peaks at the corresponding firing frequency and its harmonics, as illustrated in figure 9.14B for the gamma process of order 10.

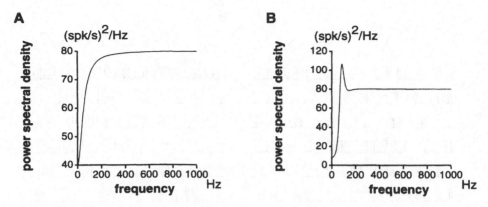

A (spk/s)^2/Hz

B (spk/s)^2/Hz

Figure 9.14
(A) Power spectrum of a renewal gamma process of order 2 (i.e., Fourier transform of the autocorrelation function of figure 9.13A). The negative correlation at short values of τ translates in a dip in the power spectral density at low frequencies. (B) For a renewal gamma process of order 10, the positive correlations at multiples of the mean ISI (see figure 9.13B) translate into a peak in power at the mean firing frequency (80 Hz).

9.6.3 Spike Train Analysis of Linear Encoding Systems

Let us now consider the response $x(t)$ of some neuronal system to an ensemble of stimuli $\{s_{mean} + s(t)\}$, where s_{mean} represents the mean stimulus (e.g., the mean luminance of a visual scene) and the ensemble $\{s(t)\}$ represents random variations around s_{mean}. We assume here that the entire system between the receptor and the neuron from which spikes are recorded can be described in the regime of interest, using a linear transfer function $K(t)$, and that the neuron encodes changes about s_{mean} by changes in its instantaneous firing rate. Using this knowledge, we would like to understand how the processing performed by the neuron on the stimulus will be reflected in the autocorrelation and power spectrum of the spike train.

We start by formulating our assumption precisely. Let $s_{mean} + s_0(t)$ be a representative stimulus drawn from the ensemble $\{s_{mean} + s(t)\}$ and let $f_{s_0}(t)$ be the changes in instantaneous firing rate,

$$f_{s_0}(t) = \langle x(t) - m \rangle_{(x|s_0)}, \tag{9.36}$$

averaged over many presentations of $s_{mean} + s_0(t)$. This average is denoted by $\langle \cdot \rangle_{(x|s_0)}$ to emphasize that $s_0(t)$ is fixed from one presentation to the next ($s_0(t)$ might be called "frozen noise"; figure 9.15). Our assumption is that changes in instantaneous firing rate are linearly related to $s_0(t)$ through a transfer function K,

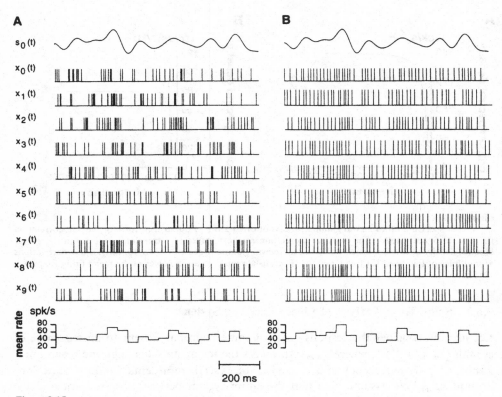

Figure 9.15
Ten spike trains of two different random threshold models in response to a single stimulus $s_0(t)$ (the "frozen noise" $s_0(t)$ is shown on top of both panels A and B). (A) Exponentially distributed threshold (corresponding to Poisson spike trains under constant inputs, figure 9.3A) leads to very irregular and varying spike trains from one presentation to the next. (B) Threshold of gamma order 10 (figure 9.3D) leads to much more regular and reproducible spike trains from one trial to the next. In spite of very different characteristics, both models encode the stimulus $s_0(t)$ in their instantaneous firing rate (see note 6), as may be seen by comparing the instantaneous firing rate (averaged over 50 msec) on the bottom of each panel to $s_0(t)$. The question of how reliably a single spike train from each one of these models encodes $s_0(t)$ will be addressed in section 9.7.3 (see figure 9.19).

$$f_{s_0}(t) = (K \star s_0)(t)$$

$$= \int_{-\infty}^{+\infty} dt_1 K(t - t_1) s_0(t_1), \tag{9.37}$$

where the symbol "$\star$" denotes convolution and where K has units of (spk/sec)/(unit stimulus/sec). This equation will hold exactly only if $(K \star s)(t) \geq -m$ (because the averaged instantaneous firing rate $m + f_{s_0}(t)$ cannot be negative), so that the effects of half-wave rectification can be neglected. To illustrate eqs. 9.36 and 9.37, consider again the random threshold models of figure 9.3 and let the constant current I be replaced by a time-varying current $i_{mean} + i_0(t)$. For each one of these models, the changes in instantaneous firing frequency averaged over many trials will be proportional to changes in the input current: $f_{i_0}(t) = \alpha i_0(t)$, with $\alpha = 1/C_m V_{th}$, so that our assumption is satisfied[6] (figure 9.15). Eq. 9.37 also holds when an arbitrary linear filter K is placed prior to the spike generation mechanism to mimic preprocessing of the stimulus before its encoding in output spike trains. An example of such a model whose mean instantaneous firing frequency reproduces the band-pass filtering properties of LGN relay cells is shown in figure 9.22.

It follows from eq. 9.37 that the correlations in instantaneous firing rate are related to correlations in the stimulus ensemble by

$$\langle f_s(t) f_s(t + \tau) \rangle_s = ((K \star \tilde{K}) \star R_{ss})(\tau), \tag{9.38}$$

where the average $\langle \cdot \rangle_s$ is over the stimulus ensemble, $R_{ss}(\tau)$ is the autocorrelation function of the stimulus, and $\tilde{K}(t) = K(-t)$. Furthermore, let us assume that correlations in the occurrence of single spikes are dominated by correlations in the stimulus

$$\langle (x(t) - m)(x(t + \tau) - m) \rangle_{(x|s_0)} = \langle x(t) - m \rangle_{(x|s_0)} \langle x(t + \tau) - m \rangle_{(x|s_0)}, \tag{9.39}$$

for $\tau \neq 0$, so that effects like those of refractoriness or regularity considered above can be neglected.[7] In the case of a leaky integrator, we expect this condition to require that the correlations in the stimulus should occur on a much longer time scale than τ_m. By taking averages over the stimulus ensemble on both sides of eq. 9.39, we obtain

$$R_{xx}^+(\tau) = \langle f_s(t) f_s(t + \tau) \rangle_s. \tag{9.40}$$

Combining eqs. 9.31, 9.38, 9.40 and Fourier-transforming results in

$$S_{xx}(\omega) = |K(\omega)|^2 S_{ss}(\omega) + m, \tag{9.41}$$

where the additive factor m originates from the δ-function at the origin in eq. 9.31. A

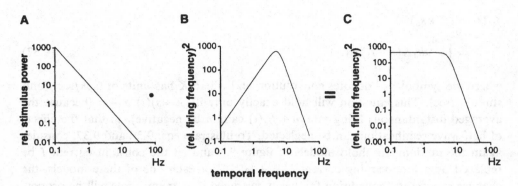

Figure 9.16
Graphical illustration of eq. 9.41 for natural visual stimuli and their processing by relay cells in the cat
lateral geniculate nucleus (LGN) in normalized units. (A) Power spectral density of natural visual scenes
has a temporal power spectrum that decays quadratically in frequency. (B) Transfer function of LGN relay
cells is band-pass in the temporal domain. (C) Multiplication of the functions in panels A and B yields an
output spike train spectrum (the constant value m has been subtracted) that is flat in temporal frequency,
thus effectively decorrelating the visual input signal. It has been argued by Dong and Atick (1995) that one
function of the LGN is to decorrelate the visual input signal, giving rise to a more effective and less re-
dundant representation of visual stimuli in cortex proper.

different derivation of this equation under the assumption of complete half-wave
rectification can be found in Gabbiani and Koch 1996 and Gabbiani 1996.

Equation 9.41 states that the power spectrum of the spike train will be related to
the power spectrum of the stimulus by multiplication with the square modulus of the
frequency response of K. One way to determine the transfer function K is to apply
the Wiener kernel method, described in section 9.7.

We consider one example illustrating possible applications of eq. 9.41. The response
of relay cells in the lateral geniculate nucleus to sinusoidal gratings of varying temporal frequencies can be used to determine their linear transfer characteristics. In the
frequency domain, the energy of the corresponding filter, $|K(\omega)|^2$, is band-pass as
illustrated in figure 9.16B (Saul and Humphrey 1990). Measurements of the temporal
power spectrum of natural images, $S_{ss}(\omega)$, show that it decays according to a power
law with temporal frequency (see figure 9.16A; Dong 1995). Therefore, multiplying
$|K(\omega)|^2$ with $S_{ss}(\omega)$ predicts that the power spectrum of LGN spike trains in response
to natural stimuli should be flat in frequency up to 10 Hz (see figure 9.16C; Dong and
Atick 1995). This encoding of temporal changes in natural images by LGN spike
trains is optimal because it amplifies the frequencies that are less well represented in
the stimulus, thus whitening the input. This prediction obtained from $S_{ss}(\omega)$, $|K(\omega)|^2$
and eq. 9.41 for the encoding of natural stimuli in spike trains of LGN relay cells has
been confirmed experimentally (Dan, Atick, and Reid 1996).

9.7   Wiener Kernels and Stimulus Estimation

Starting from the assumption of linear encoding formulated in section 9.6.3, we now explain how the transfer function characterizing the processing performed by a neuron can be computed. This is a *forward problem*, which has been extensively investigated both theoretically and experimentally. For a particular choice of the random stimulus ensemble, it is equivalent to the computation of the first-order Wiener kernel, as explained below. Next, we address the problem of how accurately a time-varying stimulus can be encoded in a single spike train. This problem is for time-varying stimuli what the problem considered in section 9.5 is for static stimuli: how accurately can single neurons convey information in their mean spike count? To solve it, we must solve the corresponding *inverse problem*, that is, we must determine how accurately a time-varying stimulus can be estimated from a single-spike train. This problem has been addressed experimentally in the fly visual system (Bialek et al. 1991), in the electrosensory system of weakly electric fish (Wessel, Koch, and Gabbiani 1996), and in the cercal system of the cricket (Theunissen et al. 1996; Roddey and Jacobs 1996). Finally, we also investigate to what extent the linear assumption of section 9.6.3 is altered by nonlinearities in the encoding.

9.7.1   First-Order Wiener Kernel and Reverse Correlation

The problem of estimating the transfer function K introduced in eq. 9.37,

$$f_{s_0}(t) = \langle x(t) - m \rangle_{(x|s_0)} = (K \star s_0)(t), \tag{9.42}$$

can be solved by correlating $s(t)$ with $x(t)$. We define the *cross-correlation* between the stimulus and spike train by

$$\begin{aligned} R_{sx}(\tau) &= \langle s(t)(x(t+\tau) - m) \rangle \\ &= \langle s(t)x(t+\tau) \rangle, \end{aligned} \tag{9.43}$$

where the second equality follows from the normalization $\langle s(t) \rangle = 0$ introduced in section 9.6.3. The cross-correlation $R_{sx}(\tau)$ is related to the autocorrelation of the stimulus through

$$R_{sx}(\tau) = (K \star R_{ss})(\tau), \tag{9.44}$$

using eq. 9.42. If we let $S_{sx}(\omega)$ denote the Fourier transform of $R_{sx}(\tau)$, we obtain $S_{sx}(\omega) = K(\omega)S_{ss}(\omega)$ after Fourier-transforming both sides of eq. 9.44. Therefore, the frequency response of K is given by

$$K(\omega) = \frac{S_{sx}(\omega)}{S_{ss}(\omega)}. \tag{9.45}$$

The computation of K is further simplified if the random stimuli $s(t)$ are chosen to have a power spectrum constant with frequency $S_{ss}(\omega) = \sigma^2$, corresponding to a *white* or uncorrelated stimulus, $R_{ss}(\tau) = \sigma^2 \delta(\tau)$ (in practice, the stimulus is chosen to be white until a cutoff frequency above the one of the system under study). Plugging the value of $S_{ss}(\omega)$ into eq. 9.45 and Fourier-transforming back to the time domain yields $K(\tau) = (1/\sigma^2) R_{sx}(\tau)$. By using eq. 9.43, the representation $x(t) = \sum_{k=1}^{N} \delta(t - t_k)$, where N is the number of recorded action potentials and $f = N/T$ the mean firing rate, we obtain

$$K(\tau) = \frac{f}{\sigma^2} \frac{1}{N} \left(\sum_{k=1}^{N} s(t_k - \tau) \right). \tag{9.46}$$

This is the celebrated *reverse-correlation formula* for K, stating that the linear transfer function of the neuron can be recovered by a simple spike-triggered average of the stimulus preceding the spikes (de Boer 1973). This technique has been applied to many different neurons at various early stages of sensory systems, for example, in cat and monkey striate visual cortex (McLean and Palmer 1989; DeAngelis, Ohzawa, and Freeman 1993; Reid and Alonso 1995). An example illustrating the computation of K from eq. 9.45 is shown in figure 9.17 for the LGN relay cell model depicted in figure 9.22.

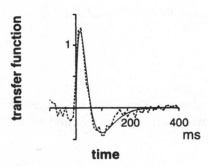

Figure 9.17
Computation of a linear transfer function using the Wiener kernel method. The solid line represents the transfer function of the model shown in the central panel of figure 9.22. The dotted line represents the estimate obtained from eq. 9.45, by cross-correlating the stimulus (shown in the right lower panel of figure 9.22 with the output spike train of the neuron (lower left panel of figure 9.22. The left axis has dimension of (spk/sec)/(unit stimulus) and has been normalized.

9.7.2 Nonlinear Encoding and Higher Kernels

If the relation between stimulus changes and instantaneous firing frequency changes is nonlinear, a transfer function $W_1(\omega)$ can still be obtained experimentally using either eq. 9.45 or 9.46, but the question of its relation to stimulus encoding by the neuron is now raised. We illustrate the significance of $W_1(\omega)$ in such cases by the following observations.

First, let us assume that the relation between stimulus and instantaneous firing frequency changes is obtained by passing $y(t) = (K \star s)(t)$ through a nonlinear function $g(y)$,

$$f_{s_0}(t) = g(y(t)), \quad y(t) = (K \star s)(t), \tag{9.47}$$

implementing half-wave rectification, compression or saturation, for instance (such a sigmoid nonlinearity is illustrated in figure 9.21A). The function g is called a "static or memoryless nonlinearity" because the output $f_{s_0}(t)$ depends only on y at time t. Because of the convolution operation with K, however, $f_{s_0}(t)$ will depend on past values of the stimulus. Let us now assume that the stimulus ensemble is *Gaussian*. By definition, this means that for arbitrary times, $t_1, \ldots, t_n$ the stimulus vector $(s(t_1), \ldots, s(t_n))$ is a jointly Gaussian random vector. This property must hold for *all* values of $n = 1, 2, 3, \ldots$.[8] Under this assumption, the cross-correlation between the stimulus and spike train can still be computed exactly:

$$R_{sx}(\tau) = c(K \star R_{ss})(\tau), \quad c = \frac{\langle yg(y) \rangle}{\sigma_y^2}, \tag{9.48}$$

where σ_y^2 is the variance of $y(t) = (K \star s)(t)$. This result is known as "Bussgang's theorem" (Bendat 1990). For example, if $y(t)$ is considered to be the somatic current driving the cell, then Bussgang's theorem states that it is possible to recover the cross-correlation between the stimulus and the somatic current from the cross-correlation between the stimulus and the output spike train (under the assumption of eq. 9.47). Up to a constant factor c, the cross-correlation of eq. 9.48 is identical to the one obtained in the linear case (eq. 9.44). Thus the effects of a static nonlinerity are *not* reflected in the time course of $W_1(\tau)$, but its presence can nevertheless be detected by using input stimuli with different variances (because c depends on the variance of the stimulus).

In the nonlinear case, the significance of $W_1(\tau)$ can be understood by considering the following question. In response to the stimulus $s(t)$, which linear function $(h \star s)(t)$ best approximates the instantaneous firing rate of the neuron in the sense that the mean square error,

$$\varepsilon^2(h) = \langle [(h \star s)(t) - f_s(t)]^2 \rangle_s, \tag{9.49}$$

is minimized when averaged over the stimulus ensemble? This equation can be solved by using the fact that at the minimum, the first-order derivative $d\varepsilon^2/dh$ has to vanish. Solving for h yields $h(\tau) = W_1(\tau)$. Thus the transfer function $W_1(\tau)$ is the best *linear estimator* for the response of the cell (in the mean square sense). The accuracy of this estimate will depend to a large extent on the nature of the nonlinearity and can fail completely in certain cases.[9]

In principle, it can be improved by considering estimators consisting of higher-order functions of the stimulus

$$g_s(\tau) = \mathbf{W_1}(s(t))(\tau) + \mathbf{W_2}(s(t_1), s(t_2))(\tau) + \cdots, \tag{9.50}$$

where $\mathbf{W_1}(s(t))(\tau) = (W_1 \star s)(\tau)$, and so on. When the stimulus ensemble used is Gaussian white noise, the functionals $\mathbf{W_n}$ are called "nth-order Wiener kernels" and procedures are known to compute them,[10] although these nonlinear methods lack the simplicity and generality of the linear case (Palm and Poggio 1977). It is, for example, unclear how the results obtained with one stimulus ensemble will generalize to other stimuli. Even for simple static nonlinearities as half-wave rectification, an infinite number of terms is needed in the series of eq. 9.50. In some cases, considerable progress has been made by combining such methods with specific assumptions on the type of nonlinearities involved (Victor 1987, 1988; Sakai, Naka, and Korenberg 1988).

9.7.3 Stimulus Estimation and Reliability of Encoding

While the first-order Wiener kernel method fully characterizes the linear encoding of time-varying stimuli by instantaneous firing rate changes, it has some shortcomings. Because it focuses on predicting the ensemble average response to the stimulus, the first-order Wiener kernel does not, for example, directly assess how much information about a time-varying stimulus is contained in a single spike train. All the models illustrated in figure 9.3 are able to encode stimulus changes by instantaneous firing rate changes (see note 6), but clearly the information contained in single spike trains will depend on the noise corrupting the encoding. In these examples, it can range from extreme (in the Poisson case) to noise-free (in the integrate-and-fire model; see figure 9.15).

The problem of how reliably a single spike train encodes a time-varying stimulus can be successfully addressed by estimating the stimulus from the spike train and characterizing the accuracy of the estimate. Such an estimate can be obtained by *Wiener-Kolmogorov filtering*, a signal-processing technique complementary to first-order Wiener kernel analysis and closely related to it (Poor 1994). We consider again a neuron encoding a stimulus by changes in its instantaneous firing rate:

$$f_s(t) = \langle x(t) - m \rangle_{(x|s)} = (K \star s)(t). \tag{9.51}$$

If we let $x_0(t)$ denote the spike train with its mean firing rate subtracted, $x_0(t) = x(t) - m$, then a linear estimate of the stimulus given the spike train can be obtained by convolving $x_0(t)$ with a filter $h(t)$, $s_{est}(t) = (h \star x_0)(t)$. Because of the discrete nature of the spike train, this amounts (up to a constant factor) to placing a copy of h around each spike,

$$s_{est}(t) = \sum_{k=1}^{N} h(t - t_k) - m \int_{-\infty}^{+\infty} h(t)\,dt, \tag{9.52}$$

to estimate deviations $s(t)$ of the stimulus from its mean value. The filter h is chosen to minimize the mean square error between the stimulus and its estimate,

$$\varepsilon^2(h) = \langle [s(t) - h \star x_0(t)]^2 \rangle, \tag{9.53}$$

and is thus the optimal linear estimator given the spike train (in the mean square sense). Eq. 9.53 is solved in the same way as eq. 9.49. Imposing the condition $d\varepsilon^2/dh = 0$ for the optimal filter and solving for h yields

$$h(\omega) = \frac{S_{sx}(-\omega)}{S_{xx}(\omega)}. \tag{9.54}$$

This formula is almost identical to the formula for $W_1(\omega)$, with $S_{xx}(\omega)$ playing the role of $S_{ss}(\omega)$. In particular, if the power spectrum of the spike train is flat, $S_{xx}(\omega) = m$ (i.e., Poisson), then $h(\omega) = (1/m)S_{sx}(-\omega)$, from which it follows that $h(\tau) = (1/m)R_{sx}(-\tau)$ is also determined by a simple spike-triggered average. This condition is usually satisfied at low firing rates, when spikes can be considered as nearly independent of each other (Gabbiani and Koch 1996; Wessel, Koch, and Gabbiani 1996). In general, the filter h computed from eq. 9.54 will not be causal in the sense that $h(t) \neq 0$ for $t > 0$, meaning that the occurrence of a spike can be used to predict the future time course of the stimulus (possible only because of the presence of correlations in the stimulus and of the response properties of the neuron). Therefore, the filter h represents a *noncausal ideal linear observer* of the spike train in the sense of section 9.5. Causal (ideal) observers and nonlinear (ideal) observers have been described in the literature (Snyder 1975; Bialek et al. 1991; Poor 1994).

If no correlations exist between $s(t)$ and $x(t)$ (i.e., $S_{sx}(\omega) = 0$ for all frequencies ω), the best linear estimator of $s(t)$ is equal to the mean value, $\langle s(t) \rangle = 0$. The maximal mean square error computed from eq. 9.53 is then equal to the variance of the stimulus, $\varepsilon_{max}^2 = \sigma_s^2$. It is therefore convenient to quantify the accuracy of stimulus encoding by normalizing the root mean square error computed from $s(t)$, $x_0(t)$, and eqs. 53–54 by its maximal value σ_s,

$$\varepsilon_r = \frac{\sqrt{\overline{\varepsilon^2}}}{\sigma_s}, \tag{9.55}$$

so that ε_r takes values between 0 and 1, with $\varepsilon_r = 0$ corresponding to perfect estimation and $\varepsilon_r = 1$ to an estimation performance not better than chance level. Equivalently, the *coding fraction*, $\gamma = 1 - \varepsilon_r$, represents the percentage of temporal stimulus fluctuations encoded, in units of the stimulus standard deviation.

The performance of stimulus encoding as a function of frequency is characterized by computing the *noise* in the stimulus estimate,

$$n(t) = s(t) - s_{est}(t), \tag{9.56}$$

and comparing the relative power of the noise and stimulus,

$$SNR(\omega) = \frac{S_{ss}(\omega)}{S_{nn}(\omega)}. \tag{9.57}$$

This signal-to-noise ratio is equal to 1 when estimation is at chance level for a given frequency (i.e., when there is as much noise as there is signal power at that frequency) and tends to infinity for perfect estimation.[11]

An example of stimulus estimation from the spike train of a Poisson model encoding a time-varying random current $i_{mean} + i_0(t)$ is shown in figure 9.18. When the correlations in single-spike occurrences are dominated by correlations in the stimulus (this condition is exactly satisfied in the Poisson model; see note 7), the power spectrum of the spike train is given by eq. 9.41 so that the linear estimation filter can be computed exactly from knowledge of the linear system's transfer function K:

$$h(\omega) = \frac{K(-\omega)S_{ss}(\omega)}{m + |K(\omega)|^2 S_{ss}(\omega)}, \tag{9.58}$$

using eqs. 9.45 and 9.54. A number of observations can be made using this result (Gabbiani and Koch 1996; Gabbiani 1996). In particular, for a fixed mean firing rate m, the fraction of the stimulus encoded, γ, will increase with the standard deviation of the stimulus σ_s (or its contrast, σ_s/s_{mean}). This is because larger values of σ_s correspond to larger fluctuations in the instantaneous firing rate $\sigma_f = \langle x_0(t)^2 \rangle$ (see eq.

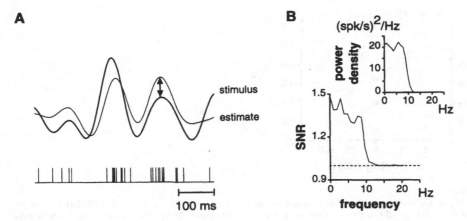

Figure 9.18
Stimulus estimation for a Poisson neuron firing at a mean rate of 50 Hz. (A) Instantaneous firing frequency of the neuron model is proportional to the stimulus (i.e., in this example, there is no filtering by the neuron model, $K(t) = \delta(t)$). In turn, the stimulus is estimated from the spike train (shown at the bottom) by placing the optimal linear filter computed from eq. 9.54 around each spike, as explained in eq. 9.52. To compute the mean square error, the difference between stimulus (thick line) and estimate (thin line) at each time point (illustrated by the double arrow) is computed and squared; the average is then taken over all time points of the observation (see eq. 9.55). Here the fraction of the stimulus encoded is only $\gamma = 0.14$. (B) Signal-to-noise ratio (SNR) for the estimation, indicating the performance of the neuron as a function of frequency (eq. 9.57). The dashed line ($SNR = 1$) indicates chance level. If we compare the SNR curve with the frequency content of the stimulus (upper graph), we see that all frequencies are equally well encoded.

9.51), which encode the stimulus more reliably. For a fixed firing rate *contrast*, σ_f/m, the fraction of the signal encoded will increase with the mean firing rate, m. This can be explained by an increased sampling of the stimulus in the spike train. Finally, the accuracy of stimulus encoding will depend on the characteristics of the stimulus. If, for instance, the frequency content of the stimulus used is not matched to the processing characteristics of the recorded cell (i.e., if there is a substantial range of frequencies for which the signal-to-noise ratio is equal to 1), then the accuracy of stimulus encoding will decrease. In such cases, it is meaningful to estimate only the range of frequencies encoded by the cell, by filtering out from the stimulus frequencies for which $SNR = 1$. The presence of such frequencies will depend on the stimulus used (through $S_{ss}(\omega)$) and the processing performed by the cell (through $K(\omega)$). Similarly, stimuli with natural statistics are expected to yield higher values of the coding fraction because they are more predictable than Gaussian stimuli.

Figure 9.19 illustrates the effect of encoding noise on the accuracy of stimulus estimation from single-spike trains. A white stimulus $s(t)$ with a cutoff frequency of

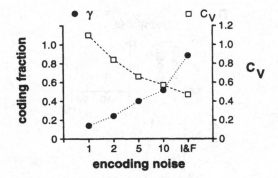

Figure 9.19
Fraction γ of the white stimulus (10 Hz cutoff frequency) shown in figures 9.18 and 9.20 that can be recovered from single-spike trains of various neuron models (mean firing rate: 50 Hz). The bottom axis shows the order of the threshold gamma distribution implementing encoding noise. These models are identical to those of figure 9.3 (except that the refractory period has been set to zero). While a Poisson neuron ($n = 1$) encodes relatively poorly the stimulus ($\gamma = 14\%$), a single perfect integrate-and-fire neuron is quite accurate ($\gamma = 88\%$).

10 Hz (figures 9.18B and 9.15) was estimated from the spike trains of the different models illustrated in figure 9.3. Examples of a single stimulus from this ensemble and the responses of two models are shown in figure 9.15. The fraction of the stimulus encoded is plotted for each one of these models in figure 9.19. A single spike train of a Poisson neuron (figure 9.15A) is able to encode $\gamma = 14\%$ of the stimulus, implying that to obtain an estimate to $\gamma = 90\%$ accuracy, an average of over $N = 74$ independent spike trains is needed (by the usual $\sqrt{N}$ argument; Shadlen and Newsome 1994; Gabbiani 1996). In contrast, an integrate-and-fire neuron firing at the same rate will encode $\gamma = 88\%$ of the stimulus, so that only $N = 2$ independent spike trains will yield an estimate with a better accuracy. Plotted on the same figure is the C_V of the spike trains used to estimate γ. The C_V goes down as stimulus estimation improves because in these models additional noise in the encoding translates into a larger variability of the spiking output. Even in the case of a perfect integrator, however the $C_V = 0.47$ amounts to half that of a Poisson spike train. This variability is not due to noise but is fully devoted to encoding the stimulus in the interspike intervals of the model spike trains. The theoretical numbers illustrated in figure 9.19 are indicative of how many neurons are needed to encode accurately a time-varying stimulus; single and multiple simultaneous recordings that take into account correlations between nerve cells are expected to settle these questions experimentally.

9.7.4 More General Estimation Techniques

It is worth emphasizing that the optimal linear filter $h(\tau)$ depends only on the cross-correlation $R_{sx}(\tau)$ and the autocorrelation $R_{xx}(\tau)$, as this has important implications. For example, one might be surprised to obtain a good estimate of $s(t)$ with the filter of eq. 9.54 because the Wiener-Kolmogorov filtering technique was originally designed to deal with a completely different situation: the recovery of $s(t)$ from continuous observations buried in Gaussian white noise. As is clear from eq. 9.54, however, any other random observation $r(t)$ that has the same cross-correlation $R_{sr}(\tau) = R_{sx}(\tau)$ with the stimulus and autocorrelation function $R_{rr}(\tau) = R_{xx}(\tau)$ as the spike train $x(t)$ will lead to exactly the same estimation problem. This will be so even if $r(t)$ is strikingly different from $x(t)$. Consider the case of a Poisson model, as in the previous paragraph. It is easy to see that if, instead of observing the spike train, we observed

$$r(t) = (K \star s)(t) + m^{1/2}w(t), \qquad\qquad (9.59)$$

where $w(t)$ is Gaussian white noise with unit variance, $R_{ww}(\tau) = \delta(\tau)$, then we would be led to the same estimation filter of eq. 9.54 and the same performance (Snyder 1975). Thus, in this case, estimation from the spike train is *equivalent* to estimation from an observation of $(K \star s)(t)$ buried in Gaussian white noise. The difference between the two signals $x(t)$ and $r(t)$ is illustrated in figure 9.20. This remark is important because it implies that improved estimation techniques developed for the additive Gaussian case can also be expected to work when applied to neuronal spike trains. These techniques include adaptive filtering, where the shape of the filter $h(\tau)$ is time-dependent to take into account firing rate adaptation, changes in the mean stimulus value, or contrast level over time. In addition, nonlinear techniques have been applied successfully to certain types of stimuli. (For examples illustrating these techniques and for further references, see Snyder 1975, chapter 6.)

9.7.5 Nonlinear Encoding and Stimulus Estimation

If the relation between stimulus changes and instantaneous firing rate changes is nonlinear, the accuracy of stimulus estimation will again depend to a large extent on the type of nonlinearity involved. A neuron that encodes specific features of a time-varying stimulus and disregards most of its time course (such as might be implemented by a static threshold nonlinearity) will yield poor estimation results (Gabbiani et al. 1996; Sheinberg and Logothetis 1997). By contrast, other nonlinearities like firing rate saturation and half-wave rectification are not expected to alter significantly

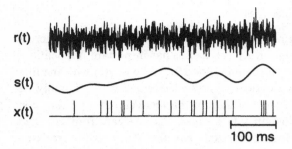

Figure 9.20
Stimulus $s(t)$ shown in the middle (thick line) can be estimated from the spike train of a Poisson neuron $x(t)$ (bottom trace, as in figure 9.18) or from the noisy continuous observation shown on top, $r(t)$. While these two estimation problems appear very different, they are in fact completely identical because the autocorrelations and cross-correlations of both observations with the stimulus are the same. As the top trace makes clear, this estimation problem is a difficult one. The fraction of the signal recovered from the noisy observation or from the spike train by linear estimation is 14% (see figure 9.18).

stimulus estimation results (Wessel, Koch, and Gabbiani 1996). Certain types of nonlinearities will even improve the encoding of time-varying stimuli in single spike trains under adequate conditions. To illustrate this point, we consider again encoding through a static nonlinearity as in eq. 9.47 and spike trains for which eq. 9.39 holds, so that the power spectrum can be computed exactly (see eq. 9.41).

Deviation from linear encoding can be assessed by computing the *magnitude coherence* between the stimulus and instantaneous firing rate,

$$|C_{sf_s}(\omega)| = \frac{|S_{sf_s}(\omega)|}{S_{ss}(\omega)^{1/2} S_{f_s f_s}(\omega)^{1/2}}, \tag{9.60}$$

where $S_{sf_s}(\omega) = S_{sx}(\omega)$ is the Fourier transform of the cross-correlation between stimulus and instantaneous firing frequency, while $S_{f_s f_s}(\omega)$ is the power spectrum of the instantaneous firing rate. The magnitude coherence is a frequency-dependent correlation coefficient measuring the extent of the linear relation between s and f_s (Carter 1987; Ljung 1987). For each frequency ω_0, $|C_{sf_s}(\omega_0)|$ takes values between 0 and 1. If $|C_{sf_s}(\omega_0)| = 0$, the relation between s and f_s is not linear (or nonexistent, $S_{sf_s}(\omega) = 0$). when $|C_{sf_s}(\omega_0)| = 1$, the stimulus s and the instantaneous firing rate f_s are perfectly linearly correlated. In the case where f_s is determined by s through eq. 9.42, it follows from eqs. 9.38 and 9.45 that $|C_{sf_s}(\omega_0)| = 1$ at all stimulus frequencies. From eq. 9.41, we know that $S_{xx}(\omega) = S_{f_s f_s}(\omega) + m > S_{f_s f_s}(\omega)$. Thus the magnitude coherence between the stimulus and spike train,

$$|C_{sx}(\omega)| = \frac{|S_{sx}(\omega)|}{S_{ss}(\omega)^{1/2} S_{xx}(\omega)^{1/2}}$$

$$= \left(\frac{SNR(\omega) - 1}{SNR(\omega)}\right)^{1/2}, \tag{9.61}$$

yields a conservative estimate of linearity between stimulus and instantaneous firing rate, $|C_{sf_s}(\omega)| \geq |C_{sx}(\omega)|$. Experimental values of $|C_{sx}(\omega)|^2$ have been reported for wind-sensitive sensory neurons in the cricket cercal system (Theunissen et al. 1996; Roddey and Jacobs 1996). While $|C_{sx}(\omega)|$ does not directly measure the linearity of stimulus encoding, it has the advantage of being directly related to the performance of stimulus estimation through eq. 9.61. This equation can be derived from the definition of the noise, $n(t)$, and of the signal-to-noise ratio, $SNR(\omega)$ (see eq. 9.57; Gabbiani 1996; Theunissen et al. 1996). In contrast, $|C_{sf_s}(\omega)|$ is not in general related to stimulus estimation performance from single-spike trains,[12] as explained below.

To illustrate the behavior of these two functions in a nonlinear situation, we return to the example of a Poisson neuron firing at a mean rate of 50 Hz and encoding a Gaussian random stimulus with a cutoff frequency of 10 Hz in its instantaneous firing rate, as in figure 9.18. This input modulates the instantaneous firing rate of the Poisson neuron between 0 and 100 spk/sec (figure 9.21A). We assume that $s(t)$ and $f_s(t)$ are related through a static sigmoid nonlinearity, $f_s(t) = g_{\alpha,l}(s(t))$ of the form

$$g_{\alpha,l}(y) = \alpha \sqrt{\frac{2}{\pi}} \frac{1}{l} \int_0^y e^{-t^2/2l^2} \, dt. \tag{9.62}$$

Two examples of such sigmoids are illustrated in figure 9.21A, together with the Gaussian distribution of the input stimulus $s(t)$ used in figure 9.18 and in the following. When the nonlinearity is of the form shown in eq. 9.62, the cross-correlation between $s(t)$ and $f_s(t)$ can be computed exactly (using Bussgang's theorem; see Bendat 1990). This is also true for the autocorrelation function of the spike train which is given by[13]

$$R_{xx}(\tau) = R_{f_s f_s}(\tau) + m\delta(\tau)$$

$$= \frac{2\alpha^2}{\pi} \sin^{-1}\left(\frac{R_{ss}(\tau)}{\sigma_s^2 + l^2}\right) + m\delta(\tau), \tag{9.63}$$

where σ_s is the standard deviation in firing rate caused by the random stimulus ($\sigma_s = 20$ Hz in the example of figure 9.21A). Thus it is possible from these equations to compute $|C_{sf_s}(\omega)|$ and $|C_{sx}(\omega)|$ numerically (by using a fast Fourier transform

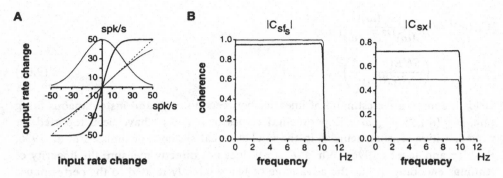

Figure 9.21
Effects of a sigmoid nonlinearity on stimulus encoding in Poisson spike trains. (A) Probability distribution of the Gaussian input is illustrated in units of firing rate changes around the mean rate of the model neuron (50 Hz). In the limit of unit sigmoid gain (the dotted line), no modification occurs between input and output rate changes; this limit is a good approximation for the weak sigmoid nonlinearity (thin line). The thick line illustrates a case where the effect of the nonlinearity is stronger. (B) Magnitude coherence between the instantaneous firing rate and the stimulus ($|C_{sf_s}|$) and between the spike train and the stimulus ($|C_{sx}|$). For $|C_{sf_s}| = 1$, the relation between the stimulus and instantaneous firing rate is a linear one. In both graphs, the thin and thick lines correspond to the thin and thick sigmoids of panel A, respectively. Note that $|C_{sf_s}|$, which measures linearity in stimulus encoding, is closer to 1 for the thin case as compared to the thick case. By contrast, the magnitude coherence $|C_{sx}|$ between stimulus and spike train shows the reversed behavior, indicating a more accurate encoding of the stimulus for the stronger nonlinearity.

algorithm, for instance). The results are shown in figure 9.21B for the two sigmoids of figure 9.21A. Note that in the case of the sigmoid with shallow slope (thin line), the magnitude coherence $|C_{sf_s}(\omega)|$ is almost equal to 1, indicative of a relation between $s(t)$ and $f_s(t)$ that is very close to linear, while the stimulus estimation performance is relatively poor ($|C_{sx}(\omega)| \cong 0.5$ corresponds to $\gamma = 0.14$; see figure 9.18). By increasing the gain of the sigmoid (figure 9.21A, thick line), the linear correlation between $s(t)$ and $f_s(t)$ is slightly diminished (the linear range is clearly reduced as compared to the compression range; see figure 9.21A), while the performance in stimulus estimation is considerably improved ($|C_{sx}(\omega)| \cong 0.72$ corresponding to $\gamma = 0.33$). This is because a large portion of the dynamic firing range of the cell is now devoted to encoding the most likely fluctuations of the stimulus (which would otherwise only cause modulations between ± 20 spk/sec; see figure 9.21A).

Acknowledgments

The research discussed here was supported by the National Science Foundation, the National Institute for Mental Health, and the Sloan Center for Theoretical Neuroscience.

Appendix A: Numerical Estimation Methods

In practice, the quantities defined in the main test, such as the C_V of the interspike interval (ISI) distribution or the power spectrum of the spike train have to be estimated from experimental or simulated data. This appendix provides a short summary of statistical and numerical methods used to obtain such estimates. We will not attempt to cover the subject in depth; extensive treatments may be found in the literature. For a classical reference devoted to the statistical analysis of point processes, see Cox and Lewis 1966; further standard textbooks and reference sources include Oppenheim and Schafer 1989, Press et al. 1992, Anderson 1994, and Ljung 1987.

Mean and Variance of the Interspike Interval Distribution

The mean of the ISI distribution is estimated by the *sample mean*,

$$\hat{\bar{t}} = \frac{1}{k}\sum_{i=1}^{k} t_i,$$ (9.64)

where $t_1,\ldots t_k$ are successively observed interspike intervals. The variance may be estimated from

$$\hat{\sigma}_t^2 = \frac{1}{k}\sum_{i=1}^{k} (t_i - \hat{\bar{t}})^2$$

$$= \left(\frac{1}{k}\sum_{i=1}^{k} t_i^2\right) - \hat{\bar{t}}^2.$$ (9.65)

In general, the accuracy of these estimates will depend on the extent of correlations between successive interspike intervals of the spike train (Cox and Lewis 1966; Anderson 1994). The most favorable case is the renewal process because successive intervals are independent. In this case, the variance of $\hat{\bar{t}}$ is given by σ_t^2/k and decreases linearly with the number of observations from an initial value equal to the variance, σ_t^2, of the ISI distribution. Typically, a few thousand spikes will be sufficient to obtain reliable estimates of $\bar{t}$ and σ_t.

Mean and Variance of the Spike Count

The simplest estimate of the spike count mean and variance on an interval of length T is obtained by subdividing an observation interval T_0 (much longer than T) into $k = T/T_0$ intervals $T_1,\ldots T_k$ of length T. If N_i is the observed count in T_i, we form the estimators

$$\hat{N}(T) = \frac{1}{k}\sum_{i=1}^{k} N_i,$$ (9.66)

$$\hat{V}(T) = \frac{1}{k}\left(\sum_{i=1}^{k} N_i - \hat{N}(T)\right)^2$$

$$= \left(\frac{1}{k}\sum_{i=1}^{k} N_i^2\right) - \hat{N}(T)^2.$$ (9.67)

Clearly, this is not the only way of subdividing T_0 into intervals of length T. The intervals $T_1 + (1/2)T,\ldots,T_{k-1} + (1/2)T$ provide $(k-1)$ further observations of N that can be used to form refined estimators for $N(T)$ and $V(T)$, although the improvement will not be as substantial as from independent observations because these new spike counts are correlated to the previous ones. A technique based on this remark consists in subdividing T_0 in $k \cdot r$ intervals $T_1^{sd},\ldots,T_{kr}^{sd}$ of length T^{sd}, such that $T = r \cdot T^{sd}$. One then computes a "moving average" estimate of the spike count in all successive intervals of length T by summing r consecutive intervals of length T^{sd}: $N_i = \sum_{j=i}^{r+i} N_j^{sd}$, where N_j^{sd} is the spike count in T_j^{sd}. As a rule of thumb, estimates obtained from eqs. 9.66–9.67 require at least ten times more data, that is, $T_0 \geq 10\,T$, than the largest interval T of interest. Moving average estimates are accurate on intervals that have a length of at most 20%–25% of T_0 (Cox and Lewis 1966).

Power Spectrum and Autocorrelation of the Spike Train

The starting point for power spectral density estimation is the *Wiener-Khinchin formula*,

$$S_{xx}(\omega) = \lim_{T \to \infty} \frac{1}{T} |X_0(\omega)|^2, \tag{9.68}$$

where

$$X_0(\omega) = \int_0^T x_0(t)e^{i\omega t}\,dt, \quad x_0(t) = x(t) - m,$$

which states that the power spectrum can be obtained directly as the squared modulus of the Fourier-transformed series $X_0(\omega)$.

In practice, the occurrence of spikes is recorded with a finite temporal resolution Δt, so that the time series of action potential events is of the form $x = \{x_1, \ldots, x_N\}$, where $x_i = x(t_i)$, $t_i = i \cdot \Delta t (i = 1, \ldots, N)$ and $T = N\Delta t$ is the recording time. The value of x_i is either 0 (if no action potential occurred in the interval $t_i \pm (1/2)\Delta t$) or $1/\Delta t$ (if an action potential occurred in the interval $t_i \pm (1/2)\Delta t$), which is the discrete approximation of the continuous δ-function. The series $\{x_0(t_i)\}_{i=1}^N$ is obtained from $\{x(t_i)\}_{i=1}^N$ by subtracting the mean firing rate, $m = (1/N)\sum_{n=1}^N x_n$.

Ideally, the sampling interval Δt should be sufficiently short to resolve the action potential waveform, thus preventing the aliasing of frequencies above the Nyquist frequency ($f_c = 1/2\Delta t$) below it. In practice, the power spectral density is of interest only for low frequencies (typically, well below 200 Hz) and a sampling interval of 0.5 msec (or even 1 msec) is amply sufficient.

The continuous Fourier transform is approximated by the discrete Fourier transform

$$\hat{X}_0(f_j) = \Delta t \tilde{X}_{0j}, \quad \tilde{X}_{0j} = \sum_{m=1}^N x_{0m}e^{2\pi i f_j t_m}, \tag{9.69}$$

where $f_j = \omega_j/2\pi$ takes values at the discrete frequencies $f_j = j/N\Delta t$, $j = -N/2, \ldots, +N/2$ (for N even). An estimator for the power spectral density is given by the *periodogram*

$$\hat{S}(f_j) = \frac{(\Delta t)^2}{T}|\tilde{X}_{0j}|^2, \quad j = -\frac{N}{2}, \ldots, \frac{N}{2}. \tag{9.70}$$

Without any form of averaging, this estimate will be very unreliable. A computationally convenient averaging procedure is to subdivide the observation series into k contiguous segments $l = 1, \ldots, k$, compute the periodogram $\hat{S}_l(f_j)$ separately over each segment, and then average:

$$\hat{S}(f_j) = \frac{1}{k}\sum_{l=1}^k \hat{S}_l(f_j). \tag{9.71}$$

A typical example would consist of a spike train sampled at $\Delta t = 0.5$ msec, for which $N = 2,048$ points (1.024 sec) are used to compute a single periodogram with a resolution of approximatively $1,000/1,024 \cong 1$ Hz in the frequency domain.[14] The number of segments needed to obtain a reliable estimate will depend on the firing frequency of the neuron; typically, averaging over 100 segments or 10,000 spikes should yield reasonably accurate results.

The estimate of eq. 9.71 is further improved by multiplying each segment of data with a *window function* prior to Fourier-transforming. This minimizes the boundary effects due to the finite size of the samples. Such a function is the Bartlett window

$$w_k = \begin{cases} \dfrac{2(k-1)}{N-1} & 1 \le k \le \dfrac{N+1}{2}, \\[2mm] 2 - \dfrac{2(k-1)}{N-1} & \dfrac{N+1}{2} \le k \le N, \end{cases} \tag{9.72}$$

which peaks at the center of the segment and decreases linearly with distance from the center. Thus, prior to Fourier-transforming, one replaces $(x_{01}, \ldots, x_{0N})$ by $(w_1 x_{01}, \ldots, w_N x_{0N})$.

Finally, the estimate of eq. 9.71 can also be improved by *overlapping* the segments on which the periodograms are computed. In other words, if the first segment consists of data points $x_{01}, \ldots x_{02,048}$, as in the previous example, the second segment should be $(x_{01,024}, \ldots, x_{03,072})$, and so on.

An estimate of the autocorrelation function is obtained from the power spectral density by a straightforward discrete inverse Fourier transformation. Similarly, estimates of cross-correlation functions are obtained using exactly the same procedure outline above, but starting from

$$S_{sx}(\omega) = \lim_{T \to \infty} \frac{1}{T} S(\omega) \bar{X}_0(\omega), \tag{9.73}$$

where the symbol "$\bar{}$" denotes complex conjugation.

First-Order Wiener Kernel, Wiener-Kolmogorov-Filtering

Although the first-order transfer functions of eqs. 9.45 and 9.54 can in principle be estimated directly from the cross-correlation and power spectral density estimates discussed above, this involves a division operation that is very sensitive to noise in the estimates of $S_{sx}(\omega)$ and $S_{ss}(\omega)$ (or $S_{xx}(\omega)$). In the case of the first-order Wiener kernel, this numerically unstable operation may be circumvented by using a white stimulus, so that division by $S_{ss}(\omega)$ at each frequency is replaced by an overall multiplicative constant (see eq. 9.46). One effective way of reducing such noise is to carefully select the sampling step Δt to exclude frequencies higher than those conveyed by the system because they only deteriorate the estimate of the transfer function. (For an example illustrating this point, see tutorial 4 of our MATLAB subroutines; more advanced techniques are discussed in Ljung 1987.) Typically, at least 10,000 spikes are needed to obtain reliable estimates of these transfer functions.

An estimator for the mean square error of eq. 9.55 is obtained from

$$\hat{\varepsilon} = \frac{1}{N} \sum_{i=1}^{N} (s_i - s_{est\,i})^2, \tag{9.74}$$

where s_i is the stimulus value at time point $i\Delta t$ and $s_{est\,i}$ is the estimate obtained by discrete convolution of the Wiener-Kolmogorov filter with $\{x_{0i}\}$. In an optimal situation, the filter h is computed from one data set and the error is estimated from a different data set to avoid a bias of the estimate $\hat{\varepsilon}^2$ toward lower values than the true value ε^2 (this technique is called the "cross-validation method"). In practice, the bias is usually negligible if a sufficiently long data record is used (typically, $|\hat{\varepsilon} - \varepsilon|/\sigma_s \le 0.01$ for data stretches longer than 100 sec) and the same data set may be used to compute the filter and the estimate $\hat{\varepsilon}^2$ (this technique is called the "resubstitution method"). However, the bias can be significant in some cases (see tutorial 6 of our MATLAB subroutines for examples).

Appendix B: MATLAB Interface and Routines

Location

The software as well as the following description may be found on the World Wide Web at http://www.klab.caltech.edu/~gabbiani/signproc.html. The software consists of compressed and archived files directly usable under Unix.

System Requirements

Our routines are written entirely using the programming commands of the MATLAB environment and are therefore independent of the particular platform used (Unix-, Windows-, or MacOS-based systems). In addition to the core MATLAB environment, some analysis routines require the Signal Processing Toolbox. The simulation routines and the graphical interface require the Simulink Toolbox. (The random number generator of the Statistics Toolbox is also used, but could be replaced by a random number generator described in Press et al. 1992.) A fast computer with plenty of memory is recommended.

Software and Data

The software consists of four different parts:

1. *Graphical interface and simulation routines.* This part of the package was written using the S-function formalism (see the Simulink reference manual) and is activated by the **startneuro** M-file (i.e., by entering the command **startneuro** at the MATLAB prompt; see figure 9.22). The subthreshold membrane voltage dynamics of the models described in the main text are linear and were implemented by numerical integration using a fixed time step. This greatly reduced the programming load but leads to relatively slow simulations. (For more sophisticated algorithms, see chapter 14, this volume.) Numerical simulation results were checked by comparison with analytical results (see part 2, "Analysis routines"), but no benchmark tests were performed to assess precisely the numerical accuracy of these routines. We would also like to caution the user that simulation results can be affected by the time step used, the properties of random number generators, and the stability of the linear system simulated.

2. *Analysis routines.* These M-files implement the analysis procedures discussed in the main text. In addition, many theoretical results described there are also implemented in the form of M-files, allowing a direct comparison between simulations and theory. References to the literature are provided in the M-files themselves or through the MATLAB help utility.

3. *Tutorials data.* The spike trains and stimuli data sets resulting from simulations of the tutorials can also be downloaded, thus avoiding having to go through the simulations themselves before performing a data analysis.

4. *Figure notes.* These describe how each figure of the main text was obtained, in the hope that this will clarify the results presented and provide starting points for further simulations.

Notes

1. This description is only accurate if two successive photon events are well separated from each other. It remains valid also for shorter separation times, but the effective number of spikes per incoming photon is reduced (for details, see Tavolacci, Teich, and Saleh, 1981; Saleh and Teich 1985; as well as tutorial 5 in our MATLAB routines).

2. A frequently used approximation uses a fixed T but varies the stimulus to obtain different (N, V) pairs. If, as a function of two variables (f, T), the stochastic properties of the neuron depend only on the product fT, varying the stimulus to increase f is equivalent to varying T. This condition is verified by the integrate-and-fire models with random threshold, provided that the refractory period is set to zero.

3. In the following we ignore the possible occurrence of ties, that is $p_0(n_t) = p_1(n_t)$. The treatment of such cases can be found, for example, in Poor 1994.

4. This terminology arose from early applications of signal detection theory to the performance of radar.

5. This result is known as the "Neyman-Pearson lemma" (Scharf 1991).

6. This result is well known for Poisson spike trains (figure 9.3A) and a general proof for gamma-distributed random threshold noise (figures 9.3B–D) can be found in Gestri 1971. For integrate-and-fire neurons

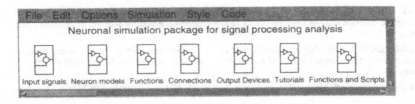

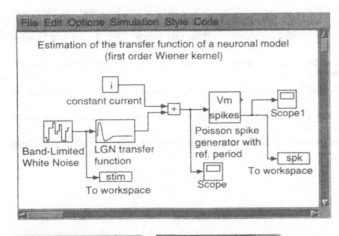

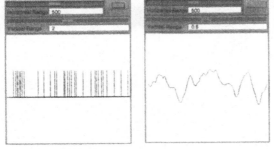

Figure 9.22
Illustration of various windows which constitute the software package for analysis of spike trains using signal processing methods. The top window can be called directly from the main MATLAB workspace window and contains several icons which can be accessed by double-clicking on them. "Input signals," "Neuron models," "Functions," "Connections," and "Output devices" contain building blocks that allow users to constitute models such as the one shown in the middle window. This window is one of the tutorials that can be accessed by double-clicking on the "Tutorials" icon, while double-clicking on the "Functions and Scripts" icon accesses help for the analysis procedures. Spike trains and stimulus vectors, such as the ones shown in the bottom two windows, can be stored directly in MATLAB variables and analyzed using the functions described by the "Functions and Scripts" icon.

(figure 9.3E), eq. 9.37 was proven in Knight 1972a. In fact, the encoding of analog time-varying signals in binary spikes of integrate-and-fire neurons is equivalent to the engineering coding scheme of *integral pulse frequency modulation* (Bayly 1968; Zeevi and Bruckstein 1977).

7. This equation holds exactly for the Poisson model of figure 9.3A (because once the mean stimulus $s_0(t)$ is specified, spikes are generated independently of each other), but will usually not be satisfied exactly by more general models.

8. This is a very strong assumption. Methods to generate such ensembles are described in Marmarelis and Marmarelis 1978.

9. An extreme (and academic) example is $g(y) = y^2$, so that $c = 0$ in eq. 9.48 and the linear estimator is at chance level.

10. Such procedures also exist for other stimulus ensembles (Palm and Poggio 1978; Victor and Shapley 1980).

11. The signal-to-noise ratio can also been normalized to take values from 0 to infinity by subtracting 1; see Bialek et al. 1991 and Gabbiani 1996.

12. The magnitude coherence $|C_{sf_t}(\omega)|$ is also difficult to measure experimentally as compared to $|C_{sx}(\omega)|$.

13. This famous result is originally due to R. F. Baum (1957). More recent derivations use a result due to Price (1958).

14. The number of points N is usually chosen to be a power of 2 so that fast Fourier transform algorithms can be applied.

10 Modeling Small Networks

Larry Abbott and Eve Marder

10.1 Introduction

Small neural networks that generate rhythmic motor patterns in invertebrates have been the subject of intense experimental and theoretical analyses designed to reveal basic dynamic principles (Getting 1989). Although there are significant differences between small invertebrate networks and large vertebrate brain structures, they share a large number of organizational and functional mechanisms. Because invertebrate pattern generators contain relatively small numbers of large, easily studied neurons, they offer the potential for uncovering some of the basic computational and functional characteristics of neural circuits in the brain.

Central pattern-generating networks are groups of neurons that produce rhythmic motor patterns even in the absence of timing signals from sensory or central inputs (Marder and Calabrese 1996). These circuits are involved in behaviors such as walking, swimming, flying, breathing, and chewing. Many central pattern generators produce fictive motor patterns when isolated in vitro, making it easy to study how behaviorally relevant neural activity is produced and controlled. For this reason, they were attractive to early integrative neuroscientists who wished to study circuits of obvious behavioral significance. The pioneers in this area set themselves the task of finding the neurons that formed these circuits and identifying the synaptic connections between them. By the mid-1980s, when "wiring diagrams" for several small pattern generating circuits first became available, it was clear that (1) networks producing similar motor patterns could differ enormously in their circuitry (Selverston and Moulins 1985; Getting 1989); (2) static connectivity diagrams did not contain all the information needed to capture the dynamics of network operation (Getting and Dekin 1985a, 1985b); and (3) the output of a given circuit could be altered dramatically by a large number of neuromodulators (Marder and Hooper 1985).

Small neural networks like central pattern generators raise the possibility of modeling neuron by neuron and synapse by synapse, something unthinkable for circuits in the vertebrate brain. Despite extensive knowledge of circuit structure and the properties of individual neurons and synapses, this is still an extraordinary challenge. As in many biological problems, moving down to what at first appears to be a simpler system means encountering a whole new level of richness, subtlety, and complexity. Experience has shown that any network capable of interesting and flexible behavior, even a small one, is still too complex for brute force modeling to be particularly successful or satisfying. Rather, as with vertebrate systems, insights arise from the creative use of models that compactly specify or describe essential features of the cellular or synaptic dynamics, and that focus on a specific issue.

The stomatogastric ganglion (STG) of the lobster *Panulirus interruptus* and the crab *Cancer borealis* is a central pattern generator that has been studied in great anatomical, physiological, and functional detail. The subcircuit of the crustacean stomatogastric nervous system that generates the pyloric rhythm provides a paradigmatic example of the conceptual problems posed by the full richness of the dynamics of a real neural circuit. In this chapter, we discuss the physiological methods, biophysical measurements, and modeling techniques employed to study this and similar neural networks. We present a number of modeling issues: models of membrane conductances based on channel models, reduction of complex conductance-based models, the dynamic clamp, activity-dependent regulation of conductances, and methods for describing synaptic dynamics. In the context of modeling the output of a small rhythmic circuit, we hope to describe them in sufficient detail so that readers can employ them in modeling other systems and analyzing other problems.

10.2   The Pyloric Network of the Stomatogastric Ganglion

The STG generates the motor patterns that move the stomach in crustacea. The crustacean stomach is a complex mechanical structure in which approximately forty sets of striated muscles move bony ossicles and teeth in response to the motor patterns produced by the STG. The crustacean stomach combines the function of the vertebrate mouth and stomach, and the complex stomatogastric motor patterns are a good model for the kinds of pattern-generating circuits found in the vertebrate spinal cord or brain stem.

In the lobster *Panulirus interruptus*, the STG contains thirty neurons, fourteen of which form the pyloric network, namely, one anterior burster (AB), two pyloric dilator (PD), one lateral pyloric (LP), one inferior cardiac (IC), one ventricular dilator (VD), and eight pyloric (PY) neurons. The pyloric rhythm is illustrated in the recordings shown in figure 10.1. The top three traces are simultaneous intracellular recordings from the somata of three STG cells, the PD, LP, and PY neurons. The next lower trace is an extracellular recording from the lateral ventricular nerve (*lvn*) showing the triphasic pyloric rhythm, in which sequential LP, PY, and PD neuron activity repeats rhythmically. The bottom trace shows an intracellular recording from one of the muscles innervated by the LP motor neuron. Each LP neuron action potential evokes an excitatory junctional potential (EJP) in the muscle. Because movement in these muscles is a graded function of intracellular depolarization, the

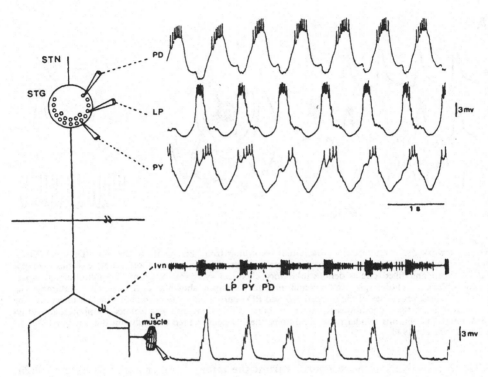

Figure 10.1
Pyloric rhythm. The stick figure shows the positions of the recordings shown on the right. All recordings were simultaneous. The top three traces are intracellular recordings from the somata of the PD, LP, and PY neurons, the next trace is an extracellular recording from the lvn, and the bottom trace is an intracellular recording from one of the muscles innervated by the LP neuron. Modified from Marder, Hooper, and Eisen 1987.

amplitude of the summed EJPs correlates with the extent of muscle contraction. Motor neurons in the STG can be identified by matching action potentials recorded intracellularly with those recorded extracellularly on nerves innervating identified muscles. Although not shown here, the IC neuron typically fires in time with the LP neuron, while the VD neuron usually fires with the PY neurons.

The AB interneuron is an important pacemaker element of the pyloric network that is electrically coupled to the two PD neurons and depolarizes synchronously with them. Recordings from the AB, PD, and LP neurons are shown in figure 10.2A. The connectivity diagram of the pyloric network (figure 10.2B) was established by exploiting the lucifer yellow photoinactivation technique (Miller and Selverston

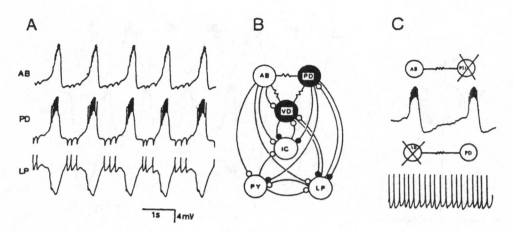

Figure 10.2
Pyloric network. (A) Simultaneous intracellular recordings from the somata of the AB, PD, and LP neurons. (B) Full connectivity diagram for the pyloric circuit. The resistor symbols denote electrical synapse and the open and filled circles denote inhibitory chemical synapses. Neurons and inhibitory synapses shown in black are cholinergic. Neurons and inhibitory synapses shown as open circles are glutamatergic. (C) The intrinsic properties of the isolated AB and PD neurons subsequent to lucifer yellow injection. The AB neuron under these conditions continued to burst. The PD neuron was isolated by photoinactivating the AB and VD neurons. Under these conditions, the PD neuron fired tonically but did not burst. Modified from Marder 1984.

1979) to selectively remove neurons from the circuit (Miller and Selverston 1982a, 1982b; Eisen and Marder 1982). An interesting feature of this circuit is that all its connections are either electrical or inhibitory; there are no excitatory chemical synapses. This provides a clear indication that more than a circuit diagram is needed to explain how this network functions. If neurons in the pyloric circuit fired only in response to synaptic drive, many would never become active. Instead, intrinsic excitability, especially rebound from inhibition, interacting with synaptic input is essential for network function.

Indeed, it was realized about twenty years ago that the synaptic connectivity diagram was only part of what was needed to understand how a network operates, and that it was essential to know the intrinsic firing properties of the neurons in the absence of their synaptic inputs (Russell and Hartline 1978; Hartline 1979). Figure 10.2C shows that the intrinsic properties of the AB and PD neurons of the pyloric network are quite different. The isolated AB neuron is a bursting neuron, while the isolated PD neuron is most often tonically active or silent, as are the other neurons in the pyloric circuit in the absence of modulatory or synaptic inputs. In the presence of modulatory inputs, isolated neurons can also display bistability, exhibiting a sustained depolarization known as a "plateau potential" after a brief depolarizing current pulse (Bal, Nagy, and Moulins 1988).

How is the pyloric rhythm generated? By the mid-1980s, we had a good, first-generation description of the operation of this pattern generator (Miller and Selverston 1982a, 1982b): the AB neuron produces a rhythmic bursting output. Because the AB neuron is electrically coupled to the PD neurons, they depolarize and fire with the AB. The AB and PD neurons inhibit the LP and PY neurons, preventing them from firing during the bursts of the AB and PD. When the AB/PD burst terminates, the LP neuron fires on rebound from the previous inhibition. Among the probable factors inducing the LP neuron to fire before the PY neurons are the strengths of the fast and slow inhibitory postsynaptic potentials (IPSPs) evoked by the AB and PD neurons, respectively (Eisen and Marder 1984), and the relative amounts of transient outward current, I_A, and hyperpolarization-activated current, I_H, in the LP and PY neurons (Hartline 1979; Tierney and Harris-Warrick 1992; Golowasch et al. 1992; Harris-Warrick et al. 1995b). Because the LP neuron strongly inhibits the PY neurons, which inhibit the LP in return, they form a reciprocally inhibitory subcircuit that contributes to the transition from LP to PY firing. There are a number of other examples of reciprocal inhibition in the pyloric circuit and these subcircuits can, under appropriate conditions, produce rhythmic activity by themselves (Miller and Selverston 1982b).

In principle, if one could measure the strengths of all synaptic connections and determine the intrinsic properties of each neuron, conventional modeling techniques could be used to construct a complete model of the pyloric circuit. It is an interesting exercise to examine what this means in practice, both experimentally and in modeling terms. There are six types of neurons and at least seventeen synaptic connections in the pyloric circuit. At present, only partial measurements of membrane conductances are available (Golowasch and Marder 1992a; Tierney and Harris-Warrick 1992; Hartline and Graubard 1992) and precise characterizations of synaptic transmission in the circuit are just beginning to appear (Harris-Warrick et al. 1992b; Johnson, Peck, and Harris-Warrick 1995; Manor et al. 1997). It is possible to build models that produce outputs similar to the pyloric rhythm (Abbott, Marder, and Hooper 1991; see Marder and Selverston 1992 for a review). While such models have been successful at reproducing specific states and activity patterns of the pyloric network and have addressed a number of interesting issues, they lack the stability, flexibility, and variability that make the real circuit interesting. Thus they cannot be viewed as complete models of the circuit. Thinking about whether modeling of a neural circuit based on measured conductances is an achievable or a desirable goal is instructive for those contemplating a similar approach to hippocampal, retinal, thalamic, or cortical circuits.

10.3   Conductance-Based Models

In 1952, Hodgkin and Huxley developed the mathematical framework that is still used to describe neuronal conductances. Each conductance is associated with a reversal or equilibrium potential E, a maximal conductance parameter $\bar{g}$, integer exponents p and q and one or two gating variables m and h (sometimes h is omitted). The membrane current carried by the conductance at membrane potential V is written as

$$I = \bar{g}m^p h^q (V - E). \tag{10.1}$$

If the exponent q is zero (as is the case for persistent or noninactivating conductances), the gating variable h is obviously not needed. The gating variables m and h, known, respectively, as the "activation" and "inactivation" variables, vary between zero and one and are described by differential equations of identical form with voltage-dependent transition rates:

$$\frac{dm}{dt} = \alpha_m(V)(1-m) - \beta_m(V)m \quad \text{and} \quad \frac{dh}{dt} = \alpha_h(V)(1-h) - \beta_h(V)h. \tag{10.2}$$

The functions $\alpha(V)$ and $\beta(V)$ are the voltage-dependent opening and closing rates for these gating variables. In other applications, the form of these equations may be modified somewhat. For example, the opening and closing rates may depend on the Ca^{2+} concentration as well as on voltage. We discuss below another modification needed to account for state-dependent inactivation. The same basic formalism can be used to describe synaptic conductances except that the opening and closing rates are functions of the amount of transmitter released. In most models, this is rewritten in terms of the Ca^{2+} concentration or voltage at the presynaptic terminal (see also chapters 4, 5 and 6, this volume).

10.3.1.   A Conductance-Based Model of the LP Neuron

Only one STG neuron, the LP neuron of the crab *Cancer borealis*, has been the subject of extensive voltage clamp measurements sufficient to characterize a majority of its membrane currents (Golowasch and Marder 1992a). The LP neuron was chosen for this study because each STG has a single LP neuron which can be isolated pharmacologically from the rest of the circuit. This work resulted in the characterization and modeling of three outward K^+ currents (a delayed rectifier, the transient current I_A, and a Ca^{2+}-activated K^+ current), a hyperpolarization-activated mixed-cation current I_H, and a partial characterization of the inward Ca^{2+} current. Because the fast Na^+ conductance that produces action potentials is not present in the somata of STG neurons, cable problems prevented it from being measured. This is a good reminder that the task of characterizing *all* the membrane conductances in a real neuron presents significant technical problems if (1) currents are distributed in a complex manner over the surface of the neuron, and therefore space clamp problems interfere with adequate voltage control; (2) adequate pharmacological tools are not available for isolating currents from one another; (3) several currents carried by the same ion have similar time or voltage dependences; or (4) some conductances are small. In the neuroscience literature, there are only a few instances where the complete set of currents used to model a neuron has actually been measured in that neuron and not taken from measurements in other cells. When the kinetics and voltage dependence of conductances are obtained from other cells, the current densities are obviously unknown. Because of this, the magnitude of the Na^+ conductance for the LP model was fit by hand to produce realistic spiking patterns.

A detailed conductance-based model, like the LP model constructed from the measurements described above, allows us to examine the role of different membrane conductances in producing the overall behavior of the neuron (Buchholtz et al. 1992; Golowasch et al. 1992). As seen in the left panel of figure 10.3, the model LP neuron, in the absence of synaptic input, fires action potentials tonically. An interesting aspect of the model revealed in figure 10.3 is that the repolarization of the neuron following an action potential is handled primarily by the Ca^{2+}-dependent K^+ current and not by the delayed rectifier, as it is in the Hodgkin-Huxley model (1952). Along with characterizing the membrane conductances, Golowasch and Marder (1992b) also measured and modeled an important modulatory conductance in the LP neuron due to the peptide proctolin. Proctolin has a strong excitatory effect on the real LP neuron. As seen in figure 10.3 (right panel), a similar increase in excitability is seen in the model when the proctolin-activated current is included. Later, we describe studies investigating the effects of proctolin on the entire pyloric network.

10.3.2   Reduction of Conductance-Based Models

Most conductance-based models, like the LP model described in section 10.3.1, involve a fairly large number of dynamic variables (thirteen for the LP model). For the mathematical analysis of these models, it is useful to reduce this number as much as possible. One method for doing this involves the use of equivalent potentials (Abbott and Kepler 1990; Kepler, Abbott, and Marder 1992) and it was applied to the LP

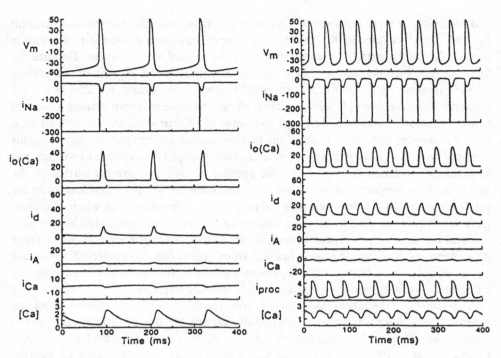

Figure 10.3
LP neuron model. The top trace in both panels is the membrane potential, V_m. Abbreviations: i_{Na}, fast Na$^+$ current; $i_{o(Ca)}$, Ca^{2+}-activated K$^+$ current; i_d, delayed rectifier K$^+$ current; i_A, transient outward current; i_{Ca}, Ca^{2+} current; [Ca], intracellular Ca^{2+} concentration; i_{proc}, proctolin current. Activity in the absence (left panel) and presence (right panel) of the proctolin current. Note that the relative contributions of the outward currents to spike depolarization change when the baseline membrane potential and spike rate are altered by the proctolin current. Modified from Golowasch et al. 1992.

model by Golomb, Guckenheimer, and Gueron (1993). We illustrate here both the general method and its application to the LP model.

The dynamic variables in conductance-based models include the membrane potential, V, and a number of gating variables like the m and h of eq. 10.2. We use a_i to represent the collection of gating variables (with i labeling their identity, for example $a_1 = m$, $a_2 = h$, etc.), and write the equations describing them in a slightly different form from eq. 10.2:

$$\tau_i(V)\frac{da_i}{dt} = \bar{a}_i(V) - a_i, \tag{10.3}$$

by defining

$$\bar{a}_i(V) = \frac{\alpha_i(V)}{\alpha_i(V) + \beta_i(V)} \tag{10.4}$$

and

$$\tau_i(V) = \frac{1}{\alpha_i(V) + \beta_i(V)}. \tag{10.5}$$

In these equations, $\bar{a}_i(V)$ and $\tau_i(V)$ have a clear functional meaning: $\bar{a}_i(V)$ is the asymptotic value that a_i approaches exponentially with time constant $\tau_i(V)$.

The idea of equivalent potentials is to make a change of variables, replacing each of the dynamic gating variables a_i by a potential U_i. The equivalent potential U_i is defined as the potential at which the gating variable a_i is equal to its asymptotic value $\bar{a}_i$. Thus U_i is defined by the equation

$$\bar{a}_i(U_i) = a_i. \tag{10.6}$$

This equation can always be solved because the $\bar{a}_i$ functions are monotonic (typically sigmoidal) and thus can be inverted. The dynamic equation governing each equivalent potential U_i can be determined from eq. 10.3 using eq. 10.6 and the chain rule of differentiation:

$$\tau_i(V)\frac{dU_i}{dt} = \frac{\bar{a}_i(V) - \bar{a}_i(U_i)}{\bar{a}_i'(U_i)}, \tag{10.7}$$

where the prime denotes a derivative. The change of variables from gating variables a_i to equivalent potentials U_i is not a reduction but an exact recasting of the model into a different form.

The advantage of this change of variables is apparent when the equivalent potentials for different gating variables are plotted and compared. This is shown for the LP model in figure 10.4, taken from the work of Golomb, Guckenheimer, and Gueron (1993). It is clear from this figure that the equivalent potentials corresponding to inactivation of the Na^+ current (U_h) and the activation of I_A (U_{aa}) are similar. Also, the equivalent potentials for the delayed-rectifier K^+ current (U_n) and the activation variable of the transient Ca^{2+} current (U_{aca1}) are quite similar (there is an approximate linear relation between them). Likewise, the equivalent potential for the inactivation of the transient Ca^{2+} current (U_{bca1}) is nearly identical to that of I_A (U_{ba}). Although not shown in this figure, the equivalent potential for the fast Na^+ activation is virtually identical to V. These similarities can be exploited by combining or averaging similar potentials in various ways (Abbott and Kepler 1990; Kepler, Abbott, and Marder 1992). The simplest procedure is to keep one of each pair

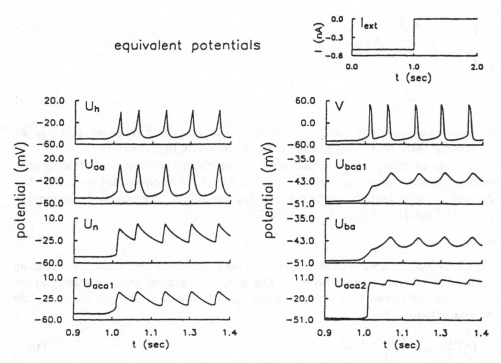

Figure 10.4
Equivalent potentials for the LP model responding to the injected current step plotted as I_{ext} at the upper right. V is the membrane potential, and the following relations hold between equivalent potentials and gating variables: U_h, Na^+ current inactivation; U_{aa}, I_A activation; U_n, delayed-rectifier K^- current activation; U_{aca1}, transient Ca^{2+} current activation; U_{bca1}, transient Ca^{2+} current inactivation; U_{ba}, I_A inactivation; U_{aca2}, persistent Ca^{2+} current activation. Taken from Golomb, Guckenheimer, and Gueron 1993.

of similar potentials as a dynamic variable and set the other potential equal to it (Golomb, Guckenheimer, and Gueron 1993). The retained equivalent potential can be computed from eq. 10.7. In this way Golomb, Guckenheimer, and Gueron (1993) reduced the LP model from thirteen dynamic variables down to seven, with little loss of accuracy. Figure 10.5 shows that the behavior of the full and reduced models is extremely close. The equivalent potential method can also be used to reduce the Hodgkin-Huxley model, which has four dynamic variables, down to a two variable system (Abbott and Kepler 1990; Kepler, Abbott, and Marder 1992) which is extremely useful for phase-plane analysis like that described in chapter 7, this volume.

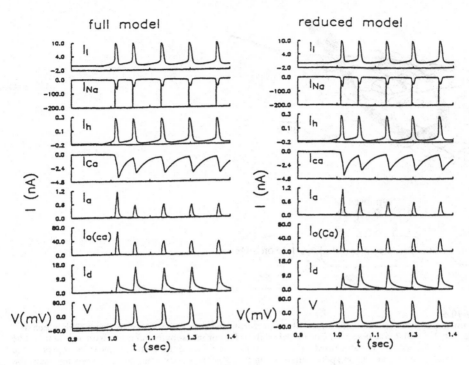

Figure 10.5
Full and reduced LP models compared. The left panel shows the full model and the right panel the reduced model. Currents are labeled as in figure 10.3, except for the membrane potential, V; the leak current
I_l and the hyperolarization activated current I_h. Taken from Golomb, Guckenheimer, and Gueron 1993.

10.3.3 Multicompartment Models

The single-compartment, conductance-based models we have been discussing, like
the LP model, provide a fairly accurate description of the total membrane current
but completely ignore the morphology of the modeled neuron. Almost all neurons
have complex shapes. While it is possible to build models with thousands of compartments that account for neuronal morphology in great detail (see chapter 3, this
volume), in many cases such a high degree of detail may be unnecessary. Figure
10.6A shows an LP neuron from the STG. There are five basic regions: (1) the soma,
(2) a neck connecting the soma to the rest of the neuron, (3) a large primary neurite,
(4) an axon, and (5) a complex branched dendritic region extending from the primary neurite. Figure 10.6B shows a three-compartment model that provides a fairly

A

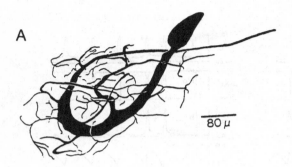

B

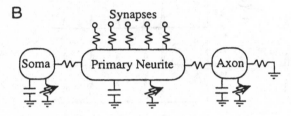

Figure 10.6
(A) Drawing of a lucifer yellow fill of an LP neuron from the crab *Cancer borealis* (from Golowasch and Marder 1992a). (B) Three-compartment model of the LP neuron. Isopotential compartments, with active conductances denoted by variable resistors and membrane capacitances shown as capacitors, represent the soma, primary neurite, and axon spike initiation regions. Resistors connecting these regions represent the neuronal cables between them. Resistors connected to synapses model the series resistances of the fine dendritic processes.

good description of this structure. The large soma, primary neurite, and spike initiation zone of the axon are approximated by equipotential compartments, while the neck, dendrites, and axon cable are represented by resistors connecting these regions.

Studies using multicompartment models like that of figure 10.6B (Liu, Marder, and Abbott 1997) have shown that the isolation of the primary neurite from the spike initiation zone on the axon is extremely important in bursting cells like the AB neuron of the STG. Bursting is produced in the AB neuron by a slowly oscillating potential generated in the primary neurite. In single-compartment models of the AB (Epstein and Marder 1990; Guckenheimer, Gueron, and Harris-Warrick 1993), this slow wave and the faster action potentials can interfere with each other. The strong depolarization following an action potential tends to disrupt the slow wave; alternatively, the steady depolarization of the slow wave can prevent deinactivation of the fast Na^+ conductance terminating the action potentials. If the slow wave and spike initiation regions are electrotonically separated, these problems disappear and much more stable behavior results (Liu, Marder, and Abbott 1997).

10.3.4   Beyond the Hodgkin-Huxley Model: Channels and Conductances

Anyone modeling a neural system must decide what level of detail to include in the model. Because neuronal modeling extends from multistate models of individual channels to binary "on/off" models of neurons, there is a huge range of levels to consider. Many researchers studying small neural networks argue that conductance-based models are appropriate for these systems. To explore this issue further, we will examine the transition from channel models to conductance models.

Studies of single ion channels have greatly expanded our understanding of membrane conductances at both microscopic and macroscopic levels (Hille 1992). Detailed knowledge of single-channel dynamics has confirmed some of the assumptions made in Hodgkin-Huxley descriptions of macroscopic currents, but in other instances discrepancies between the two levels of description have arisen. For example, the Na^+ channel modeled so successfully by Hodgkin and Huxley (1952) does not actually function in a manner consistent with their model (see Armstrong and Bezanilla 1977; Bean 1981; Aldrich, Corey, and Stevens 1983; Hille 1992). By basing the macroscopic conductance description on the underlying channel dynamics, it is possible to build a modified model of the Na^+ channel that is more faithful to the actual functional mechanisms and that fits data in situations where the Hodgkin-Huxley model fails (Marom and Abbott 1994). Here we illustrate the same technique for linking channel models to macroscopic conductance descriptions by applying it to a slowly inactivating K^+ channel, Kv1.3.

Kv1.3 is a voltage-dependent K^+ channel found in rat brain that exhibits a form of state-dependent cumulative inactivation (Aldrich 1981; Decoursey 1990; Marom and Levitan 1994). The conventional Hodgkin-Huxley description implies that the inactivation process is controlled only by the membrane potential and is unaffected by the activation state of the channel. Data on the dynamics of the Kv1.3 channel are in direct disagreement with this basic assumption of the Hodgkin-Huxley model. Transition rates to the inactivated state of the Kv1.3 channel (like those of the Na^+ channel) appear to be voltage-independent, and the inactivated state can only be reached from the fully activated open state (Marom and Levitan 1994). Inactivation occurs slowly and recovery from inactivation is slower still. The multisecond time scale for recovery from inactivation suggests that this conductance might play a role in behaviorally relevant phenomena. This idea will be explored after we build a macroscopic description of the Kv1.3 conductance.

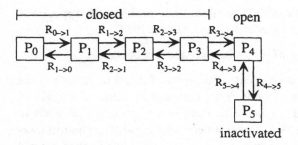

Figure 10.7
State diagram for the Kv1.3 channel. The open state of the channel is reached through a sequence of four states. The probability of the channel being in state i is denoted by P_i, and the transition rate between state i and state j is $R_{i \to j}$. The single inactivated state can be reached only be passing through the open state.

10.3.5   State-Dependent Inactivation of the Kv1.3 Conductance

Ion channels open and close by passing through a sequence of different conformational states. By observing how channels open and close and measuring the movement of gating charges during state transitions, a state diagram can be constructed describing the dynamics of a given channel. Figure 10.7 shows a somewhat simplified state diagram of the Kv1.3 channel inferred from experimental data (Marom and Levitan 1994). The channel opens by passing through a sequence of four closed states, numbered 0, 1, 2, 3, ultimately reaching the open state labeled 4. State 5 is an inactivated state that can only be reached from the open state. A microscopic model of the Kv1.3 channel can be built directly from the state diagram of Figure 10.7. We denote the probability that the channel is in state i by P_i. The rate constant for transitions from state i to state j is denoted by $R_{i \to j}$. The probabilities for being in the various states satisfy the following kinetic equations (see also chapter 1, this volume):

$$\frac{dP_0}{dt} = R_{1 \to 0} P_1 - R_{0 \to 1} P_0 \tag{10.8}$$

$$\frac{dP_i}{dt} = R_{i-1 \to i} P_{i-1} + R_{i+1 \to i} P_{i+1} - (R_{i \to i-1} + R_{i \to i+1}) P_i, \tag{10.9}$$

for $i = 1, 2, 3$, and 4, and

$$\frac{dP_5}{dt} = R_{4 \to 5} P_4 - R_{5 \to 4} P_5. \tag{10.10}$$

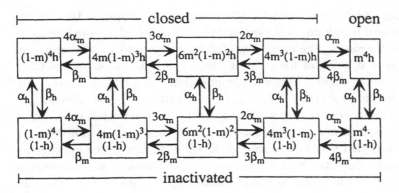

Figure 10.8
State diagram for a Hodgkin-Huxley model of an inactivating K^+ channel. The top row of states form an activation sequence leading to opening of the channel. The bottom row is a duplicate set of states except that these are inactivated. The probabilities for the channel to be in the various states are given in terms of the Hodgkin-Huxley activation and inactivation variables m and h. The rates for transitions between these states are given by the appropriate α and β functions from eq. 10.2.

The membrane conductance per unit area of membrane for a large number of channels is the product of the open channel conductance and the density of channels (a factor denoted by $\bar{g}$) times the probability of the channels being in the open state. Thus the membrane current is $I = \bar{g}P_4(V - E_K)$.

While the above equations provide a microscopic description of the Kv1.3 channel, they are not in a form familiar to most neural modelers. Modeling using a full, multistate channel description like this is certainly possible, but it requires a significantly larger number of dynamic variables than the Hodgkin-Huxley approach. For example, Kv1.3 is described by six dynamic variables in the above equations, whereas a Hodgkin-Huxley model of an inactivating current requires only two variables. Furthermore, a multistate description contains much more information than we normally require in a conductance-based model. The only state probability that enters into the membrane current is P_4; the other state probabilities are extraneous additional variables. To build a more compact description, we will present a technique for reducing such a multistate channel model to a new state-dependent form of the Hodgkin-Huxley equations (Marom and Abbott 1994).

In the Hodgkin-Huxley model (1952), an inactivating K^+ current would typically be expressed in the form of eqs. 10.1–10.2, with $p = 4$ and $q = 1$. The state diagram corresponding to the Hodgkin-Huxley description of an inactivating conductance with these parameters is shown in figure 10.8. The complexity of figure 10.8 is a bit of a shock for those who have not seen Hodgkin-Huxley state diagrams before. The multitude of states and transitions is caused by the assumption of state-independent processes built into the model. The upper row of states in figure 10.8 is the activation sequence that leads to opening of the channel. Because $p = 4$, four separate gating events must occur for the channel to open. The probability of a gating event having occurred is m while the probability that it has not occurred is $1 - m$. Similarly, a single gating event (since $q = 1$) causes a transition to the inactivated sequence of states shown in the bottom row. The probability that the inactivation transition has occurred is $1 - h$, and that it has not occurred, h. The first state in the opening sequence, represented by the upper left box in figure 10.8, corresponds to no activation gatings and no inactivation gating so it has probability $(1 - m)^4 h$. This state can make a transition to the next state in the opening sequence by activating any one of its four activation gates. The rate for this process is four times the basic voltage-dependent activation gating rate in the model, α_m. The probability for the state with a single activated gate is $4m(1 - m)^3 h$ because there is one activated m gate and this can be any one of four possible gates, three nonactivated m gates and a noninactivated h gate. The next transition in the opening sequence has a rate $3\alpha_m$ because there are now three possible gating processes that can occur. Similar arguments can be used to fill in all of the state probabilities and transition rates in figure 10.8. For the deactivation cascade from the open state back down through the closed states, the gate opening rate α_m is replaced by the closing rate β_m, and the combinatorial factors are reversed. Note that the probability of being in the open state is $m^4 h$, so that the total current arising from a large number of channels is $I = \bar{g} m^4 h (V - E_K)$.

How can we reconcile the descriptions provided by the two very different state diagrams shown in figures 10.7 and 10.8? First, note that the sequence of transitions leading to the open state in the two diagrams is similar. Indeed, if the transition rates $R_{i \rightarrow j}$ in the opening sequence of figure 10.7 match those given in figure 10.8 in terms of the functions α_m and β_m, the two series of states would be identical in the absence of inactivation. Experimental data (Marom and Levitan 1994) indicate that an acceptable fit can be obtained by assuming that the transition rates for the activation and deactivation of the channel are given by those of the Hodgkin-Huxley model shown in figure 10.8. This means that we can write $P_4 = m^4 h$ and use the Hodgkin-Huxley equation for m (eq. 10.2), rather than the set of equations given above describing P_0 to P_4. However, this does not resolve the problem of how to describe the inactivation process represented by the variable h. The inactivation transitions in figures 10.7 and 10.8 are so different that it is necessary to modify the equation for h to obtain a compact description of the multistate channel model.

Fortunately, the appropriate equation for h can be extracted from figure 10.7 combined with the state probabilities shown in figure 10.8. The novel feature in figure 10.7, not in accordance with the Hodgkin-Huxley description, is the presence of a single inactivated state that can only be reached from the open state. Moreover, the transition rate is completely independent of voltage. The rates for inactivation, $R_{4\to5} = 1/0.7$ sec and for recovery from inactivation (or deinactivation), $R_{5\to4} = 1/10$ sec are both constant (Marom and Levitan 1994). The trick for constructing an approximate description of the state transitions in figure 10.7 is to combine the transition structure of this figure with the state probabilities of the Hodgkin-Huxley description. Recall that in the Hodgkin-Huxley model $1 - h$ is the probability that the channel is in the inactivated state and m^4h the probability that it is in the open state. We thus set $P_4 = m^4h$ and $P_5 = 1 - h$ and substitute these expressions into eq. 10.10 describing the time evolution of P_5. The result is an equation for h,

$$\frac{dh}{dt} = R_{5\to4}(1 - h) - R_{4\to5}m^4h, \tag{10.11}$$

that is similar in form to the usual Hodgkin-Huxley equation and yet is significantly different from it. In contrast to the usual form of the inactivation equation (eq. 10.2), the membrane potential does not appear anywhere in eq. 10.11. Rather, the activation variable m appears in the equation and it, not the voltage, drives the transitions that change the value of h. The macroscopic description of eq. 10.11 is not completely equivalent to the model of figure 10.7, but it captures the essential features of the microscopic model and provides an accurate description of the Kv1.3 current (Marom and Abbott 1994). We will make use of this description to study the effects of the Kv1.3 conductance on a real neuron in a later section.

10.4   Problems with Conductance-Based Models

Despite their successes, it is difficult to view conductance-based models of single neurons, whether single or multiple compartment, with unbridled enthusiasm. While in some ways conductance-based modeling of neurons and small circuits has been gratifying, in other ways it has disappointed. Ironically, the source of these reservations is closely related to the rich dynamics that makes these models interesting. Complex, conductance-based neuron models exhibit what mathematicians call "structural instability" and physicists call "unnaturalness." This means that the behavior of any given model can change dramatically when relatively small modifications are made in its parameter values. For example, small changes in the parameters that control the strength, voltage dependence, or temporal dynamics of any single conductance in a model may dramatically alter the model's pattern of activity. Likewise, the addition of even a small conductance can dramatically change the model's dynamics (see, for example, Canavier et al. 1993). The behavior of a multi-compartmental model is also highly sensitive to the way different conductances are distributed over its extended spatial structure (Mainen and Sejnowski 1996 and chapter 5, this volume). Of course, these features would not be problematic if we could determine from experiments the exact values of all the relevant parameters, that is, if we were sure that all the conductances in a neuron had been measured and if we knew their spatial distributions. Unfortunately, this is rarely, if ever, the case. The extended structure of most neurons severely limits the accuracy with which conductances can be measured accurately, especially those with fast dynamics. Some conductances may only appear under modulatory conditions that are different from those of the experimental preparation. Data about the spatial distribution of some conductances have only recently become available (Stuart and Sakmann 1994) and are not yet complete enough to establish conductance distributions in model cells.

Because of these limitations, a detailed model of a given neuron cannot be viewed as a unique description of it, even if the behavior of the model accurately matches that of the biological cell under some conditions. Nevertheless, the goal of understanding the behavior of a neuron or small neural circuit in terms of its underlying conductances is central to neuroscience. Only by doing this will we be able to understand how circuit function and, ultimately, behavior are affected by modifications of membrane and synaptic conductances due to neuromodulators, toxins or drugs, long-term potentiation and depression, and other activity-dependent processes. The basic problem is one of incomplete knowledge amplified by the structural instability of the models. To overcome it we must either get around the limitation of incomplete knowledge or eliminate the structural instabilities. We have developed techniques for doing both of these.

For most neurons and neural circuits, a subset of the conductances can be modeled with great accuracy, and for some of these (typically those with relatively slow dynamics), knowledge of the exact spatial distribution of conductances may not be essential. However, conductances that are not as well measured and modeled and for which there is a high degree of sensitivity to spatial distribution make it impossible to develop a convincing model of the entire neuron or circuit. To overcome these problems, we have developed a technique for building hybrid computer/biological models of neurons and neural circuits (Sharp et al. 1993a, 1993b). With this tool, known as the "dynamic clamp," conductances that have been described accurately can be simulated computationally, while biological neurons "simulate" all the elements we are less confident about describing mathematically.

Another way to resolve the problems of conductance-based modeling is to build neuron models that do not exhibit structural instabilities. To this end, we have constructed models in which the parameters regulating individual conductances and the distribution of conductances are not fixed, but are dynamic elements of the model (LeMasson, Marder, and Abbott 1993; Abbott and LeMasson 1993; Siegel, Marder, and Abbott 1994; Liu, Golowasch, Marder, and Abbott 1998), as described below.

10.4.1 The Dynamic Clamp Technique

Given the membrane potential, the membrane current carried by any modeled conductance can be computed by integrating eq. 10.2 and substituting the result into eq. 10.1. The use of efficient numerical integration techniques (see chapter 14, this volume), coupled with the power of present-day computers, allows this calculation to be performed in real time or faster. This means that the current due to any modeled conductance can be reproduced and added to a real, biological neuron, provided its membrane potential can be monitored continuously and the computed current can be injected into the cell. Standard techniques of electrophysiology allow for both of these, either through two electrodes, one to measure voltage and the other to inject current, or through a single electrode, using a time-sharing technique known as "discontinuous current clamp."

Figure 10.9 shows the basic dynamic clamp setup. The arrangement shown, with two impaled neurons allows the addition of simulated membrane currents into each

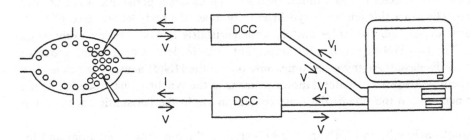

Figure 10.9
Dynamic clamp. Either synaptic or intrinsic conductances are modeled by conventional methods and intracellular recordings are made from either one or two neurons (as shown here) using discontinuous current clamp (DCC). The voltage is sent to the computer, which then computes the current that would flow through the modeled conductance at that membrane potential. This current is converted to a command voltage signal that instructs the current clamp to inject the current into the neuron. Modified from Sharp, Skinner, and Marder 1996.

individual cell and of synaptic connections in either or both directions between the cells. The dynamic clamp computer software runs in discrete time steps of submilli-second duration. At each time step, the recorded membrane potential is converted to digital form and fed into the computer. The computer is programmed to integrate the equations describing the conductance to be duplicated and then output the value of the membrane current carried by the modeled conductance as a function of the recorded membrane potential and of time. The computer output is converted back into analog form and used to control an amplifier that injects the computed amount of current through the microelectrode into the cell.

It is important to appreciate that the dynamic clamp modifies the conductance of the target neuron, even though it injects a computed current. This is because, unlike a conventional current clamp, the amount of current injected depends on the membrane potential of the target neuron and the computed dependence of this potential on the injected current exactly matches the voltage dependence of the current through a membrane conductance. In addition to this Ohmic dependence on membrane potential, the current injected for an active membrane conductance includes the nonlinear dependence on voltage and time arising from eqs. 10.1–10.2. For a synaptic conductance, the current injected into the postsynaptic neuron depends both on the postsynaptic potential and on the voltage of the presynaptic neuron.

The dynamic clamp can be used to confirm that a measured change in a conductance is sufficient to explain a given function. This is illustrated in Gramoll, Schmidt, and Calabrese's (1994) use of the dynamic clamp to study the role of a leakage current in mode switches of the leech heartbeat system. In this system, the two sides of the animal operate in different modes. One side generates a rear-to-front progression of activity in heart motor neurons that causes a peristaltic wave of contraction. The other side contracts synchronously down the body length. Every 20–40 heartbeat cycles, the two sides switch, with peristalsis and synchrony exchanging places. The two HN(5) neurons are important links in determining which mode of activity is displayed. At any given time, only one of the HN(5) neurons is active. The active neuron keeps its ipsilateral motor neurons in the synchronous mode, while the motor neurons on the side of the inactive neuron are in the peristaltic coordination mode.

Gramoll, Schmidt, and Calabrese (1994) studied the membrane potential and input impedance of HN(5) neurons during switches from inactive to active states and concluded that the activation of a voltage-independent leakage current was responsible for the difference in the activity of the neurons in the two modes. Using the dynamic clamp, they were able to replicate the membrane potential recordings of an inactive neuron by adding the appropriate leak to an active neuron. In this way, the dynamic clamp was used to show that the amplitude and reversal potential of a measured current were sufficient to account for the properties attributed to it. This example highlights the fact that modulation of a leakage current can have extremely significant effects on the behavior of a neuron.

Hutcheon, Miura, and Puil (1996) have used a similar dynamic clamp approach they developed independently to study the effects of changing the strength of an I_H conductance in cortical neurons. This current plays a central role in producing a subthreshold resonance oscillation in neurons of sensorimotor cortical slices from rat brain. The dynamic clamp has also been used to study changes in action potential waveform kinetics during repetitive spiking. In the R20 neurons of *Aplysia*, the duration of the falling phase phase of the action potential increases from two- to tenfold during a spike train (Ma and Koester 1995). Because spike broadening is thought to play an important role in determining how much transmitter is released, considerable attention has been given to analyzing the relative contribution of different K^+ currents to spike repolarization and spike broadening. Prior to dynamic clamp analyses, the conventional methods available were pharmacological blockade of ionic currents and the construction of conventional conductance-based simulations. Ma and Koester (1995) used these conventional methods to study frequency-dependent spike broadening in R20 neurons and concluded that a fast transient A-type current, I_{adepol}, is the major outward current contributing to spike repolarization of nonbroadened spikes. They argued that this current undergoes pronounced cumulative inactivation, which produces spike broadening. They also argued that activity-dependent changes in a delayed rectifier I_{K-V}, and in two other K^+ currents had additional effects on the extent and kinetics of spike broadening. However, in this study the authors were hampered in their analyses by the lack of specific blockers that could pharmacologically dissect the K^+ currents.

This problem was overcome by using the dynamic clamp to block specific currents and to modify their inactivation (Ma and Koester 1996). First, conventional two-electrode voltage clamp experiments were used to build mathematical models of the ionic currents. This allowed the authors to remove the characterized currents from the cells using the dynamic clamp and to modify their inactivation and activation kinetics. (Conductances can be removed using the dynamic clamp by adding an effective negative conductance.) In addition, outward currents could be pharmacologically blocked and added back separately with the dynamic clamp. Together, these methods gave Ma and Koester (1996) the ability to study the effect of inactivation of I_{adepol} on spike broadening and on the development of I_{K-V}. These methods demonstrate that inactivation of I_{adepol} is necessary for the initiation of the spike-broadening process. Longer duration spikes later in a train cause the other K^+ currents to activate more fully so the contribution of the different currents to spike broadening changes during the course of a train.

There are three primary limitations of the dynamic clamp method. One is a problem shared by voltage and current clamp methods: measuring and controlling the potential in situations where the neuron is not electrotonically compact. Because the dynamic clamp simulates a point source of conductance, it does not accurately describe the normal distribution of channels in the membrane. Instead, the added conductance acts as if it were entirely concentrated at the tip of the electrode. In an extended neuron, this may limit the utility of the technique, especially for fast currents. Currents that cannot be accurately simulated due to this problem will also be difficult to characterize because of the same space clamp limitations. On the other hand, if the neuron is reasonably compact and if the modeled conductance is fairly slow, the dynamic clamp will provide a good simulation.

Another issue arises because ions that enter a cell may produce secondary effects. This is particularly true of Ca^{2+} ions, which can activate Ca^{2+}-dependent K^+ currents and a variety of signal transduction pathways. Ca^{2+} entry through Ca^{2+} channels could be simulated by using Ca^{2+} containing electrodes. However, this is unlikely to duplicate the secondary effects of Ca^{2+} because the dynamic clamp injects current at the site of the electrode tip rather than where the Ca^{2+} channels are located. In this case, testing whether the dynamic clamp can replicate the effects of a Ca^{2+} conductance can help determine whether its primary effect is to change the membrane conductance or to activate other currents or transduction pathways.

Finally, because the membrane potential is the only variable being measured electrophysiologically, it is not possible for the dynamic clamp to compute Ca^{2+}-dependent membrane or synaptic conductances directly. Rather, the computational description must contain a model of the relationship between intracellular Ca^{2+} and membrane potential. For synaptic conductances (see below), we do this by writing the postsynaptic conductance directly in terms of the presynaptic membrane potential, rather than the intracellular Ca^{2+} concentration in the presynaptic terminal.

10.4.2 Single-Neuron "Short-Term Memory" Effects from Kv1.3

In section 10.3.5, we developed a model of the Kv1.3 conductance and noted some of its characteristics. How do the unusual inactivation properties of the Kv1.3 channel affect the behavior of a neuron? Conventional modeling studies indicated that the relatively slow deactivation of the Kv1.3 current significantly reduces the firing rate of a model neuron (Marom and Abbott 1994). Conversely, inactivation of the Kv1.3 conductance removes this effect, allowing the neuron to fire more rapidly. Because the recovery from inactivation for Kv1.3 is exceptionally slow (10–20 sec), this effect can last a significant amount of time, producing a short-term "memory" effect. As is often the case, this theoretical work was done within the context of a simplified neuronal model. To test whether these effects could occur in real neurons, we used the dynamic clamp to add the Kv1.3 conductance to cultured neurons from the STG (Turrigiano, Marder, and Abbott 1996).

Figure 10.10 shows two effects of artificially adding a Kv1.3 conductance to a cultured STG neuron that fired tonic spikes when depolarized. In Figure 10.10A, three depolarizing current pulses were delivered to a neuron without any Kv1.3 conductance added. The first and third pulses were of identical magnitude and produced a subthreshold depolarization, but no spiking. Pulses of this magnitude did not produce firing, no matter how long they lasted. The middle pulse was slightly larger and evoked tonic spiking with little latency or change in spike frequency. In figure 10.10B, the same protocol was followed except that all three current pulses had identical magnitude and a Kv1.3 conductance was added using the dynamic clamp. As in figure 10.10A, the first pulse caused depolarization but no firing. The second, longer pulse, however, produced firing after a long latency of about 4 sec. After that, the firing frequency increased over time. This is the effect of the slow inactivation of the Kv1.3 conductance. A similar phenomenon has been observed in hippocampal neurons (Storm 1988). After a 4 sec pause, a third, identical pulse depolarized the neuron and, in this case, induced firing. The first and third pulses in figure 10.10B are identical, but one produced firing, while the other did not. The difference is due to inactivation of the Kv1.3 conductance during the long, second depolarization. The effect of the long depolarization lasts for many seconds because of the very slow recovery from inactivation of the Kv1.3 conductance.

Figures 10.10C and 10.10D show that the Kv1.3 conductance can cause transitions between tonic firing and bursting behavior. In the absence of Kv1.3, the neuron seen in figure 10.10C displayed bursting when depolarized (this is a different neuron than the tonically firing neuron shown in figure 10.10A and 10.10B). After Kv1.3 was added, the neuron switched to tonic firing activity (figure 10.10D, first pulse). Over the course of a long depolarization, the behavior switched from tonic firing to bursting as the Kv1.3 conductance inactivated (middle pulse of figure 10.10D). Because the slow-wave depolarization during bursting is sufficient to keep the Kv1.3 conductance inactivated, once bursting starts it continues as long as the neuron is depolarized. Furthermore, due to the slow recovery from inactivation, there is a "memory" effect. A third current pulse, identical to the first, caused bursting, not tonic firing (third pulse of figure 10.10D). Thus a relatively small Kv1.3 conductance is able to make this neuron essentially bistable. Its response to repeated short depolarizations can be either tonic firing or bursting. Long periods of depolarization

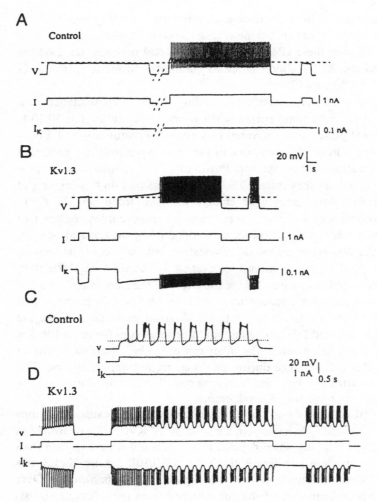

Figure 10.10
Effect of introducing a Kv1.3 conductance into cultured STG neurons. Notation: V, membrane potential; I, imposed current; I_K, dynamic clamp current resulting from modeled Kv1.3 conductance. (A) Control, in the absence of added Kv1.3. (B) Same cell as in panel A but after turning on 1 µS maximal conductance of Kv1.3. (C) Different neuron in control conditions with no added Kv1.3. (D) Same neuron as in panel C but after the addition of a 10 µS maximal conductance of Kv1.3. Modified from Turrigiano, Marder, and Abbott 1996.

switch it into bursting mode and long periods of silence change it back to tonic mode.

It is impressive that a single K^+ conductance added to a neuron expressing numerous other conductances can have such a profound effect on its activity. This is not due to the magnitude of the added conductance; it was quite modest, but rather to its slow dynamics. The multisecond time scale for recovery of inactivation of Kv1.3 is reflected in the memory effects we found. Such memory and bistability phenomena are often ascribed to complex neural circuits. It is interesting to note that they can arise not only as single-neuron phenomena but from the effects of a single conductance (Marder et al. 1996).

10.4.3 Activity-Dependent Conductances

Realistic conductance-based neuron models, like the LP model described above, involve a large number of free parameters that must be set either by experimental measurement or by adjusting them until the model performs properly. In addition to the parameters that control the voltage and time dependence of the conductance gating variables, each current has a maximal conductance parameter $\bar{g}$ that is proportional to the density of its ion channels. Experience has shown that the adjustment of these parameters is tedious because there are so many of them, because the behavior of models is extremely sensitive to their values, and because, as they are adjusted, they interact with each other in complex ways. Along with the general level of aggravation that this causes, there are compelling biophysical reasons to believe that laboriously searching for the "correct" values of these parameters may be misguided.

Ion channels in neurons are continually being synthesized, transported to various parts of the cell, and inserted into the membrane while old channels are removed and disassembled. In the membrane, channels are subject to a variety of modulatory influences. The molecular mechanisms responsible for ion channel synthesis, modulation, and degradation are typically ignored in neuron models because it is assumed that these processes maintain the densities of ion channels over the surface of the cell membrane at constant levels. As a result, channel densities are treated as fixed parameters in most models. We suggest, instead, that the cell biology of the neuron might be geared to maintaining constant average activity, rather than constant channel densities. It is difficult to see how a neuron could actually monitor the densities of its ion channels other than through the effect they have on electrical activity. Furthermore, it seems more likely that the processes controlling channel density would have evolved to maintain the neuronal activity needed for a specific task, rather than to maintain the specific numbers of channels present and active in the membrane. We have constructed and studied models that incorporate this alternate conception of the role of the molecular machinery of the cell (LeMasson, Marder, and Abbott 1993; Abbott and LeMasson 1993; Siegel, Marder, and Abbott 1994; Liu, Golowasch, Marder, and Abbott 1998). In addition, we have conducted a series of experiments that support this viewpoint (Turrigiano, Abbott, and Marder 1994; Turrigiano, LeMasson, and Marder 1995).

Modeling the mechanisms by which ion channels are constructed, transported, inserted into the cell membrane, modulated, and degraded would be an enormously complicated undertaking. Fortunately, we can learn about the role of these processes and, in particular, the effect of their dependence on activity without constructing a detailed mechanistic model. Two features help to simplify the construction of such models. First, the essential element needed to understand the impact of activity-dependent intrinsic properties is the feedback mechanism that links a neuron's electrical characteristics to its activity. Second, channel synthesis, insertion, modulation, and removal are much slower than the usual voltage- and ligand-dependent processes that open and close channels. Thus activity-dependent regulation of conductances introduces a new, slower dynamic time scale into modeling neural excitability. Because activity-dependent changes are so much slower than the processes responsible for action potentials, bursting, and other similar phenomena, the dynamics splits into two widely different temporal scales, which simplifies the analysis of activity-dependent models (Abbott and LeMasson 1993).

The basic idea of activity-dependent conductances is that the electrical activity of a neuron plays a feedback role in regulating its currents. The feedback element giving rise to activity-dependent conductances should be sensitive to activity and must be capable of regulating numerous biochemical processes. Intracellular Ca^{2+} is a prime candidate for such an element. The rate of Ca^{2+} entry into a neuron is well correlated with its level of electrical activity (Ross 1989; LeMasson, Marder, and Abbott 1993). Ca^{2+} is a ubiquitous regulator of biochemical pathways and it appears to play a role in many processes affecting membrane conductances. Changes in the intracellular Ca^{2+} concentration are associated with both modifications of channel properties (Chad and Eckert 1986; Gruol, Deal, and Yool 1992; Kaczmarek and Levitan 1987) and long-term changes in gene expression (Murphy, Worley, and Baraban 1991). The models we have constructed to study activity-dependent conductances use Ca^{2+} entry as the feedback element linking neuronal characteristics to electrical activity.

In the most recent version of these models (Liu, Golowasch, Marder, and Abbott 1998), the maximal conductances of membrane currents are regulated by the activity of the neuron through a number of Ca^{2+} "sensors." We label the different membrane currents with an index i and denote the maximal conductance for current i by $\bar{g}_i$. The maximal conductances are not fixed parameters as in conventional models, but instead can change over time, governed by the Ca^{2+} sensors. We assume that this is a slow process, occurring over hours or even days. The Ca^{2+} sensors are integrators of the Ca^{2+} current entering the cell. In general, there are multiple Ca^{2+} sensors with different integration time constants. These will be discussed in more detail below. We denote the value of a Ca^{2+} sensor by S_a, where the index a indicates the identity of the particular sensor. We assume that these sensors are coupled to pathways that modulate channel conductances and densities. At a particular sensor value, when $S_a = \bar{S}_a$, the pathway coupled to sensor a is assumed to be in equilibrium, and as a result, it produces no net change in membrane conductances. However, when the sensor variable S_a deviates from its equilibrium value $\bar{S}_a$, the pathway acts to change the maximal conductances of membrane currents. For simplicity, we assume a linear dependence between the value of a Ca^{2+} sensor and the rate at which maximal conductances change, and we assume that the different sensors act additively. As a result, the time evolution of the maximal conductance $\bar{g}_i$ is determined by the equation (Liu, Golowasch, Marder, and Abbott 1998).

$$\tau \frac{d\bar{g}_i}{dt} = \sum_a B_{ia}(S_a - \bar{S}_a), \tag{10.12}$$

where τ is a time constant that reflects the slow dynamics of the activity-dependent processes. The parameter B_{ia} determines how sensor a affects conductance i, may be positive, negative, or zero, and may depend on the $\bar{g}_i$.

In conventional neuron models, the maximal conductances $\bar{g}_i$ are parameters that are carefully adjusted until the model produces a pattern of activity that matches the biological neuron being studied. In our models, the maximal conductances are dynamic variables and they take whatever values eq. 10.12 assigns to them. The pattern of activity that the model neuron exhibits is controlled by setting the equilibrium points for the sensors, the $\bar{S}_a$ parameters, to appropriate values. When the model is running, eq. 10.12 acts as a self-consistency condition. The maximal conductances determine the type of electrical activity that the neuron will produce. This activity affects Ca^{2+} entry and thus the values of the Ca^{2+} sensors. The Ca^{2+} sensors in turn modify the maximal conductances through eq. 10.12. The entire system will come to equilibrium when the maximal conductances take steady-state values that produce a level of Ca^{2+} entry that sets all of the Ca^{2+} sensors to their equilibrium values, that is, $S_a = \bar{S}_a$ for all a. If the B_{ia} parameters are chosen appropriately, any deviations from this equilibrium activity will result in changes of maximal conductances that restore the equilibrium behavior. In these models, the set of maximal conductances that a given neuron develops depends not only on the level and time course of Ca^{2+} entry but also on the past history of the cell.

Because the parameters B reflect the actions of the complex mechanisms and pathways responsible for the effects of activity on neuronal conductances, they are fairly unconstrained. The basic guiding principle used to establish their values is stability. As an example, we will discuss the Ca^{2+} sensors and B values in a model of a bursting neuron that we have studied that has seven activity-regulated conductances (Liu, Golowasch, Marder, and Abbott 1998). Three Ca^{2+} sensors are used in this model, and they act as band-pass filters integrating the Ca^{2+} current over three different time scales. Specifically, the sensors are constructed in a similar manner to Hodgkin-Huxley conductances; each has an activation and inactivation variable that is controlled through equations like eq. 10.2 except that the rate constants α and β depend on the Ca^{2+} current rather than on voltage. The values of these rate constants determine the frequency range over which a particular sensor is sensitive to changes in the Ca^{2+} current. By operating in different frequency ranges, the sensors can monitor activity occurring at different time scales and can target the specific conductances that control various aspects of neuronal activity. For example, the fastest sensor registers Ca^{2+} entry over single action potentials. A drop in its value typically indicates that the neuron has stopped firing action potentials. As a result, we couple this fast sensor to the Na^+ and delayed-rectifier K^+ maximal conductances responsible for spiking and choose the signs of the B parameters so that low sensor values increase their values. Similarly, we couple a slower sensor to the maximal conductances of currents that control bursts, Ca^{2+} currents for example. Again, the signs of the B parameters are chosen to assure that a low sensor signal, corresponding to the loss of bursting activity, will act to restore bursts. A third, DC sensor monitors and regulates the long-term average membrane potential and prevents latching of the model neuron into a chronically depolarized state.

The model neuron discussed above is self-assembling. In other words, starting with any set of maximal conductances, the model will reach an equilibrium point exhibiting a certain type of activity. Figure 10.11 illustrates an interesting feature of self-assembly. Here the model has spontaneously developed a set of maximal conductances that result in bursting behavior, starting from two different initial conditions. Although the final activity shown in figures 10.11A and 10.11B is similar, the maximal conductances established by the model are quite different. The view that a given neuron has a fixed set of conductances uniquely tied to its behavior is therefore not supported by the model. An internal mechanism that guides the construction and modulation of membrane channels can produce the required behavior in a number

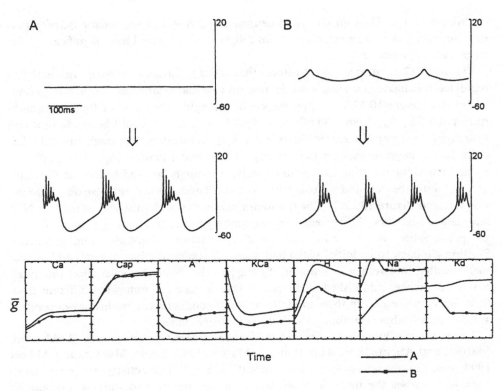

Figure 10.11
Spontaneous development of bursting in a model neuron with activity-dependent conductances. The
model neuron started with the two sets of initial conditions shown in the top traces. In panel A, the neuron
was initially silent. In panel B, the neuron initially showed small depolarizing potentials but no spikes. In
both cases the model evolved to generate the bursting mode of activity seen in the second row of traces.
The plots at the bottom show the changes in the maximal conductances as a function of time as the model
evolved. Conductances represented: *Ca*, transient calcium; *Ca$_p$*, persistent Ca^{2+}; *A*, transient outward
conductance; *K$_{Ca}$*, Ca^{2+}-activated K$^+$; *H*, hyperpolarization-activated inward conductance; *Na*, Na$^+$
conductance; *Kd*, delayed-rectifier K$^+$. (Unpublished figure of Z. Liu)

of different ways. Thus an identified neuron displaying a characteristic activity pattern measured in two animals, or at two different times, could have significantly different sets of conductances.

Figure 10.12 illustrates the robustness that is the hallmark of models with activity-regulated conductances. Here a model neuron that had established a bursting pattern of activity (figure 10.12A) was perturbed by changing the value of the K^+ equilibrium potential, E_K, from -80 mV to -60 mV. Such a shift could be made in a real system by changing the extracellular K^+ ion concentration. Although this shift initially had a large impact on the activity of the model neuron (figure 10.12B), the model sensed the resulting change in its activity through the modification in the entry of Ca^{2+} into the cell and adjusted its maximal conductances until strong bursting was restored (figure 10.12C). The dominant conductance change was in the fast Na^+ and delayed-rectifier K^+ currents, corresponding to the fact that the main effect of the perturbation was to reduce the number of action potentials being generated. Shifting E_K back to its initial value had a similar transient effect (figure 10.11D) and then resulted in a return to bursting (figure 10.11E). Note, however, that the maximal conductances established at the end of this exercise are somewhat different from those initially present. In these models, maximal conductances are history-dependent and highly variable even though activity is robustly stable.

These models have a number of additional interesting properties (LeMasson, Marder, and Abbott 1993; Abbott and LeMasson 1993; Siegel, Marder, and Abbott 1994; Liu, Golowasch, Marder, and Abbott 1998). (1) The activity-dependent feedback loop causes the intrinsic properties of model neurons to shift in response to stimulation and to the presence of other neurons in a network. (2) Coupled neurons can differentiate spontaneously, so that model neurons described by the same underlying equations can develop different sets of conductances and play different roles in the functioning of a network. (3) A nonuniform distribution of membrane currents can arise in a spatially extended model neuron in response to spatial variations of the intracellular Ca^{2+} concentration related both to the morphology of the cell and to the pattern of synaptic input it receives. (4) Synaptically driven shifts in the distribution of membrane currents tend to equalize synaptic inputs that are nonuniform over a dendritic tree. (5) Activity-dependent conductances can modify the level of excitability of a neuron to compensate for changes in the strengths of its synaptic inputs.

One of the most significant messages provided by models of conductance regulation is that the same mechanisms that develop and maintain membrane conductances are likely to modify these conductances in response to long-lasting changes in the activity of the neuron. An interesting variant of the perturbation shown in figure 10.12 is to study what happens when two neurons make synaptic connections. Be-

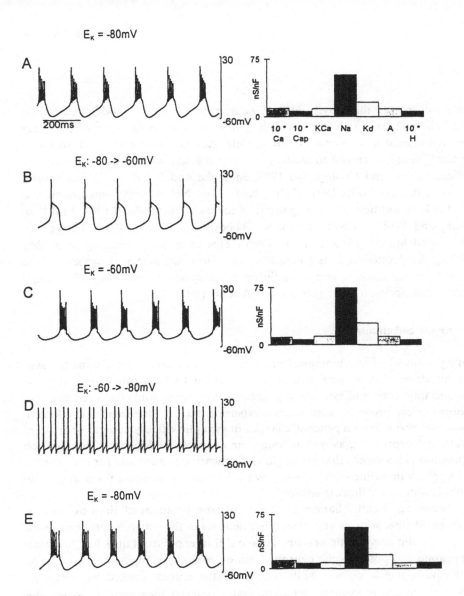

Figure 10.12
Response of the activity-dependent model to changes in E_K. The left-hand plots show the membrane potential as a function of time, and the right-hand histograms give the maximal conductances in the model. Abbreviations for the conductances are the same as in figure 10.11. (A) Model was initially in a bursting mode with $E_K = -80$ mV. (B) Model behavior immediately after shifting E_K from -80 mV to -60 mV. (C) After sufficient time with $E_K = -60$ mV, the model neuron restored bursting activity. The histograms at the right show that the Na$^+$ and delayed rectifier K$^+$ conductances were up-regulated, and this was associated with the resumption of full bursting. (D) Activity immediately after setting E_K back to -80 mV from -60 mV. (E) After sufficient time at -80 mV, the model resumed bursting and the Na$^+$ and delayed rectifier K$^+$ conductances had decreased. From Liu, Golowasch, Marder, and Abbott 1998.

cause this will modify the activity of each neuron, it will, in the model, cause their maximal conductances to shift. This adds a new element to the type of plasticity normally considered in neuronal circuit models. Activity, acting through an intracellular Ca^{2+} signal, is known to mediate many processes, including changes in synaptic efficacy (Bliss and Collingridge 1993; Malenka and Nicoll 1993) and neurite outgrowth (Kater and Mills 1991; Fields, Neale, and Nelson 1990; van Ooyen and van Pelt 1994) in addition to the magnitude of ionic currents (Alkon 1984; Franklin, Fickbohm, and Willard 1992; Turrigiano, Abbott, and Marder 1994; Turrigiano, LeMasson, and Marder 1995; Li et al. 1996). This raises the interesting possibility of modeling the development and maintenance of intrinsic neuronal properties, the growth of neuronal circuits, and the adjustment of synaptic strengths—all through the effects of intracellular Ca^{2+} (Jensen and Abbott 1997).

10.5 Synaptic Subcircuits

In building a model of any biological network, it is necessary to determine the synaptic architecture, that is, how neurons are coupled to each other, and also the strength and time course of synaptic interactions. Measuring and characterizing synaptic transmission presents considerable experimental and theoretical challenges. Most synapses show time-dependent changes in synaptic efficacy such as short-term facilitation and depression, as well as long term changes like long-term potentiation and depression. This means that no single static measure is adequate for defining the synaptic strength in a functioning circuit. We will discuss techniques for dealing with this complication in a following section.

In an operating circuit, changes in the membrane potential of the postsynaptic neuron from intrinsic sources and from other neurons in the network can obscure the effects of a specific presynaptic neuron. To avoid this, experimentalists like to isolate the presynaptic and postsynaptic neurons from other synaptic inputs and to voltage-clamp the postsynaptic neuron while measuring the current evoked by presynaptic activation. Studying synaptic strength under optimal measurement conditions usually means suppressing the activity levels of the network, but most synapses are subject to activity-dependent modulation. Therefore, measurements are often made under conditions that do not apply when the network is actually operating.

In addition to adding membrane conductances to neurons, the dynamic clamp can be used to create artificial synapses between neurons, either electrical (Joyner, Sugiwara, and Tau 1991; Sharp, Abbott, and Marder 1992) or chemical (Robinson and Kawai 1993; Sharp et al. 1993a, 1993b; Sharp, Skinner, and Marder 1996). To construct an artificial chemical synapse, for example, the conductance of the postsynaptic neuron is modified by an amount that depends on the membrane potential of the presynaptic neuron. By building an artificial synapse in parallel with a real synapse, the synaptic strength can be increased or decreased in a controlled manner and the effect on network activity can be observed. Alternately, artificial synapses with precisely controlled characteristics can be used to form novel circuits from otherwise unconnected neurons. The following sections describe the theoretical methods needed to characterize synaptic transmission mathematically, and then present examples of the use of the dynamic clamp to construct artificial synapses and hybrid circuits.

10.5.1 Modeling Electrical Synapses

Electrical synapses formed by gap junctions are a common feature in many neural circuits. Although they would appear to have the effect of bringing the membrane potentials of the pre- and postsynaptic neurons closer to each other, electrical synapses can have more exotic and counterintuitive impacts on circuit activity (Sherman and Rinzel 1992). The synaptic current of the postsynaptic neuron due to an electrical synapse is given by

$$I_s = \bar{g}_e(V_{post} - V_{pre}). \tag{10.13}$$

If the electrical synapse is nonrectifying, the synaptic current for the two cells is of equal magnitude but opposite sign. If, however, the electrical synapse is rectifying, the coefficient $\bar{g}_e$ takes different values for the two directions of synaptic coupling.

10.5.2 Modeling Chemical Synaptic Transmission

At a chemical synapse, presynaptic firing results in the release of transmitter, which induces a change in the membrane conductance of the postsynaptic neuron at the site of the synapse. The synaptic current for the postsynaptic neuron can be written as

$$I_s = \bar{g}_s s(V_{post} - E_s), \tag{10.14}$$

where E_s is the synaptic reversal potential and $\bar{g}_s$ scales the magnitude of the current. The variable s here plays exactly the same role as the variable m in eq. 10.1. Like m, s is a dynamic variable in the range $0 \leq s \leq 1$; it corresponds to the probability that a synaptic receptor channel is in an open, conducting state. This probability depends on the presence and concentration of neurotransmitter released by the presynaptic neuron. Let us assume that the transmitter released by the presynaptic terminal interacts with a receptor through a binding reaction of the form

$$\text{closed receptor} + n \text{ transmitter molecules} \rightleftharpoons \text{open receptor.} \tag{10.15}$$

This assumes a direct binding to the channel as opposed to second-messenger activation of the channel. If we denote the forward rate constant by k_+ and the backward rate constant by k_-, the open probability for the receptor s satisfies the first-order chemical kinetic equation

$$\frac{ds}{dt} = k_+ T^n (1 - s) - k_- s, \tag{10.16}$$

with T the transmitter concentration. The steady-state open probability given by this equation is

$$\bar{s} = \frac{k_+ T^n}{k_- + k_+ T^n}. \tag{10.17}$$

If we assume that the amount of transmitter released is a function of the presynaptic voltage (through the intracellular Ca^{2+} concentration), we can express $\bar{s}$ as a function of the presynaptic potential, $\bar{s}(V_{pre})$. Then, with a little algebraic rearrangement, eq. 10.16 can be rewritten as

$$\left(\frac{1 - \bar{s}(V_{pre})}{k_-} \right) \frac{ds}{dt} = \bar{s}(V_{pre}) - s, \tag{10.18}$$

which shows that s approaches the value $\bar{s}$ asymptotically and that the time constant for this process is $(1 - \bar{s})/k_-$. As a result, synaptic activation, when $\bar{s}$ is near one, is a much faster process than deactivation, when $\bar{s}$ is near zero. This suggests that the time course of the postsynaptic conductance can probably be fit by a sum of two exponentials, something that is commonly done.

A number of different equations can be used to model the function $\bar{s}(V_{pre})$, which controls the synaptic current in this model. It can be written as a sigmoidal function of the presynaptic potential,

$$\bar{s}(V_{pre}) = \frac{1}{1 + \exp((V_{th} - V_{pre})/\Delta)}, \tag{10.19}$$

where Δ and V_{th} are constants that determine the threshold voltage of the synapse and the slope of its voltage sensitivity. Alternately, if synaptic transmission rises sharply from zero at the threshold value, we can use the expression

$$\bar{s}(V_{pre}) = [\tanh((V_{pre} - V_{th})/\Delta)]_+, \tag{10.20}$$

where, for any quantity x, the notation $[x]_+$ is equal to x if $x \geq 0$ and is zero otherwise.

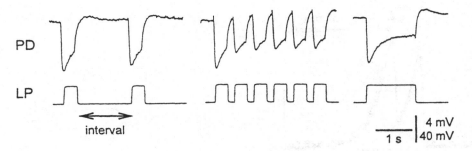

PD

LP

interval

4 mV
1 s   40 mV

Figure 10.13
Graded synaptic transmission in the STG shows depression. The LP neuron was voltage-clamped, and the graded synaptic potential evoked in the PD neuron in response to LP neuron depolarization was recorded. The preparation was placed in 10^{-7} M TTX to block all action potentials. Square-wave depolarizations of the LP evoked a graded IPSP with rapid onset and slow attenuation. The amplitude of the IPSP decreased over time for repetitive pulses. From Manor et al. 1997.

At most synapses, action potentials trigger the release of neurotransmitter, and the threshold for transmitter release may be quite depolarized if there are high-threshold Ca^{2+} channels in the presynaptic terminal. At other synapses, transmitter release may not require action potentials, presumably because there are low-threshold Ca^{2+} channels at the presynaptic terminal. The synapses of the pyloric network exhibit such non-spike-mediated, graded release. For example, figure 10.13 shows graded synaptic transmission between the LP and PD neurons of the STG (Manor et al. 1997). To generate this figure, action potentials were pharmacologically blocked. The LP neuron was depolarized by injecting current into it in a series of square pulses (lower trace), which produced a series of graded IPSPs in the PD neuron (upper trace). Figure 10.13 reveals that the description given above for graded synaptic transmission is not complete for this synapse. Both during individual pulses, and across the sequence of pulses, the IPSP amplitude decreases or depresses over time. Other synapses, such as the neuromuscular junction shown in figure 10.14, display the opposite phenomenon, synaptic facilitation. We will discuss the modeling of these important effects within the context of spike-mediated synaptic transmission, where the analysis is considerably simpler.

10.5.3 Modeling Facilitation and Depression

The postsynaptic conductance at a spike-mediated synapse depends on the temporal sequence of action potentials arriving at the presynaptic terminal. An isolated action potential evokes a pulse of postsynaptic current (PSC) and a resulting postsynaptic

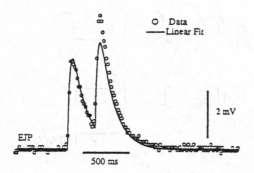

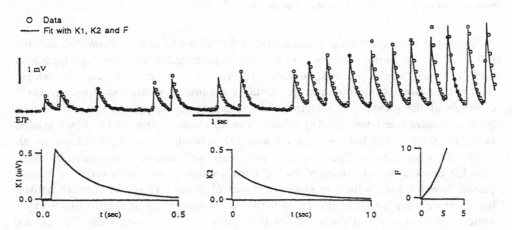

Figure 10.14
Modeling spike mediated synaptic transmission to an STG muscle. Fit of EJPs arising from nerve stimulation and recorded from the gm8 muscle. In the upper plot, the open circles show the recorded response to two presynaptic action potentials. The solid line was obtained by summing the response to two isolated action potentials. The middle plot shows data recorded in response to a random presynaptic spike train (open circles) and the solid line fit obtained from the additive model described in the text. The functions used in the model, K_1, K_2 and F are plotted at the bottom. Modified from Sen et al. 1996.

potential (PSP) that can be modeled in a variety of ways: by a linear rise and exponential decay, by an α-function, $t \exp(-\alpha t)$, or by the difference of two exponentials. Let K_1 denote the function that fits the shape of the postsynaptic response to an isolated presynaptic action potential. If an isolated presynaptic spike arrives at time t_i, the postsynaptic response (either a PSC or PSP depending on which is being modeled) at a later time t is $R(t) = K_1(t - t_i)$.

As a crude approximation, we might try summing individual responses to model the postsynaptic response arising from a train of action potentials. In other words, we might write the response at time t to a series of action potentials occurring at earlier times t_i as $R(t) = \sum_{t_i < t} K_1(t - t_i)$. For most synapses, such a simple description will not work. For example, the upper panel of figure 10.14 shows an unsuccessful attempt to fit the potential of an STG muscle fiber responding to a pair of spikes from a motor neuron by using a simple sum of this form. Processes such as synaptic facilitation and short-term depression cause the amplitude of the response to depend on the previous history of presynaptic firing. To describe postsynaptic responses (either PSCs or PSPs) accurately, we need a formalism that accounts for these history-dependent effects (Krausz and Friesen 1977; Magleby and Zengel 1975; Zengel and Magleby 1982; Sen et al. 1996). This can be done by introducing an amplitude factor that appropriately adjusts the magnitude of the single-spike response, K_1:

$$R(t) = \sum_{t_i < t} A(t_i) K_1(t - t_i). \tag{10.21}$$

The factor $A(t_i)$ scales the response evoked by a single spike at time t_i by an amount that depends on the timing of this spike relative to others in the train. For an isolated spike, or if no history dependence is present, A takes the value one.

We will begin by showing how the amplitude A can be modeled when only a moderate amount of a single form of either depression or facilitation is present. We will then discuss the changes that can be made to deal with more complex cases. A simple way to model the amplitude of the postsynaptic response to a presynaptic spike is to imagine that each spike modifies A but that between spikes A returns to its equilibrium value of one. The recovery process is modeled as exponential,

$$\tau_A \frac{dA}{dt} = 1 - A, \tag{10.22}$$

with a time constant τ_A fit to the particular case being studied. When a presynaptic spike occurs, A must be increased in the case of facilitation and decreased in the case of depression. This can be done in either an additive or a multiplicative manner. In other words, whenever a presynaptic spike occurs, we either make the replacement $A \to fA$ (multiplicative) or $A \to A + (f - 1)$ (additive). If $f > 1$ in either case, the amplitude grows corresponding to facilitation. If $f < 1$, the amplitude decreases, corresponding to depression. There is a strong theoretical reason to favor an additive description for facilitation and a multiplicative description for depression. We can uncover this reason by computing the steady-state amplitude for the response to a spike train firing at a steady rate r, which is

$$A_{\infty}(r) = \frac{1 + (f - 2) \exp(-1/r\tau_A)}{1 - \exp(-1/r\tau_A)} \tag{10.23}$$

in the additive case and

$$A_{\infty}(r) = \frac{1 - \exp(-1/r\tau_A)}{1 - f \exp(-1/r\tau_A)} \tag{10.24}$$

in the multiplicative. If $f < 1$, the amplitude for the additive case displays the awkward feature of becoming negative at high rates. For $f > 1$, the multiplicative amplitude displays the equally unrealistic feature of diverging at a finite rate. For these reasons, it is a good idea to use a multiplicative description for depression ($f < 1$) and an additive description for facilitation ($f > 1$).

In the case of an additive description of facilitation, a closed expression for the amplitude factor A can be derived by integrating the equations given above. Thus we can write

$$A(t) = 1 + S(t), \tag{10.25}$$

where

$$S(t) = \sum_{t_i < t} K_2(t - t_i) \tag{10.26}$$

and

$$K_2(t) = (f - 1)\exp(-t/\tau_A). \tag{10.27}$$

This integrated form, which is completely equivalent to the additive differential form given above, is convenient for determining the best values of f and τ_A from data (Sen et al. 1996). It also opens up the possibility of making modifications to improve the accuracy of the description. First, nothing restricts the function K_2 to being an exponential. Any function can be used and finding the optimal function is somewhat similar to finding the optimal filter for decoding spike trains of sensory neurons

(Bialek et al. 1991). Second, we can introduce a nonlinear dependence of the amplitude A on the sum S by writing

$$A = 1 + F(S), \tag{10.28}$$

rather than using eq. 10.25. We have found that the quality of the fit to high-frequency trains is improved by including such a nonlinear function (Sen et al. 1996). We have used this procedure to describe excitatory junctional currents (EJCs) in crab muscle fibers responding to motor neuron spike trains. The middle trace in figure 10.14 shows one such fit. In this case, the best fitting K_2 had $\tau_A = 2.7\,\text{sec}$, and the nonlinear function F was a quadratic polynomial. These functions are shown at the bottom of figure 10.14.

For many synapses, a number of different processes may affect the amplitude of the postsynaptic response. For example, recent measurements of layer-4 to layer-2/3 synapses in the primary visual cortex of rats (Abbott et al. 1997; Varela et al. 1997) revealed facilitation and two forms of depression acting at different time scales. Such multiple processes can be modeled by expressing the total postsynaptic response amplitude as the product of several separate amplitude factors, each described as above. Sometimes the fit can be improved by raising these individual factors to various powers so that the general expression (Zengel and Magleby 1982; Varela et al. 1997) is

$$A = A_1^{p_1} A_2^{p_2} A_3^{p_3} \cdots . \tag{10.29}$$

10.5.4 Study of a Reciprocally Inhibitory Oscillator

Reciprocal inhibition is important in the generation of many rhythmic motor patterns and appears to be the critical mechanism for providing circuit rhythmicity in some central pattern generators, such as the leech heartbeat system and the *Clione* swim system (Marder and Calabrese 1996). In motor systems, it was long assumed that reciprocal inhibition is a circuit design that only supports out of phase activity. However, recent theoretical work has shown that reciprocal inhibition can produce either synchrony or asynchrony, depending primarily on the relationship of the time course of the synaptic conductance relative to the time course of the depolarization (Wang and Rinzel 1992; Hansel, Mato, and Meunier 1993; van Vreeswijk, Abbott, and Ermentrout 1994). Figure 10.15 shows this phenomenon in dynamic clamp experiments using crab stomatogastric ganglion neurons (Sharp, Skinner, and Marder 1996). In these experiments, gastric mill (GM) neurons were used because they do not make synaptic connections between themselves or with other STG neurons.

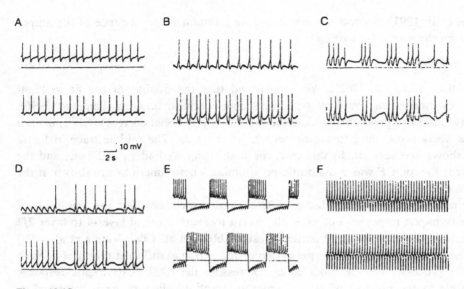

Figure 10.15
Reciprocal inhibition can produce a wide variety of circuit activity patterns. In all panels, two GM neurons of the crab STG were connected by mutual inhibition using the dynamic clamp. The horizontal lines indicate the threshold for transmitter release for the graded synaptic potential used. (A) The two cells fire almost synchronously because both are above the threshold for transmitter release and the continuous release produces an effectively slow synaptic potential. (B) The two cells fire somewhat differently, but in the same phase. (C) The two cells fire almost synchronous bursts. (D) Disjointed pattern of activity, with alternation between asynchrony and sychrony. (E) Stable alternations of bursting activity. (F) Stable pattern of single spike alternation. Further details can be found in Sharp, Skinner, and Marder 1996, from which this figure is reproduced.

Picrotoxin was applied to block most other synaptic connections within the ganglion. Under these conditions the GM neurons are essentially isolated. The dynamic clamp was then used to create artificial inhibitory connections between these neurons, and to apply additional I_H conductances. Figure 10.15 shows some of the different circuit activities that arose as the parameters controlling the synaptic potentials were modified. Note that stable alternating bursts of activity are only one of many different possible circuit outputs.

The dynamic clamp was used to determine how the oscillation period of the reciprocally inhibitory circuit depended on a variety of parameters including synaptic threshold, conductance and time course, as well as on the voltage dependence and maximal conductance of I_H (Sharp, Skinner, and Marder 1996). Not surprisingly, each of these parameters influenced the period of circuit oscillations. Most interesting are several parameter variations that produce nonmonotonic changes in the

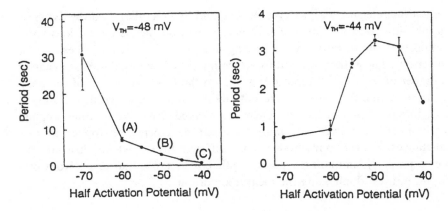

Figure 10.16
Period of a reciprocal oscillator is a function of the synaptic and intrinsic properties of the cells. An alternating oscillator (as in figure 10.15E) was formed by creating reciprocal inhibitory synapses between two GM neurons of the STG of the crab. With the threshold for synaptic transmitter release set at −48 mV, the half activation potential of a dynamic clamp added I_H current was moved from −70 mV to −40 mV. The left-hand plot shows the oscillation period as a function of this half activation potential. The right-hand plot shows the period with the threshold for synaptic transmitter release set at −44 mV. Note that changing the threshold for synaptic transmitter release alters the effect of changing the half activation potential of I_H. Modified from Sharp, Skinner, and Marder 1996.

oscillation period. The effects of altering the voltage dependence of I_H are shown in figure 10.16. When the threshold for synaptic release was −48 mV and the half activation potential of I_H was shifted in the depolarizing direction, the period decreased monotonically (figure 10.16, left). When the threshold for transmitter release was −44 mV, however, the same shift in the half activation of I_H had an entirely different effect on period (figure 10.16, right). Thus the modulation of one current may have an entirely different effect on a network, depending on the other currents relevant for network dynamics.

10.5.5 Other Examples of Simulated Synaptic Conductances

The dynamic clamp has been used in a number of other studies to explore the role of synaptic conductances in shaping network behavior. Robinson and Kawai (1993) independently developed a related approach and used it to introduce prerecorded sequences of synaptic conductances into neurons. Jaeger and Bower (1996) used the method to study the effects of balanced excitatory and inhibitory inputs to cerebellar Purkinje cells. Ulrich and Huguenard (1996) studied the role of $GABA_B$ synapses on burst firing of thalamic neurons by simulating $GABA_B$ mediated conductance changes. In another elegant study, Reyes, Rubel, and Spain (1996) used the dynamic clamp to apply simulated synaptic conductances to neurons in the the nucleus laminaris, an important site in birds for processing interaural time delays necessary for sound localization. The authors wished to determine the effect of changes in synaptic strength, number of inputs, and input firing rate on the firing frequency of the postsynaptic neurons. Synaptic currents were initially measured under voltage clamp as the stimulus intensity was increased. Then the evoked PSCs were either applied directly to the neurons as imposed synaptic current waveforms, or applied as synaptic conductances. These two methods yielded different results, which illustrates the importance of properly simulating a postsynaptic conductance that arises from presynaptic input, not just duplicating the measured current.

10.6   Neuromodulation of Central Pattern Generators

The stomatogastric ganglion is modulated by at least twenty different amines and peptides released by sensory and modulatory neurons that project into the STG (figure 10.17). Some of these modulatory projection neurons are known to be activated by sensory input (e.g., Meyrand, Simmers, and Moulins 1991, 1994), and it is presumed that all are activated at one time or another in various behavioral circumstances. Figure 10.18 demonstrates that these modulatory substances can profoundly alter the intrinsic properties of individual STG neurons and their synaptic interactions.

Modulatory substances can activate burst generating mechanisms in STG neurons, as illustrated by the response of an isolated AB neuron to the muscarinic agonist, pilocarpine (figure 10.18A). In this experiment, the AB neuron was silent in the control recordings, and the slow time base recordings demonstrate that the pilocarpine elicited oscillatory bursts in the AB neuron. Note that the amplitude and the frequency of the oscillation increased in a graded fashion during the pilocarpine application. Figure 10.18B illustrates that a modulatory substance can evoke plateau-generating mechanisms in neurons. In control saline, the dorsal gastric (DG) neuron only fired during depolarizations. In the presence of the peptide SDRNFLRFamide, however, short depolarizations evoked long-lasting plateau potentials that could be terminated by short hyperpolarizing current pulses. These plateau potentials will alter appreciably the responses of a neuron to synaptic inputs because they maintain a "memory" of the sign of prior synaptic input.

There are numerous examples of modulatory substances that alter synaptic strength (e.g., Dickinson, Mecsas, and Marder 1990; Johnson, Peck, and Harris-

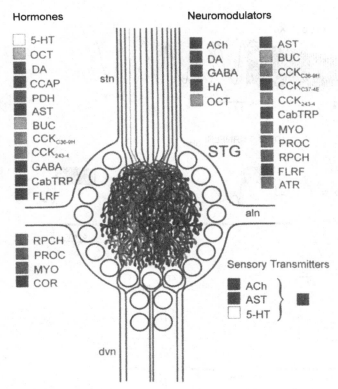

Figure 10.17
Neuromodulatory control of the STG of the crab *Cancer borealis*, as of the summer of 1996. A large number of substances are released into the circulation by neurosecretory structures and act hormonally to regulate the networks and neuromuscular junctions of the stomatogastric nervous system. Many of these same substances are found in modulatory projection fibers or peripheral sensory neurons that release these substances into the neuropil of the STG. See Christie, Skiebe, and Marder 1995 and Marder, Christie, and Kilman 1995 for abbreviations, references, and further details.

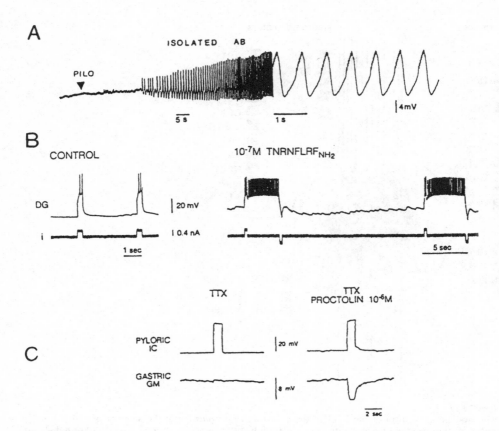

Figure 10.18
Modulators can alter intrinsic membrane properties and synaptic strength. (A) Intracellular recording
from an isolated AB neuron of the STG of the lobster *Panulirus interruptus*. At the downward arrowhead,
10^{-4} M pilocarpine (pilo) was added to the bath. Shortly thereafter, the AB neuron started to generate
slow bursts, which increased in amplitude and frequency. The faster time base recording at the right illustrates the bursts. Modified from Marder et al. 1987. (B) Intracellular recording from the DG neuron of
the crab *Cancer borealis*. Under control conditions a short depolarizing current pulse (i) elicited action
potentials only during the pulse. In the presence of 10^{-7} M TNRNFLRFamide, a short current pulse
evoked a plateau potential in which firing persisted until the plateau was terminated by a short pulse of
hyperpolarizing current. Modified from Weimann et al. 1993. (C) Simultaneous intracellular recordings
from the IC and GM neurons of the crab *C. borealis* in the presence of TTX to block spike-mediated
transmitter release. This allows the study of graded transmitter release between the neurons. Depolarization of the IC (left) evokes no synaptic potential in the GM neuron. In the presence of proctolin (right),
depolarization of the IC neuron evokes a large graded IPSP in the GM neuron. Modified from Marder et
al. 1997.

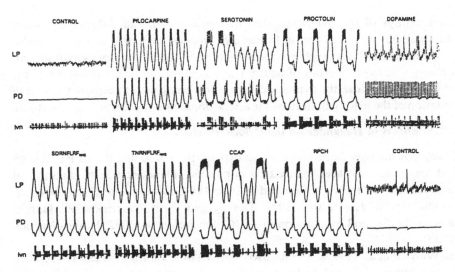

Figure 10.19
Multiple forms of the pyloric rhythm induced by different neuromodulatory substances in an isolated STG from the crab *Cancer borealis*. In all panels, the top trace is an intracellular recording from the lateral pyloric (LP) neuron, the second trace is an intracellular recording from the pyloric dilator (PD) neuron and the third trace is an extracellular recording from the *lvn*. The preparation was extensively washed between each modulator application and it returned to control levels of activity before each new application. Concentrations: pilocarpine, 10^{-5} M; serotonin, 10^{-4} M; proctolin, 10^{-6} M; dopamine, 10^{-6} M; SDRNFLRFamide, 10^{-7} M; TNRNFLRFamide, 10^{-7} M; CCAP, 10^{-6} M; RPCH, 10^{-6} M. Taken from Marder and Weimann 1992.

Warrick 1995). In some cases, these changes are relatively modest, while in others, modulation can be functionally equivalent to turning a synapse "off" and "on," as illustrated in figure 10.18C. In control saline, there is no evidence of a synaptic contact between the IC and GM neurons of the STG. In the presence of proctolin, however, depolarization of the IC neuron evokes a large IPSP in the GM neuron (Marder et al. 1997). This synapse is thus functionally part of the connectivity diagram only in the appropriate modulatory environment, and is functionally absent in other modulatory environments.

Abundant data (Hooper and Marder 1987; Flamm and Harris-Warrick 1986; Bal, Nagy, and Moulins 1994; Johnson, Peck, and Harris-Warrick 1995), such as that shown in figure 10.18, lead us to conclude that the connectivity diagram in figure 10.2 is a shorthand representation "standing in" for a large set of possible circuit configurations that can support a range of different outputs. Figure 10.19 shows that each of a number of different modulatory substances can alter the frequency and phase relationships of the pyloric rhythm in characteristic and different manners. Computational models must account for the dynamics of the circuit in a given modulatory environment and also explain how alterations in the modulatory environment, causing changes in the properties of neurons and synapses, modify the output of the circuit. As described below, the dynamic clamp is now being used to explore features of the modulation of the pyloric rhythm by the amine dopamine and the peptide proctolin.

10.6.1   The Effects of Dopamine on the Pyloric Rhythm

Several mechanisms have been proposed to explain the phase of LP and PY neuron firing and the phase advances induced by dopamine. These include modulation of PD neuron transmitter release (Eisen and Marder 1984; Johnson and Harris-Warrick 1990), modulation of I_A (Hartline 1979; Tierney and Harris-Warrick 1992; Harris-Warrick et al. 1995a) and modulation of I_H (Golowasch et al. 1992; Harris-Warrick et al. 1995b).

Harris-Warrick et al. (1995a, 1995b) used the dynamic clamp to assess the relative roles of modulation of I_A and I_H by dopamine in determining the postinhibitory rebound properties of LP neurons in response to hyperpolarization. In these experiments, the endogenous I_H was blocked by Cs^+, the dynamic clamp was used to add back I_H, and the latency to the first spike after a hyperpolarization was studied. The effects of altering the voltage dependence and inactivation rate of I_H were then examined. When the authors applied dopamine, they were able to assess the effects of its modulation of I_A with and without its effect on I_H (which was simulated with the dynamic clamp). These experiments explored the role of several currents in producing postinhibitory rebound after long, DC hyperpolarizations. It would be interesting to study the effects of modulating I_A and I_H in conjunction with simulated PD/AB synaptic currents to determine if the same results hold for physiologically realistic trajectories.

10.6.2   Dynamic Clamp Modeling of the Effects of Proctolin

When bath-applied to preparations that are either silent or slowly active, the peptide proctolin strongly activates the pyloric rhythm (figure 10.19). As a first step in understanding how proctolin affects the pyloric network, Hooper and Marder (1987) studied the actions of proctolin on each cell type individually. Proctolin increases the frequency and amplitude of the bursts in the isolated AB neuron and depolarizes the isolated LP neuron, causing it to fire tonically at high frequency. These data suggested that the activation of the AB neuron by proctolin could account for its ability to activate the pyloric rhythm, and that the effect of proctolin on the isolated LP neuron could explain the enhanced LP bursts evoked by proctolin in the ganglion.

Understanding the modulatory actions of proctolin on the pyloric rhythm required characterization of the proctolin-activated current. Proctolin evokes a nonspecific cation conductance that is maximal at membrane potentials close to the resting potential but decreases at hyperpolarized potentials due to a voltage-dependent block by extracellular Ca^{2+} (Golowasch and Marder 1992b). This current was modeled using conventional methods, and studied in the conductance-based model of the LP neuron described above. The model suggested that the proctolin-evoked current was sufficient to account for the effects of proctolin on the LP neuron (figure 10.3), although the impact of this result was somewhat compromised because, as with almost all conventional conductance-based models, some aspects of the model were necessarily fudged. This problem was overcome by using the dynamic clamp to add the modeled proctolin current to a real LP neuron simulating the effects of the endogenous peptide (Sharp 1994). The artificial proctolin current produced a depolarization and induced tonic firing that matched the effects of real proctolin.

The proctolin current has been characterized only in the LP neuron, but the AB neuron is an important additional target for proctolin action. We used the dynamic clamp to investigate whether the proctolin current measured in the LP neuron could account for the effects of proctolin on the AB neuron (Sharp et al. 1993b). As figure 10.20 illustrates, the voltage dependence of the proctolin current is critical for its action on the AB neuron. If the midpoint of the activation of the proctolin current is too hyperpolarized with respect to the AB neuron oscillation, the effect of the proctolin current is similar to that of the constant depolarizing current shown in figure 10.20 (right). This occurs because the neuron does not hyperpolarize to membrane

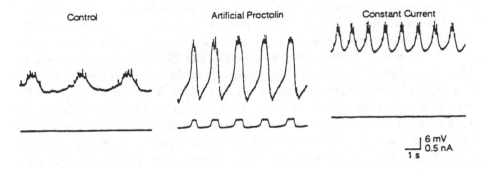

Figure 10.20
Effect of an artificial proctolin conductance on the AB neuron. The left-hand panel shows an intracellular recording from a crab AB neuron in control saline. The middle panel shows the effect of adding 20 nS of simulated proctolin current to the cell. The right-hand panel shows the very different effect of depolarization by a constant current. Modified from Sharp et al. 1993b.

potentials at which the proctolin current turns off. On the other hand, if the midpoint of the proctolin current activation curve is situated approximately at the midpoint of the AB neuron oscillation, the membrane potential swings of the AB oscillation take advantage of the voltage dependence of the proctolin current. This increases the amplitude and frequency of the AB oscillations, two essential features of the effects of real proctolin on the AB neuron.

Two important points are made by the dynamic clamp studies of the effects of the proctolin current on the AB neuron. First, proctolin evokes a small current when measured in the LP neuron. However, the voltage dependence of this small current, interacting with the voltage dependence of the other intrinsic currents of both the LP and the AB neurons, can produce significant changes in their activity. Second, the voltage dependence of the proctolin current must be properly matched to the voltage dependence of all of the other currents in the AB neuron, specifically those responsible for generating the slow wave oscillations. The dynamic clamp experiments on the AB neuron required that the voltage dependence of the proctolin current be adjusted individually for each AB neuron to ensure that it was within the envelope of the slow wave oscillations. This suggests that neurons may have mechanisms that allow them to regulate or tune the activation curves of their voltage-dependent currents.

Can the effects of proctolin on the intact pyloric network be explained by the proctolin-evoked current in the LP and AB neurons? To answer this question, Sharp (1994) compared the effects of bath application of proctolin at a variety of concentrations to the effects of adding the proctolin current to the LP neuron alone, to the AB neuron alone, and to both the AB and LP neurons (figure 10.21). In this experiment, the modulatory inputs to the STG were removed and, under control conditions, the preparation generated only a very weak and infrequent pyloric rhythm. Bath application of proctolin increased the frequency of the pyloric rhythm, and the number of LP action potentials in each burst in a dose-dependent manner (figure 10.21, left). When the dynamic clamp was used to add 20 nS of proctolin current to the AB neuron (figure 10.21, right), the amplitude of the AB oscillations increased significantly, but their frequency only increased slightly. When 20 nS of proctolin current was added to the LP neuron alone, it depolarized and fired tonically but no rhythmic bursting was produced. However, when 20 nS of proctolin current was applied to both the AB and LP neurons, a full pyloric rhythm was elicited. Interestingly, the frequency of the network rhythm was significantly greater than that seen when the proctolin current was added only to the AB neuron. Presumably, this occurred because the LP inhibition of the PD neurons (and thus indirectly of the AB neuron) causes them to burst earlier due to their postinhibitory rebound properties. Under these conditions, the frequency of the pyloric rhythm increased because of the action of the proctolin current on both the AB and LP neurons.

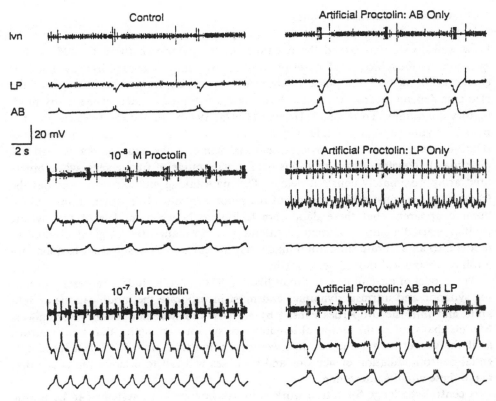

Figure 10.21
Effect of real and dynamic clamp applied proctolin on the pyloric network. Both panels show simultaneous extracellular recording from the *lvn* and intracellular recordings from the LP and AB neurons of the crab STG. The left plots show the control pyloric rhythm, the activity in 10^{-8} M proctolin and in 10^{-7} M proctolin. The right plots show a 20 nS proctolin conductance added with the dynamic clamp to the AB neuron alone, then 20 nS proctolin current added to the LP neuron alone, and, in the bottom panel, the effect of adding 20 nS of proctolin current to both the LP and AB neurons. Taken from Sharp 1994.

10.7   Current Problems and Issues

How well do we understand the dynamics of the pyloric rhythm? To address this question, we must have a full description of the dynamics of the pyloric rhythm. This entails knowing how the phase relationships and firing frequencies of each of the elements depend on frequency, and how these are altered in each of the many modulatory conditions. To this end, Hooper (1997a, 1997b) altered the frequency of the pyloric rhythm by current injection into the AB neuron and measured the phase relationships of each of the pyloric neurons. Some of the neurons maintained approximately constant phase relations over a wide range of frequencies, while others fired at approximately constant delays. This painstaking analysis now provides the framework for constraining models of the pyloric rhythm. It is worth noting that it became apparent that these data were lacking only when models of the pyloric rhythm started being constructed. Attempts to formalize the original qualitative model into an accurate simulation made that it clear that data sufficient to constrain a full mathematical model were lacking.

Any model of a small neural circuit like the STG must include a representation of the synaptic and intrinsic dynamics and must incorporate the modifications of synaptic and intrinsic properties caused by activity and neuromodulatory substances. Models that neglect the temporal dynamics of synaptic strengths, that treat neurons as if the slower membrane currents were not important, or that neglect the differential neuromodulation of neurons and synapses will fail to address the issues that make these circuits interesting.

A central challenge for future work is to ask how nervous systems can be plastic and susceptible to modulation and learning—and yet stable. There are so many biological mechanisms for short-, medium-, and long-term modulation, adaptation, and learning, that it is amazing that nervous systems manage to function stably for the lifetime of an organism. The next generation of models must not only explain the full range of network dynamics but also give us a deeper understanding of how such numerous plasticity mechanisms are balanced by mechanisms that ensure the fundamental stability of neural circuits.

Acknowledgments

We thank the many colleagues with whom we have worked on these topics. Our research was supported by the Sloan Center for Theoretical Neurobiology at Brandeis University, the W. M. Keck Foundation, the McKnight Foundation, National Institute of Mental Health grant MH-46742 and National Science Foundation grant DMS-95032.

11 Spatial and Temporal Processing in Central Auditory Networks

Shihab Shamma

11.1 Introduction

A fundamental organizational principle of the nervous system is that neurons are interconnected to form purposeful networks. This is especially relevant in higher animals, where nervous function depends primarily on the patterns of interconnections among large numbers of neurons rather than on elaborate specializations of individual neurons. Thus, to understand brain function, the focus of our investigations must expand from the detailed responses and structure of single cells to include unit responses to the activity of other cells, and how of these responses are distributed over a population of similar cells as well as across populations of different cell types.

Computational neurobiology plays a particularly critical role in the study of neural networks. In part, this is due to the lack of adequate experimental methods between the patch clamp, intracellular, and extracellular recordings appropriate to single cells, on the one hand, and the relatively coarse evoked potential recordings, EEGs, and 2-deoxyglucose labeling methods, on the other. The technology of multicellular recordings on a moderate scale is still at its infancy. Consequently, studies of neural networks have relied heavily on theoretical models to relate and explain experimental data derived from finer and coarser levels of experimentation.

Neural network models typically exhibit three distinct and equally important flavors: biological, algorithmic, and phenomenological (Marr 1982). All styles serve to relate relatively peripheral measures (e.g., environmental signals and outputs of sensory organs) to higher-level functions and percepts, thus providing varied descriptions of brain function. These approaches differ mainly in the overall objectives and constraints they assume. Thus, in the biologically oriented models, the goal most often is to provide a concise mathematical description relating directly to neurophysiological and anatomical data. In the phenomenological models, abstract and "black box" models of the network components are commonly used, and the emphasis shifts to descriptions of higher functions and psychophysical percepts, very often within a computational framework. Algorithmic formulations are intermediate in that computational structures replace "black boxes," but little or no attempt is made to relate them to the actual biological substrate.

In this chapter, we shall illustrate the interactions between the biological and algorithmic approaches in the study of neuronal processing in the mammalian auditory system, which consists of several parallel pathways, beginning at the hair cells of the inner ear, passing through up to six major nuclear subcortical groups, and ending at the auditory cortex. Considerable information has been gathered over the last two decades from the peripheral levels of the cochlea and the VIII (auditory) nerve, which gives a fairly accurate picture of the patterns of neural activity at the input of the auditory system (Young and Sachs 1979). Although at its "output," the system derives many perceptually important measures of the sound signal such as its spectrum and pitch (primarily monaural tasks, critical for speech and music perception) and its binaural attributes (important for sound localization and signal-in-noise enhancement), considerably less is known about the topology and function of the intermediate neural structures responsible for these transformations, despite the substantial body of anatomical and neurophysiological data available (Clarey, Barone, and Imig 1992; Webster 1992).

Therefore, in understanding auditory function, network modeling provides the pivotal link between signal and perception and will be demonstrated with regard to the spectral estimation and analysis problems in monaural audition. Specifically, we shall analyze critically how three different computational algorithms are motivated and implemented as neural network models so as to extract the acoustic spectrum at the early auditory stages. Later in the chapter, we shall illustrate how linear systems analysis methods can be used to model the function of primary auditory cortex. Many general themes and conclusions will emerge that also apply to the modeling of other sensory sytems. We first review some basic organizational principles of the mammalian auditory system. Three possible strategies for the central auditory processing of sound are then discussed in relation to their performance and the details of their neural network formulations. The details and results of simulating these networks are illustrated in section 11.5. We conclude with the cortical model and its implications in section 11.7.

11.2 The Mammalian Auditory System

An important function of the mammalian auditory system is to discriminate and recognize complex sounds based on their spectral composition. The basic underlying processing steps occur early in the auditory system at the cochlea of the inner ear (see schematic of figure 11.1). The pressure waves of an incoming sound signal cause vibrations of the tympanic membrane (eardrum) and ossicles of the middle ear, which in turn excite mechanical vibrations in the form of waves that travel along the length of the basilar membrane of the inner ear. Because of the unique spatially distributed geometry and mechanical properties of the basilar membrane, the traveling waves acquire distinctive properties that reflect the amplitudes and frequencies of the sound stimulus.

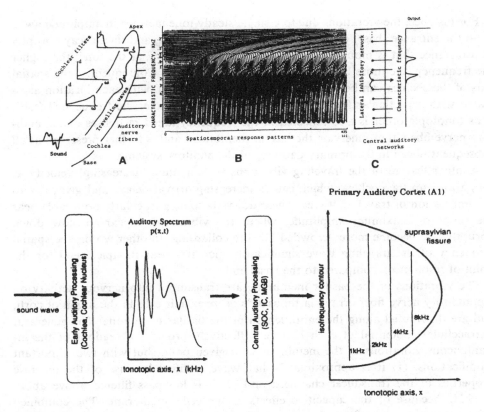

Figure 11.1

(Top) Schematic of early stages in monaural auditory processing. (a) Two-tone stimulus (600 Hz, 2,000 Hz) is analyzed by a detailed multistage biophysical model of the cochlea (Holmes and Cole 1984; Shamma et al. 1986). The responses are computed by a model composed of a bank of 128 filters, representing the effective transfer functions between the stimulus and the outputs at different cochlear locations. Schematic transfer functions, $d(\omega)$, of three such filters are shown in the figure. Note the shift in the "center frequency" of the filters from low frequencies (at the apex) to high frequencies (at the base). Each filter output is processed by a model of inner hair cell function (Shamma et al. 1986) and the response is interpreted as the instantaneous probability of firing of the auditory nerve fiber that innervates that location (Shamma 1985a). For frequencies below 3–4 kHz, the responses are phase-locked, that is, they approximately reflect the waveform of the underlying movement of the basilar membrane. For higher frequencies, only the amplitude of the membrane's displacements (i.e., proportional to the power output of the filter) is encoded. (b) Hair cell responses are organized spatially according to their tonotopic order. The characteristic frequency (CF) of each hair cell or fiber is indicated on the spatial axis of the responses. The resulting total spatiotemporal pattern of responses reflects the two-tone stimulus, with each tone dominating the activity of a different group of fibers along the tonotopic axis. (c) Neural networks of the central auditory system (e.g., the lateral inhibitory network) generate an estimate of the spectrum of the stimulus. (Bottom) Schematic of central stages in monaural auditory processing. Overview of the auditory nervous pathway includes cochlea, cochlear nucleus, superior olivary complex (SOC), lateral limniscus, inferior colliculus (IC), the medial geniculate body (MGB), and the tonotopically organized primary auditory cortex and other cortical fields.

For instance, the vibrations due to a single steady tone increase in amplitude away from the entrance (base) of the cochlea, reach a maximum, and then decay abruptly at a distance that is monotonically related to the frequency of the tone; the higher the frequency, the more basal is the location of the peak. Consequently, the spatial axis of the cochlea can be viewed as tonotopically ordered, with each location associated with a particular frequency, also called the "characteristic frequency" (CF). This tonotopic order is also reflected in the frequency-tuned responses of the auditory nerve fibers that innervate the basilar membrane, and is further preserved at all subsequent nuclei in the primary pathway of the auditory system.

Another feature of the traveling vibrations is their finite (decreasing) velocity as they travel up the cochlea, which causes increasing arrival delays and gives rise to the impression of traveling waves. These delays become particularly noticeable near the point of maximum amplitude, where the vibrations appear to slow down abruptly and become more "crowded" before collapsing. In other words, the spatial frequency of the traveling wave significantly increases near its apical end (or the point of resonance), compared to the basal end.

The vibrations of the basilar membrane are transduced into nervous activity on the auditory nerve fiber array via thousands of inner hair cells in the organ of corti, and are distributed along the entire length of the basilar membrane. The generator (intracellular) potential of each hair cell effectively provides a readout of the instantaneous vibrations of the membrane at a given point, but with two important modifications: (1) it is approximately half-wave rectified because of the intrinsic properties of the transducer channels; and (2) it is low-pass filtered above about 3–4 kHz because of the capacitive effects of the cell's membrane. The combined effect of these two transformations causes the higher frequency tones to produce only constant intracellular potential at their CF locations.

Figure 11.1 illustrates the spatiotemporal response patterns of an array of hair cells (128) in response to a two-tone stimulus (600 Hz, 2,000 Hz), computed using detailed biophysical models of basilar membrane and hair cell function (Holmes and Cole 1984; Shamma et al. 1986). The outputs are plotted as they would project onto the auditory nerve, that is, they are spatially organized according to their point of origin, and thus tonotopic order is preserved. The resulting responses display the fundamental properties of the basilar membrane traveling wave discussed earlier. In particular, note the (frequency-dependent) spatial segregation of the responses to the two tones, and the rapid changes (both in the amplitude and phase) of the response waves near the CF locations corresponding to the tones. The responses compare well with those recorded from a large population of cat auditory nerve fibers (Miller and Sachs 1983; Young and Sachs 1979), and reconstructed in the same format of the above figure (Shamma 1985a).

Each inner hair cell is connected to several independent and stochastically firing auditory nerve fibers that encode the intracellular potential by their instantaneous firing rates. Experimentally, a poststimulus histogram of many repetitions of a fiber's extracellular response record provides an approximate measure of the time course of the underlying hair cell potential.[1] Central auditory neurons, receiving inputs from several converging auditory nerve fibers (of approximately equal CFs), can also reproduce the hair cell potential by integrating the independent firing patterns. Therefore, the stochastic firing of auditory nerve fibers can be viewed primarily as a means for conveying hair cell potentials to the central auditory networks, rather than as an information-processing stage; and as such, modeling the synaptic transformations at the peripheral and central terminals of the nerve fiber array and the stochastic nature of their firings can often be bypassed in a first-order approximation. As we shall elaborate later, similar simplifications can be applied to the modeling of neuronal interactions in a network.

11.2.1 The Spectral Estimation Problem

The composition of the frequency spectrum of an acoustic stimulus is a primary cue for its identification. A basic issue in central auditory processing has been the question of how the system makes an estimate of this spectrum from the responses of the auditory nerve. In principle, there are two sources of information in the responses that can be utilized: spatial and temporal. The spatial aspect refers to the use of the response distribution along the tonotopic axis, while the temporal aspect refers to the information available in the synchronized (or phase-locked) components of the response. As we shall elaborate in sections 11.4 and 11.5, using one or both of these response properties has profound implications for the topology and characteristics of the central auditory networks presumed to estimate the spectrum. In the following sections, we shall illustrate the kind of considerations that arise in constructing different types of neural networks to implement three distinct algorithmic hypotheses for the spectral estimation problem: the mean rate (purely spatial) hypothesis, the periodicity (primarily temporal) hypothesis, and the spatiotemporal hypothesis. In each case, we shall first outline the specific computational algorithm, then make the appropriate models and approximations, and finally discuss the physiological relevence of the results.

11.2.2 The Spectral Analysis Problem

The spectral pattern extracted early in the auditory pathway (the cochlea and cochlear nucleus) is relayed to the auditory cortex through several stages of processing, which may include the superior olivery complex, nuclei of the lateral limniscus, the inferior colliculus (IC or ICC), and the medial geniculate body (MGB) (Webster 1992). The core of this pathway, passing through the central nucleus of the IC and the ventral division of the MGB, and ending in the primary auditory cortex (AI), remains strictly tonotopically organized, indicating the importance of this axis as an organizational feature. Unlike its essentially one-dimensional spread along the length of the cochlea, however, the tonotopic axis takes on an ordered two-dimensional structure in the AI forming arrays of neurons with similar CFs (called "isofrequency planes") across the cortical surface (figure 11.1; Merzenich, Knight and Roth 1975). Similarly organized areas (or auditory fields) surround the AI, possibly reflecting the functional segregation of different auditory tasks into the various auditory fields (Clarey, Barone, and Imig 1992; Irvine 1986; Reale and Imig 1980).

Within the AI, however, the creation of the isofrequency axis suggests that additional features of the auditory spectral pattern are perhaps explicitly analyzed and mapped out. Such an analysis occurs in the visual and other sensory systems and has been a powerful inspiration for the search for auditory analogues. For example, an image induces retinal response patterns that roughly preserve the form of the image or the outlines of its edges. This representation, however, becomes much more elaborate in the primary visual cortex (VI) and beyond, where edges with different orientations, asymmetry, and widths are extracted and neurally represented. Does this kind of an analysis of the spectral pattern occur in AI and other auditory fields?

This question is addressed in section 11.7, where we present a model representation of the spectral profile in AI. We then illustrate how a mathematical formulation of this model can be related to experimental data, and specifically how notions of linear systems theory can be used to define and interpret measurements of receptive field width, asymmetry, and CF location.

11.3 The Single-Neuron Model

The first and perhaps most critical step in modeling a neural network is the choice of its constituent neural elements. The level at which a single neuron is described mathematically (i.e., the amount of detail and the degree of abstraction) depends primarily on the nature of the application at hand. Thus, at one extreme, modeling a small circuit of morphologically and functionally different neurons may require significant detail to capture the characteristics of each neuron. At the other extreme, it may be advantageous to bypass the single-neuron model entirely, using instead a continuum model to describe the activity of a dense and homogenous neural tissue. Both levels are useful in modeling intermediate neural networks; gravitating toward one extreme or the other would then serve to highlight different aspects of the response or, as is often the case, to facilitate analytical treatments or computer simulations.

The basic single-neuron model we shall use, shown in figure 11.2a, is viewed as a processor with multiple, differently weighted inputs and a single output. In many cases, such a description should be considered merely "functional" and not necessarily corresponding to specific anatomical structures (e.g., dendrites and axons). Let $q_j(t)$ represent the train of spikes arriving from the jth neuron to the ith neuron. A single spike at time τ_k is modeled by a delta function, $\delta(t - \tau_k)$. The influence of this spike at the soma of the postsynaptic cell (i.e., the excitatory or inhibitory postsynaptic potential, EPSP or IPSP) is modeled by a linear time-invariant transformation with impulse response, $h_{ij}(t)$. Thus $h_{ij}(t)$ includes the efficacy, sign, and temporal properties of the synaptic response, the time constants of the cell membranes, and the effective spatial transformations due to dendritic branching and the location of the synapse relative to the cell body. Assuming that synaptic inputs do not interact with each other in any way and that they behave largely in a linear fashion, the overall intracellular potential due to N such inputs is given by

$$y_i(t) = \sum_{j=0}^{N} \int_{-\infty}^{t} h_j(v)q_j(t - v)\, dv = \sum_{j=0}^{N} h_{ij}(t) * q_j(t), \tag{11.1}$$

where $q_j(t) = \sum_k \delta(t - \tau_k)$, and $(*)$ denotes the convolution operation. This highly abstract and simplified description of synaptic interactions should not, of course, be viewed at the same level of detail as that involving, say, the physical nonlinear processes of transmitter release and conductance changes (see chapters 3 and 4, this volume). The impulse response $h_{ij}(t)$ is meant to embody the salient aspects of these processes at a purely phenomenological level.

We next assume that the instantaneous firing rate, $z_i(t)$, of the postsynaptic cell is a monotonically increasing function of the intracellular potential $y_i(t)$, with two important nonlinear deviations: saturation and threshold. The first, due to the refractory period of axonal firing, limits the maximum rates at which a neuron can fire (z_{max}). The second reflects the fact that the firing rate cannot be negative and that the production of an action potential requires a significant EPSP. One simple way to approximate this relation between $y_i(t)$ and $z_i(t)$ is given by the following sigmoidal function:

$$z_i(t) = g(y_i(t)) = \frac{z_{max}}{1 + e^{-b(y_i(t)-y_0)}}, \tag{11.2}$$

where b, y_0 are constants to be chosen appropriately to reflect the spontaneous firing of the cell and its maximum rate of change as a function of the input.

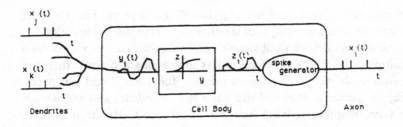

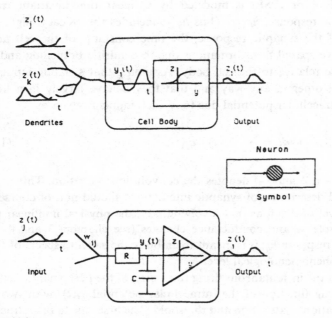

Figure 11.2
Models of a single neuron. (a) Model of a single neuron, using stochastic spike input and output descriptions. (b) Simplified version of the neuron model, using instantaneous firing rates as the input and output variables. (c) Minimal model of the single neuron using a simple first-order decription of the membrane impulse response, $h(t) = (1/\tau)e^{-(t/\tau)}$. The "neuron symbol" indicates the input and output ports and their directions.

Finally, an important simplification often used in network models concerns the description of the stochastic firing of the cells. The output of the ith neuron is a train of spikes $q_i(t)$ similar to those impinging on it, $q_j(t)$. A particularly useful idealization is to model the stochastic behavior of the neuron, $q_i(t)$, as a nonstationary point process (see note 1), with its instantaneous rate $z_i(t)$ given by $E(q_i(t))$, where $E(\cdot)$ denotes the expectation operator (Snyder 1975; chapter 9, this volume). Consequently, explicit references to the stochastic firings of all cells, $q_j(t)$, can now be eliminated if we redefine $y_i(t)$ as the ensemble mean of the instantaneous intracellular potential:

$$y_i(t) = E\left[\sum_{j=0}^{N} h_{ij}(t) * q_j(t)\right] = \sum_{j=0}^{N} h_{ij}(t) * E(q_j(t))$$

$$= \sum_{j=0}^{N} h_{ij}(t) * z_j(t), \tag{11.3}$$

where $h_{ij}(t)$ is assumed to be a deterministic function (see Sejnowski 1977 for more examples). Note that the interchange of the expectation, convolution, and summation is possible because of their linearity. The variables $y_i(t)$ and $z_i(t)$ can in principle be measured experimentally from poststimulus histograms of intracellular and extracellular records, respectively. The resulting simplified neuron model is shown in figure 11.2b.

The choice of the exact form of $h_{ij}(t)$ depends critically on the objectives of the modeling and the computational costs involved. For instance, if the details of the dendritic branching and function are important, then $h_{ij}(t)$ may take elaborate forms that reflect the effects of the spatial spread and attenuation of the potential from the synapse to the soma (Rall 1964; Segev et al. 1985; see also chapters 2 and 3, this volume). In other cases, such effects may be simplified to a scaling parameter that determines both the sign and efficacy of a typical synaptic "impulse response," that is, $h_{ij}(t) = w_{ij} \cdot h_o(t)$ for all i and j, where $h_o(t)$ models the temporal characteristics of a typical postsynaptic potential, and w_{ij} is a scalar that determines its sign (excitatory or inhibitory) and the overall strength of the connection between neurons i and j. Once again, $h_o(t)$ can take many forms depending on the amount of detail required, for example, $h_o(t) = (t/t_{peak})e^{-t/t_{peak}}$ (the so-called α function), $h_o(t) = (1/\tau)e^{-t/\tau}$ (a leaky integrator with time constant τ), or $h_o(t) = \delta(t - t_o)$ (a pure t_o time delay). In many situations, ignoring the entire temporal component of the responses, $h_o(t) = \delta(t)$, can lead to further simplifications and valuable insights into the role of the w_{ij} interconnection profiles in the network function.

We shall consider here the intermediate case of $h_o(t) = (1/\tau)e^{-t/\tau}$ as an example that can be extended or reduced to other forms. Substituting into eq. 11.3, we get

$$y_i(t) = \sum_{j=0}^{N} \dot{h}_{ij}(t) * z_j(t) = \sum_{j=0}^{N} w_{ij} \int_{-\infty}^{t} h_o(t-v)z_j(v)\, dv$$

$$= \sum_{j=0}^{N} w_{ij} \int_{-\infty}^{t} \frac{1}{\tau}\, e^{-(t-v/\tau)} z_j(v)\, dv. \tag{11.4}$$

Taking the time derivative, d/dt, of the above equation, a set of coupled, nonlinear, first-order differential equations results that describes the dependence of the intracellular potential of each neuron, $y_i(t)$, on the activities of all other neurons in the network (figure 11.2c):

$$\tau \frac{dy_i}{dt} + y_i = \sum_{j=0}^{N} w_{ij}z_j, \tag{11.5}$$

for all i, where the explicit dependence of $y_i(t)$ and $z_i(t)$ on time has been dropped for notational convenience. Furthermore, the influences of an array of external inputs $e_j(t)$, with synaptic weights v_{ij} onto neuron i, can be readily incorporated into the above equation to give

$$\tau \frac{dy_i}{dt} + y_i = \sum_{j=0}^{N} w_{ij}z_j + \sum_{j=0}^{M} v_{ij}e_j. \tag{11.6}$$

This equation can be written in many equivalent forms, for example, the vector notation in terms of $\mathbf{y}$;

$$\tau\dot{\mathbf{y}}(t) = \mathbf{W} \cdot g(\mathbf{y}(t)) + \mathbf{V} \cdot e(t) - \mathbf{y} = \mathbf{F}(\mathbf{y}, e; \mathbf{V}, \mathbf{W}, t), \tag{11.7}$$

where $\mathbf{g}(\mathbf{y}) = (g(y_0), g(y_1), \ldots, g(y_i), \ldots, g(y_N))^T$.

The neuronal model of eq. 11.6 can now be used to construct a variety of neuronal networks to perform a wide range of functions. The principal task that remains is the choice of the connectivities of the network, w_{ij} and v_{ij}, so as to achieve specific goals or to describe certain topologies. This process will be illustrated in the network implementation of three algorithms. The first two (section 11.4) derive their computational properties from the temporal characteristics of the constituent neural elements, rather than from the spatial patterns of interconnections among them (as in the case of the third algorithm; section 11.5).

11.4   Neural Networks for Spectral Estimation

In illustrating the two networks that perform the monaural spectral estimation task, the computational algorithm will be discussed first, then its neural network implementation, based on the single-neuron model derived above. Only the outlines of the method will be presented, with more emphasis placed on the general class of computations that the resulting neural network can perform.

11.4.1   The Mean Rate Hypothesis

According to this hypothesis, the spectrum of an acoustic stimulus is encoded in the spatial profile of the mean firing rates of the auditory nerve fibers. Thus the amplitude and frequency of a stimulus component is reflected by a relative increase in the average activity of a fiber population located at the appropriate characteristic frequency (CF) along the tonotopic axis. Such a profile essentially reflects the envelope of the basilar membrane vibrations (i.e., the amplitude) and ignores completely the fine structure of the traveling waves (i.e., the phase).

The computations a central auditory network needs to perform in order to estimate this profile are rather simple. For each fiber, a running average of the firing rate is estimated over a short time interval (typically, 10–20 msec), which is then plotted against the CF of the fiber (i.e., its location along the tonotopic axis). A simple network model to implement these computations would consist of a tonotopically organized array of neurons. Each neuron receives an excitatory input from a spatially restricted set of fibers, and integrates the activity with a membrane time constant of the order of a few milliseconds. Conceptually, there are no interconnections required in this network, and hence the neuron model of figue 11.2c and eq. 11.6 (with $v_{ij} = 0, w_{ij} = 0, i \neq j$) can readily perform this operation, given the appropriate values of τ.

Although the simplicity of such a "network" is appealing, there are several complications, most important among them being the dynamic range issue (a problem common to other sensory systems; Koch and Poggio 1987). In order for a neuron to encode the typical range of intensities seen in environmental sounds, the dynamic range of its response (between the threshold of response and its saturation) has to exceed 70–80 dB. The dynamic range of auditory nerve fiber responses rarely exceeds 30–40 dB (Sachs and Young 1979). Furthermore, experimental recordings (Sachs and Young 1979) show that at moderate sound levels, most fibers' responses are saturated and thus are incapable of encoding the relative height of the different frequency components in the signal.[2] Consequently, for such a network to be a viable scheme for central auditory processing, additional hypotheses are needed to resolve the dynamic range problem. These include the proposition that most information at moderate and high sound levels is encoded in the firings of unsaturated high-threshold fibers (less than 20%), or that the experimental data are an inaccurate reflection of the situation in the normally behaving animal.

11.4.2 The Periodicity Hypothesis: Neural Networks for Temporal Processing

In the second view of cochlear processing, the responses of the auditory nerve are presumed to encode the stimulus spectrum primarily through the temporal modulations of their instantaneous firing rates. Consequently, in order to derive the spectral estimate, the central auditory networks would have to process the detailed temporal structure of the nerve responses, rather than the simple average measures as in the above case. Although it has long been observed experimentally that the firing patterns of mammalian auditory nerve fibers can phase-lock to the temporal waveform of their input stimulus for frequencies up to 3–4 kHz, not until the series of experiments by Sachs and Young (Miller and Sachs 1983; Young and Sachs 1979) were the importance and richness of the temporal aspects of the nerve responses fully appreciated. In recordings from large populations of nerve fibers responding to speechlike stimuli, they demonstrated that the temporal structure of the responses can robustly encode the spectrum of the stimulus over large dynamic ranges and background noise levels. This work pushed to the forefront the questions of what type of computations are needed to exploit the temporal response patterns to derive the spectrum, and how they are to be implemented in the neural networks of the central nervous system.

Many computational algorithms have subsequently been suggested to tackle these questions (Delgutte 1984; Seneff 1984; Sinex and Geisler 1983; Young and Sachs 1979). Common to all of them is the use of some form of frequency analysis to measure the periodicities in the response waveforms, either explicitly through Fourier transform methods, or implicitly through computing autocorrelation functions in the time domain. Operating on the time history of the nerve firing rate, these algorithms need to store and to combine in various ways the response waveform over a finite interval. In order for such computations to occur in the nervous system, neural networks would have to exhibit precise series of time delays organized in a regular topology. Such delays might arise through systematic variations in the morphological features of the network neurons, for example, axons or dendrites with regularly changing lengths, diameters, or membrane time constants.

An Example of a Network Implementation Consider the "neural" implementation of a particularly simple example of such algorithms—called the "cosinusoidal comb filter." The algorithm presented here is similar to one proposed earlier by Young and Sachs (1979) and Delgutte (1984). The basic idea behind this scheme is to estimate the spectrum by measuring the degree of phase-locking exhibited by the synchronized responses of the fiber array to a bank of band-pass filters with center frequencies organized according to the CF of each fiber. The output of such a filter array would then reflect the spectrum of the input stimulus. A neural circuit that approximately achieves the band-pass transfer function of each filter is shown in figure 11.3a, where the central auditory neuron receives the responses of one fiber, and in addition a delayed version through a longer axon collateral or an excitatory interneuron. The exact amount of delay (τ_c) is critical and must be consistent with the CF of the input fiber, that is, $\tau_c = 1/(2\pi f_c)$, where f_c is the CF of the fiber. Using the neuron model of eq. 11.6, and assuming no interconnections among the central neurons ($w_{ij} = 0$) and no divergence in the inputs ($v_{ij} = 0, i \neq j$), the intracellular potential of the receiving cell is then given by

$$\tau \frac{dy_i}{dt} + y_i = e_i + e_i(t - \tau_c), \qquad (11.8)$$

for all i, where, to simplify, we have arbitrarily assumed unity input weights ($v_{ii} = 1$). Because eq. 11.8 is linear, it is particularly convenient to use the frequency domain to illustrate the transfer characteristics of the neuron. Taking the Fourier transform on both sides and collecting the resulting terms, we obtain

$$Y(\omega) = E(\omega) \cdot (1 + e^{-j\omega\tau_c}) \cdot \frac{1}{1 + j\omega\tau}, \qquad (11.9)$$

where $Y(\omega)$ and $E(\omega)$ are the transformed variables, and $\omega = 2\pi f$ is angular frequency. The output power spectrum is therefore given by (see figure 11.3b)

$$P_Y(\omega) = P_E(\omega) \cdot 2(1 + \cos(\omega\tau_c)) \cdot \frac{1}{1 + \omega^2\tau^2}. \qquad (11.10)$$

The input spectrum, P_E, is therefore modified by two terms in the above transfer function. The first is due to the delayed pathway (τ_c), which emphasizes the frequency components at f_c and its harmonics relative to other frequencies (thus the name "comb filter"). Note also that the input DC component ($\omega = 0$) is also retained in the output. The second term is the low-pass filter due to the time constant (τ) of the cell membranes. If $\omega_c \approx 1/\tau$, the low-pass filter will further attenuate the harmonics of f_c passed through by the first (comb) filter. Thus the remaining output signal $y(t)$ will reflect primarily the input fiber responses in the neigborhood of f_c,

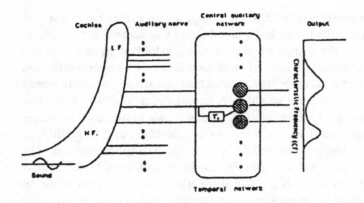

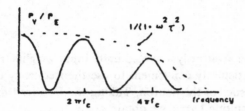

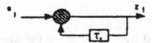

Figure 11.3
Schematic of the auditory processing stages according to the temporal processing hypothesis. (a) Non-recurrent network for measuring the periodicities of auditory nerve responses. Each central neuron receives as input the instantaneous firing rate of an auditory nerve fiber, and a second delayed version (τ_c delay). The amount of delay varies along the network and is equal to $1/CF$, where CF = characteristic frequency of the fiber. (b) Transfer function of each neuron in the temporal network. (c) Alternate recurrent implementation of the temporal network elements.

and a DC component that can be easily removed through such mechanisms as adaptation or self-inhibition. The final output, $z_i(t)$, is a compressed version of $y_i(t)$.

In this manner, a neural circuit can approximately perform frequency measurements, a fundamental operation in a large class of temporal algorithms (Seneff 1984; Sinex and Geisler 1983; Young and Sachs 1979). Furthermore, with minor modifications on the scheme outlined above, finer control can be achieved over many of the parameters of the filters, such as their band widths and sharpness (Delgutte 1984). It is also possible to show that somewhat different operations and connectivities can result in essentially equivalent transfer characteristics, for example, using multiplication (rather than addition) at the cell's input (Delgutte 1984), or substituting the delayed input with a delayed feedback from the output (figure 11.3c). The latter modification contrasts two basic arrangements of neural interactions that will be discussed in detail in section 11.5: the recurrent versus nonrecurrent topologies.

Finally, an important question that arises here concerns the biological feasibility of such neural circuits. To measure a range of frequencies, f_c, a corresponding range of delays, τ_c, needs to exist via regular changes in axonal lengths or membrane time constants along the tonotopic axis. The anatomical and physiological evidence in support of such models at present can only be found in the medial superior olivary (MSO) nucleus, a structure clearly involved in binaural processing and sound localization. Evidence of the existence of ordered neural delays along the major monaural pathway is at present weak. Furthermore, there are few examples of such arrangements from other mammalian sensory systems. This raises the real possibility that, despite the richness and robustness of the information carried in the temporal modulations of the auditory nerve responses, it may be irrelevant as far as the central auditory system is concerned. There is, therefore, a powerful incentive to formulate and test more biologically realistic algorithms that are capable of extracting the temporal cues.

11.5   Neural Networks for Spatial Processing: Lateral Inhibitory Networks

A simple alternative strategy for the central auditory processing of temporal cues emerges if we examine the detailed spatiotemporal structure of the responses of the auditory nerve. Such a natural view of the auditory nerve (and, indeed, of any other neural tissue) has been lacking primarily because of the immense technical difficulties in obtaining recordings from large populations of nerve cells. Figure 11.1b illustrates this view of the responses of the ordered array of auditory nerve fibers to a two-tone stimulus (600 Hz and 2,000 Hz). As mentioned earlier, each tone generates a traveling wave on the basilar membrane that synchronizes the responses of a different band of fibers along the tonotopic (spatial) axis. The responses reflect two fundamental properties of the traveling waves—namely, the abrupt decay of the amplitude and the rapid accumulation of phase lag near the point of resonance (Shamma 1985a).These features are in turn manifested in the spatiotemporal response patterns as edges or sharp discontinuities between the response regions phase-locked to different frequencies (figure 11.1a). Because the saliency and location of these edges along the spatial tonotopic axis are dependent on the amplitude and frequency of each stimulating tone, a spectral estimate of the underlying complex stimulus can be readily derived by detecting these edges, using algorithms such as those performed by the lateral inhibitory networks of the retina (Hartline 1974; Shamma 1985b).

As we shall elaborate below, the processing that a lateral inhibitory network performs is primarily spatial in character and therefore depends on the patterns of interconnections that exist among the network elements. To illustrate this and other aspects of the network operation, we shall review the analysis of models of two possible lateral inhibitory network topologies: recurrent and nonrecurrent (see figure 11.4).[3] These terms refer to the presence or absence of feedback from the neural outputs. Thus, in figure 11.4a, the inputs to the nonrecursive lateral inhibitory network $(e_i, i = 1 \ldots N)$ are combined to compute the final outputs $(z_i(t), i = 1 \ldots N)$ without any recurrent connections, that is, only feedforward computations are performed. Recurrent networks are shown in figure 11.4b, where the output of each neuron is fed back to the input of neighboring neurons. These two types of networks can serve equivalent functions, but may also diverge considerably depending on the strength and profile of the network interconnections.

11.5.1 Analysis of the Nonrecurrent Lateral Inhibitory Network

Using the neuron model of eq. 11.6, the nonrecurrent lateral inhibitory network can be described by the following system of linear equations:

$$\tau \frac{dy_i}{dt} + y_i = \sum_{j=0}^{N} v_{ij} e_j, \qquad\qquad (11.11)$$

for $i = 1 \ldots N$. To simplify the later comparison of this network with recurrent lateral inhibitory networks, we rewrite the matrix of input weights (v_{ij}) into two parts: the $v_{ii} = 1$ term, which represents the weight of the excitatory input that spatially coincides with neuron i, and the v_{ij} terms, which represent all other inhibitory input influences (see figure 11.4a):

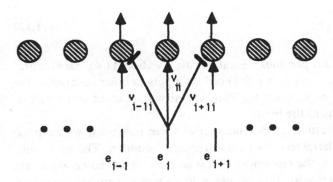

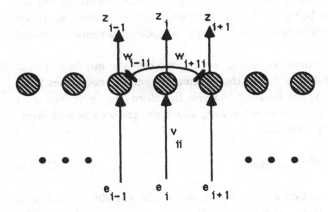

Figure 11.4
Two types of lateral inhibitory networks. (a) Nonrecurrent lateral inhibitory network. (b) Recurrent lateral inhibitory network. Excitatory and inhibitory "synapses" are indicated by arrows and bars, respectively.

$$\tau \frac{dy_i}{dt} + y_i = e_i - \sum_{j=0,\dots,N, j \neq i} v_{ij} e_j. \tag{11.12}$$

Note that here, unlike the two previous neural circuits (section 11.4), each neural output y_i (or, equivalently, $z_i = g(y_i)$) is influenced by inputs to other neurons in the network through the matrix of weights, v_{ij}. Thus the network output is a result of processing the spatial patterns of the input.

In order to gain better intuition of the function of these networks, we examine their input-output transfer characteristics in the frequency domain. The main simplifying assumption adopted in the remainder of this section is that the networks are either infinitely long or are circular, thus allowing us to ignore network boundary effects. The frequency domain analysis can be carried out using the network description discussed above as a system of discrete, coupled differential equations or, alternatively, using a continuum description of the network. While in the following, we shall adopt the continuum formalism along the spatial axis, it should be clear that the discrete analysis (corresponding to a sampled spatial axis) yields analogous formulas, the main difference being in the interpretation of the spatial variables as sampled functions, and their transforms as being periodic functions of spatial frequency.

To develop the continuous system equations, we assume that the number of neurons, N, is large and that the differences in the parameters and connectivities from one neuron, i, to another, $i + 1$, are small. A neuron therefore can be viewed as a member of a continuum—a large, densely packed, and homogeneous neural layer. The discrete equations (eq. 11.12) become

$$\tau \frac{dy(x, t)}{dt} + y(x, t) = e(x, t) - v(x) *_x e(x, t), \tag{11.13}$$

where x is the spatial (or tonotopic) axis of the network, the variables $y(x, t)$ and $e(x, t)$ become continuous functions of time as well as space, and $(*_x)$ denotes the spatial convolution between the input spatial pattern at time t and the profile of inhibitory connectivities, $v(x)$. We shall assume here that the network is homogeneous (i.e., that at any point x', a neuron "sees" the same weight profile, $v(x - x')$) around it, and that the spatial Fourier transform of $v(x)$ exists. Taking the Fourier transforms with respect to both the spatial and temporal axes, we obtain the transfer function of the network:

$$Y(\Omega, \omega) = E(\Omega, \omega) \cdot (1 - V(\Omega)) \cdot \frac{1}{1 + j\omega\tau}, \tag{11.14}$$

where Ω and ω represent the spatial and temporal frequency variables, and E and Y represent the transformed variables.

The above equations indicate that the input is modified by two separate terms. The first, $1 - V(\Omega)$, is purely spatial and is related to the Fourier transform of the input connectivity profile, $v(x)$. The second is purely temporal and reflects the low-pass filtering due to the cell membranes. Before discussing the properties of the network and illustrating the outputs that result from applying the spatiotemporal patterns of the auditory nerve to this network, we examine and compare the processing in its recurrent version.

11.5.2 Analysis of the Recurrent Lateral Inhibitory Network

The recurrent lateral inhibitory network (figure 11.4b) can be thought of as consisting of a single layer of neurons that are mutually inhibited, either directly through axon collaterals (i.e., the neurons are inhibitory), or indirectly through a second layer of inhibitory interneurons. We consider first a single-layer network of N inhibitory neurons. The dynamics can be described by the following set of equations:

$$\tau \frac{dy_i}{dt} + y_i = \sum_{j=0}^{N} v_{ij} e_j - \sum_{j=0}^{N} w_{ij} g(y_j), \tag{11.15}$$

where the w_{ij} values represent the inhibitory recurrent interconnections among the network elements. Due to the presence of the nonlinear function $g(\cdot)$, the above system of equations is nonlinear and thus has the potential for considerably more complex and interesting dynamics than the linear system of the nonrecursive lateral inhibitory network above. To compare the two networks, we consider first the linear behavior of this lateral inhibitory network around a steady-state potential y_i^* and input e_i^*, where (from eq. 11.15)

$$y_i^* = \sum_{j=0}^{N} v_{ij} e_j^* - \sum_{j=0}^{N} w_{ij} g(y_j^*).$$

Let $y_i = y_i^* + \tilde{y}_i$ and $e_i = e_i^* + \tilde{e}_i$, where $\tilde{y}_i$ and $\tilde{e}_i$ are small-signal fluctuations around the steady states, then

$$\tau \frac{d\tilde{y}_i}{dt} + \tilde{y}_i = \tilde{e}_i - \sum_{j=0}^{N} w_{ij} \tilde{y}_j, \tag{11.16}$$

where the slope of $g(\cdot)$ around y^* has been absorbed in w_{ij}, and we have assumed that each neuron is driven externally only by its coincident input, that is, $v_{ij} = 0$, for $i \neq j$, and $v_{ii} = 1$.

These equations can be written in the continuum form as before:

$$\tau \frac{d\tilde{y}(x,t)}{dt} + \tilde{y}(x,t) = \tilde{e}(x,t) - w(x) *_x \tilde{y}(x,t), \tag{11.17}$$

with the same assumptions as in the nonrecurrent case applying to $w(x)$ and its Fourier transform. Taking the spatial and temporal Fourier transforms, we obtain

$$\tilde{Y}(\Omega,\omega) = \tilde{E}(\Omega,\omega) \cdot \frac{1}{1 + j\omega\tau + W(\Omega)}, \tag{11.18}$$

where $\tilde{Y}$, $\tilde{E}$, and W are the transformed variables.

11.5.3 Spatial Processing with the Lateral Inhibitory Network: Edge Detection and Peak Selection

Eqs. 11.14 and 11.18 represent the linear transfer characteristics of the two lateral inhibitory networks. We concentrate first on the spatial transformations that these networks apply to their input patterns, that is, we assume that the temporal variations of the input are slow relative to the time constant of the network (τ). To compare the two networks directly, we consider identical profiles of inhibitory connectivities, that is, $w_{ij} = v_{ij}$ (and hence $W(\Omega) = V(\Omega)$). Then eqs. 11.14 and 11.18 become

$$\tilde{Y}(\Omega,0) = \tilde{E}(\Omega,0) \cdot (1 - W(\Omega)),$$

for the nonrecurrent network, and

$$\tilde{Y}(\Omega,0) = \tilde{E}(\Omega,0) \cdot \frac{1}{1 + W(\Omega)},$$

for the recurrent network.

For small $W(\Omega)$, the latter equation can be expanded and approximated by the nonrecurrent equation, which suggests that the two networks can perform essentially similar functions in the spatial domain (in the case of weak recurrent connections). To understand how the profile of connectivities, $W(\Omega)$, is chosen, we recall that the lateral inhibitory network was initially invoked to detect the "edges" created by the rapid amplitude and phase changes of the traveling waves. These edge regions are (by definition) regions of rapid change that exhibit high spatial frequencies, Ω, compared to the flat (low spatial frequency) regions in between. Consequently, to enhance these edges and thus sharpen the input patterns, the network transfer function, $\frac{\tilde{Y}}{E}(\Omega, 0)$, should have spatial high-pass transfer characteristics, as illustrated in figure 11.5b. Figure 11.5a illustrates the profiles of inhibitory connections, $w(x)$, needed for both lateral inhibitory networks, and the way the strength of these connections falls off gradually with distance. For either network, the patterns of connectivity can be simply described as follows: each neuron requires a central excitatory input and an inhibitory surround. In the recursive lateral inhibitory network, the inhibition is derived from the outputs of surrounding neurons, whereas in the nonrecurrent case, it is derived from the inputs to surrounding neurons. The exact shape (strength or spread) of the $w(x)$ profile determines the effectiveness of the lateral inhibitory network in sharpening the input profiles. For instance, a narrow $w(x)$ generally allows only the highest spatial frequencies to pass; similarly, a stronger $w(x)$ further attenuates the lower spatial frequencies.

A major difference between the two networks concerns their stability properties. Unlike the nonrecurrent network, which is always stable, the recurrent lateral inhibitory network may become unstable for certain $w(x)$ profiles. Specifically, when $W(\Omega) = -1$, the denominator of eq. 11.18 is equal to zero, and the output is ill defined. This occurs generally when the self-inhibition of each neuron of the network is small compared to the mutual inhibition.[4] The linear model of the lateral inhibitory network cannot serve a useful purpose when it becomes unstable. If, on the other hand, the nonlinearities of threshold and saturation are retained in the model (eq. 11.15), then it can be shown that the instability leads to hysteresis phenomena, to the generation of spatial periodic patterns, and to other interesting and complex phenomena that may serve as models of various perceptual experiences (Ermentrout and Cowan 1980; Morishita and Yajima 1972).

One particularly useful function that the nonlinear lateral inhibitory network can serve is in local or global peak selection—also known as the "winner-take-all" function. It is easy to see intuitively how the pattern sharpening of the linear network gives way with increasing inhibition to the all-or-none outputs of the nonlinear network, as illustrated schematically in figure 11.5 (bottom). Consider first the situation where each neuron in the network inhibits equally all other neurons, but not itself (i.e., in eq. 11.15, let $w_{ij} = w$, for $i \neq j$ and $w_{ii} = 0$). For small w, the inhibition is weak enough that no neuron is shut off or saturated, and the network sharpens the input according to the linear analysis discussed above. With stronger inhibition, neurons representing the output activity due to the valleys of the input pattern become more suppressed and only neurons driven by the peaks of the input pattern continue to fire. At the strongest inhibition, only one neuron can survive—that representing the largest peak of the pattern—while all others are suppressed. In effect, the lateral inhibitory network has selected the largest peak in the entire input pattern

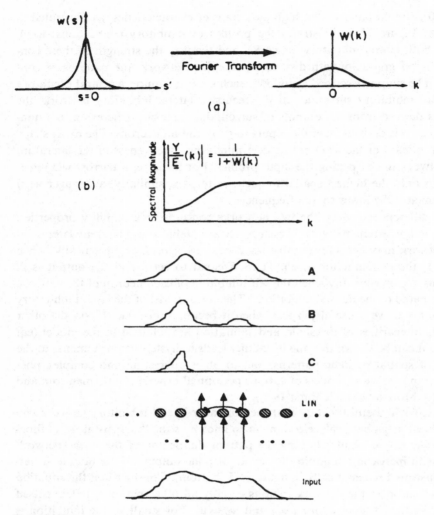

Figure 11.5
(Top) Transfer characteristics of the linear lateral inhibitory networks. (a) The profile of inhibitory connectivities and its spatial Fourier transform. (b) The spatial transfer function of the linear recurrent lateral inhibitory network. (Bottom) The winner-take-all function of the nonlinear lateral inhibitory networks. Progressive sharpening of the output patterns occurs with increasing lateral inhibition (from panel A to panel C).

(the global peak) and signaled its location by the activity of the appropriate neuron. The lateral inhibitory network can perform the same function locally if the inhibitory profile, w_{ij}, is spatially limited (e.g., $w_{ij} = w$, for $|i - j| \leq c$, and $w_{ii} = 0$). In this case, the same peak selection (or suppression) is observed for peaks that are less than c neurons apart (Sellami 1988). Such processing is valuable in simulating the feature extraction and recognition of contaminated input patterns.

From a biological point of view, both types of lateral inhibitor networks appear feasible. The recurrent lateral inhibitory network was first found in the compound eye of the horseshoe crab, *Limulus* (Hartline 1974). Extensive elegant experiments and theoretical studies of this network (Hartline 1974) have demonstrated its role in sharpening visual images by highlighting their spatial edges and peaks and by detecting and emphasizing their temporal changes. The ON-center/OFF-surround responses of the retinas of many animals can be seen as functionally equivalent to the lateral inhibitory network in *Limulus*, although they may exhibit additional more complex responses. Nonrecurrent lateral inhibition can be mediated via many possible anatomical arrangements, for example, inhibitory interneurons or dendrodendritic synapses. Indeed, a combination of these two possibilities has been found in the olfactory bulb (Rall 1970).

11.5.4 Temporal Processing with Lateral Inhibitory Network: Onset Sharpening and Oscillations

In the nonrecurrent (feedforward) lateral inhibitory network, the processing of the temporal fluctuations of the input pattern is decoupled from the spatial component and consists of simple low-pass filtering, as seen in eq. 11.14. In the recurrent network, the processing of the spatial and temporal components is closely coupled. This becomes more apparent if we rewrite eq. 11.18 as

$$\tilde{Y}(\Omega, \omega) = \tilde{E}(\Omega, \omega) \cdot \frac{1}{(1 + j\omega\tau_{eff})} \cdot \frac{1}{(1 + W(\Omega))}, \tag{11.19}$$

where $\tau_{eff} = \tau/(1 + W(\Omega))$ is now the effective time constant of the low-pass filter represented by the first term of the transfer function. The value of τ_{eff} depends on the value of $W(\Omega)$; thus, for higher spatial frequencies, $W(\Omega) \rightarrow 0$ (see figure 11.5), the time constant increases and the output is attenuated at lower temporal frequencies. This can be understood intuitively by observing that for the recurrent inhibition to be effective, sufficient time is required for it to be fed back. For fast-changing inputs, the inhibition may not keep up, and thus the sharpening of the instantaneous input patterns may deteriorate significantly. For the processing of auditory nerve response periodicities of $\approx 1\text{--}2\,\text{kHz}$, the lateral inhibitory network should act with time constants (τ) of the order of 0.1–0.2 msec. Note that although the single-layer lateral inhibitory network is first-order with respect to time, it is still capable of simulating periodic oscillatory phenomena if, for example, asymmetrical inhibitory profiles of connectivities are used.[5]

11.5.5   Processing with More Elaborate Lateral Inhibitory Network Models

The above linear analysis of the lateral inhibitory network can be extended to many more complex situations and topologies. The most common is the double-layer lateral inhibitory network, where the inhibition among the excitatory cells of the first layer is mediated by inhibitory interneurons of a second layer (see Cannon, Robinson, and Shamma 1983; Morishita and Yajima 1972). In this case, a system of second-order nonlinear differential equations results that can be used to simulate damped or periodic oscillatory responses. More elaborate single-neuron models can also be used to account for such higher-order properties as adaptation (Stein et al. 1974), axonal transmission delays (Oguztoreli 1979), shunting inhibition (Grossberg 1976), and dendritic processing (Poggio, Torre, and Koch 1985; Rall 1964; Segev et al. 1985). For instance, if we assume that recurrent inhibition exhibits an absolute transmission delay, τ_a, from one neuron to another, then eq. 11.17 becomes

$$\tau \frac{d\tilde{y}(x,t)}{dt} + \tilde{y}(x,t) = \tilde{e}(x,t) - w(x) *_x \tilde{y}(x, t - \tau_a), \tag{11.20}$$

with the spatial and temporal Fourier transforms given by

$$\tilde{Y}(\Omega, \omega) = \tilde{E}(\Omega, \omega) \cdot \frac{1}{1 + j\omega\tau - W(\Omega)e^{-j\omega\tau_a}}. \tag{11.21}$$

This lateral inhibitory network is capable of simulating considerably richer modes of temporal processing.

Introducing these or other details into the lateral inhibitory network models is often accompanied by heavy computational costs and stability problems. Therefore, it is best to use initially the simplest minimal model, and to modify its structure gradually when secondary details are necessary. Clearly, the choice of the minimal model is closely tied to the objectives of the problem. For instance, because including the temporal components would introduce "predictable" effects in the responses and significantly increase the complexity of the simulations, we shall sometimes forgo computation of the temporal dynamics of the responses of the nonlinear lateral inhibitory network in order to highlight the network's peak selection property.

11.5.6 Other Formulations for Early Auditory Processing

The neural models discussed thus far are intermediate in their biological details in that they attempt to describe discrete "neuronal entities" and employ variables that can be approximately identified with membrane potentials or firing rates, but do not take into account specific structural details of any particular neuron. Often, more abstract descriptions derived from these models are mathematically more tractable and lend more insight into the functional significance of the processing stages. For instance, lateral inhibitory networks detect or enhance edges and peaks in their input patterns, a "function" that is equivalently accomplished by a first- (or higher-) order derivative operation with respect to the tonotopic axis of the input pattern. Similarly, detailed models of cochlear mechanics and the biophysics of the inner hair cells can be reduced to a succession of simple stages which include linear filtering of the sound signal followed by a compressive nonlinearity with high gain (or a limited dynamic range) (Yang, Wang, and Shamma 1992). Combining these stages turns out to produce an effective and simple model can be used to clarify the roles played by different stages of the auditory periphery in the spectral estimation problem, and to analyze the relationship between the lateral inhibitory network (LIN) and other estimation algorithms. (For detailed reviews of these model formulations and their analyses, see Lyon and Shamma 1996 and Yang, Wang, and Shamma 1992.) Further abstraction of the discussed models employing stochastic formulations has proven invaluable in explaining the origin of noise robustness and of the enhancement of perceptually significant features of the extracted auditory spectrum (Wang and Shamma 1994). These findings have potentially profound implications and benefits in many engineering systems such as in the design of front-end stages in automatic speech recognition systems.

11.6 Implementations of Lateral Inhibitory Networks

We now consider the issues that arise in simulating two examples of the lateral inhibitory network models: a linear nonrecurrent and a nonlinear recurrent lateral inhibitory network. The first lateral inhibitory network, **LIN.I**, processes the auditory nerve responses directly to generate an estimate of the acoustic spectrum; the second lateral inhibitory network, **LIN.II**, selects and thus highlights the local peaks of the **LIN.I** outputs. In both cases, the discrete rather than the continuous version of the models are simulated (eqs. 11.12 and 11.15).

In general, simulations of linear networks or transfer functions are considerably faster than their nonlinear counterparts, mostly because of the availability of analytical solutions or fast algorithms to perform the forward and inverse Fourier transforms (so-called fast Fourier transforms—FFTs; Oppenheim and Schafer 1976). When analytical solutions are not available, numerical methods to integrate the differential equations can be used, which are almost always computationally very expensive in a moderate system of tens of neurons. Several computational packages are available, ranging from standard integration routines (e.g., the well-known DGEAR) to circuit simulation programs that compute various input-output transfer characteristics of the equivalent electrical circuit diagram of the network (e.g., NEURON or GENESIS; see chapter 3, this volume, for more details).

11.6.1   Simulating Nonrecurrent Lateral Inhibitory Networks

As discussed in section 11.5, an estimate of the acoustic spectrum can be extracted from the responses of the auditory nerve by detecting the peaks and edges created by the traveling wave patterns due to the different components of the stimulus. To demonstrate this, the response patterns of the two-tone stimulus shown in figure 11.1 and the spoken word "magnanimous" of figure 11.6 were applied to the nonrecurrent lateral inhibitory network model of eq. 11.12. Although recurrent lateral inhibitory network topologies can also be used, this lateral inhibitory network was chosen both for biological and computational reasons:

1. Because the edges of the auditory nerve responses are created by phase or frequency mismatches between the response waveforms of neighboring fibers that are synchronized to relatively high frequencies (up to 2–3 kHz), it is essential that the

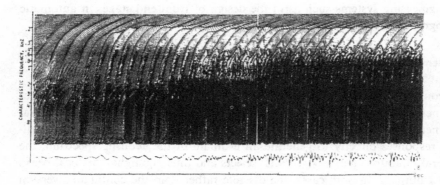

Figure 11.6
Auditory processing of cochlear outputs: spatiotemporal outputs of the spoken word /magnanimous/ processed using the cochlear model described in figure 11.1. Only responses to the initial part of the word are shown (i.e., the segment /ma/), together with the input waveform fed into the model.

network cells have fast inhibitory time constants (≈ 0.1–0.2 msec) so as to detect and sharpen these edges. Recurrent inhibition is likely to be slow compared to non-recurrent inhibitory dendrodendritic synapses.

2. The nonrecurrent lateral inhibitory network can be simulated rapidly. If we assume that the time constant of the lateral inhibitory network neurons (τ) is small relative to the uppermost frequency of phase-locking on the auditory nerve, eq. 11.12 simplifies further to

$$y_i = e_i - \sum_{j=0,\dots,N; j \neq i} v_{ij} e_j, \qquad (11.22)$$

where v_{ij} is the profile of inhibition around the ith neuron. The remaining action of this lateral inhibitory network is therefore intuitively simple and computationally fast: to compute the output trace at the ith location, y_i, subtract from the ith input trace, e_i, a weighted sum of its neighbors.

There remain two important parameters to be determined before such a simulation can be run: the number of inhibitory neurons, N, and the exact inhibitory profile, v_{ij}. The number of neurons in this network was determined by the prior choice of 128 as the number of auditory nerve fibers. For different applications, this number varies depending on the desired spatial resolution of the input patterns. Using a 128-neuron network here and in other later simulations places a high premium on using the simplest and computationally most efficient network realizations. The choice of the inhibitory profile, v_{ij}, is not critical provided that its spatial extent reflects the slopes and the spatial resolution of the edges and peaks to be detected in the input patterns. In the auditory system, the spatial resolution of the different, simultaneously presented frequency components is on the order of one-third of an octave, that is, a spatial distance on the tonotopic axis of the network layer of approximately six neurons. The v_{ij} profile was thus chosen to be symmetrical, five coefficients long (two on either side of the central excitatory unit input), and with values that produce zero outputs for a locally flat input (e.g., the profile used for the computations of the output in figure 11.1c and figure 11.7a is $+0.25$, -0.75, 0, -0.75, $+0.25$, with $v_{ii} = 1$). Finally, the resulting trace from each neuron, $y_i(t)$, is rectified to generate the output $z_i(t) = g(y_i(t))$. For plotting purposes, this output is averaged with a relatively long moving window (e.g., 10 msec, every 3 msec),[6] and the entire array is then displayed in one of two ways: (1) in the case of stationary signals where the location of the edges does not change with time (e.g., the two steady tones of figure 11.1b), only one cross section is plotted; (2) for nonstationary stimuli, where the stimulus spectrum (and hence the edge and peak locations)

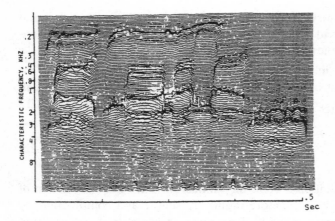

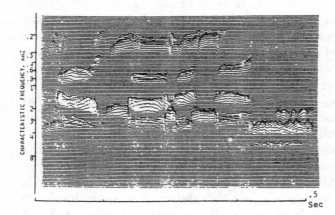

Figure 11.7
Auditory processing of cochlear outputs. (a) Output patterns generated by the LIN.I nonrecurrent network. The peaks represent perceptually significant features of the stimulus spectrum. Note the change in these features with time corresponding to the different phonemes. (b) Further sharpening of the LIN.I outputs using the recurrent LIN.II network.

changes with time, the entire averaged spatiotemporal output is plotted (see figure 11.7a).

In either case, the outputs clearly mark the locations and saliency of the edges of the input auditory nerve patterns, which in turn represent the main spectral components of the acoustic stimulus. In this manner, the auditory system can easily generate an estimate of the stimulus spectrum without recourse to Fourier analysis or other temporal correlation schemes (see section 11.4.2).

11.6.2 Simulating Nonlinear Recurrent Lateral Inhibitory Networks

The recurrent lateral inhibitory network model is used here to further sharpen the spectral peaks generated by the **LIN.I** (see figure 11.7a). The network performs this function by implementing a winner-take-all strategy over local regions of the input pattern. The exact behavior of the network is primarily determined by the parameters of the inhibitory profile, w_{ij}. Specifically, the strength (magnitude) of the weights controls the amount of suppression the winning peak applies to the rest of the network, while the width of the profile determines the resolution of the selected peaks (or the extent of the local regions).

Because the nonlinearities of neuronal transmission play a critical role in mediating the function of this network, the simplest equations we can use are those of eq. 11.15. A fundamental difference between these equations and those of **LIN.I** (e.g., eq. 11.12) is that, in the recurrent case, the computations of all neuron outputs has to proceed in parallel because the value of $y_i(t)$ depends on the concurrent outputs, $y_j(t)$, of other neurons, whereas the computation of $y_i(t)$ in the feedforward **LIN.I** topology depends only on present and past inputs and not on the outputs of the other neurons, $y_j(t)$. Therefore, in solving eq. 11.15, the whole system has to be integrated simultaneously, which is computationally very expensive. One way to simplify the task is to ignore the settling behavior (the dynamics) of the network, and instead to compute the equilibrium states achieved by the network for each input pattern, that is, to find all the $y_i(t)$, for $i = 0 \cdots N$, that satisfy the following equations:

$$y_i = \sum_{j=0}^{N} v_{ij} e_j - \sum_{j=0}^{N} w_{ij} g(y_j) \qquad (11.23)$$

or, equivalently, in terms of $z_i = g(y_i)$:

$$z_i = g \left(\sum_{j=0}^{N} v_{ij} e_j - \sum_{j=0}^{N} w_{ij} z_j \right) \qquad (11.24)$$

These equations are solved for each new input pattern $\mathbf{e}(t)$.

An easy way to perform these calculations is to initiate first the **z** vector, then compute a new value using the right side of eq. 11.24, and finally iterate until a fixed point of the mapping is achieved (**z***). The iteration can be done in one of two ways: synchronously, where the entire vector **z** is updated at each iteration; or asynchronously, where only one element of the vector is randomly chosen and updated at each iteration. In either case, the iterations are stopped when the updated vectors cease changing. This process is then repeated for each new input vector.

Two complicating factors have to be considered when performing the above computations: hysteresis and limit cycles. An inherent property of the winner-take-all function of the recurrent lateral inhibitory network (Morishita and Yajima 1972), hysteresis is manifested in eq. 11.24 by the fact that for a given input pattern, e, different initial states may lead to different final outputs **z***. The hysteresis property may or may not be desirable, depending on the details of the task modeled. Limit cycles occur in the network iterations in rare circumstances, mostly when using the synchronous method of updating the vectors. In these situations, the updated vector usually oscillates between two states (rarely longer cycles).

An example of the recursive network output is shown in figure 11.7b, where the output of **LIN.I** was applied to the network as described by eq. 11.15, with network connectivities w_{ij} given by the following symmetric inhibitory profile: 0 (midpoint), 0.02, 0.05, 0.1, 0.15, 0.2, 0.25, 0.25, 0.2, 0.15, 0.1, 0.05, and its reflection. All other $w_{ij} = 0$; $v_{ij} = 0$, for $i \neq j$, and $v_{ii} = 1$. There are two important regions in the inhibitory profile: the central "weakly coupled" region, and the strongly inhibitory surround. The width of the central region was chosen so as to allow the selected output peaks to be approximately equal to the typical width of the input peaks. The width and strength of the inhibitory surround were chosen such that a selected winner output peak suppresses the peaks and activity of all neighboring neurons (within ≈ 20 neurons). All computations were performed using the asynchronous updating method, and the output evaluated for each input profile, starting at zero output initial conditions. It should be emphasized that, in principle, the recursive network could have been applied directly to the spatiotemporal patterns of the cochlea (figure 11.6) with similar results. Because the **LIN.II** simulations are computationally expensive compared to those of **LIN.I**, however, it is much more effective to use first the **LIN.I** to process the cochlear outputs and thus reduce the sampling rate of the patterns from the 20,000 patterns/sec at the **LIN.I** input, to the 200 patterns/sec at their output. Performing the **LIN.II** computations on 20,000 patterns directly is computationally not practical.

11.6.3 Summary of the Lateral Inhibitory Network Processing of Auditory Patterns

In vision, as in the somatosensory system, the traditional role of the lateral inhibitory network has been to detect and highlight the edges and peaks in the spatial patterns defined by the mean firing rates of the sensory epithelium. This is exactly the case in the auditory system for sound stimuli where no phase-locking is present, such as for high-frequency stimuli (>4 kHz). For the important lower frequencies, however, the edges are primarily expressed as borders between response regions that are phase-locked to different frequencies. These edges are particularly stable with respect to sound level variations because, despite the limited dynamic range of the auditory nerve fibers and the saturation of their mean response rates at high stimulus levels, the temporal course of their instantaneous firing rates remains relatively intact (Shamma 1985b, 1986). Consequently, the overall texture of the responses, particularly the sharp discontinuities between the different response regions, is largely preserved, and thus can be exploited by the lateral inhibitory network at all sound levels (Shamma 1986).

In postulating lateral inhibitory networks as computational algorithms for monaural spectral estimation, the temporal structure of auditory nerve responses is seen to play an indirect role in encoding the sound spectrum, being only a "carrier of" the spatial features the network detects. This view is fundamentally different from that of the purely temporal algorithms (as in section 11.4.2) designed to derive direct temporal response measures (e.g., the absolute frequency of phase-locking), and consequently requiring for their implementation such neural structures as the organized time delays.

11.7 Cortical Representation of the Spectral Profile: The Spectral Analysis Problem

As mentioned earlier, the spectral pattern extracted early in the auditory pathway (the cochlea and cochlear nucleus) is relayed to the auditory cortex through several stages of processing. On the basis of neurophysiological and psychoacoustical data collected over the last decade, it is believed that the auditory spectrum is repeatedly represented in AI at various degrees of resolution. As we shall elaborate below, this *multiscale* or multiresolution representation is mathematically equivalent to the visual representation of images based on the orientation and other feature maps. The basic outlines of this representation are illustrated in figure 11.8, where the spectral profile of the vowel /aa/ (as in "bat") is shown at the top (figure 11.8A). Several versions of this profile are displayed in figure 11.8B, with various degrees of resolution from the coarsest (smoothest or the most averaged) at the bottom, to the finest

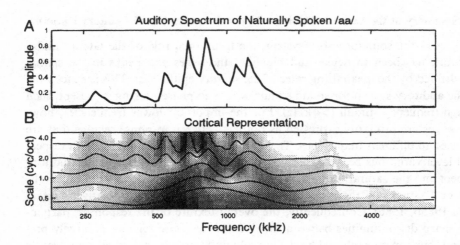

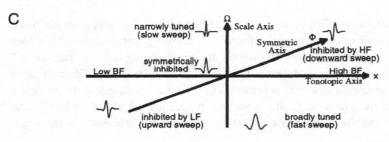

Figure 11.8
Multiscale representation of spectral profiles in the auditory cortex. (A) Spectral profile of a naturally spoken vowel /aa/. (B) Cortical representations of the spectral profile of the naturally spoken vowel /aa/. The tonotopic axis is given in kilohertz. The ordinate is the scale axis (cycles/octaves), which reflects the width of the response field (RF) and is labled by the ripple frequency to which the RF at each scale is most responsive. The strength of the response (reflected by the intensity of the color) at several scales is also shown by the solid profiles superimposed upon this figure. The fine structure of the spectral profiles is seen only at the highest scales, whereas its coarse overall outlines are seen at the lower scales. The local asymmetry of the RF is encoded by the color: responses in yellow indicate that the most responsive RF at that location is symmetric ($\phi_o = 0$); red (blue) indicate filters that are odd-symmetric ($\phi_o = \pm \pi/2$); and purple is an inverted RF. The color provides a description of the local energy distribution in the spectrum. For example, the tonotopic locations at which the spectrum is locally symmetric (yellow) closely reflect the positions of the peaks in the auditory spectrum; red (blue) indicate whether the local spectral slope is rising (falling) or if the nearest spectral peak is at a higher (lower) frequency. (C) Schematic of the three RF organizational axes that give rise to the cortical representation: the best frequency (tonotopic axis), the bandwidth (the scale axis), and the asymmetry (the phase axis).

(most detailed) at the top. One way to generate this pattern of cortical activation is through repeated layers of tonotopically ordered neurons with receptive fields of decreasing widths, in effect forming a two-dimensional sheet of AI neurons with the receptive field widths gradually changing along the isofrequency axis.

The spectral representation in AI is more complex, however, with the addition of a third dimension encoding the local shape (or asymmetry) of the spectrum. Thus receptive fields occur with a range of asymmetries as shown in figure 11.8D, forming an axis which maps out explicitly the local skewness (or tilt) of the spectrum at each CF. The combined three-dimensional cortical representation is illustrated in figure 11.8C for the vowel /aa/, where the most prominant features of the spectral profile—its formant peaks (labled F1–F4) and the closely spaced harmonic peaks in the low CF region (< 1 kHz)—are encoded in terms of their local width (scale) and asymmetry (Wang and Shamma 1995).

11.7.1   Mathematical Formulation of the Cortical Model

The response patterns illustrated in figure 11.8 are computed from a mathematical model that relates spectral profile analysis in the auditory cortex to the characteristic frequency, scale, and asymmetry of the ripple frequencies. A similar theoretical framework for multiscale representations was initially developed in the context of image analysis in the visual system to describe well-known organizational features such as the orientation columns, discovered using the very intuitive, but mathematically ill-defined stimuli of oriented bars and edges with different widths (DeValois and DeValois 1990; Hubel and Wiesel 1962). The multiscale visual models relied on linear systems concepts and analysis methods, and hence utilized an alternate stimulus to provide the basic experimental data—namely, the sinusoidal grating (DeValois and DeValois 1990). Applying these methods, gratings could be used to determine the linearity of unit responses, as in the distinction between simple (linear) and complex (nonlinear) cells, and to measure the receptive field of simple cells from their transfer functions, that is, the magnitude and phase of the responses as a function of grating density (better known as the "spatial frequency"). Furthermore, a unit's response properties to different parameters of the grating (e.g., their selectivity to a spatial frequency or phase) was directly related to the bandwidth, asymmetry, and orientation of its two-dimensional receptive field. Consequently, response maps such as the orientation columns generated using the oriented bar stimulus could be equivalently characterized in terms of parameters of the grating. For example, a cell's selectivity to a specific bar orientation is equivalent to its selectivity to a specific combination of spatial frequencies along the horizontal and vertical axes of the grating.

In applying these ideas to the auditory system, the spectral profile can be thought of as a one-dimensional image similar to a one-dimensional cross section of the gratings. After reviewing the mathematical framework for the multiscale analysis, we shall investigate its utility to the understanding of spectral profile analysis in the auditory system.

The Cortical Model   Let $p(x, t)$ denote the dynamic spectrum at the input of the cortical model. This could be the acoustic spectrum on a logarithmic frequency axis, the auditory spectrum at the output of the cochlear nucleus, $y(s, t)$, or some slightly modified version of these two. For stationary profiles, the t index can be dropped; later, this index will be reintroduced to include the case of dynamic input spectra. The Fourier transform of $p(x)$ is defined as

$$P(\Omega) = \int_{\mathscr{R}} p(x)e^{-j\Omega x}\, dx$$

$$p(x) = \frac{1}{2\pi} \int_{\mathscr{R}} P(\Omega)e^{j\Omega x}\, d\Omega.$$

Note that the tonotopic x-axis is analogous in vision to the spatial axis, hence Ω can be thought of as a "spatial frequency." A spectral pattern that has a sinusoidal shape along the logarithmic frequency axis is also known in the psychoacoustical literature as a "ripple." Therefore, Ω is referred to in the following as the "ripple frequency" and $P(\Omega)$ as the "ripple spectrum." Finally, as throughout this chapter, functions in the signal space and the Fourier domain are denoted in small and capital letters, respectively.

The receptive field of a neuron is defined as $w_s(x; x_o, \phi_o)$, located at $CF = x_o$ and whose asymmetry and width are parametrized by ϕ_o and s, respectively. A family of such response fields (RFs), varying gradually in symmetry (along the symmetry axis in figure 11.8D) can be generated by sinusoidally interpolating a symmetric (with respect to x_o) seed function $h_s(x)$ and its Hilbert transform, $\hat{h}_s(x) = \frac{1}{\pi} \int_{\mathscr{R}} \frac{h_s(v)}{x-v}\, dv$:

$$w_s(x; x_o, \phi_o) = h_s(x - x_o) \cos \phi_o - \hat{h}_s(x - x_o) \sin \phi_o. \tag{11.25}$$

For reasons that will become clear later, ϕ_o will be referred to as the "characteristic phase." Figure 11.8E illustrates RFs with different values of ϕ_o; For instance, the values of $w_s(x; x_o, \pm\pi/2)$ are antisymmetric, and the symmetry gradually changes toward the center, where $w_s(x; x_o, 0)$ is symmetric. An experimentally important quantity is the Fourier transform of the RF, $W_s(\Omega; x_o, \phi_o)$, which has a constant phase $-\phi_o \operatorname{sgn}(\Omega)$ (with respect to x_o). This family of functions also have the same magnitude since

$$|W_s(\Omega; x_o, \phi_o)| = |H_s(\Omega)e^{j(\Omega x_o + \phi_o)}| = H_s(\Omega), \tag{11.26}$$

for all Ω and ϕ_o.

Linearity of the Cortical Model A major assumption of this model, one we shall critically examine later, is that cortical cells analyze their input spectral profiles in a linear manner; That is, unit reaponses satisfy the superposition principle, whereby the response to a complex spectrum composed of a sum of several profiles is the same as the sum of the responses to the individual profiles. Therefore, given an input spectrum $p(x)$, the response of a unit located at x is computed as

$$r_s(x, \phi) = \langle p(v), w_s(v; x, \phi) \rangle_v = \int_{\mathscr{R}} p(v)w_s(v; x, \phi)\, dv. \tag{11.27}$$

Because in the Fourier domain

$$R_s(\Omega; x, \phi) = P(\Omega)W_s(\Omega; x, \phi) = P(\Omega)H_s(\Omega)e^{j\phi\, \mathrm{sgn}(\Omega)},$$

we then have

$$r_s(x, \phi) = \langle P(\Omega)e^{j\Omega x}, W_s^*(\Omega; x, \phi) \rangle_\Omega$$
$$= \langle \Re\{P(\Omega)e^{j\Omega x}\}, H_s(\Omega) \rangle_\Omega \cos\phi - \langle \Im\{P(\Omega)e^{j\Omega x}\}, H_s(\Omega)\, \mathrm{sgn}(\Omega) \rangle_\Omega \sin\phi$$
$$= a_s(x)\cos(\phi - \psi_s(x)), \tag{11.28}$$

where $\Re\{P\}, \Im\{P\}$ indicate the real and imaginary part of P, respectively, and

$$a_s(x) = |\langle P(\Omega)e^{j\Omega x}, H_s(\Omega)(1 - j\,\mathrm{sgn}(\Omega)) \rangle_\Omega| \tag{11.29}$$

$$\psi_s(x) = \tan^{-1} \frac{\langle \Im\{Pe^{j\Omega x}\}, H_s\,\mathrm{sgn}(\Omega) \rangle_\Omega}{\langle \Re\{Pe^{j\Omega x}\}, H_s \rangle_\Omega}. \tag{11.30}$$

The two functions $a_s(x)$ and $\psi_s(x)$ can be thought of as the "windowed" estimates of the magnitude and phase of the Fourier transform of the input auditory spectrum $P(\Omega)e^{j\Omega x}$.

Finally, as discussed earlier, the RF widths (or bandwidths) change significantly, creating the multiscale representation of the profile. This change can be modeled by a systematic dilation of the seed function $h_s(\cdot)$ as

$$H(k, s) = H_s(k) = H_m(k/\alpha^s), \tag{11.31}$$

for some *mother function* $h_m(\cdot)$ and dilation factor α. The multiscale RF can therefore be modeled as $w(x; x_o, \phi_o, s_o) = w_{s_o}(x; x_o, \phi_o)$. Following the previous derivation, the multiscale cortical selectivity $r(x, \phi, s) = r_s(x, \phi)$ can therefore be described by the local magnitude response $a(x, s) = a_s(x)$ and local phase response $\psi(x, s) = \psi_s(x)$, respectively.

The Dynamic Cortical Model   The cortical model developed thus far can be used to compute the responses to complex sound stimuli such as the speech vowels in figure 11.8. This formulation can be further extended to represent dynamic spectra—spectral profiles that change in time. Such spectra can be conceptually considered as a weighted sum of ripples moving in time at various speeds and directions, that is, a two-dimensional Fourier decomposition:

$$p(x, t) = \iint_{\mathscr{R}} P(\omega, \Omega) e^{j2\pi(\omega t + \Omega x)} \, d\omega \, d\Omega. \tag{11.32}$$

Once again, assuming linearity of responses, all response measures previously defined remain valid and similarly relevant, the only difference being the extra time-dimension. For instance, the response of a unit at x to a dynamic spectrum can be computed from a modified form of eq. 11.3 as

$$r_{s,l}(x, t, \phi, \theta) = \langle p(v, t), w_{s,l}(v, t; x, \phi, \theta) \rangle_{v,t} = \iint_{\mathscr{R}} p(v, t) w_{s,l}(v, t; x, \phi, \theta) \, dv \, dt, \tag{11.33}$$

where l is a *temporal scale* variable reflecting the range of dynamic properties the RF may possess, and θ is a phase factor that affects the polarity and symmetry of the temporal course of the RF (exactly analogous to the role of ϕ along the spatial axis). Because in the Fourier domain

$$R_{s,l}(\Omega, \omega; x, \phi, \theta) = P(\Omega, \omega) W_{s,l}(\Omega, \omega; x, \phi, \theta), \tag{11.34}$$

where ω is temporal frequency, then the response is given by

$$r_{s,l}(x, t, \phi, \theta) = \iint_{\mathscr{R}} P(\Omega, \omega) \exp^{j2\pi(+\omega t + \Omega x)} W_{s,l}^*(\Omega, \omega; x, \phi, \theta) \, d\omega \, d\Omega. \tag{11.35}$$

The same magnitude and phase functions described earlier can now be computed with an added temporal dimension.

11.7.2   Measuring the Response Field with Stationary Ripples

The model equations above suggest ways to measure RFs using single stationary ripple profiles. Let the input profile be the rippled spectrum illustrated in figure 11.9, with frequency Ω' defined as $p(x) = \cos(2\pi\Omega' x)$ (or $P(\Omega) = \frac{1}{2}(\delta(\Omega - \Omega') + \delta(\Omega + \Omega'))$).

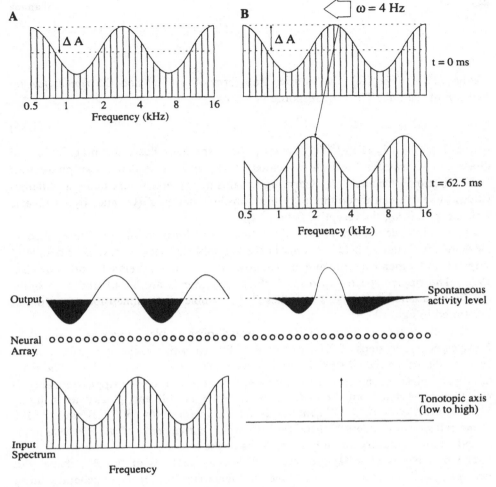

Figure 11.9
(Top) Stationary (left) and moving (right) ripple spectra. The ripple spectrum is a sinusoidal spectral profile defined against a logarithmic frequency axis x. The carrier of the profile can be broadband noise or a series of equally spaced tones (as shown). The ripples shown have an overall intensity (dB), a ripple modulation amplitude ($\Delta A = 0.5$), a ripple density of frequency ($\Omega = 0.5$ cycles/octave), and a ripple phase ($\Phi = \pi/2$ radians). These parameters define the amplitude of each component in the ripple spectrum as $p(x) = 1 + \Delta A \cdot \sin(2\pi\Omega \log_2 x + \Phi)$. The moving ripple spectrum travels to the left at a constant velocity ω in units of cycles/second. The amplitude of each component in the ripple spectrum is therefore given by $p(x, t) = 1 + \Delta A \cdot \sin(2\pi(\omega t + \Omega x) + \Phi)$. (Bottom) Schematic of presumed responses of an array of AI cells uniformly distributed along the tonotopic axis. The response pattern to the left is evoked by a rippled spectrum stimulus. The output is an alternating (sinusoidal) pattern of excitation and inhibition, which is amplified or attenuated in amplitude and phase-shifted relative to the input pattern. A transfer function can be measured by noting the amplitude and phase of the output relative to the input ripple at various ripple frequencies. The responses to the right are due to a single tone, represented by an impulse stimulus along the tonotopic axis. The tone evokes a response pattern along the axis that is a mirror image of the RF of the cells in the layer (which is asymmetric in this example).

Define $T_s(\Omega) \overset{\text{def}}{=} W_s^*(\Omega)$, the Fourier transform of $w_s(-x)$ and the *ripple transfer function* of the unit. Then the response becomes

$$r_s(x) = |T_s(\Omega')| \cos(\Phi(\Omega') - 2\pi\Omega' x) \tag{11.36}$$

where $T_s(\Omega') = |T_s(\Omega')| e^{j\Phi(\Omega')}$. That is, the response reflects the magnitude and phase of the transfer function evaluated at Ω', with an added linear phase shift $2\pi\Omega' x$ (bottom of figure 11.9). Carrying out this measurement repeatedly at different values of Ω, we can determine fully the transfer function $T_s(\Omega)$ and, by an inverse Fourier transform, the receptive field $w_s(x)$.

Figure 11.10 demonstrates how these theoretical formulations can be applied to measure the receptive fields of units in the primary auditory cortex. (For details of surgical and other experimental procedures, see Shamma, Versnel, and Kowalski 1995.) The rippled spectra used in all these experiments are broadband with sinusoidally modulated envelopes or profiles that resemble a one-dimensional grating, as illustrated in figure 11.9.

The cell shown in figure 11.10 was tested over ripple frequencies from 0 to 2 cycles/octave in steps of 0.4 cycles/octave. For each ripple, the responses to a full cycle of the ripple (i.e., 2π phase change) were measured (figure 11.10A). The magnitude and phase of the primary component synchronized to each ripple frequency Ω was then extracted from the histograms in figure 11.10B and plotted as in figure 11.10C: $T(\Omega) = |T(\Omega)| e^{j\Phi(\Omega)}$. Inverse Fourier transformation of $T(\Omega)$ gave the RF of the cell shown in figure 11.10D. Positive and negative peaks of the RF were interpreted as the excitatory and inhibitory fields of the cell.

The parameters of $T(\Omega)$ are related to specific features of the RF shape. For example, $|T(\Omega)|$ that are broad or tuned to higher ripple frequencies generally imply narrower RFs (Shamma, Versnel, and Kowalski 1995). Similarly, the phase function $\Phi(\Omega)$, which can be fit by the straight line $(2\pi x_o \Omega + \phi_o)$ in almost all units recorded (Shamma, Versnel, and Kowalski 1995), reflects both the CF and asymmetry of the RF through its slope and intercept (x_o and ϕ_o) (figure 11.10C). For instance, the RF is even and odd symmetric about its center for $\phi_o = 0$ and $\pm 90°$, respectively.

Validating the Linear Cortical Model The transfer function and RF derived in figure 11.10 are typical of data collected from hundreds of units in the primary and anterior auditory cortical fields. The data validate two features of the cortical multiscale model: (1) The RFs exhibit a wide range of widths and asymmetries at all CFs as illustrated in figure 11.10E. Furthermore, these properties are topographically organized across the surface of the AI (Versnel, Shamma, and Kowalski 1995). These results indicate that the cortex as a whole is capable of analyzing the spectral profile so

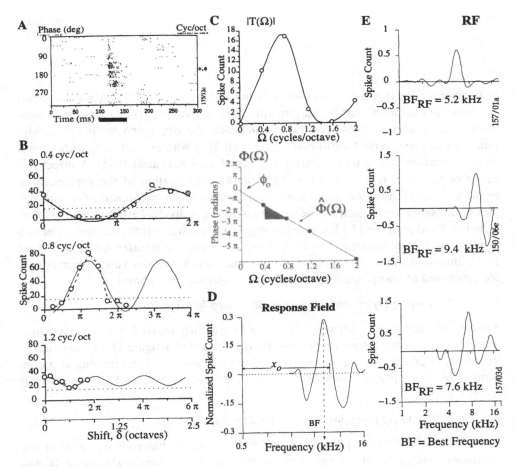

Figure 11.10

Analysis of responses to stationary ripples. (A) Raster responses of an AI unit to the various phases of a ripple spectrum ($\Omega = 0.8$ cycle/octave) at various ripple phases (0°–315° in steps of 45°). The stimulus lasts from 100 msec to 150 msec, and is repeated twenty times for each ripple phase. Spike counts are computed over a 50 msec window, as indicated by the bar below the figure. (B) Measured and fitted responses to single-ripple profiles at various ripple frequencies. In each plot, the response is measured at various phases of the ripple (eight $\pi/4$ steps per cycle) as indicated by the circles. The solid curve is the best sinusoidal fit to the data. For the 0.4 cycle/octave ripple, a full cycle of the response is equivalent to a 2.5-octave shift (or translation) of the stimulus profile, as indicated by the two axes at the bottom. The axis labeled δ (octaves) indicates the equivalent amount of shift each ripple pattern undergoes at each phase step. For ripples 0.8–1.6 cycles/octave, the full cycle corresponds to progressively smaller shifts of the profiles. Thus the response curves are simply repeated in the plots to indicate what they would look like if the full 2.5-octave shift had been applied to each ripple. (C) Ripple transfer function $T(\Omega)$. Top plot represents the weighted amplitude of the fitted sinusoids (as in panel B) as a function of ripple frequency Ω. Bottom plot represents the phases of the fitted sinusoids as a function of ripple frequency. The straight line fit $\hat{\Phi}(\Omega)$ has a slope x_o and intercept ϕ_o, which reflect the CF and asymmetry of the RF, respectively. (D) Response field (RF) of the unit, computed as the inverse Fourier transform of the ripple transfer function. (Shamma et al. 1995a, 1995b). (E) Examples of RFs with different shapes.

as to generate the representation shown earlier in figure 11.8C. (2) Cortical responses are linear in character, that is, one can apply linear systems ideas and response measures and obtain reasonable results. For instance, the ripple and temporal transfer functions can be inverse-transformed to generate RFs with properties consistent with what is measured using tones (Shamma, Versnel, and Kowalski 1995). A direct evidence of linearity, however, is the experimental confirmation of the superposition principle, namely, that the response to a complex spectrum composed of several ripples is the same as the sum of the responses to the individual ripples. This is illustrated in detail in figure 11.11, where the responses to simple profiles composed of two rippled spectra are compared to those predicted from the transfer function. Figure 11.12 illustrates the same principle, using a much more complex vowel spectral profile composed of many ripples with different amplitudes and phases.

11.7.3 Measuring Dynamic Response Fields Using Moving Ripples

Theoretical Framework   Dynamic RFs can be similarly derived from transfer functions measured using the moving ripple spectra illustrated in figure 11.13. Specifically, let the input profile be a rippled spectrum with frequency Ω', and moving at a constant velocity $\omega' : p(x, t) = \cos(2\pi(\Omega'x + \omega't))$. Substituting into eq.11.9, the response is given by

$$r_{s,l}(x, t) = |T_{s,l}(\Omega', \omega')| \cos(\Phi(\Omega', \omega') - 2\pi(\Omega'x + \omega't), \tag{11.37}$$

where $T_{s,l}(\cdot) \stackrel{\text{def}}{=} W^*_{s,l}(\cdot) = |T_{s,l}(\Omega', \omega')|e^{j\Phi(\Omega', \omega')}$. That is, the response reflects the magnitude and phase of the two-dimensional transfer function evaluated at Ω' and ω'. Repeating this kind of a measurement at different Ω' and ω' fully determines the transfer function and (by an inverse Fourier transform) the dynamic RF, $w_{s,l}(x, t)$. In the remainder of this section, the scale variables s, l (subscripts) will be dropped to simplify the notation.

Figures 11.13 and 11.14 illustrate the responses and the analysis methods used to derive the RF. In figure 11.13, the transfer function $T(\Omega, \omega)$ is measured as a function of ω, that is, a *temporal transfer function*, $T_\Omega(\omega)$. The complementary test is shown in figure 11.14, where the transfer function is measured as a function of Ω, that is, a *ripple transfer function*, $T_\omega(\Omega)$.

The raster responses in figure 11.13A were elicited by a rippled spectrum traveling at a range of velocities, $\omega = 4–32$ Hz. Following a transient portion near the onset of the stimulus, responses become more steady and periodic, reflecting the ripple velocity. The amplitude and phase of the synchronized response component is extracted from period histograms constructed at each ω (figure 11.13B), and plotted as the

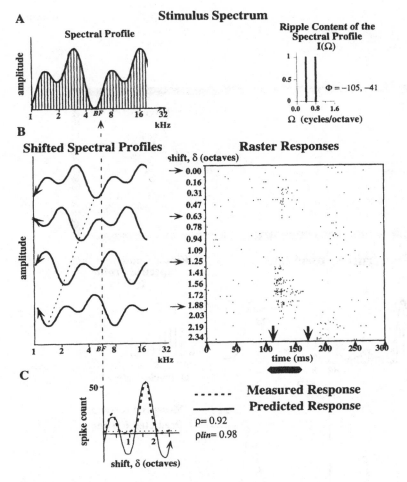

A
Stimulus Spectrum

Spectral Profile

amplitude

1   2   4 *BF* 8   16   32
kHz

Ripple Content of the Spectral Profile
$I(\Omega)$

1

0.5

$\Phi = -105, -41$

0

0.0   0.8   1.6
Ω (cycles/octave)

B
Shifted Spectral Profiles   **Raster Responses**

shift, δ (octaves)

amplitude

1   2   4 *BF* 8   16   32
kHz

→ 0.00
   0.16
   0.31
   0.47
→ 0.63
   0.78
   0.94
   1.09
→ 1.25
   1.41
   1.56
   1.72
→ 1.88
   2.03
   2.19
   2.34

0   50   100   150   200   250   300
time (ms)

C

50

spike count

1   2

shift, δ (octaves)

- - - - - **Measured Response**
_____ **Predicted Response**

$\rho = 0.92$
$\rho lin = 0.98$

Figure 11.11
Linearity of cortical responses to stationary spectra. (A) Spectral profile of a stimulus (left plot) composed of two ripples; schematic illustration of the amplitude and phases of the two ripples (right plot). (B) Spectral profile of the stimulus with increasing amount of shift (from top to bottom, as indicated by the dashed line). The profile is periodic against the tonotopic axis with a period of 2.5 octaves. The underlying tones of the stimulus complex are omitted in these plots. The raster to the right illustrates the nature of the responses obtained as a function of profile shift. The profile is always shifted by a total amount equal to its period (i.e., 2.5 octaves for this profile), and with a resolution corresponding to at least eight samples of the maximum ripple frequency in the complex. In this example, the maximum ripple frequency is 0.8 cycles/octave, and hence to sample it in eight steps, requires each shift to be 0.156 octaves. The stimulus burst is indicated by the bar below the raster. The arrows define the window over which the response spike counts are made. (C) Response spike counts to different shifts are indicated by the dashed curve as a function of profile shift. The solid line is the response predicted from the ripple transfer function and the stimulus profile. The scale of the solid curve is in arbitrary linear units. The dotted horizontal line is the spike count of the flat spectral profile; it is used as the baseline for the predicted response curve, $r_p(\delta)$. The whole plot is aligned with the stimulus profile according the *BF* of the unit (determined from its RF). The correlation coefficient ρ s a measure of the match between the two waveforms (Shamma, Versnel, and Kowalski 1995).

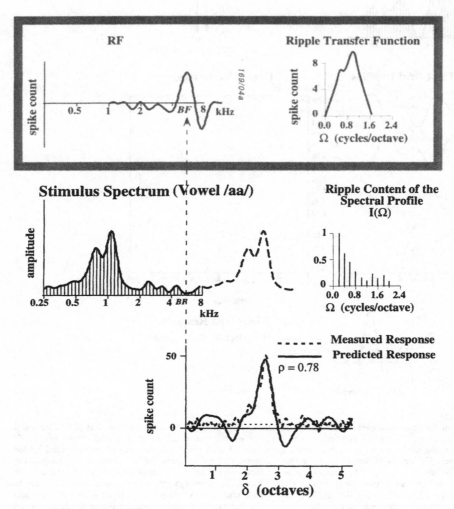

Figure 11.12
Measured and predicted responses to naturally spoken vowel /aa/ profile. All details are as in figure 11.11.

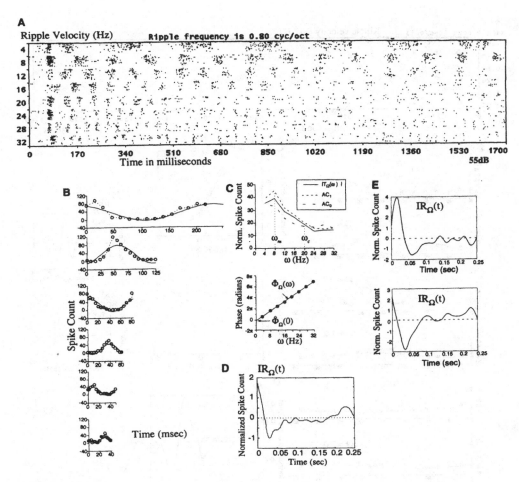

Figure 11.13
Analysis of responses to ripples moving at different velocities (temporal transfer function). (A) Raster responses to a ripple ($\Omega = 0.8$ cycle/octave) moving at different velocities ω. Period histograms are constructed from responses starting at $t = 120$ msec (indicated by the arrow). The stimulus lasted up to 1.7 sec with similar rise/fall times. At the onset of the sweep, the ripple spectrum was started in a sine phase (defined as $0°$) as depicted in figure 11.3B ($t = 0$). The ripple begins immediately moving to the left at a specific constant velocity for the duration of the stimulus. The stimulus is turned on at 50 msec. (B) Period histograms (16 bin) constructed at each ω. The best fit to the spike counts (circles) in each histogram is indicated by the solid lines. (C) Amplitude (dashed line in top plot) and phase (bottom data points) of the best fit curves are plotted as a function of ω. Also shown in the top plot is the normalized transfer function magnitude ($|T_\Omega(\omega)|$) and the average spike count as functions of ω. A straight line fit of the phase data points is also shown in the lower plot. (D) Inverse Fourier transform of the temporal transfer function $T_\Omega(\omega)$ gives the impulse response function of the cell ($IR_\Omega(t)$). (E) Examples of $IR_\Omega(t)$ measured from different cells.

Shamma

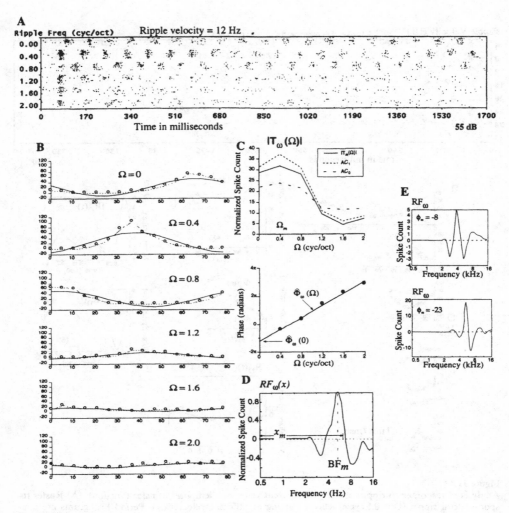

Figure 11.14
Analysis of responses to moving ripples with different ripple frequencies (ripple transfer function). (A)
Raster responses to a ripple moving at $\omega = 12\,\text{Hz}$, with different ripple frequencies $\Omega = 0$–2 cycle/octave.
The stimulus is turned on at 50 msec. Period histograms are constructed from responses starting at $t =$
120 msec (indicated by the arrow). (B) Period histograms (16 bin) constructed at each Ω. The best fit to the
spike counts (circles) in each histogram is indicated by the solid lines. (C) Amplitude (dashed line in top
plot) and phase (bottom data points) of the best fit curves are plotted as a function of Ω. Also shown in the
top plot is the normalized transfer function magnitude ($|T_\omega(\Omega)|$ and the average spike count as functions
of Ω. A straight line fit of the phase data points is also shown in the lower plot. (D) Inverse Fourier
transform of the ripple transfer function $T_\omega(\Omega)$ gives the response field of the cell ($RF_\omega(x)$). (E) Examples
of $RF_\omega(x)$ measured from different cells.

transfer function $T_\Omega(\omega)$ (figure 11.13C). Similar data analysis methods lead to the complementary transfer function $T_\omega(\Omega)$ illustrated in figure 11.14. Although these transfer functions are measured at a single Ω and ω, extensive measurements have revealed that they remain stable for a given unit, apart from a scale change, over a wide range of Ω and ω frequencies, including the stationary ($\omega = 0$) and the flat ($\Omega = 0$) spectra (Kowalski, Depireux, and Shamma 1996). To characterize a unit's dynamic RF, it is thus sufficient to carry out the measurements at one ripple frequency and velocity (usually the most effective ones), implying that the two-dimensional transfer function $T(\Omega, \omega)$ is separable into the product of a purely temporal and a purely ripple transfer function. Consequently, the dynamic RF derived from the inverse Fourier transform of $T(\Omega, \omega)$ becomes the convolution of purely spatial and temporal functions, $\mathscr{RF}$ and $\mathscr{IR}$, which are derived from the inverse Fourier transforms of the corresponding ripple and temporal transfer functions.

As expected, parameters of the transfer functions are related to the shape of their inverse Fourier transforms, the $\mathscr{RF}$, and the temporal impulse response, $\mathscr{IR}$. For instance, a narrowly tuned temporal transfer function implies a prolonged "ringing" impulse response (see examples in Kowalski, Depireux, and Shamma 1996). The phase functions (or their linear fits in particular) reveal much information about the shapes of $\mathscr{RF}$ and $\mathscr{IR}$. For example, let $\hat{\Phi}_\omega(\Omega) = 2\pi\omega\tau_d + \hat{\Phi}_\Omega(0)$ and $\hat{\Phi}_\Omega(\omega) = 2\pi\Omega\tau_d + \hat{\Phi}_\omega(0)$ be the linear phase fits, then the slopes and intercepts reflect the following features:

1. $\hat{\Phi}_\omega(\Omega)$: The slope, x_m, reflects the location of the RF relative to the left edge of the stimulus spectrum. The intercept $\hat{\Phi}_\omega(0)$ represents the contributions due to three factors: ϕ_m, due to dynamic RF asymmetry; $2\pi\omega\tau_d$, due to the absolute time delay or response latency; and θ, a temporal constant phase shift that reflects the polarity of the $\mathscr{IR}$. Therefore,

$$\hat{\Phi}_\omega(0) = 2\pi\omega\tau_d + \theta + \phi_m. \tag{11.38}$$

2. $\hat{\Phi}_\Omega(\omega)$: The slope τ_d reflects the absolute time delay between stimulus and response. The intercept is due to the other three phase shifts:

$$\hat{\Phi}_\Omega(0) = 2\pi\Omega x_m + \theta + \phi_m. \tag{11.39}$$

Validating the Dynamic Cortical Model   The $\mathscr{RF}$ functions measured from many single units in the primary and anterior auditory cortical field exhibit a wide variety of shapes—widths, asymmetries, and best frequencies (BFs) similar to those shown in figure 11.8 for stationary ripples—a finding that supports the hypothesis that they can analyze locally the spectral profile into its constituent ripple components, generating a multiscale representation similar to the one described in figure 11.8. The same observations hold for the $\mathscr{IR}$, suggesting that a multiscale analysis might be taking place in time as well.

As with stationary ripples, it is important to recognize that the utility of the transfer function measurements and the decomposition of dynamic spectral profiles into moving ripples are valid conceptually only if linearity of the responses can be established or, equivalently, if the superposition principle can be shown to hold. That this is the case is demonstrated in figure 11.15, which compares responses to spectral profiles composed of mulitple moving ripples to those predicted from the transfer functions (or the $\mathscr{RF}$ and $\mathscr{IR}$) of the units. In the first test (top), a three-ripple combination stimulus is depicted in the form of a spectrogram (panel A). The stimulus (and hence all responses) is periodic with a fundamental period of 250 msec. The $\mathscr{RF}$ of the cell is shown in panel B oriented (vertically) along the frequency (tonotopic) axis, with CF of approximately 3 kHz. Panel C illustrates the product of the $\mathscr{RF}$ with the stimulus profile as a function of time, which represents the response of the unit due to the $\mathscr{RF}$ alone. This (periodic) function is then modified by the dynamic response properties of the cell through a convolution with the $\mathscr{IR}$ shown in panel D. One fundamental period of the final predicted response of the unit is illustrated in panel E (solid line), superimposed (with an arbitrary scale) against the measured response of the cell to the stimulus (dashed line). More complex spectral profiles are predicted in the other plots. Note that in all examples, the temporal course of the responses (in panel E) does not resemble the response predicted from the $\mathscr{RF}$ alone (panel C) because the $\mathscr{IR}$ is sufficiently complicated so as to influence significantly the final shape of the response.

11.7.4   Response Nonlinearities

It is evident from the data illustrated in all figures above that cortical units respond largely linearly to the spectral profile of the stimulus, although, strictly speaking, "linear" here should be qualified in two ways. The first is that the "linear" responses are measured to within a scale factor and are taken relative to a baseline activity (defined as the responses to a flat spectrum). In this sense, we consider the response to be "linear" if it changes relative to the baseline in a manner that resembles the shape of the predicted response. The second qualification on the meaning of "linearity" concerns such response nonlinearities as saturation and rectification of the firing rates. These nonlinearities distort ("clip") the response waveforms in understandable ways that can in principle be relatively easily removed (Shamma and

Versnel 1995). In other words, "linearity" as used here is meant to apply to the responses *prior to* or *without* these obvious distortions.

It remains, however, a valid question as to why despite these nonlinearities at the cortex and at every prior auditory stage, the responses remain linear in the sense defined above? Although a satisfying theoretical answer is probably unattainable at present, given the complexity of the neural processing along the auditory pathway, one may gain insights and intuition from a variety of similar phenomena. For instance, rectification and saturation of auditory nerve fiber firing rates do not invalidate measurements of the cochlear filter transfer functions using the reverse correlation and other methods that imply the linearity of the underlying system (DeBoer and DeJongh 1975). In fact, experiments using stimuli with broadband spectra have repeatedly demonstrated the linear character of the auditory nerve responses (Deng, Geisler, and Greenberg 1988). In VI, reverse correlation procedures for measuring the two-dimensional receptive fields have been effectively used despite the prevalence of the same nonlinearities (Jones and Palmer 1987). It should be noted here that rectification, saturation, and other instantaneous nonlinear deformation of a waveform do not necessarily imply a loss of information provided the zero-crossings of the waveform are preserved (Logan 1977). In the context of the auditory system, this means that the representation of a spectral profile remains unique despite the distortions it undergoes through the successive stages.

11.7.5 Summary

We have demonstrated how an abstract mathematical model of cortical processing is developed and used to interpret physiological recordings of single-unit responses in the auditory cortex. In particular, linear systems analysis methods were adapted and applied to derive unit RFs and to explore and understand the functional significance and organization of their properties. Perhaps the most surprising finding here is the degree to which apparently complex responses of the cortex can be faithfully captured by the relatively simple mathematical tools of linear analysis (DeValois and DeValois 1990; Shamma and Versnel 1995). In fact, even in these cases where linearity clearly does not hold, for example, responses of complex cells in VI, linear systems terminology, and tests can still provide concrete ways to describe and classify their nonlinear behavior.

11.8 The Biological Plausibility of a Neural Network Model

A critical element in the design process of any neural network is the nature of the available constraints. Often, these constraints are formulated only as an input-output

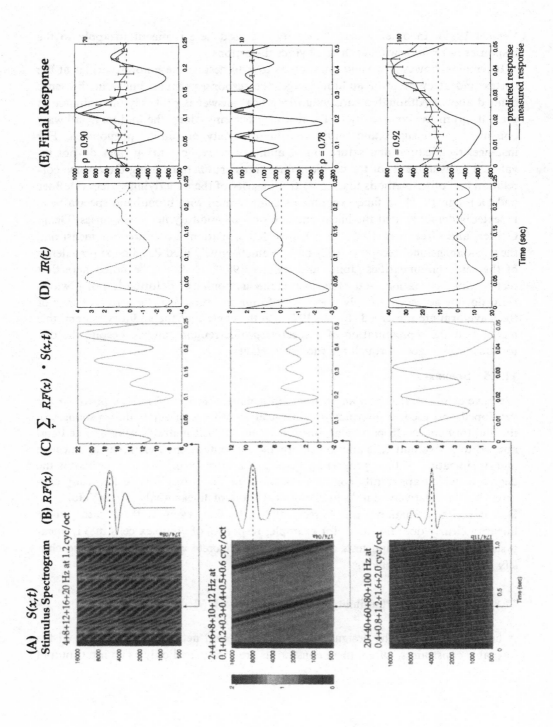

(A) $S(x,t)$ Stimulus Spectrogram (B) $RF(x)$ (C) $\sum_r RF(x) \cdot S(x,t)$ (D) $IR(t)$ (E) Final Response

map that defines the transfer characteristics of the desired network, but not its implementation. For instance, in the case of the auditory spectral estimation problem discussed earlier, both the auditory nerve responses (input) and the hypothetical perceived spectrum (output) are known, and the objective is to design the network (algorithm) that performs the desired mapping. There are literally countless network topologies and algorithms that can perform this task, of which two classes were contrasted: the temporally based and the spatially based. Consequently, the following question arises: How is one to compare and select critically among these networks?

This question is important when the objective of the modeling is to discover the underlying biological neural substrate that performs the computations. It is relatively easy in general to come up with a network that can perform any desired task, given enough complex neuron models (systems of nonlinear differential equations) with arbitrary connectivities (arbitrary coupling). It is a different matter altogether to come up with a biologically plausible network to perform the task. Unfortunately, there are no definitive rules that lead to such network designs; rather, there are intuitive guidelines that are based on our current understanding of the function and anatomy of the central nervous system. For instance, electrophysiological studies have provided detailed results of the kind of computations and the range of speeds expected of typical mammalian neurons. Thus a neuron cannot compute at nanosecond speeds, nor does it have access to precisely synchronized clocks. Neurons do, however, form elaborate dendritic trees and axonal arborizations, and are thus capable of establishing finely tuned connectivities with other neurons. These findings suggest that, in the absence of specific evidence to the contrary, neural networks are more likely to utilize and process input patterns that are distributed in space rather than in time.

Figure 11.15
Predicting the responses to multiple moving ripple stimuli. (Top row) (A) Spectrogram of the stimulus $(p(x, t))$, along with its ripple content (three moving ripples in this case, all at $\Phi = 0$). The gray-scale indicates relative amplitude of the spectrogram. (B) $\mathcal{RF}$ of the cell with $BF = 3\,\text{kHz}$. The function is plotted sideways, that is, aligned to the logarithmic frequency axis of the spectrogram (which also represents the tonotopic axis). (C) Product of the stimulus spectrogram and its $\mathcal{RF}$ generates a time function which is the response of the unit due to the $\mathcal{RF}$ alone. (D) $\mathcal{IR}$ of the cell, convolved with the function in panel C to produce the final response shown in panel E. (E) Final predicted response of the cell (solid line) superimposed the measured spike count (dotted curve). The error bars for the measured response curve and the correlation between measured and predicted responses are also shown. The dashed line is the zero spike count. All abscissas measure time in seconds; all y-axes are normalized spike counts. Arrows indicate the location of $t = 0$ of the periodic functions in panels C–E, relative a corresponding period of the stimulus. (Second row) Measured and predicted responses to temporal noise stimulus generated with five random phase moving ripples all at $\Omega = 1.2$ cycles/octave. (Third row) Predictions for a simulated FM stimulus composed of five ripples to produce effectively a single peak with velocity 20 octaves/sec. (Bottom row) Predictions for ripple noise stimulus generated by adding five ripples with different values of Ω and random phases.

Another important source of information for neuronal modeling concerns the representational primitives of the particular nervous system under study. Such knowledge, usually derived from psychophysical or neurophysiological studies, provides valuable constraints on the type of computations that the network models perform and the output measures they seek to extract. A particularly good example of such primitives are the oriented edge and motion detectors of the mammalian visual system. The discovery of these organizational features has restricted significantly the range of plausible network models involved in vision processing, which in turn has led to the design of more focused and fruitful physiological and anatomical studies of the visual system. By contrast, the situation in the auditory system is considerably vaguer; indeed, no comparable primitives have emerged. Consequently, only a few constraints exist in the formulation of auditory processing algorithms and network implementations, and one is forced to rely on more general plausibility arguments, such as those outlined above. Nevertheless, the example of the visual system remains as a powerful source of inspiration for similar networks in other sensory systems.

Notes

1. There are many detailed models of various aspects of hair cell/nerve fiber transformations (see, for example, Deng, Geisler, and Greenberg 1988; Westerman and Smith 1984). Auditory nerve fiber responses are most often modeled as a nonstationary point process whose instantaneous rate is approximately given by the hair cell's intracellular potential (for details, see Siebert 1970).

2. Decibels (dB) are logarithmic units used often in amplitude comparisons of ratios r_1 and r_2 ($20 \cdot \log(r_1/r_2)$). A 6 dB increase in the ratio of two quantities then corresponds roughly to a doubling of the ratio of their amplitudes. Therefore, an 84 dB dynamic range is roughly equal to a 16,000-fold change in the sound amplitude between threshold and saturation.

3. See Hartline 1974 for an excellent review of the physiology and mathematics of such networks in the retina.

4. More precise statements can be made given specific profiles. For instance, for a symmetric positive $w(x)$ profile (and hence $W(\Omega)$ is maximum at $W(0)$), the area under the profile of inhibition, $\int_{-\infty}^{\infty} w(x)\, dx$, should be ≤ 1 for stability.

5. Asymmetrical profiles of $w(x)$ give rise to complex forms of $W(\Omega)$ in eq. 11.19, and hence to complex poles that result in oscillatory behavior (Morishita and Yajima 1972; Matsuoka 1985).

6. In the case of the auditory system, the moving window averaging step has an important physiological interpretation based on the well-established observation that phase-locking deteriorates significantly in the responses of central auditory neurons. These neurons can only encode the averaged outputs of the LIN.I, such as those of figure 11.7a.

12 Simulating Large Networks of Neurons

Alexander D. Protopapas, Michael Vanier, and James M. Bower

12.1 Introduction

The behavior of the nervous system is the outcome of processes at multiple levels of organization. Learning mechanisms, for example, are most likely manifested at all levels from gene expression to synaptic plasticity to changes in behavior. Thus large numbers of neurobiologists interested in learning focus their efforts on the molecular level, while others focus on the single cell, the network, the system, and behavioral levels (Baudry and Davis 1994).

Although investigations at specific levels of scale provide important information about brain organization, it is likely that a complete understanding of the functional organization of the nervous system will require connecting these levels. It is our contention that computer models will increasingly allow us to make just such connections. Indeed, models based on the real anatomy and physiology of the nervous system already constitute what is, in effect, a compact and self-correcting database of neurobiological facts and functional relationships (Bower 1996). We believe that, more and more, laboratories and researchers will rely on such models and modeling software to check the significance and accuracy of their data as well as to further collaboration and communication within neuroscience as a whole.

This chapter serves to document the iterative, multilevel modeling approach we have taken in investigating the functional organization of the mammalian olfactory system. Our work, which started with a network-level simulation of the olfactory, or piriform, cortex originally constructed by Matt Wilson (Wilson and Bower 1992), led to numerous questions regarding the effects of network dynamics on more physiologically realistic cells. Because the original network simulations were based on quite simplified neurons, pursuing this new direction required that we construct much more detailed single-cell simulations, which can then provide a means of upgrading the realism of the cells in the network simulation. In the final section of the chapter, we describe the approach we have taken to improve the network simulation based on the single-cell model.

12.2 General Issues

12.2.1 The GENESIS Neural Simulator

The models described in this chapter were all generated using the GENESIS neural simulator developed in our laboratory (Wilson et al. 1989) and specifically designed to allow modeling at many different levels of neural organization (Bower and Beeman 1995). Although other simulation systems support the construction of models at one or another level (see De Schutter 1992), GENESIS remains one of the few that, in principle, support all levels. For example, GENESIS-based models currently exist at the systems (Morissette 1996), network (Wilson and Bower 1989), single-cell (Jaeger, De Schutter, and Bower 1997), and subcellular (Bhalla 1997) levels. A number of key GENESIS features as well as some of the mathematical methods utilized by GENESIS are discussed in appendixes A–E. Additional information about GENESIS can be obtained on the World Wide Web at http://www.bbb.caltech.edu/GENESIS. This site also contains a tutorial based on the network simulation described in this chapter (tutorial name: "piriform") which can be downloaded.

12.2.2 Realistic Modeling and Questions of Scale

Our models are all of the sort we have referred to previously as "realistic" (Bower 1990), namely, models primarily based on the actual anatomy and physiology of the nervous system and designed to discover as yet unknown relationships between the structure of the nervous system and its function. *Realistic models* can be contrasted with what we have termed *demonstration models*, which are primarily intended to provide support for a particular preexisting theory or functional point of view. While most theoretical models published to date are of the demonstration type, it is our view that realistic models will become increasingly prominent because they have the greatest chance of discovering new functional relationships. Typically, realistic models are also more closely linked to experimentally testable predictions and therefore of greater use in guiding experimental efforts.

One question that immediately arises in realistic modeling concerns which data to include and which to leave out; this will be specifically addressed in several sections below. In general, however, because realistic models are specifically intended to discover function from structure, they should contain more rather than less biological detail. In addition, the more realistic the model, the more likely it will generate realistic physiological data for comparison with real experiments.

While, in principle, realistic models should include as much biological detail as possible, in practice, there are often real-world limitations on what can be included. The most obvious limitation is computing resources, especially in the case of network modeling, where even complex single-cell models can tax the most sophisticated computers (De Schutter and Bower 1994a, 1994b).

A second, and perhaps more important, limitation on model complexity is the lack of available biological data. Realistic modelers usually discover during the initial stage of model construction that there are large gaps in the information necessary to construct a model. Although identifying such gaps can serve as a valuable means of directing experimental investigation, the lack of quantitative data often means that information must either be imported from another system, included as a best guess, or excluded from the model altogether.

Finally, the complexity of a model is also a matter of scale and objectives. For example, if the purpose of a network model is to understand the oscillatory structure of the electroencephalogram (EEG), it is both impractical and probably unnecessary to simulate the three-dimensional diffusion of calcium within the network's neurons. Accordingly, all modeling efforts involve some level of abstraction and require initial decisions regarding the level of detail to include in the model. Yet despite the necessity of this type of abstraction, one almost inevitably finds that a model generated at one level of scale raises questions that can only be addressed at another level.

12.2.3 The Piriform Cortex Network Model

We developed our modeling methods in the course of our ongoing efforts to understand the mammalian olfactory system (Bower 1995b). Because these methods can be understood only in the context of scientific objectives, we must briefly describe the scientific motivation for our work.

The basis of our first modeling efforts (and of this chapter) is a network model of the piriform cortex constructed several years ago by Matthew Wilson in our laboratory (Wilson and Bower 1989, 1992; Wilson 1990). Piriform cortex is the largest region of primary olfactory cortex and is assumed to be directly involved in olfactory object recognition (Haberly and Bower 1989). Figure 12.1 shows the piriform cortex in the context of the rest of the olfactory system. Odorants arrive at the nasal epithelium, where they activate olfactory receptor neurons. These cells send their axons to the olfactory bulb, which in turn connects to the piriform cortex via the lateral olfactory tract (LOT). The LOT then sends collateral fibers into the piriform cortex, which projects to the entorhinal cortex, which then feeds into the hippocampus,

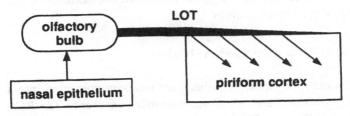

Figure 12.1
Olfactory input to the piriform cortex.

believed to be involved in long-term memory. This is likely to account for the powerful memory-evoking effect of olfactory stimuli (Eichenbaum et al. 1991).

12.3 Modeling Objectives

Our ultimate interest in modeling the olfactory cortex is to understand how the piriform cortex network supports the process of olfactory object recognition (Wilson and Bower 1989, Hasselmo et al. 1990). Because our modeling philosophy is to let the structure of the brain tell us something about its function, in constructing realistic models we first identify some physiological feature of the structure to be modeled that is not obviously related to the function of interest, but that can be used to tune model parameters (Bower 1995a, 1996). This exercise builds confidence in the overall structure of the model and also assures us that the model is generating realistic physiological responses for later comparisons to experimental data; it is far more satisfying and reassuring if the model generates interesting behavior without being specifically tuned to do so. In general, we prefer that the functional properties of interest be an emergent property of the simulation rather than a built-in feature.

In the case of the piriform cortex network model, we (M. A. Wilson and J. M. Bower) first focused on replicating the spatial and temporal patterns of activity evoked by artificially stimulating the primary afferent pathway to this network, the lateral olfactory tract (LOT). Evoked potential responses to LOT stimulation are well described (Ketchum and Haberly 1993a) and characteristic of this cortex. Having established the appropriate response patterns to this artificial stimulus, we froze our model parameters and provided a more realistic LOT stimulus. We wanted to determine whether a model tuned on evoked potentials could generate the principal features of the electroencephalogram (EEG), which had been well described previously (Freeman 1960). As demonstrated in later sections, we found that this was the case. Furthermore, the cellular mechanisms revealed by the model to underlie the EEG patterns suggested several novel ideas concerning the functional implications of this network-level behavior for single-cell physiology.

12.4 Overall Structure of Piriform Cortex and the Model

A simplified version of the network model described here has been converted into a computer tutorial with a graphical interface and accompanying chapter in *The Book of GENESIS* (Protopapas and Bower 1995). The tutorial is freely available as part of the standard GENESIS release through http://www.bbb.caltech.edu/GENESIS. The reader is encouraged to obtain and examine the tutorial while reading this section of the chapter.

Because the initial focus of our modeling efforts was on what could be considered the "aggregate" activity of the piriform cortex (evoked potentials and the EEG), we elected to base the model on large numbers of relatively simplified neurons. Because experimental data (Haberly and Bower 1984) suggested that the laminar organization of synaptic inputs in this cortex was important in generating the evoked potential responses, we modeled cortical pyramidal cells using five electrical compartments (figure 12.2), each representing a different cortical lamina. These five compartments also correspond to the origins of five distinctly different types of synaptic input to the pyramidal cell. Inhibitory neurons were modeled more simply, as single compartments, because their spherical geometry is unlikely to contribute to electrical responses, and because much less is known about their physiological and synaptic organization. What is known is that there are at least two types of inhibitory neurons, one activated by afferents directly and responsible for feedforward inhibition onto pyramidal cells, and a second receiving pyramidal cell inputs and mediating a feedback inhibition (Tseng and Haberly 1988). Both types were included in the model.

The other critical component in any network model is the connectivity to and within the model. The network connectivity for this model is summarized in the circuit diagram in figure 12.2. Lateral olfactory tract (LOT) input is modeled as a set of independent fibers that make sparse connections with pyramidal cells and both types of inhibitory interneurons. Because previous experimental data had suggested that the conduction velocities of the afferent axons had an important effect on evoked potentials in different regions of the cortex, we took care to include the correct velocities for each axonal type (Haberly 1978). Signals travel along the LOT rostrally to caudally, and are distributed across the cortex via many small collaterals (Devor 1976). In the model, as in the brain, signals proceed along the LOT toward cortex at a speed of 7.0 m/sec. Collaterals leave the main fiber tract at a 45° angle and travel across the cortex at a speed of 1.6 m/sec (Haberly 1973b). Finally, there is anatomical (Price 1973; Schwob and Price 1978) and physiological (Haberly 1973b) evidence that the effects of the afferent fiber system are greater in rostral than caudal cortex. To simulate this effect in the model, the strength of synaptic input due to afferent signals was exponentially attenuated with increased distance from the rostral site of stimulation.

Piriform cortex is also characterized by an extensive set of intrinsic excitatory connections originating in its own pyramidal cells (Luskin and Price 1983). Physiological data suggested that these intrinsic axonal connections made an important contribution to evoked potentials (Haberly and Bower 1984). These so-called

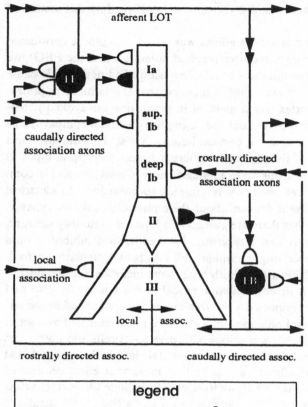

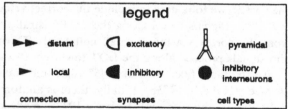

Figure 12.2
Schematic diagram of pyramidal cell and network circuitry. The pyramidal cell consists of five distinct electrical compartments. FF and FB label feedforward and feedback inhibitory cells, respectively. Pyramidal cell axons originate in the layer II (somatic) compartment of the cell. Different compartments are labeled by their layer (Ia, superficial Ib, etc.). The legend explains the symbols in the schematic.

association fibers terminate on the layer-Ib compartments of the pyramidal cells, with the superficial Ib compartment acting as a termination point for caudally directed axons from rostral pyramidal cells in the network. Input from the rostrally directed axons of caudal pyramidal cell is located in deep Ib compartments. Fibers appear to spread out radially from the originating cell and travel rostrally at a speed of 1.0 m/sec, and caudally at a speed of 0.5 m/sec (Haberly 1973b, 1978). Local connections are made on the basal dendrite (Haberly and Presto 1986). These conduction velocities are used in the model to calculate axonal delays. Simulation scaling considerations additionally require that association fiber interconnectivity be greatly increased as compared to that of the actual cortex. As with afferent input, intrinsic excitatory connections are attenuated exponentially with distance from the originating cell.

In general, the pattern of inputs to and outputs from inhibitory neurons is much less well understood biologically. In this model, feedforward inhibitory neurons are activated primarily by the afferent pathway (with some feedback from pyramidal cells) and then form synapses on the Ia compartment of the pyramidal neuron. In contrast, the feedback inhibitory interneurons are activated primarily by pyramidal cell axons (with minor feedforward activation) and form synapses on the somata (layer II) of the pyramidal neuron. Feedforward inhibition is a slow $GABA_B$ K^+-mediated conductance while feedback inhibition is a fast $GABA_A$ Cl^--mediated conductance. Support for the inhibitory architecture of the model comes from a variety of experimental sources (Biedenbach and Stevens 1969a, 1969b; Haberly 1973a; Satou et al. 1982; Haberly and Bower 1984; Tseng and Haberly 1986).

12.5 Simplifying Network Components

We have shown how the structure of our model resembles the general structure of the olfactory cortex, and how model components were included in accordance with our initial objective: to generate the evoked potential and EEG response patterns seen in the real cortex. Many specific decisions remain to be made before our model can actually generate output. Indeed, a distinct advantage of constructing realistic models is that you are forced to confront the details, although, as we shall see in the next section, you are also forced to reduce the number of details, or to guess about details for which no biological data are yet available.

12.5.1 Connections between Individual Neurons

Having sketched out in general terms the circuitry of our piriform cortex network model, we need to formulate rules that determine the connections between individual neurons. In the biological network, connections are determined by complex rules for self-organization, which determine the extent of connections and the strength of individual synapses, and which have been shown to be governed by a variety of factors ranging from growth factors to activity-dependent synaptic modification (Purves and Lichtman 1985). Because the biological details for these processes in the piriform cortex are not well understood, the model's network connections were established to conform to general anatomical constraints, but may not necessarily reflect the precise structure of the biological network. Thus, our initial focus on the reconstruction of aggregate electrical activity allowed us to ignore the details of biological connectivity. As our future modeling efforts expand to include learning and memory, we will have to become more concerned with precise patterns of neural interconnectivity.

Since we do not know the biological rules that determine precise connections, we have formulated statistical rules that are within reasonable anatomical constraints. For example, the maximum spatial extent of a pyramidal cell's connection to a feedback inhibitory cell is 1 mm. The probability that the pyramidal cell will connect to any one feedback inhibitory neuron is 0.2. The space constant for the exponential decay in connection strength from the pyramidal cell to the interneuron is 5 mm. As we shall see in later sections, these simple statistical rules are sufficient for generating realistic behavior in the network model. (Specifics on connection parameters for all synaptic pathways can be found in chapter appendix F).

12.5.2 Numbers of Neurons

The simplification needed to construct our realistic model involves not only the complexity of the modeled neurons and interneuronal connections but also the number of neurons being simulated. The piriform cortex of the rat contains on the order of 10^6 neurons and covers an area that is roughly 10 mm by 6 mm (Haberly 1990). However, the model described here consists of only 4,500 cells, representing three populations of neurons (1,500 each of superficial pyramidal, feedforward inhibitory, and feedback inhibitory neurons). One way of thinking about this simplification is that individual simulated neurons really represent the average responses of a much larger set of neurons in their immediate vicinity. Thus, although single neurons are modeled to have cellular properties like those of real individual cells (see below), we adjust for the neurons missing in the simulation by artificially increasing the strength of synaptic connections between cells. In this sense, a single modeled cell integrates information as a single neuron, but communicates the results as if it represented the average output of multiple neurons.

12.5.3 Types of Neurons

Although our network model of piriform cortex comprises three types of neurons, there are many more than three types in the real cortex (Haberly 1983). For example, two different types of pyramidal neurons have been identified, each with somewhat different physiological properties (Tseng and Haberly 1989). Moreover, there is an additional excitatory cell type that is nonpyramidal in structure, the so-called multipolar cell (Tseng and Haberly 1989; Hoffman and Haberly 1989), which also has distinct and interesting physiological properties (although there are far fewer multipolar cells than pyramidal neurons). Again, for the sake of simplicity these cell types were not included in the original model. Later iterations of the network model will likely include members of these other neuron classes.

12.5.4 Biophysical Properties

Another level of simplification at the single-cell level involves the membrane properties of the modeled neurons. Although our model includes Hodgkin and Huxley–like currents, many additional types of voltage-gated conductances known to exist in piriform pyramidal neurons (Banks, Haberly, and Jackson 1996; Constanti and Sim 1987a; Constanti et al. 1985, Constanti and Galvan 1983a, 1983b) are not included. Instead, we modeled only those currents associated with the fast sodium and potassium currents responsible for spike generation. To avoid the computationally expensive calculations associated with the Hodgkin-Huxley equation, the modeled currents were further simplified by activating the sodium and potassium currents only when the membrane potential crossed a fixed threshold. At that point, a very fast Na^+ current would activate, followed by a slower K^+ current, thus accurately re-creating the currents and membrane potentials associated with real action potentials, but without the computational overhead of a full Hodgkin-Huxley current. A serious shortcoming of this approach, however, is that it eliminates the contribution of voltage-gated currents to subthreshold activity, which recent studies have suggested is important to neural computation (Protopapas and Bower 1998b). Faster computers no longer make these compromises with conductances as necessary.

As with voltage-gated currents, synaptic conductances are modeled neglecting computationally expensive details like the kinetics of ligand binding, neurotransmitter uptake, and so on. Instead, changes in synaptic conductance are modeled as the difference of exponential functions, which approximates the shape of EPSPs seen in experimental studies (see "Synaptic Currents" in chapter appendix B).

12.6 Modeling Results

Our primary modeling objective was to generate the characteristic pattern of the electroencephelogram (EEG; see chapter appendix A for definition) seen in piriform cortex (Freeman and Schneider 1982; Freeman 1960). Because the shape of the EEG is presumably directly related to the interaction of many network components, we thought that it would provide a good measure of the basic validity of the model's structure. In accordance with our approach to modeling, we initially tuned our model on a physiological measure not directly or obviously related to our specific modeling objective, in this case, the surface evoked responses of the network to direct LOT stimulation. At the time, we were not aware of any direct relationship between these responses and the activity patterns seen in the EEG. As will become clear in later sections, the model suggested that there was indeed a direct relationship.

12.6.1 Tuning Network Parameters

The response of piriform cortex to LOT stimulation is very well described experimentally as this is one of the ways in which experimentalists have traditionally probed the organization of this structure (Haberly 1973a; Haberly and Bower 1984; Bower and Haberly 1986; Freeman 1968a, 1968b). This makes the evoked potential responses a good measure for model tuning. It has also been demonstrated that small changes in the strength of the LOT shock result in distinctly different spatial and temporal patterns of surface evoked potentials (Freeman 1968b). Specifically, as shown in figure 12.3, a weak shock to the LOT produces a prolonged damped oscillatory response, while a strong shock produces a short-duration biphasic response. From the point of view of modeling, this means that different model results can be compared by changing only a single parameter, in this case, the strength of the stimulus presented to the model's LOT. When tuning any model, it is an advantage to be able to test the results by changing a single stimulus variable. Our model has the added advantage that the stimulus strength dependence of the actual cortex is somewhat unusual because a weak shock generates more sustained activity than a strong shock.

Figure 12.3 demonstrates that the simulation replicates quite well the shock strength dependence of cortical evoked potentials. Furthermore, as described in more detail in Wilson and Bower 1992, the model accounted for the shock strength dependence of the cortex in a way that was not expected prior to the simulation results. For example, the simulations suggested that the reactivation of the rostral part of the cortex at the beginning of the second phase of oscillation of the network

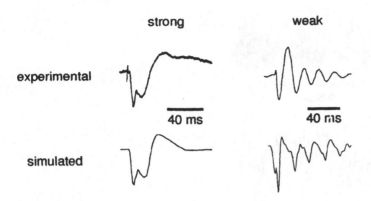

Figure 12.3
Comparison of field potential responses of simulated and biological piriform cortex to strong and weak
shocks of the LOT. Experimental data for strong shock are taken from Haberly 1973, while experimental
data for weak shock results are taken from Freeman 1968. All simulation data come from Wilson and
Bower 1992.

was a result of the interaction between the spread of activity throughout the whole
network and the time constants of locally activated inhibitory neurons. The role of
inhibitory neurons in cortical oscillations has since been proposed by numerous other
modelers (Bush and Sejnowski 1996; Jefferys, Traub, and Whittington 1996) and
recently demonstrated physiologically for olfactory structures in insects (MacLeod
and Laurent 1996). At the time, however, it was unexpected.

12.6.2   Simulating the Electroencephalogram

Once the network was tuned to produce the evoked potential responses characteristic
of real piriform cortex, model parameters were fixed and a more natural pattern of
afferent input was applied. Because it is known that olfactory bulb field potentials
oscillate at similar frequencies to those seen in the olfactory cortex (Bressler 1984;
Freeman and Schneider 1982), the model was initially presented with low levels of
phasic afferent input. Under these conditions, and without any change in model
parameters, the modeled cortex generated an EEG with both the high-frequency
(40–60 Hz) and low-frequency (5–12 Hz) components characteristic of the real cortex
(see figure 12.4), although it was perhaps not terribly surprising since the input pattern had similar frequencies. What we did not expect was that the cortex produced
the same shape EEG even without a temporally patterned input. The fact that this
simulation replicates both principal frequency components of the EEG, given either
phasic or tonic input, suggested that these oscillatory patterns may be intrinsic

experimental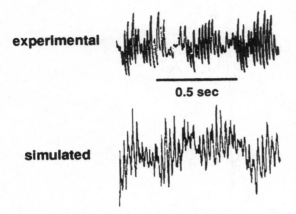

Figure 12.4
Comparison of EEG results from physiological experiments and the network model. Fast oscillations
constitute the gamma rhythm (40–60 Hz), while the modulation of gamma oscillations represents the theta
rhythm (5–12 Hz). Simulation data come from Wilson and Bower 1992 and experimental data from
Bressler 1984.

properties of the circuitry itself. Freeman reached the same conclusion from experiments where the LOT was cut and low levels of stimulation given to the cortical side of the cut tract (Freeman 1968a). Thus experimental and simulation results both support the idea that the piriform cortex oscillates intrinsically at frequencies appropriate to the phasic patterns of afferent activity it would naturally receive during the active sniffing cycle of the animal.

12.6.3 Functional Significance

The simulation experiments described here were the first step in our efforts to use modeling techniques to explore how the olfactory cortex might contribute to recognizing odors. Although our intention was to use the simulation of network dynamics to test the validity of the model's basic structure, even at this initial stage, the simulations led to several new and unexpected ideas about the possible significance of the dynamical behavior of piriform cortex.

One of the surprises of this early modeling effort was that the cortex itself seemed to oscillate intrinsically, even when presented with continuous random patterns of input, and even though the cells from which the model was built had no intrinsic oscillatory properties of their own. Thus the oscillations emerged from the structure of the network itself. This observation led us to examine more carefully which aspects of network structure underlie oscillations, although a detailed answer to this question is beyond the scope of the present chapter (see Bower 1995b). In short, what we found was that the periodicity in the EEG was reflected in a periodicity in the synaptic influences impinging on the pyramidal cell dendrites during each phase of the oscillation. For example, oscillations in the fast component (40–60 Hz) of the EEG were reflected in waves of synaptic activity moving back and forth across the cortex at these frequencies. Furthermore, the timings of the different synaptic inputs were regular and reproducible in each 40 Hz cycle of the oscillation. For example, the excitatory influences of the afferent and association fiber synapses and the synapses of the feedback inhibitory neurons all appeared to peak at different phases of the 40 Hz cycle. The spiking output of pyramidal cells and inhibitory neurons also occurred at different phases of the intrinsic 40 Hz oscillations. Given that theta bursts are correlated with the sniffing rate of the animal (Bressler 1984; Freeman and Schneider 1982), this suggested that the theta oscillations reflect an iterative computational process leading to odor recognition (Bower 1995b).

Whatever the computational significance of the oscillations, the most immediate implication of these results was that the oscillations arise indirectly from network-based mechanisms that control the timing of information arriving on the dendrites of cortical pyramidal cells (Bower 1990). In this view, the oscillations themselves are an epiphenomenon, reflecting more complex mechanisms that serve to control the timing of synaptic influences throughout the network. This in turn suggested that pyramidal cells might require that synaptic inputs of different sorts arrive at particular times with respect to each other, a conclusion also implied in current-source-density studies by Ketchum and Haberly (1993b). Pyramidal cells might therefore work something like internal combustion engines in which the cylinders need to be sparked in the right time and in the right sequence for proper functioning. Exploring this question, however, required the development of a much more realistic model of single pyramidal cell dendrites.

12.7 Detailed Model of a Single Pyramidal Cell

12.7.1 Structure of the Pyramidal Cell Model

To explore the sensitivity of pyramidal cell responses to different patterns of synaptic input, we needed to construct a model cell with realistic dendritic morphology and the proper passive and active membrane properties. Because several other chapters (3, 4, and 5) in this book deal with constructing single-cell models, we shall only summarize the approach taken here (additional details can be found in Protopapas and Bower 1998a, 1998b).

12.7.2 Passive Properties

As is often the case with realistic single-cell models, the morphology of the model was taken from the anatomical reconstruction of a real neuron (anatomy performed by Mark Domroese of the University of Wisconsin). The next step was to establish the passive properties of the model, using experimentally obtained values for input resistance, R_{in}, the membrane time constant, τ_0, and the first equalizing time constant, τ_1, from traces of membrane potential in response to constant current injection. Experimental values for these passive properties were obtained in our laboratory from whole-cell recordings in piriform cortex slices bathed in Cs^+ (nonspecific K^+ channel blocker) and TTX (Na^+ channel blocker). Using experimental values for R_{in}, τ_0, and τ_1 and standard methods, we were able to calculate values for the model parameters R_m (specific transmembrane resistance), R_a (specific axial resistance), and C_m (specific membrane capacitance; Protopapas and Bower 1998b; Rapp, Segev, and Yarom 1994; Major et al. 1994). See table 12.1 for parameter values.

Table 12.1
Parameter values for full and reduced models of piriform cortex pyramidal cell

	Full model	Reduced model
Number of compartments	1,089	15
Voltage-gated conductances	Fast Na^+	Fast Na^+
	Persistent Na^+	Persistent Na^+
	Delayed-rectifier K^+	Delayed-rectifier K^+
	M-current K^+	M-current K^+
	Slow AHP K^+	Slow AHP K^+
	A K^+	A K^+
	Slow Ca^+	Slow Ca^+
	Fast Ca^+	Fast Ca^+
Synaptic conductances	Non-NMDA	Non-NMDA
	NMDA	NMDA
	$GABA_A$	$GABA_A$
	$GABA_B$	$GABA_B$
Average electrotonic length of compartment (λ)	0.0184	0.0916
R_{IN} (MΩ)	47.6	58.1
R_m (k$\Omega \cdot$ cm^2)	30.0	5.0
R_a (k$\Omega \cdot$ cm)	0.350	58
C_m (μF/cm^2)	0.80	4.36
τ_0 (msec)	23.6	22.0
τ_1 (msec)	2.10	2.15

12.7.3   Active Conductances

Any model of realistic single-cell behavior must include active membrane properties. In the case of piriform cortex pyramidal cells, a number of voltage-gated currents have been characterized in the pyramidal cell, including at least one Ca^{2+} current (Constanti et al. 1985) and several potassium currents: a fast inward rectifier (Constanti and Galvan 1983a), a noninactivating muscarinic (M) current (Constanti and Galvan 1983b; Constanti and Sim 1987a), a slow Ca^{2+}-activated afterhyperpolarization (AHP) current (Constanti and Sim 1987a), and an A-current (Banks, Haberly, and Jackson 1996). Because piriform pyramidal neurons are known to have fast spikes, we assume the presence of fast sodium and delayed-rectifier potassium currents. Furthermore, we found that the addition of a persistent sodium current greatly improved the behavior of the model. Although there is no direct evidence that this current exists in the piriform pyramidal cell, it has been shown to exist in pyramidal neurons from the hippocampus (French et al. 1990). When voltage clamp data were available for piriform currents, we used these in our model; otherwise, we borrowed hippocampal voltage clamp data from previously modeled currents (Traub et al. 1991; McCormick and Huguenard 1992). The internal calcium dynamics used to activate the AHP current were a simplified model of the one used by Sala and Hernandez-Cruz (1990; see also chapter 6, this volume).

12.7.4   Synaptic Conductances

To examine the effect of patterns of synaptic inputs on the dendrites of the pyramidal cell, we needed to add realistic distributions of synaptic conductances to the modeled dendrite. As shown in figure 12.2, the synaptic input to piriform pyramidal cells is organized in a laminar fashion. Afferent projections from the olfactory bulb arrive via the LOT and terminate on the most distal part of the apical dendrite (Heimer 1968; Rodriguez and Haberly 1989; Ketchum and Haberly 1993a; Price 1973; Haberly and Behan 1983), while excitatory projections originating within the cortex terminate on more proximal regions of the dendrite (Bower and Haberly 1986; Haberly and Bower 1984).

   We also had to provide the synapses themselves with realistic kinetic properties. Pharmacological experiments performed in rat piriform cortex slices show that LOT-induced excitation of pyramidal neurons is mediated by both NMDA and non-NMDA receptors in layer Ia (Kanter and Haberly 1990; Jung, Larson, and Lynch 1990). A slow-acting $GABA_B$ K^+-mediated inhibition present in layer Ia is believed to originate in feedforward inhibitory neurons also excited by LOT afferents (Tseng and Haberly 1988). In the model, afferent excitation (with NMDA and non-NMDA components) and GABA$_B$ inhibition are restricted to layer Ia. The layer-Ib portion of the dendrite has also been shown to contain both NMDA and non-NMDA type receptors (Kanter and Haberly 1990) and, as in the network model, GABA$_A$-type receptors are present in the layer-II portion of the dendrite and also the soma (Tseng and Haberly 1988).

The time constants for the non-NMDA synapses were chosen to fit experimental data on the time course of non-NMDA conductances in hippocampal pyramidal cells (Mason, Nicoll, and Stratford 1991). Our model of NMDA-mediated synapses was identical to that used by Holmes and Levy (1990; see also chapter 6, this volume). Time constants for GABA$_B$ synapses were chosen to match experimental data on the time course of GABA$_B$ responses in rat hippocampal neurons (Ling and Benardo 1994). Time constants for GABA$_A$ responses were taken from Pearce 1993. In the model, the parameters for NMDA and non-NMDA synapses in layer Ib were identical to those used in layer Ia, except that channel densities were varied. Specifically, to account for the stronger NMDA response in layer Ib seen experimentally (Kanter and Haberly 1990), the channel density of the NMDA receptors was made twice as large in layer Ib.

12.7.5 Simplifying Cellular Components

To conform to computational constraints, and because of a lack of experimental data, a number of simplifications to the single-cell model had to be made. Dendritic spines were not modeled explicitly, but rather were included as an increase in dendritic membrane area. Similarly, second-messenger pathways for metabotropic synaptic receptors and complex calcium dynamics (e.g., Ca^{2+} release from intracellular stores) were not included in the model, even though they are known to exist (Tseng and Haberly 1988; Sah 1996). These omissions were permitted primarily in the name of computational efficiency. Fortunately, the model still exhibits reasonable approximations to real behavior (see below).

A further simplification was the absence of voltage-gated channels in the dendritic tree. Although numerous recent reports have shown the existence of voltage-gated channels in the dendritic trees of neocortical and hippocampal pyramidal cells (Stuart and Sakmann 1994; Magee and Johnston 1995), adequate data do not yet exist for the neuron we are modeling, and there is evidence to suggest that some voltage-gated channels that exist in the dendrites of neocortical and hippocampal pyramidal neurons may not exist in the dendrites of piriform pyramidal cells (Westenbroek et al. 1992). Furthermore, evidence in hippocampal pyramidal neurons suggests that active dendritic properties may primarily serve a role in synaptic plasticity and additionally may only come into·play when a somatic spike has already been elicited (Magee and Johnston 1997; Markram et al. 1997). Because the present single-cell model does not address issues of plasticity, we felt that we could neglect the active properties of the dendrite. Future iterations of the single-cell and network models will almost certainly have to include active dendritic conductances.

12.7.6 Tuning Neuronal Parameters

As with the network model, the process of tuning the single-cell model involved identifying a physiological response that could be well characterized but that was not directly linked to the neural behavior the model was eventually intended to study. The measure chosen was in vitro responses to somatic current injection (Protopapas and Bower 1998b; Barkai and Hasselmo 1994). Because this nonphysiological stimulus generates characteristic cellular responses, intracellular current injection is comparable to the electrical LOT shock used to tune the network model.

In most realistic single-cell models, the most poorly constrained parameters are the densities of the active channels. In the present case, this set of important parameters was tuned by matching the spiking behavior of the model to experimental F/I (frequency against current injection) plots obtained with different levels of somatic current injection (Barkai and Hasselmo 1994). In addition, the ability of the model to match subthreshold events and the actual spike shapes seen in experimental traces were also quantified. When simulated and experimental spiking behavior are compared (figure 12.5), much of the behavior seen in the real spike train can also be seen in the model spike train, for example, the two fast spikes at the beginning of the train and the subthreshold oscillations following the last spike.

12.7.7 Response to Synaptic Input

Once the model was tuned, synaptic input was applied to the dendrite of the cell and the responses measured. Because we were interested in exploring how synaptic activity patterns suggested by the network model and experimental studies (Ketchum and Haberly 1993a, 1993b, 1993c) might influence the information-processing properties of this neuron, we applied a synaptic input pattern believed to underlie the 40 Hz oscillations seen in the EEG (Ketchum and Haberly 1993b, 1993c), and then examined the effect of this pattern on the intracellular response of the pyramidal cell. Figure 12.6A shows how a change in the synaptic input underlying a single 40 Hz oscillation can affect subsequent oscillations during the course of a theta (5–12 Hz) oscillation. This suggests that the activity induced during the course of a single 40 Hz oscillation is not independent of the activity underlying nearby oscillations. Therefore, the computations that the neuron performs during the course of a single theta

EXPERIMENT

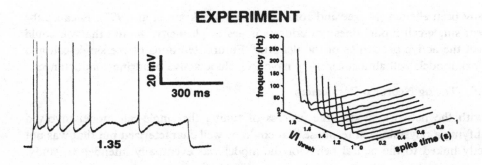

FULL MODEL

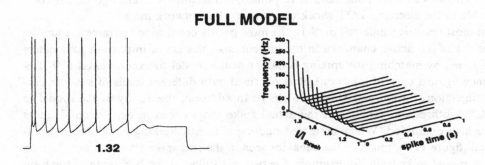

REDUCED MODEL

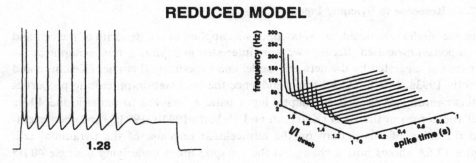

Figure 12.5
Comparison of full and reduced models to experimental response to current injection. The numbers below the voltage traces indicate the threshold normalized current injection used in each case. $I_{threshold} = 1$.

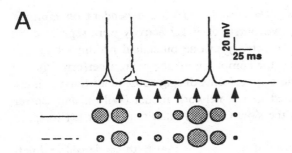

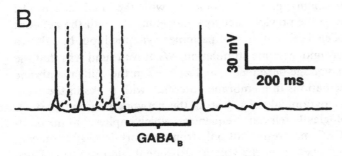

Figure 12.6
Effects of the input underlying a single 40 Hz oscillation during subsequent 40 Hz oscillations. Two intra-cellular traces from the detailed single-cell model are shown. The input underlying each trace is identical except that the input for the first 40 Hz oscillation is much smaller for the dotted trace than for the solid. The divergence between the two traces lasts approximately 90 msec showing that the effects of the input underlying a single 40 Hz oscillation can last much longer than the 25 msec duration of single oscillation. (B) Two bursts of 40 Hz activity (believed to represent activity underlying single theta oscillations) are separated by 200 msec. Again, the figure shows two overlapping traces; in this case, the input underlying the two traces is identical except in the first burst of 40 Hz activity. As can be seen, despite the difference in the initial burst, the second set of bursts is identical, suggesting that activity in the previous burst has little impact on subsequent bursts provided they are separated by 200 msec. Such a separation in time can be accounted for biologically by the presence of a slow $GABA_B$ inhibition.

oscillation (consisting of a burst of 40 Hz oscillations) are dependent on multiple 40 Hz oscillations. When, however, two bursts of 40 Hz activity were separated by 200 msec or more, we found that the activity in one burst had no impact on the activity of the second, suggesting that the computations the neuron performs during one burst may be independent of those it performs during subsequent bursts (figure 12.6B). This result was first predicted in the network model (Wilson and Bower 1992), where it was speculated that the slow $GABA_B$ inhibition might act to space out theta activity.

Perhaps the most encouraging aspect of this work is that both single-cell and network models imply similar computational features, although at quite different levels of scale. Both models suggest that cortical oscillations reflect an iterative computational process operating at 40 Hz packed into oscillations at the theta frequency. There is, however, another unanticipated phenomenon with the single-cell model that is immediately relevant to the previous network modeling. As with the network model, we subjected the modeled cell not only to patterned synaptic input but also to random, unpatterned background synaptic stimulation. What we found was that the interaction of the particular voltage-dependent conductances in the cell's membrane resulted in subthreshold fluctuations in membrane potential, with peaks in the theta range. Thus it appears that pyramidal cells, just as the network they are part of, naturally oscillate at physiologically relevant frequencies, which implies that the oscillatory patterns seen in the EEG may result not only from network-level phenomena, but also from the emergent properties of the voltage-dependent conductances. Thus, there also appears to be a resonance between network and single cell properties.

To study this relationship further, and to pursue our computational interpretation of cortical oscillations, we had reconstitute a network-level simulation based on neurons with more realistic biophysical properties. Accordingly, just as our original network models led us to single-cell modeling, now our single-cell modeling has led us back to network simulations.

12.8   Refining the Network Model

The specific objective of our third stage of modeling of olfactory cortex is to construct a network model based on more sophisticated pyramidal cell simulations. While computers are dramatically more powerful now than they were when we built our first network model twelve years ago (on an IBM XT!), they are still not powerful enough to construct a large-scale network model out of full-scale single-cell simulations. It is therefore necessary to reduce the complexity of the single-cell models.

12.8.1   Reducing the Single-Cell Model

In simplifying our detailed pyramidal cell model, we wanted to preserve as many of the physiological properties of the original full-scale single-cell model as possible, in particular, the model's dynamical properties. To accomplish this task, we have chosen to reduce the full model using a method that conserves axial resistance but that treats unit membrane resistance and capacitance as free parameters (cf. Bush and Sejnowski 1993). This method, which reduces two cylinders located at the end of a dendritic tree into one equivalent cylinder (whose radius is the geometric mean of the radii of the two original cylinders and whose length is the sum of the lengths of the two cylinders), can be applied iteratively to reduce the original model as much as one desires. When any two cylinders have widely differing lengths, we simply remove the smaller dendrite to avoid distorting the geometry of the cell. Because this method does not conserve total cell area, R_M and C_M of the model are rescaled until the input resistance R_{in} and input time constant τ_0 are roughly the same in both models. To ensure accurate numerical results, it is also necessary that each compartment have an electrotonic length of less than 0.1 λ (Segev et al. 1985).

To be more specific, the cell model is simplified as follows:

1. Unbranched chains of compartments are reduced to a single compartment having the same electrotonic length and physical length. This is done by calculating the total electrotonic length of the branch and then adjusting the diameter of the new compartment to give the same total electrotonic length.

2. Branches are collapsed into single compartments, starting from the distal end and proceeding inward, according to the Bush and Sejnowski (1993) algorithm described above. This is repeated until only five compartments remain: a basal dendritic compartment, the soma compartment, and an apical dendrite in three compartments (proximal layer 1b, distal layer 1b, and layer 1a). The apical dendrite compartments, which can be joined together, are kept separate because the connection topology of the model requires separate compartments. At this point, we have five compartments.

3. Because the basal and apical dendritic compartments are considerably longer than the 0.1 lambda limit normally considered to be the maximum length compatible with numerical accuracy, we subdivide each of the dendritic compartments into two to six compartments, which results in fifteen compartments all less than 0.1 lambda in length. One thing to note is that this method assumes a passive dendritic tree and is therefore not likely to be valid with active dendrites. In the current version of our model, however, all the active conductances are located in the soma.

The fact that the full and reduced models both contain the same voltage-gated channel types in roughly equal proportions implies that they will have very similar active properties. As with all our models, however, we first test the reduced model's performance with a functionally neutral response pattern, in this case, the same measure we applied to the full single-cell model: the response of the cell to somatic current injections. In figure 12.5, we have plotted the spike frequency against current injection during a series of increasing current steps for the two models. The results demonstrate almost identical performances, which is not surprising given that the reduced model was tuned to have an input resistance, as well as membrane and equalizing time constants τ_0 and τ_1, similar to those of the full model. Table 12.1 compares the behavior and parameters of the two models for several additional measures. The only significant differences are seen in the number of compartments, the specific transmembrane resistance, R_m, the specific axial resistance, R_a, the specific membrane capacitance, C_m, and, most important, the execution time (2.22 min for the full model vs. 3 sec for the reduced model for simulation of 100 msec on a 200 MHz PC running Linux). The astute reader may additionally note that the average electrotonic length of compartments in the full and reduced models suggests that total electrotonic length is not conserved between the full and reduced models. This may be unavoidable because many individual dendrites are collapsed into single dendrites during the reduction process.

12.8.2 The Costs of Model Simplification

Given that the transient responses of the complex and simplified models are essentially the same, it is likely that under many conditions both models will respond almost identically to individual synaptic inputs. Because the geometrical complexity of the neuron has been dramatically decreased, however, some patterns of single-cell response will no longer be possible. For example, in the reduced model multiple dendritic branches are represented by single compartments or strings of compartments. Because a small high-resistance compartment in the detailed model will be represented by a lower-resistance compartment in the reduced model, synaptic inputs will see different input resistances in the different models. Perhaps more important, it will not be possible with the reduced model to study how particular spatial patterns of synaptic inputs on individual dendrites might functionally affect cellular or network output. This means, for example, that in the network model we will not be able to study the consequences of synaptic segregation on individual dendritic branches. Furthermore, even though particular spatial patterns of synaptic input on single branches are important, as has been suggested (Koch, Poggio and Torre 1982), they will not figure in our network simulations. Because these questions can be studied using our existing single-cell simulation, our research will almost certainly continue to be based on the iterative use of the single-cell and network models.

12.9 Discussion

One of the most basic assumptions underlying the construction of realistic simulations is that the structure of the nervous system, if we respect it, will lead us to ideas about its function. In this chapter, we have attempted to illustrate how our simulations of olfactory cortex have led us to new and unanticipated functional ideas as well as to new simulations at different levels of scale with which to test them. This is the power and excitement of realistic modeling. For several fortuitous reasons, our work in the olfactory system has also allowed us to demonstrate the process of extracting functional ideas from neural structure without the problem of imposing ad hoc theoretical interpretations on neural data.

At the time our simulations were first completed (Wilson and Bower 1987), there was little interest outside of the olfactory community in cerebral cortical oscillations. Indeed, a paper submitted to *Science* in 1988 describing the implications of our network simulations for the origins of cortical oscillations was rejected without review as being "not interesting to a broad audience." In 1989 however, *Science* published a report describing oscillations of similar frequencies in visual cortex (Gray et al. 1989). Since that time, there has been tremendous interest in cortical oscillations involving the visual system.

The primary reason for this interest was that changes in the oscillatory structure of the response seemed to be directly related to changes in the visual stimulus presented. While, by itself, this was probably not too exciting, several years earlier it had been proposed on theoretical grounds that synchronous neuronal firing might provide the means of solving what is known in the machine vision and artificial intelligence fields as "the binding problem," the presumed difficulty that feature detection–based systems have in assigning multiple attributes (e.g., color, texture, etc.) to the same object. It was proposed that by synchronized neuronal firing, multiple attributes could be represented together (von der Malsburg and Schneider 1986) and Gray et al. (1989) had found synchronous oscillations in visual cortex that seemed to be related to the nature of the stimulus.

What has happened since that 1989 report was published is nothing short of remarkable. Large numbers of meetings have been held and models generated to look at the mechanisms and functional significance of cortical oscillations. Not only have oscillations been linked to the binding problem, but other authors have extended their applicability to models of visual attention (Niebur, Koch, and Rosin 1993) and even consciousness (Crick and Koch 1990). These ideas continue to have a substantial influence on both experimental (Whittington, Traub, and Jefferys 1995) and theoretical (Traub et al. 1996) neurobiology. Most of the models used to investigate these phenomena, however, have been "demonstration models," intended, with greater or fewer real "neural features," to support the plausibility of a particular functional idea.

Our own interpretation of the significance of oscillations in olfactory cortex is very different from the interpretation applied to the visual system. That the model we used to investigate oscillations was firmly based on real biology led us to suspect the interpretation of the oscillations applied to the visual system for several practical reasons (Wilson and Bower 1991). First, as in our models of olfactory cortex, the oscillations recorded in the visual system were of the EEG/evoked potential type. Unfortunately, most theorists assumed that the timing of evoked potentials and EEGs directly reflected the timing of pyramidal cell spiking. From our models, we knew that these field potential effects were actually related to synaptic inputs on dendrites, and not necessarily to spike outputs. Accordingly, the actual patterns of spikes could not be directly inferred from the EEG or evoked potential patterns. Second, from our simulations of a more visual cortex–like structure (based on the olfactory cortex simulation; Wilson and Bower 1991), we predicted that the oscillations would not be instantaneous, continuous, or even very regular, as was implied by simple versions of the binding/attention hypothesis. Finally, it seemed quite unlikely to us, given the duration of the effects of the synaptic input underlying a single 40 Hz oscillation, that these neurons would do a good job of detecting millisecond coincidences in firing (Protopapas and Bower 1998a).

For each of these reasons, we are skeptical about a direct role for oscillations in neural coding. Instead, as we suggested many years ago, based on our realistic network models (Wilson and Bower 1991), cortical oscillations are more likely to indirectly reflect network and single-cell processes involved in regulating the timing of synaptic activity in and between networks. Recent experiments demonstrating that different structures within the somatosensory system start to oscillate synchronously prior to the onset of sensory or motor behavior (Nicolelis et al. 1995) are consistent with the idea that the oscillations reflect the control of synaptic timing and the flow of information. Furthermore, we have suspected for many years that oscillatory activity patterns also indirectly reflect the timing and organization of computational cycles within cortical circuits. Finally, whatever the functional role of oscillations in cortical networks, we believe it is more useful to develop theories based on realistic models than to try to squeeze brain circuits into ad hoc theories, where once the model has demonstrated plausibility, the modeling is done. As demonstrated in this chapter, realistic modeling is never done. There are always more interesting relationships to discover.

Acknowledgments

We wish to thank Fidel Santamaria and Jenny Forss for their helpful comments on the text; Mark Domroese for providing us with an anatomically stained pyramidal cell for our single-cell modeling work; and John Miller and Gwen Jacobs for their generous help in digitizing the cell's anatomy. Chris Assad was also very helpful in generating the contour plots that are basis for figure 12.7. Finally, we wish to thank Matt Wilson, who wrote the network modeling chapter in the first edition of this volume, on which this chapter is based.

Appendix A: Using the Model to Generate Field Potential Events

This appendix describes how evoked potential and EEG responses were derived from model activity. While both kinds of responses fall under the category of field potential recording, what differentiates them is the experimental context in which the field potentials are recorded. *Evoked potential* refers to a change in the extracellularly recorded field potential in response to a specific stimulus (e.g., a shock to the LOT). By contrast, *EEG*, a more general term, refers to field potential recordings taken at the cortical surface or even the scalp, often in the absence of a well-characterized stimulus and almost always over a large area of the brain. For example, EEG recordings are often made while an animal is freely exploring its surroundings, rather than in response to a well-timed shock. The neuronal origin of field potentials is not easy to elucidate, and efforts to do so are still an active area of research (Ketchum and Haberly 1993a, 1993b, 1993c). As we shall see shortly, this difficulty arises from the physics underlying field potentials.

To simulate field potentials in the model, we first calculated the extracellular currents expected to flow through the cortex due to neuronal activity. Neurons, like any electrical entity, must obey Kirchoff's current law, which states that the sum of all currents entering and leaving a circuit node must equal zero. In the case of a neuron, this means that if synaptic current, for example, enters the cell at one point, it must leak from another, thereby generating an extracellular current (see figure 12.7). Because compartmental modeling deals with lumped representations of neurons (i.e., electrical compartments are discrete), field potentials can be calculated using the following equation:

$$\Phi(\vec{d}, t) = \frac{1}{4\pi\sigma} \sum_{i=1}^{n} \frac{I_i(t)}{d_i}, \qquad (12.1)$$

where Φ is the field potential in volts, I_i (equivalent to the transmembrane current in a single compartment) is the total current (in amperes) from the ith current source into brain tissue of conductivity σ (in Ohms^{-1}meters^{-1}), and d_i (in meters) is the distance of the ith current source from the recording site (Nunez 1981). Note that this equation assumes the extracellular medium is a noncapacitative homogeneous conductor, which is only an approximation to biological reality (Ketchum and Haberly 1993b).

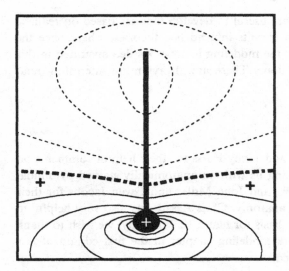

Figure 12.7
A model cell is shown as it is receiving synchronous excitatory synaptic input along its dendrite. The opening of synaptic channels generates current sinks along the dendrite, while a current source is generated at the soma where current is leaking out of the cell. The current sinks (minus signs) generate negative field potentials shown by the thin dotted isopotential contour lines. Conversely, the current source at the soma is responsible for generating the positive field potentials indicated by the thin solid lines. The thick dotted line represents the region where the field potential has a value of zero. For a more detailed study of field potentials generated by single neurons, specifically during the course of an action potential, see Rall 1962. The figure shown here was inspired by that work.

A brief examination of eq. 12.1 indicates why it is difficult to ascertain which types of physiological activity underlie real field potentials. Specifically, the equation tells us that the size of the field potential increases in amplitude with the magnitude of transmembrane current and decreases with distance between the current source and electrode. Therefore, although neither the position of the electrode nor the magnitude of a transmembrane current can uniquely explain the magnitude of a field potential signal, anatomical constraints such as those imposed by the network model can reduce the number of physiologically plausible explanations for different field potential patterns. Indeed, this was one of the primary motivations in performing the original network modeling study.

In the model, both evoked potentials and the EEG were calculated at positions corresponding to those where physiological measurements had previously been made by other researchers. In the case of the evoked potentials, calculations were made at single surface locations at varying depths. By contrast, the field potentials calculated from forty evenly spaced recording sites on the surface of the simulated cortex were averaged to produce an estimate of the EEG in response to patterned and unpatterned input.

Appendix B: Neuronal Objects in GENESIS

This appendix briefly discusses the mathematical representation of a number of common neuronal objects in GENESIS. (For a more complete description, see Bower and Beeman 1995.)

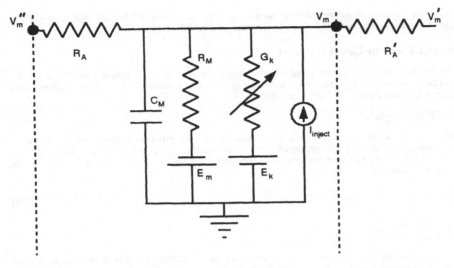

Figure 12.8
Circuit representation of a GENESIS compartment. V_m'', V_m, and V_m' are the membrane potentials for the left, center, and right compartments demarcated by the dotted lines. R_A and R_A' are the axial resistances for the center and right compartments, respectively. C_M, R_M, and E_m are the membrane capacitance, membrane resistance, and leak current reversal potential, respectively. G_k is a variable conductance representing synaptic or voltage-gated conductances, and E_k is the reversal potential associated with the particular conductance. I_{inject} represents current being injected into the compartment (e.g., current injection through an intracellular electrode).

Compartmental Representation

Figure 12.8 shows a circuit diagram of a typical GENESIS compartment (chapters 3, 4, and 5, this volume, describe the theoretical basis for compartmental modeling). Values for membrane resistance, R_M, capacitance, C_M, and axial resistance, R_A, are automatically calculated for the compartment object by the "readcell" command. Users set values for specific membrane resistance (R_m, in $\Omega \cdot m^2$), specific membrane capacitance (C_m, in Farads per square meter), and specific axial resistance (R_a, in Ohms times meter). Values for R_M, C_M, and R_A are calculated using the following relations:

$$C_M = \pi\, dl\, C_m \tag{12.2}$$

$$R_M = \frac{R_m}{\pi\, dl} \tag{12.3}$$

$$R_A = \frac{4l R_a}{\pi d^2}, \tag{12.4}$$

where d is the diameter and l is the length of the morphological compartment.

The membrane potential of a compartment is calculated from the following differential equation:

$$C_M \frac{dV_m}{dt} = \frac{(E_m - V_m)}{R_M} + \sum_k [G_k(E_k - V_m)] + \frac{(V_m' - V_m)}{R_a'} + \frac{(V_m'' - V_m)}{R_A} + I_{inject}, \tag{12.5}$$

where all variables are defined in figure 12.8.

Compartments may be organized into a parameter text file within GENESIS that specifies the morphology, channel distribution, and passive properties of a model neuron.

Voltage- and Calcium-Gated Currents

The GENESIS voltage- and calcium-gated current objects used in these simulations are based on the Hodgkin-Huxley formalism. Typically, the current coming through a particular voltage- or calcium-gated conductance is calculated from the following equation:

$$I(V, t) = m^p h^q \bar{g}(E_{rev} - V_m),$$
(12.6)

where $I(V, t)$ is the current passing through the voltage- or calcium-gated conductance, m the activation gate, h the inactivation gate, $\bar{g}$ the maximum possible conductance, E_{rev} the reversal potential for the channel, V_m the membrane potential, and p and q exponents for m and h. Activation and inactivation are governed by the equations:

$$\frac{dm}{dt} = \frac{m_\infty - m}{\tau_m}$$
(12.7a)

idem for h, $\frac{dh}{dt} = \frac{h_\infty - h}{\tau_h}$
(12.7b)

where m_∞ is steady-state activation and τ_m is the time constant of activation and both m_∞ and τ_m depend on voltage. Users may define m_∞ and τ_m explicitly or by defining the voltage-dependent rate constants α and β, which take the following form:

$$\alpha = \frac{A_\alpha + B_\alpha V_m}{C_\alpha + \exp\left(\frac{V_m + D_\alpha}{F}\right)}$$
(12.8a)

$$\beta = \frac{A_\beta + B_\beta V_m}{C_\beta + \exp\left(\frac{V_m + D_\beta}{F_\beta}\right)},$$
(12.8b)

where A, B, C, D, and F are user-defined parameters. In this case, α and β may be related to m_∞ and τ_m in the following way:

$$m_\infty = \frac{\alpha_m}{\alpha_m + \beta_m}$$
(12.9a)

$$h_\infty = \frac{\alpha_h}{\alpha_h + \beta_h}$$
(12.9b)

$$\tau_m = \frac{1}{\alpha_m + \beta_m}$$
(12.10a)

$$\tau_h = \frac{1}{\alpha_h + \beta_h}.$$
(12.10b)

Calcium-activated currents are modeled in an identical fashion except that rate constants and activation parameters are calcium-dependent instead of voltage-dependent. Using this formalism, one may also combine voltage and calcium activation to create a current that is dependent on both.

Typically, the simulation of Hodgkin and Huxley–type currents is computationally expensive because exponential functions must be calculated at each time step. GENESIS avoids this problem by giving the user the opportunity to create lookup tables that contain precalculated values of rate parameters. Values for rate parameters are evaluated by interpolating from entries contained in the lookup table. This method greatly increases the speed of simulations.

Synaptic Currents

In order to simulate synaptic currents, spike trains from presynaptic neurons must be converted into time-varying conductances in postsynaptic cells. The most general way to do this is to use a convolution operation:

$$\hat{g}(t) = \int_0^{t_d} G(\lambda)S(t - \lambda - t_t)\,d\lambda, \tag{12.11}$$

where $\hat{g}(t)$ is the actual conductance elicited by synaptic activation in the postsynaptic cell, $G(t)$ the synaptic conductance waveform for the postsynaptic cell, $S(t)$ the spike signal from the presynaptic cell, t_d the time interval over which incoming spikes are convolved with the conductance waveform, and t_t the propagation delay from the presynaptic to the postsynaptic cell. The convolution approach has the advantage that $G(t)$ can be arbitrarily defined. Unfortunately, it requires significant computational or storage overhead because a history of spiking must be maintained in order to calculate synaptic conductance at every time step. To increase the efficiency of synaptic current simulations, GENESIS models a synaptic input as the impulse response of a damped oscillator; this approach uses a second-order differential equation to model synaptic input and does not require a history of spike events that is necessary when using the convolution approach. The general form of this equation is

$$\ddot{G} + \alpha\dot{G} + \beta G = x(t), \tag{12.12}$$

with

$$\alpha = \frac{\tau_1 + \tau_2}{\tau_1 \tau_2}, \quad \beta = \frac{1}{\tau_1 \tau_2}. \tag{12.13}$$

The impulse response of this system ($x(t) = \delta(t)$) with initial conditions of $G(0)$ has the following dual exponential form:

$$G(t) = \frac{\tau_1 \tau_2}{\tau_1 - \tau_2}\left(e^{-t/\tau_1} - e^{-t/\tau_2}\right), \tag{12.14}$$

with time to peak given by

$$t_{peak} = \frac{\tau_1 \tau_2}{\tau_1 - \tau_2} \ln\left(\frac{\tau_1}{\tau_2}\right). \tag{12.15}$$

When $t_1 = t_2$, the dual exponential form takes the form of an alpha function:

$$G(t) = te^{-t/\tau}, \tag{12.16}$$

where $t = t_1 = t_2$. In this case $t_{peak} = \tau$.

To calculate synaptic conductance at every time step, the second-order system is described by two first-order equations:

$$\dot{z} = -\frac{1}{\tau_1}z + x(t) \tag{12.17}$$

$$\dot{G} = -\frac{1}{\tau_2}G + z. \tag{12.18}$$

These equations can then be numerically integrated to yield $G(t)$. The net conductance can then be calculated by

$$\hat{g}(t) = \frac{g_{max}}{G_{peak}}G(t)w(t), \tag{12.19}$$

where g_{max} is the maximal possible synaptic conductance as determined by the modeler and $w(t)$ is the synaptic weight.

Appendix C: Numerical Methods

GENESIS users may select from a number of different numerical methods based on their specific simulation needs. As discussed in greater detail in chapter 14 of this volume, the choice of numerical method is critical for the fast and accurate solution of the differential equations that make up any neural simulation. Given the importance of this issue, we will briefly describe the methods available to GENESIS users. The models described in this chapter made use of the exponential Euler (network model) and backward Euler (single-cell simulations) methods.

Explicit Methods

Forward Euler The forward Euler method is the simplest numerical method for approximating solutions to differential equations of the form

$$\frac{dy}{dt} = f(t). \tag{12.20}$$

At time Δt, we can approximate $y(t + \Delta t)$ with

$$y(t + \Delta t) = y(t) + f(t)\Delta t. \tag{12.21}$$

Although forward Euler method allows for quick calculation at each time step, it is very unstable and therefore requires very small time steps for accurate results, which makes it quite unsuitable for most neural simulations.

Adams-Bashforth Adams-Bashforth methods, although more accurate than forward Euler, are still relatively unstable. These methods take the form

$$y(t + \Delta t) = y(t) + \Delta t(a_0 f(t) + a_1 f(t - \Delta t) + a_2 f(t - 2\Delta t) + \cdots + a_n f(t - n\Delta t)), \tag{12.22}$$

where a_n coefficients may be found by expanding $f(t - n\Delta t)$ in a Taylor series. An Adams-Bashforth method is said to be of the $(n + 1)$th order when $f(t)$ is evaluated at n previous time steps. GENESIS allows users to choose from second- to fifth-order Adams-Bashforth methods.

Exponential Euler This method is applicable in the case of neural simulations because the differential equations used in neural simulations (e.g., eqs. 12.5 and 12.7) are generally of the form

$$\frac{dy}{dt} = A - By. \tag{12.23}$$

In which case, we can approximate a solution at time $t + \Delta t$ with

$$y(t + \Delta t) = y(t)e^{-B\Delta t} + \frac{A}{B}(1 - e^{-B\Delta t}) \tag{12.24}$$

Although, under most circumstances, A and B are not constants, if they change little over the course of a time step, this method gives a reasonable approximation. For simulations where neurons consist of only a few compartments and active channels, this method appears to work better than the two previously mentioned.

Implicit Methods

Although implicit methods tend to have greater accuracy for a given time step size than explicit methods, because they are dependent on the value of $f(t + \Delta t)$, the solution process is more complex and thus the computational cost per time step is greater. In general, the greater accuracy permits the use of a much larger time step, leading to greater computational efficiency with implicit methods. Two implicit methods are available to GENESIS users.

Backward Euler   Backward Euler is identical in form to forward Euler, except that $y(t + \Delta t)$ is defined implicitly as

$$y(t + \Delta t) = y(t) + f(t + \Delta t)\Delta t. \tag{12.25}$$

This method is first-order correct in Δt and always stable.

Crank-Nicholson   The Crank-Nicholson method averages forward and backward Euler methods to achieve a partial cancellation of errors. The method has the following form:

$$y(t + \Delta t) = y(t) + \frac{(f(t) + f(t + \Delta t))\Delta t}{2}. \tag{12.26}$$

This method is second-order correct in Δt and is usually stable except for very small Δt.

Hines Method for Solving Branched Dendritic Trees   For single-cell simulations, GENESIS uses a method developed by Michael Hines (1984) to number compartments in a branched dendritic tree in such a way that they can be organized into a tridiagonal matrix, where each row represents the difference equation for the membrane potential in a compartment. This greatly facilitates the use of implicit methods because the matrix represents a series of coupled equations that can easily be solved by Gaussian elimination. (For a more detailed discussion of the Hines method and numerical methods in general, see chapter 14, this volume.)

Appendix D: Network Connections

As we have stressed many times throughout this chapter, realistic neural models can easily exceed available computer power. For this reason, simulation systems like GENESIS seek to find simplifications that reduce computational overhead without compromising model structure too severely. In the case of network simulations, one such simplification involves representing the connections between neurons as delay lines that carry simple impulses with the duration of a single time step and a unit amplitude, which makes it unnecessary to explicitly model axonal action potentials. In GENESIS, a threshold is set in the presynaptic neuron to determine when a spike is to be transmitted to a postsynaptic cell, which receives the spike at a fixed time delay determined by the delay line. The spike is then converted into a synaptic conductance at the postsynaptic neuron. Numerous GENESIS commands exist to specify connectivity patterns, delay distributions, strength of interneuronal connections, and so on (see Bower and Beeman 1995 for further details).

Appendix E: Additional Features of GENESIS

Simulating Synaptic Plasticity

GENESIS simulations can also include the effects of synaptic plasticity using the *hebbsynchan* object, which works exactly like the standard synaptic object, except that the weight value of the synapses are adjusted based on a product of the pre- and postsynaptic activities. The presynaptic activity measure is calculated by having each spike generate an alpha-function waveform with a slow time constant (representing NMDA kinetics, which are much slower than AMPA kinetics). These alpha-functions do not directly control the channel conductance; they are only summed to generate the presynaptic activity measure. The postsynaptic activity measure is simply a low-pass-filtered version of the postsynaptic membrane potential. The time constants of this filtering and of the presynaptic alpha-function waveform are adjustable parameters of the object. Synaptic weights increase when pre- and postsynaptic activities are above user-defined thresholds and decrease when one of the activities is below its threshold. When both activities are below threshold, no change in weights occurs. Arbitrary weight change algorithms can be incorporated into this object by making minor modifications to the object's C code.

Although this object is a tremendous simplification of the complex electrical and biochemical events that underlie processes like long-term potentiation (LTP), computational efficiency in network modeling often requires that such processes be modeled as simply as possible.

Parameter Search Routines

One of the most tedious aspects of constructing realistic models is searching through large parameter spaces to find models that produce outputs matching experimental data. GENESIS contains a library of parameter search routines that can automate this process to a large degree, in some cases reducing months of painstaking manual searches to a few days of automated searching. Several different parameter search methods have been implemented thus far, including conjugate gradient descent, stochastic search, genetic algorithms, and a continuous version of simulated annealing. (For a comparison of these methods on some simple models, see Vanier and Bower 1996.) These methods are most useful in two cases: (1) for fine-tuning a model that already generates output qualitatively similar to that of the real system, and (2) for determining whether a reasonable match to data is possible, given the model. Case 2 is especially important in that it can suggest that the model is insufficiently detailed to capture the behavior of the real system, and may suggest how it might be extended to better match the data.

Parallel GENESIS

Parallel GENESIS was developed by Nigel Goddard and Greg Hood (1997) of the Pittsburgh Supercomputing Center to allow GENESIS to run on any platform that supports Parallel Virtual Machine (PVM), a software package developed to allow the computing resources of multiple workstations and PCs to be pooled together and used like a parallel machine. Parallel GENESIS can therefore be run on everything from multiple PCs running Linux to a CRAY supercomputer.

Certain problems in computational neuroscience are particularly well suited to parallel implementations. Parameter searches often require running a single simulation hundreds or even thousands of times while varying individual parameters. By farming out individual simulation runs to different processors, the user can perform searches that would have taken an unbearably long time on a serial machine. Similarly, large networks can be implemented in such a way that individual neurons or groups of neurons can be simulated on single processors. Parallel GENESIS commands have been tailored to facilitate these two applications.

Chemical Kinetics

In general, electrical signals in the nervous system are mediated by four mechanisms: (1) gap junctions, (2) voltage-gated channels, (3) ligand-gated channels, and (4) metabotropic receptors. Almost all of the neural models of the past decade have focused on the first three of these mechanisms, with special emphasis on the second and third, although increasing experimental evidence shows that metabotropic receptors play a major role in neural computation. These receptors are activated by an extracellular molecule (typically, a neurotransmitter or neuromodulator), which then triggers a biochemical cascade inside the neuron. This cascade then generates molecules (typically, activated G-proteins or cyclic nucleotides), which activate channels by binding to intracellular sites.

Biochemical pathways are additionally important in neural computation because they are at the root of the synaptic plasticity observed in the nervous system. The pathways underlying long-term potentiation

(LTP) are controlled by multiple factors, which makes the use of a kinetic modeling system ideal for the study of this phenomenon.

For these reasons, Upinder Bhalla (1997) developed a GENESIS library for the simulation of biochemical pathways. Simulation of biochemical reactions requires that one formulate a rate equation. If we have a reaction

$$A + B \underset{k_b}{\overset{k_f}{\rightleftharpoons}} C + D, \tag{12.27}$$

where $A, B, C,$ and D are biologically important molecules, k_f the forward rate constant, and k_b the backward rate constant, we can describe this with the differential equation

$$\frac{d[A]}{dt} = k_b[C][D] - k_f[A][B]. \tag{12.28}$$

Parameters such as k_f and k_b can be approximated from data found in the literature. (For a more detailed discussion of the issues and methodologies involved in the modeling of biochemical pathways, see Bower and Beeman (1997).)

Appendix F: Model Parameters

Parameters for Full and Reduced Single-Cell Models

Both full and reduced models use the same voltage-gated and synaptic currents. The voltage-gated currents are described using the Hodgkin-Huxley formalism set forth in "Voltage- and Calcium-Gated Currents," chapter appendix B, and synaptic currents are parameterized according to the equations in "Synaptic Currents," chapter appendix B. (For a more detailed justification of the parameters shown here, see Protopapas and Bower 1998b.) For all of the following equations, time is in milliseconds and membrane potential is in millivolts.

Fast Sodium Current Parameters for this current were obtained from a study by Traub et al. (1991). Slight modifications were made to conform to experimental data.

$$I = m^2 h\bar{g}(E_{rev} - V_m), \quad E_{rev} = 55\,\text{mV}; \tag{12.29}$$

for m_∞ and τ_m:

$$\alpha = \frac{0.32(36.2 + V)}{1.0 - \exp\left(\frac{36.2+V}{-4.0}\right)}, \quad \beta = \frac{0.28(9.2 + V)}{\exp\left(\frac{9.2+V}{5.0}\right) - 1.0}; \tag{12.30}$$

for h_∞ and τ_h:

$$\alpha = 0.128\exp\left(\frac{32.3 + V}{-18.0}\right), \quad \beta = \frac{4.0}{1.0 + \exp\left(\frac{9.3+V}{-5.0}\right)} \tag{12.31}$$

Persistent Sodium Current Although there has been no direct evidence for the presence of this current in piriform pyramidal cells, it is known to exist in pyramidal neurons from other areas (French et al. 1990) and when added to our model, it greatly improved active behavior. Kinetic parameters come from a model by McCormick and Huguenard (1992) with the activation curve shifted slightly to the right to match experimental data from piriform cortex.

$$I = m\bar{g}(E_{rev} - V_m), \quad E_{rev} = 55\,\text{mV}; \tag{12.32}$$

for m_∞ and τ_m (no inactivation):

$$\alpha = \frac{0.091(V + 48.0)}{1.0 - \exp\left(\frac{-(V+48.0)}{5.0}\right)}, \quad \beta = \frac{-0.062(V + 48.0)}{1.0 - \exp\left(\frac{V+48.0}{5.0}\right)} \tag{12.33}$$

$$m_\infty = \frac{1.0}{1.0 + \exp\left(\frac{43.0+V}{-5.0}\right)}, \quad \tau_m = \frac{1.0}{\alpha + \beta} \tag{12.34}$$

Potassium Delayed Rectifier   Parameters for this current are identical to those used in a study by Traub et al. (1991).

$$I = m\bar{g}(E_{rev} - V_m), \quad E_{rev} = -90\,\text{mV}; \tag{12.35}$$

for m_∞ and τ_m (no inactivation):

$$\alpha = \frac{0.016(-39.2 - V)}{\exp\left(\frac{-39.2-V}{5.0}\right) - 1.0}, \quad \beta = 0.25 \exp\left(\frac{-54.3 - V}{40.0}\right) \tag{12.36}$$

Potassium A-Current   This current has been studied experimentally by Banks, Haberly, and Jackson (1996) in piriform pyramidal neurons. We use the parameters obtained in that study.

$$I = m^3 h\bar{g}(E_{rev} - V_m), \quad E_{rev} = -90\,\text{mV}; \tag{12.37}$$

for m_∞ and τ_m:

$$\alpha = 0.5 \exp\left(\frac{0.5V + 19.65}{15.4}\right), \quad \beta = 0.5 \exp\left(\frac{0.5V + 19.65}{-15.4}\right); \tag{12.38}$$

for h_∞ and τ_h:

$$\alpha = 0.04 \exp\left(\frac{0.9V + 59.13}{-6.86}\right), \quad \beta = 0.04 \exp\left(\frac{0.1V + 6.57}{6.86}\right) \tag{12.39}$$

Potassium M-Current   Although there is experimental evidence for the existence of the M-current in piriform pyramidal neurons (Constanti and Galvan 1983a; Constanti and Sim 1987a, 1987b), its exact parameters have not been well described. Therefore, we use an M-current much like the one described by Yamada, Koch, and Adams (see chapter 4, this volume) except that the kinetics are approximately three times as fast. This current does not inactivate.

$$I = m\bar{g}(E_{rev} - V_m), \quad E_{rev} = -96\,\text{mV} \tag{12.40}$$

$$m_\infty = \frac{1.0}{1.0 + \exp\left(\frac{35.0+V}{-10.0}\right)} \tag{12.41}$$

$$\tau_m = \frac{330.0}{11.3\left(\exp\left(\frac{V+35.0}{20.0}\right) + \exp\left(\frac{V+35.0}{-10.0}\right)\right)} + 10.89 \tag{12.42}$$

Potassium Slow AHP Current   Voltage clamp and pharmacological evidence support the existence of a slow AHP current in piriform pyramidal neurons (Constanti and Sim 1987a). Because the precise kinetics and calcium dynamics underlying this current are not well described, we constructed a phenomenological model based on the best fit we could obtain with the simple calcium dynamics described in equation 6.1. We use the Hodgkin-Huxley formalism to model this calcium-dependent current, except that the voltage-dependent gate m is replaced by the calcium-dependent gate z as follows. All concentrations are in micro-molar and times are in milliseconds.

$$I = z\bar{g}(E_{rev} - V_m), \quad E_{rev} = -96\,\text{mV} \tag{12.43}$$

$$\frac{\partial z}{\partial t} = \frac{z_\infty - z}{\tau_z} \tag{12.44}$$

$$\alpha = \min\left(\frac{[Ca^{2+}]}{0.52\,\mu M}, 0.01\right) \tag{12.45}$$

$$\beta = 0.0005 \tag{12.46}$$

$$z_\infty = \frac{\alpha}{\alpha + \beta}, \quad \tau_z = \frac{1.0}{\alpha + \beta}. \tag{12.47}$$

Fast Calcium Current Although a voltage-gated calcium current has been observed in piriform pyramidal neurons (Constanti et al. 1985), it has not been parameterized, nor have there been any efforts to determine the individual calcium currents that may underlie the more general voltage-gated calcium current observed by Constanti et al. (1985). Therefore, we constructed a phenomenological model of the voltage clamp data obtained for the calcium current in the study by Constanti et al. (1985). To accurately replicate the voltage clamp data, we found it necessary to use two calcium current components, one fast, and one slow. Because of the enormous calcium concentration gradient that exists across the membrane, it is not possible to use the standard Hodgkin-Huxley model of voltage-gated currents; instead, we must utilize the Goldman-Hodgkin-Katz equation (discussed in greater detail in chapters 4, 5, and 6, this volume). This equation calculates transmembrane current and is dependent on a variable representing the Ca^{2+} permeability of the membrane. We use the gating concept from the Hodgkin-Huxley model to develop an expression for calcium permeability due to the fast calcium current:

$$I = I_{CaF} = P_{CaF}z_{Ca}^2 \frac{VF^2}{RT} \frac{[Ca^{2+}]_i - [Ca^{2+}]_o \exp\left(\frac{-z_{Ca}FV}{RT}\right)}{1.0 - \exp\left(\frac{-z_{Ca}FV}{RT}\right)}, \tag{12.48}$$

where P_{CaF} is the Ca^{2+} permeability due to the fast calcium current, z_{Ca} is the valency of the calcium ion, and V, R, F, and T are the membrane potential, gas constant, Faraday constant, and temperature (in Kelvins), respectively. To calculate permeability, we use the following expression:

$$P_{CaF} = m^2 h \bar{P}, \tag{12.49}$$

where m and h are activation and inactivation gates, as before, and $\bar{P}$ the maximum permeability due to the fast calcium current.

$$m_\infty = \frac{1.0}{1.0 + \exp\left(\frac{42.0+V}{-2.0}\right)} \tag{12.50}$$

$$\tau_m = \frac{1.0}{\exp\left(\frac{162.0+V}{-26.7}\right) + \exp\left(\frac{26.8+V}{18.2}\right)} + 1.0 \tag{12.51}$$

$$h_\infty = \frac{1.0}{1.0 + \exp\left(\frac{54.0+V}{2.0}\right)} \tag{12.52}$$

$$\tau_h = \frac{18.0}{\exp\left(\frac{82.0+V}{-2.7}\right) + \exp\left(\frac{28.0+V}{28.0}\right)} + 3.0 \tag{12.53}$$

Slow Calcium Current The slow component of the calcium current is described by the following equation:

$$P_{CaS} = mh\bar{P} \tag{12.54}$$

$$m_\infty = \frac{1.0}{1.0 + \exp\left(\frac{32.0+V}{-10.0}\right)} \tag{12.55}$$

Table 12.2
Synaptic channel parameters for full and reduced models of piriform cortex pyramidal cell

Type	Location	τ_1	τ_2	E_{rev}
Non-NMDA (excitatory)	Ia, Ib	1.50 msec	3.00 msec	0.0 mV
NMDA	Ia, Ib	(see text)		0.0 mV
GABA$_A$	II	1.00 msec	5.50 msec	−60 mV
GABA$_B$	Ia	150 msec	180 msec	−90 mV

Table 12.3
Neuronal parameters for piriform cortex network model

C_m	Specific membrane capacitance	2.0 μF/cm²
$R_{m(p)}$	Pyramidal-specific membrane resistance	4.0 kΩ · cm²
$R_{(m(i)}$	Interneuron-specific membrane resistance	2.0 kΩ · cm²
R_a	Specific axial resistance	100 Ω · cm
R_e	Extracellular resistance	100 Ω/cm
R_{IN}	Pyramidal input resistance	38 MΩ
E_m	Resting membrane potential	−70 mV
t_r	Absolute refractory period	10 ms
t_e	Synaptic delay	0.8 ms
$t_{e(ff)}$	Feedforward inhibitory delay	8 ms

Synaptic conductances

	τ_1	τ_2	g_{peak}	Reversal potential
excitatory	1 msec	3 msec	200 pS/synapse	0 mV
GABA$_A$(Cl⁻)	1 msec	7 msec	500 pS/synapse	−65 mV
GABA$_B$(K⁺)	10 msec	100 msec	50 pS/synapse	−90 mV

Action potential conductances

	τ_1	τ_2	$g_{peak\text{-}pyr}$	$g_{peak\text{-}fb}$	$g_{peak\text{-}ff}$	E_{rev}
Na⁺	0.2 msec	0.2 msec	450 nS	75 nS	35 nS	55 mV
K⁺	1.0 msec	1.0 msec	50 nS	8 nS	4 nS	−90 mV

Cellular dimensions

	Length	Diameter
Pyramidal soma	70 μm	20 μm
Pyramidal dendrites (4)	120 μm	4 μm
Feedforward interneuron soma	10 μm	10 μm
Feedback interneuron soma	15 μm	15 μm

Table 12.4
Connection parameters for piriform cortex network model

	Pathway velocities
Main afferent LOT	7.00 m/sec (SD = 0.06, max/min = 7.20/6.80)
Afferent collateral	1.60 m/sec (SD = 0.06, max/min = 1.80/1.40)
Rostrally directed	0.85 m/sec (SD = 0.13, max/min = 1.25/0.45)
Caudally directed	0.37 m/sec (SD = 0.03, max/min = 0.48/0.25)
Inhibitory pathways	1.00 m/sec (SD = 0.06, max/min = 0.80/1.20)

	Pathway extents
Local pyramidal to pyramidal	0.5 mm
Distant pyramidal to pyramidal	10.0 mm
Pyramidal to feedback interneuron	2.0 mm
Pyramidal to feedforward interneuron	0.5 mm
Feedback interneuron to pyramidal	1.0 mm
Feedforward interneuron to pyramidal	1.0 mm

	Pathway space constants
Pyramidal to pyramidal	5 mm
Pyramidal to interneurons	5 mm
Interneurons to pyramidal	5 mm
Main LOT	20 mm
LOT collaterals	10 mm

	Connection probabilities
LOT to pyramidal/interneurons	0.10
Local pyramidal to pyramidal	0.20
Distant pyramidal to pyramidal	0.02
Pyramidal to interneurons	0.20
Interneurons to pyramidal	1.00

	Synapses onto pyramidal cells
From LOT	1,500
From local pyramidal	750
From distant caudal pyramidal	1,200
From distant rostral pyramidal	2,200
From feedback interneurons	1,500
From feedforward interneurons	500

	Synapses onto feedback interneurons
From LOT	50
From pyramidal	300

	Synapses onto feedforward interneurons
From LOT	130
From pyramidal	50

$$\tau_m = \frac{1.0}{\exp\left(\frac{3.2+V}{-6.7}\right) + \exp\left(\frac{16.8+V}{18.2}\right)} + 3.0 \tag{12.56}$$

$$h_\infty = \frac{1.0}{1.0 + \exp\left(\frac{40.0+V}{35.0}\right)} \tag{12.57}$$

$$\tau_h = \frac{350.0}{\exp\left(\frac{35.0+V}{12.0}\right) + \exp\left(\frac{25.0+V}{-12.0}\right)} + 10.0. \tag{12.58}$$

Synaptic Currents   Table 12.2 lists the parameters for the synaptic currents in the single-cell models that were described by the dual exponential form (see "Synaptic Currents," chapter appendix B; the Holmes-Levy 1990 model of NMDA conductance is described in chapter 6, this volume).

Parameters for the Piriform Cortex Network Model

Tables 12.3 and 12.4 list all of the parameters for the network model. The "space constants" referred to in table 12.4 show the space constant for the exponential decay in connection strength along different synaptic pathways.

13 Modeling Feature Selectivity in Local Cortical Circuits

David Hansel and Haim Sompolinsky

13.1 Introduction

Neuronal representations of the external world are often based on the selectivity of the responses of individual neurons to external features. For example, many neurons in visual cortex respond preferentially to visual stimuli that have a specific orientation (Hubel and Wiesel 1959), spatial frequency (Campbell et al. 1969), color (Hubel and Wiesel 1968), velocity and direction of motion (Orban 1984). In motor systems, neuronal activities are tuned to parameters of a planned action such as the direction of an arm reaching movement (Georgopoulos, Taira, and Lukashin 1993), or the direction of a saccadic eye movement (for a review, see Sparks and Mays 1990). It is often assumed that the primary mechanism underlying the response properties of a neuron resides in the transformations of sensory signals by feedforward filtering along afferent pathways (e.g., Hubel and Wiesel 1962). Although, in some cases, the feedforward model is consistent with our understanding of the nature of afferent inputs (Reid and Alonso 1995; Chapman, Zahs, and Stryker 1991), in others, particularly in motor areas, the relation between afferent inputs and cortical neuronal response properties is not obvious. Moreover, neurons in cortex, even in the input stages of primary sensory areas, receive most of their excitatory inputs from *cortical* sources rather than from afferent thalamic nuclei (Levay and Gilbert 1976; Peters and Payne 1993; Ahmed et al. 1994; Pei et al. 1994; Douglas et al. 1995). Cortical responses are also modulated by strong inputs from inhibitory cortical interneurons (Sillito 1977; Tsumoto, Eckart, and Creutzfeldt 1979; Sillito et al. 1980; Ferster and Koch 1987; Hata et al. 1988; Nelson et al. 1994). These facts and other experimental and theoretical considerations suggest that local cortical circuits may play an important role is shaping neuronal responses in cortex.

In this chapter we review the theoretical study of the function of local networks in cortex in relation to feature selectivity. By "local network" we mean an ensemble of neurons that respond to the same patch of the external world and are interconnected by recurrent synaptic connections. Typically, a local network spans roughly 1 mm^2 of cortical surface and is assumed to consist of subgroups of neurons each of which is tuned to a particular feature of an external stimulus. These subgroups will be called "feature columns" and the whole network a "hypercolumn," in analogy with the "ice cube" model of primary visual cortex (Hubel 1988; for a review of local cortical circuitry, see Martin 1988; Gilbert 1992; Abeles 1991).

The complexity of neuronal dynamics and circuitry in cortex precludes systematic investigation of the properties of realistic large-scale neuronal models of local cortical circuits within a reasonable range of their parameter space (see chapter 12, this volume). Therefore simplified abstract models offer very valuable theoretical tools to gain insight into the working of these systems. Not only is the reduced parameter space of these simplified models significantly easier to search, but many are amenable to analytical investigations. Analytical solutions are extremely useful in that they often explicitly reveal the important relationships between a dynamic property of the network and some of its parameters. A primary goal of this chapter is to describe the application of analytical methods to simplified network models and their solutions. We will study models known as "neuronal rate models" or "neuronal population dynamics" (Wilson and Cowan 1972; Ginzburg and Sompolinsky 1994), in which the state of each neuron is characterized by a single continuous variable representing its activity level averaged over a short period of time. Similar models are the analog circuit equations for neural networks (Hopfield 1984). Although these models obviously cannot exhibit the complex dynamics of real neurons and circuits, they can account for some of the emergent cooperative properties that are either stationary or evolve on relatively slow time scales. To demonstrate the relevance of the simplified models to realistic situations, we will also describe in detail numerical simulations of networks consisting of conductance-based models of cortical neurons and synapses. (See also chapters 5 and 10, this volume.)

The present study focuses on networks that code the value of a single feature variable of the external stimulus, and thus have a one-dimensional functional architecture. The spectrum of possible spatiotemporal patterns of activity in such networks can be rich. We will restrict our attention to relatively simple spatial patterns consisting of a single domain of high activity, sometimes called an "activity hill." We will also consider the cases of 'moving hills' of activity, where the activity profile is not static but propagates across the network, successively activating neighboring columns. We will study the conditions for the emergence of these patterns and analyze which of their properties depend on the intrinsic circuit parameters and which, on the properties of the external stimulus.

Modeling of neuronal functions by static and moving *localized* spatial patterns in one-dimensional nonlinear neural networks dates back to Didday's model on the frog tectal bug detection system (Didday 1976) and the reticular formation model for behavioral mode selection of Kilmer, McCulloch and Blum (1969); (see Amari and Arbib 1977; and Montalvo 1975 for reviews of these and other models). Theoretical analysis of these patterns has been pioneered by Amari (1977). The difference between Amari's theory and the present work will be elucidated in section 13.8. *Global* spatiotemporal patterns in one- (and two-) dimensional networks have been studied also by Ermentrout and Cowan (see Ermentrout 1982 for review). More recently, localized patterns in one- and two-dimensional neuronal rate models have been studied in relation to orientation selectivity in primary visual cortex (Ben-Yishai, Lev Bar-Or, and Sompolinsky 1995; Ben-Yishai, Hansel, and Sompolinsky 1997), the coding of direction of arm movements in motor cortex (Lukashin and Georgopoulos 1993; Lukashin et al. 1996), head direction tuning in the limbic systems (Redish, Elga, and Touretzky 1996; Zhang 1996), and the control of saccadic eye movements (Droulez and Berthoz 1991; Schierwagen and Werner 1996; Kopecz and Schöner 1995). The mechanisms underlying the emergence of spatiotemporal patterns of the types described above are quite universal. For this reason, here these models will be studied in the general context of coding of a one-dimensional feature (detailed applications to concrete cortical systems can be found in the recent literature devoted to these models).

The network models examined here are characterized by a strong internal recurrency, which gives rise to intrinsic stable static or dynamic patterns, called "attractors" (for a review of dynamical systems theory see, for example, Strogatz 1994). Computation by attractors has been studied in recent years in relation to associative memory and optimization problems (Hopfield 1982, 1984; Hopfield and Tank 1986; Amit, Gutfreund, and Sompolinsky 1985; Amit 1989). The models we will be examining differ in that their intrinsic stable states are not isolated points in configuration space (the space of all possible instantaneous states of the system) but form a continuous line in this space. Recently a network model with line attractor has been studied as a mechanism for gaze holding by Seung (1996) and by Lee et al. (1996). We will briefly compare these models in section 13.8.

Section 13.2 describes our network model's basic architecture and defines the network's rate dynamics of excitatory and inhibitory populations in a hypercolumn. Section 13.3 further simplifies the model by collapsing the excitatory and inhibitory populations into a single "equivalent" population; this one-population rate model serves as the basis of our subsequent analytical investigations. Section 13.4 explores the properties of static activity profiles that emerge in the case of a uniform external stimulus and in response to a spatially tuned stimulus. We will analyze in detail how cortical feedback shapes the emergent activity profile.

Section 13.5 examines, first, the network response to a "moving" external stimulus (one whose feature value changes with time), where an interesting issue is the network's ability to lock to the moving stimulus. Our investigation also illustrates the usefulness of phase dynamics (see chapter 7, this volume) in describing how a spatiotemporal pattern is phase- and frequency-locked to an external force. We next discuss the emergence of *intrinsic* moving profiles in networks with static uniform stimulus. Propagating pulses are known to exist in excitable one-dimensional media, such as the propagation of action potential along a nerve's axon (Hodgkin and

Huxley 1952; Rinzel and Keller 1973; Tuckwell 1988). Here we study a mechanism for generating moving localized activity profiles in neural networks which is based on neuronal adaptation. We incorporate neuronal adaptation current into the one-population rate model by a simple phenomenological model of a slow, local negative linear feedback, showing that, for sufficiently strong adaptation, the static hills become destabilized and that propagating hills of activity become the stable states of the system instead. We briefly discuss the interaction between the intrinsic moving hills and an external tuned static stimulus.

A central issue of this chapter is the relation between the spatial modulation of the external input, as well as the cortical interactions, and the emergent tuning of the network responses. In the model studied in sections 13.2–13.5, the spatial modulations of the internal and external inputs are characterized by their spatial modulation *depth*. Their range, however, is assumed to be long and fixed. An important question is the role of the spatial *width* of the synaptic interactions or of the external input on the emergent spatial activity profile. This is the topic of section 13.6, which presents a solution to a model where both the excitatory interactions and the external input are exponentially decreasing functions of distance. Although more complex, this model can still be solved analytically, and it enables us to elucidate the role of both the spatial modulation depth and the spatial range of the synaptic inputs.

Section 13.7 considers a network model that incorporates realistic conductance-based dynamics appropriate for cortical neurons, whose architecture is similar to the rate models, except that the network consists of separate excitatory and inhibitory populations. Many aspects of the simulations, including the size dependence of the network behavior and the classification of its synchrony and temporal variability, are described in detail in Hansel and Sompolinsky (1996). Here we focus mainly on results directly relevant to the comparison with the predictions of the rate model. We first show that under certain conditions the state of these networks can also be described by self-consistent rate equations. We then proceed to present the results of numerical simulations of this model, and compare them with the predictions of the rate model. The results are also briefly discussed in our conclusion, section 13.8.

13.2 Model of a Cortical Hypercolumn

13.2.1 Network Architecture

We consider a network of neurons that code for a sensory or movement feature. The feature is assumed to be a scalar denoted by θ, with a finite range of values (in most of this chapter, $-\pi/2 \leq \theta < \pi/2$). For simplicity, we will assume periodic boundary conditions, so that θ can be considered an angle, and all functions of θ will be periodic functions with period π. In section 13.6 we will consider the more general case where θ is not an angle variable, so that the boundary conditions are not periodic.

Each neuron in the hypercolumn is selective to a particular range of feature values, and fires maximally when a feature with a particular value is present. This value is called the "preferred feature" (PF) of the neuron. The network consists of N_E excitatory neurons and N_I inhibitory neurons, parametrized by a coordinate θ, which denotes their PF. The PFs are assumed to be distributed uniformly between $-\pi/2$ and $+\pi/2$. An additional N_0 neuron provides external input to the network. These external sources are typically excitatory afferent currents induced by sensory stimulation. We will refer to this input as the "stimulus input" of the network. We denote an excitatory neuron by an index E and an inhibitory one by I. The external excitatory neurons are denoted by 0.

Each neuron receives a synaptic current, $I^\alpha(\theta, t)$, where $\alpha = E, I$ denotes the type of the neuron, θ its PF, and t denotes time. This current consists of three components:

$$I^\alpha(\theta,\ t) = I^{\alpha E}(\theta, t) + I^{\alpha I}(\theta, t) + I^{\alpha 0}(\theta, t), \tag{13.1}$$

where $I^{\alpha\beta}(\theta, t)$ is the synaptic current on a θ neuron in the αth population generated by the activity of the βth population, and $I^{\alpha 0}(\theta,\ t)$ stands for synaptic currents from the external neurons. The synaptic currents $I^{\alpha\beta}$ are each a sum of synaptic inputs from individual neurons mediated by pairwise synaptic interactions. The synaptic efficacy between a presynaptic *excitatory* neuron, θ', and a postsynaptic neuron, θ of type α, is denoted by $(1/N_E)J^{\alpha E}(|\theta - \theta'|)$. The interaction strength between a presynaptic *inhibitory* neuron, θ', and a postsynaptic neuron, θ of type α, is denoted by $(1/N_I)J^{\alpha I}(|\theta - \theta'|)$. The functions $J^{\alpha\beta}(\theta)$ represent the dependence of the interaction between neurons on the similarity of their PFs. Both excitatory and the inhibitory interactions are assumed to be strongest in magnitude for neurons that have identical PFs. This hypothesis is consistent with the anatomical and physiological evidence available in primary visual cortex (Ferster 1986; Ts'o, Gilbert, and Wiesel 1986; Martin 1988). The factors of N_E and N_I are introduced in order to facilitate the analysis of the size of the inputs from the above three sources in a large, highly connected network. It is assumed that each neuron is connected to a significant fraction of neurons of both subpopulations. Thus, with the above normalization, the *total* inputs $I^{\alpha\beta}$ from each of the populations are proportional in scale to the functions $J^{\alpha\beta}$ (for a detailed discussion of this scaling, see Hansel and Sompolinsky 1996; for alternative scaling of connections in large networks, see Van Vreeswijk and Sompolinsky 1996).

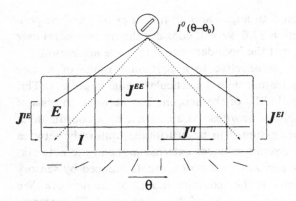

Figure 13.1
Architecture of the network.

To model the information carried by the stimulus about the external features, the input to the neuron θ of type α is taken to be of the form $I^{\alpha 0}(\theta - \theta_0)$, where θ_0 denotes the feature for which the external input is maximal. Thus θ_0 represents the feature value selected by the external input, or simply the stimulus feature. The network architecture is shown in figure 13.1.

A simple model of the interactions and of the external stimulus is given by retaining only the first Fourier components of their feature dependence. Thus

$$J^{\alpha\beta}(\theta - \theta') = J_0^{\alpha\beta} + J_2 \cos(2(\theta - \theta')), \qquad (13.2)$$

where $J_0^{\alpha E} \geq J_2^{\alpha E} \geq 0$ and $J_0^{\alpha I} \leq J_2^{\alpha I} \leq 0$. These inequalities are consistent with the above assumption that both excitatory and inhibitory interactions are maximal for neurons with similar PFs. Likewise,

$$I^{\alpha 0}(\theta - \theta_0) = C_\alpha (1 - \varepsilon + \varepsilon \cos(2(\theta - \theta_0))), \quad 0 \leq \varepsilon \leq 0.5. \qquad (13.3)$$

The above functions are depicted in figure 13.2A and figure 13.2B. The parameters C_α are assumed to be positive. They denote the maximal amplitude of the external inputs to the two populations. We will refer to them simply as the "stimulus intensity." The parameter ε measures the degree of modulation of the input to the cortical neurons. In the limit $\varepsilon = 0.5$, the external input to neurons farthest away from the stimulus feature, namely, neurons with $\theta = \theta_0 \pm \pi/2$, is zero. For $\varepsilon = 0$, the external input to all neurons in the same population is identical. We will refer to ε as the "stimulus tuning;" it is important to note that this parameter is determined both by the degree of tuning of the sensory stimulus itself and by the organization of

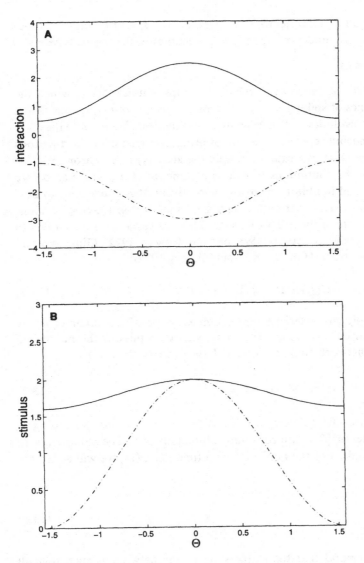

Figure 13.2
(A) Interactions as given in eq. 13.2. Solid line: excitatory interaction, with $J_0^{\alpha E} = 1.5$ and $J_2^{\alpha E} = 1$; dash-dotted line: inhibitory interaction, with $J_0^{\alpha I} = -2$ and $J_2^{\alpha I} = -1$. (B) Example of a stimulus given by eq. 13.3, with $C_\alpha = 2$. Solid line: $\varepsilon = 0.1$; dash-dotted line $\varepsilon = 0.5$.

the afferents to individual cortical neurons. In general, C_α, ε, and θ_0 may be time-dependent. To complete the model, we specify the dynamics of the network below.

13.2.2 Network Dynamics

Our theoretical study will be based on a relatively simple rate model in which the highly nonlinear dynamics of spiking neurons is replaced by smooth equations which describe the temporal evolution of the neuronal activities. These activities are smooth functions of time and represent the rate of firing averaged over short periods of time. In the present context, the rate (or simply the activity) of a neuron (α, θ) at time t is represented by the continuous functions of time, $m_\alpha(\theta, t)$, where as before $\alpha = E, I$, for excitatory and inhibitory neurons, respectively. It is convenient to normalize the rates by appropriate saturation levels so that $0 \le m^\alpha(\theta, t) \le 1$. Thus, $m^\alpha = 1$ represents firing rate of the order of 1 kHz. The rate variables are assumed to obey the following dynamic equations (Wilson and Cowan 1972; Ginzburg and Sompolinsky 1994; Ben-Yishai, Hansel, and Sompolinsky 1997):

$$\tau_0 \frac{d}{dt} m^\alpha(\theta, t) = -m^\alpha(\theta, t) + G(I^\alpha(\theta, t) - T_\alpha), \quad \alpha = E, I, \tag{13.4}$$

where τ_0 is a microscopic characteristic time assumed to be of the order of a few milliseconds. The quantities $I^\alpha(\theta, t)$ are the total synaptic inputs to the neuron $\alpha\theta$ (see eq. 13.1). The two network contributions to $I^\alpha(\theta, t)$ are of the form

$$I^{\alpha\beta}(\theta, t) = \int_{-\pi/2}^{+\pi/2} \frac{d\theta'}{\pi} J^{\alpha\beta}(\theta - \theta') m^\beta(\theta', t), \quad \beta = E, I. \tag{13.5}$$

Here we have used a mean field description, valid for large networks, according to which the activity profiles $m^\alpha(\theta, t)$ are continuous functions of θ. The parameters T_α are the neuronal thresholds. For the nonlinear gain function $G(I)$, we will adopt the simple semilinear form

$$G(I) = \begin{cases} 0 & I < 0 \\ I & 0 < I < 1 \\ 1 & I > 1. \end{cases} \tag{13.6}$$

Furthermore, we will demand that the stable state of the network is such that all the neurons are far from their saturation level. Therefore in practice the only nonlinearity we will consider is a threshold nonlinearity,

$$G(I) = [I]_+, \tag{13.7}$$

where $[X]_+ = X$ for $X > 0$, and zero otherwise.

In the case of time-independent external inputs, the dynamics of the rate model may converge to a fixed point. The fixed point equations are

$$m^\alpha(\theta) = [I^\alpha(\theta) - T_\alpha]_+, \quad \alpha = E, I, \tag{13.8}$$

where $I^\alpha(\theta)$ depends on the network activity profiles $m^\alpha(\theta)$ through

$$I^\alpha(\theta) = \sum_{\beta=E,I} \int_{-\pi/2}^{+\pi/2} \frac{d\theta'}{\pi} J^{\alpha\beta}(\theta - \theta')m^\beta(\theta') + I^{\alpha 0}(\theta - \theta_0). \tag{13.9}$$

If we linearize eq. 13.4 with respect to a small perturbation near the above fixed point, we find that the criterion of the linear stability of the fixed point is that all the eigenvalues of the stability matrix

$$M_{\alpha\beta}(\theta, \theta') = -\delta(\theta - \theta')\delta_{\alpha\beta} + \Theta(I_\alpha(\theta))J^{\alpha\beta}(\theta - \theta') \tag{13.10}$$

have negative real parts. The function $\Theta(x)$ is the step function, that is, $\Theta(x) = 1$, for $x > 0$, and zero otherwise.

12.3 One-Population Rate Model

The solution of the above two-population rate model is discussed in detail in Ben-Yishai, Hansel, and Sompolinsky (1997). Here we will study a simpler model, in which the excitatory and the inhibitory populations are collapsed into a single equivalent population. This reduces substantially the number of parameters and greatly facilitates the analysis of the system behavior (the justification of this reduction will be discussed in section 13.7). The one population model is described in terms of a single rate variable $m(\theta, t)$ which represents the activity of the population of neurons in the column θ at time t. The rate dynamics are defined by

$$\tau_0 \frac{d}{dt} m(\theta, t) = -m(\theta, t) + [I(\theta, t) - T]_+, \tag{13.11}$$

where

$$I(\theta, t) = \int_{-\pi/2}^{+\pi/2} \frac{d\theta'}{\pi} J(\theta - \theta')m(\theta', t) + I^0(\theta - \theta_0) \tag{13.12}$$

and T is the neuronal threshold.

Adopting the additional simplification of retaining only the first two Fourier components in the interaction and external input spatial dependencies as in eqs. 13.2

and 13.3, we have

$$J(\theta - \theta') = J_0 + J_2 \cos(2(\theta - \theta')), \quad J_2 \geq 0, -J_0 \tag{13.13}$$

and

$$I^0(\theta - \theta_0) = C(1 - \varepsilon + \varepsilon \cos(2(\theta - \theta_0))). \tag{13.14}$$

Substituting eqs. 13.13 and 13.14 into eq. 13.12 yields

$$I(\theta, t) = C(1 - \varepsilon) + J_0 r_0(t) + C\varepsilon \cos(2(\theta - \theta_0)) + J_2 r_2(t) \cos(2(\theta - \Psi(t))), \tag{13.15}$$

where

$$r_0(t) = \int_{-\pi/2}^{+\pi/2} \frac{d\theta}{\pi} \, m(\theta, t) \tag{13.16}$$

$$r_2(t) = \int_{-\pi/2}^{+\pi/2} \frac{d\theta}{\pi} \, m(\theta, t) \exp(2i(\theta - \Psi(t))). \tag{13.17}$$

The phase $\Psi(t)$ is defined by the requirement that $r_2(t)$ is a nonnegative real number. The quantities $r_0(t)$, $r_2(t)$, and $\Psi(t)$ are global measures of the activity profiles and are called the "order parameters" of the network. The first-order parameter r_0 measures the activity of the neurons averaged over the entire network. The second-order parameter $r_2(t)$ measures the degree of "spatial modulation" in the activity profile. The complex number $r_2(t) \exp(2i\Psi(t))$ represents a vector in two dimensions, which corresponds to the *population vector* of the system, evaluated by summing unit vectors pointed in the PFs of the neurons, weighted by their instantaneous activities (Georgopoulos, Taira, and Lukashin 1993; Schwartz 1993). The phase $\Psi(t)$ denotes the angle of the population vector and r_2 denotes its length, that is, the strength of the spatial modulation of the population. From a functional point of view, $\Psi(t)$ may represent the population coding of the stimulus feature (Seung and Sompolinsky 1993).

Fourier transforming of eq. 13.11 yields self-consistent equations for the temporal evolution of the order parameters, which in turn determines the dynamics of $m(\theta, t)$ (these equations are derived in chapter appendix A). In the following we study the properties of the fixed-point solutions. We first assume that, at the fixed point, the population profile $m(\theta)$ is centered at the peak of the external input, that is, at $\theta = \theta_0$, hence

$$\Psi = \theta_0. \tag{13.18}$$

Substituting eq. 13.18 in eq. 13.15, we observe that the fixed-point solution for eq. 13.11 has the form

$$m(\theta) = M(\theta - \theta_0), \tag{13.19}$$

where

$$M(\theta) = [I_0 + I_2 \cos(2\theta)]_+. \tag{13.20}$$

The coefficients I_0 and I_2 are

$$I_0 = C(1 - \varepsilon) + J_0 r_0 - T \tag{13.21a}$$

$$I_2 = C\varepsilon + J_2 r_2. \tag{13.21b}$$

Eq. 13.20 shows that eq. 13.18 is indeed self-consistent. The fixed-point values of the r_0 and r_2 are given by the self-consistent equations

$$r_0 = \int_{-\pi/2}^{+\pi/2} \frac{d\theta}{\pi} M(\theta) \tag{13.22}$$

$$r_2 = \int_{-\pi/2}^{+\pi/2} \frac{d\theta}{\pi} M(\theta) \cos(2\theta), \tag{13.23}$$

which will be analyzed below. An interesting quantity is the network gain, G, defined as the ratio between the activity of the maximally active neuron and the stimulus intensity relative to threshold:

$$G \equiv \frac{M(0)}{C - T}. \tag{13.24}$$

Note that, by definition, $G = 1$ for an isolated neuron.

The stability of the above fixed point is determined by the following equation for the linear perturbation $\delta m(\theta, t) = m(\theta, t) - m(\theta)$:

$$\tau_0 \frac{d}{dt} \delta m(\theta, t) = -\delta m(\theta, t) + \Theta(m(\theta))(J_0 \delta r_0(t) + J_2 \delta(\cos 2(\theta - \Psi(t)) r_2(t))). \tag{13.25}$$

As usual, stability requires that the solutions for $\delta m(\theta, t)$ decay to zero. (This stability analysis can also be reduced to the study of the stability of the order parameters, as described in chapter appendix B.)

13.4 Stationary Activity Profiles

To solve eqs. 13.20–13.23, we have to distinguish between broad and narrow profiles. We say that the activity profile is "broad" when all the neurons are above threshold for all stimulus angles, that is, $M(\theta)$ is positive, for all θ. Conversely, a "narrow" profile is characterized by $M(\theta)$ that vanishes at and beyond a certain angle θ_C. Of course, whether the profile is broad or narrow depends both on the stimulus inhomogeneity and on the cortical interaction parameters, as will be shown below. Note that $m(\theta)$'s being a function of the difference between θ and θ_0 implies that the form of the activity profile $M(\theta)$ is identical to the form of the output tuning curve of a single neuron. Thus a narrow (broad) profile corresponds to a narrow (broad) output tuning curve.

13.4.1   Broad Activity Profile

We first consider the relatively simple case of a broad $M(\theta)$, where all the neurons are above threshold. Thus eq. 13.20 simply reads

$$M(\theta) = I_0 + I_2 \cos(2\theta). \tag{13.26}$$

Substituting this expression in eqs. 13.22–13.23 yields $r_0 = I_0$; $r_2 = I_2/2$. Substituting in eqs. 13.21a–13.21b results in

$$r_0 = \frac{C(1 - \varepsilon) - T}{1 - J_0} \tag{13.27}$$

$$r_2 = \frac{C\varepsilon}{1 - \frac{1}{2}J_2}. \tag{13.28}$$

In the case of a homogeneous input, $\varepsilon = 0$, the above solution reduces to a homogeneous state:

$$M(\theta) = \frac{C - T}{1 - J_0}, \quad \varepsilon = 0. \tag{13.29}$$

For $\varepsilon > 0$, the gain is

$$G = \frac{1 - \Upsilon}{1 - J_0} + \frac{2\Upsilon}{1 - \frac{1}{2}J_2}, \tag{13.30}$$

where the *effective stimulus tuning* is defined as

$$\Upsilon = \frac{\varepsilon C}{C - T} \tag{13.31}$$

As expected, positive feedback generated by positive J_0 or J_2 enhances the system's gain, whereas negative feedback suppresses it. As we will see below, the parameter Υ is an important measure of stimulus tuning: it takes into account the potential enhancement of the tuning of cortical neuron activity by the effect of its threshold.

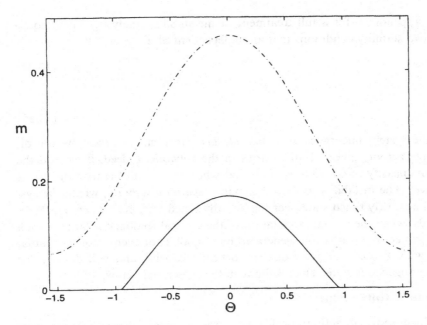

Figure 13.3
Activity profile in the one-population rate model for $J_0 = -2$ and $J_2 = 0$. The tuning of the input is
$\varepsilon = 0.1$. The profile of activity is broad for a contrast $C = 2$ (dash-dotted line). For a lower contrast, here
$C = 1.3$ (solid line) the profile is narrow.

When the stimulus intensity is close to threshold, a weak stimulus tuning will cause a
relatively narrow output tuning because the neuron will be active only if it is maximally stimulated. It should be noted, however, that Υ is a single-neuron property. It
does not take into account the potential modification of the threshold by the cortical
network. An example of a broad profile is shown in figure 13.3.

Eqs. 13.26–13.28 are a self-consistent solution of eq. 13.20, provided that the gain
given by eq. 13.30 is positive. This depends on the value of Υ. For sufficiently large values of Υ, G becomes negative and the broad solution is not valid any
more. In addition, one has to consider the stability of this solution. The stability
analysis is performed by Fourier transforming eq. 13.25 (taking into account that
here $\Theta(m(\theta)) = 1$, for all θ), yielding

$$\tau_0 \frac{d}{dt} \delta r_0(t) = -(1 - J_0)\delta r_0(t) \tag{13.32}$$

$$\tau_0 \frac{d}{dt} \delta r_2(t) = -\left(1 - \frac{J_2}{2}\right)\delta r_2(t). \tag{13.33}$$

(See chapter appendix B for a full treatment of the stability analysis.) These equations define two stability conditions that are independent of Υ:

$$J_0 < 1 \tag{13.34}$$

and

$$J_2 < 2. \tag{13.35}$$

At $J_0 = 1$, the system undergoes an *amplitude instability* characterized by the divergence of the activity levels of all neurons in the network. Indeed, if we add the saturation nonlinearity of eq. 13.6, we find that when $J_0 = 1$, all the neurons fire at saturation level. The instability at $J_2 = 2$ signals a *spatial instability*, where the system prefers a narrowly tuned state over the broadly tuned one, even when Υ is zero. In other words, when the spatial modulation of the cortical feedback is large, even a small inhomogeneous perturbation (generated by a small Υ, or even a nonzero initial value of r_2, with $\Upsilon = 0$) will grow due to cortical feedback, and will destroy the underlying homogeneous state. The resultant state is described below.

13.4.2 Narrow Activity Profile

We have defined above an activity profile as *narrowly tuned* if there exists an angle θ_C such that $M(\theta)$ vanishes for $|\theta| \geq \theta_C$. In this case, eq. 13.20 is no more linear. It can be written as

$$M(\theta) = I_2[\cos(2\theta) - \cos(2\theta_C)]_+, \tag{13.36}$$

where

$$\cos(2\theta_C) = \frac{-I_0}{I_2}. \tag{13.37}$$

The angle θ_C denotes the width of the tuning curve. Substituting in eqs. 13.22–13.23 yields, after some algebra, the following self-consistent equation for θ_C:

$$1 - \frac{1}{\Upsilon} = \frac{J_0 f_0(\theta_C) + \cos(2\theta_C)}{1 - J_2 f_2(\theta_C)}, \tag{13.38}$$

where

$$f_0(\theta_C) = \frac{1}{\pi}(\sin(2\theta_C) - 2\theta_C \cos(2\theta_C)) \tag{13.39}$$

$$f_2(\theta_C) = \frac{1}{\pi}\left(\theta_C - \frac{1}{4}\sin(4\theta_C)\right). \tag{13.40}$$

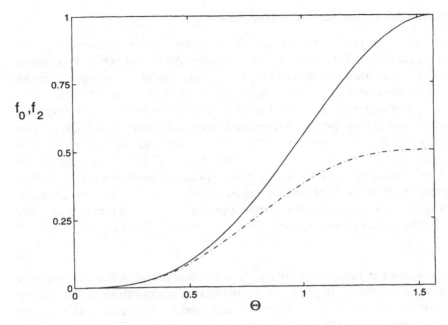

Figure 13.4
Function $f_0(\theta)$ (solid line) and $f_2(\theta)$ (dashed-dotted line).

These functions are plotted in figure 13.4. The gain of the network

$$G = \frac{I_2(1 - \cos(2\theta_C))}{C - T} \tag{13.41}$$

is given by

$$G = \Upsilon\left(\frac{1 - \cos(2\theta_C)}{1 - J_2 f_2(\theta_C)}\right). \tag{13.42}$$

These equations (derived in chapter appendix A) are a valid solution for the fixed point provided G is positive and eq. 13.38 has a solution; otherwise, the only solution is a broadly tuned one, as described above. Finally, the stability of this solution has to be determined by linearizing the dynamics around this fixed point (the resultant stability conditions are derived in chapter appendix B). An example of a narrow profile is shown in figure 13.3. We discuss below the interaction parameters where the broad or the narrow solutions are the stable states of the system.

13.4.3 Weakly Modulated Cortical Interactions

When the tuning of the input is large, that is, $\Upsilon \gg 1$, the cortical interactions may have little effect on the shape of the activity profile. On the other hand, when the stimulus tuning is weak, the cortical interactions may play a large role in the emergent network tuning. Thus a convenient way to characterize the effect of the cortical interactions is to calculate the influence on the critical value of Υ, denoted as Υ_c, below which the system has a broad activity profile. According to our analysis above, we suspect that Υ_c is positive for $J_2 < 2$, whereas $\Upsilon_c = 0$ for $J_2 > 2$. The role of J_0 is different: it may affect the value of Υ_c, but it will not drive it to *zero* if $J_2 < 2$. In addition, the value of J_0 may affect the overall stability of the system. A large positive value of J_0 signals strong positive feedback, which causes an instability of the network state. The above qualitative considerations are borne out by our detailed results below. We first consider the regime of weakly modulated interactions defined by

$$J_2 < 2, \quad J_0 < 1. \tag{13.43}$$

Afferent Mechanism of Feature Selectivity   The classical model of feature selectivity assumes that the selectivity is generated by the spatial organization of the afferent input to the cortical neurons. In the context of our model, this implies that Υ is large and that the contribution of the cortical interactions is not essential, namely,

$$J_0, \quad J_2 \approx 0. \tag{13.44}$$

In this case, the narrow profile described by eq. 13.20 reduces to

$$M(\theta) = \varepsilon C [\cos(2\theta) - \cos(2\theta_C)]_+, \tag{13.45}$$

where θ_C is

$$\theta_C = \frac{1}{2} \arccos(1 - \Upsilon^{-1}), \quad \Upsilon > \Upsilon_c. \tag{13.46}$$

The lowest value of Υ for which this solution exists is

$$\Upsilon_c = \frac{1}{2}. \tag{13.47}$$

For $\Upsilon < \Upsilon_c$, the system is in a broadly tuned state, where

$$M(\theta) = C(1 - \varepsilon) - T + \varepsilon C \cos(2(\theta - \theta_0)), \quad \text{for } all \ \theta \tag{13.48}$$

These results are shown in figure 13.5. Finally, in the absence of cortical interactions, the gain of the system is the same as that of a single neuron, namely, $G = 1$.

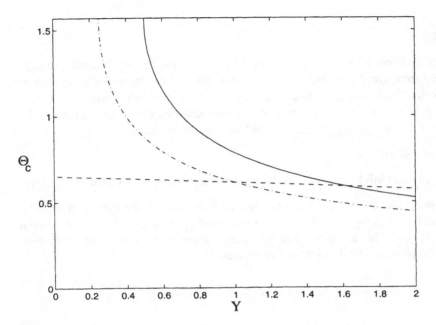

Figure 13.5
Width of the tuning curve, Θ_c, as a function of Υ. Solid line; afferent mechanism; dash-dotted line: uniform cortical inhibition, $J_0 = -2$; dashed line: marginal phase, $J_0 = -2$ and $J_2 = 6$.

Uniform Cortical Inhibition   The previous feedforward scenario has an obvious drawback. If the input tuning ε is smaller than $1/2$, sharply tuned profile exists only if the intensity is near the single-neuron threshold. A stimulus with $\varepsilon < 1/2$ and a high intensity relative to T will necessarily generate broad profiles of activity. A simple mechanism for sharpening the tuning invokes global cortical inhibition. Within our model, this scenario corresponds to the parameter regime

$$J_0 = -|J_0| < 0, \quad J_2 \approx 0. \tag{13.49}$$

In the presence of this inhibition, the external input of each neuron has to overcome an effective threshold given by $\pi + |J_0|r_0$. This effective threshold increases linearly with r_0 and therefore also with C. Thus, even for $C \gg 1$ and small ε, the uniform inhibition can provide a sufficiently potent threshold to sharpen the tuning width. In particular, substituting eq. 13.49 in eq. 13.38 and noting that the maximal value of θ_C is $\pi/2$, we see that a narrow profile exists as long as Υ is bigger than

$$\Upsilon_c = \frac{1}{2 + |J_0|}.\tag{13.50}$$

The effect of J_0 on θ_C is shown in figure 13.5, which shows clearly that although the inhibition sharpens the orientation tuning, the value of θ_C depends strongly on Υ, hence on both C and ε. This highlights the fact that uniform inhibition is incapable of generating feature tuning on its own; it can only sharpen the tuning generated by the modulated input. Finally, from eq. 13.42 we have in the present case

$$G = \Upsilon(1 - \cos(2\theta_C)).\tag{13.51}$$

Because the cortical inhibition reduces θ_C, it suppresses the system's gain as expected.

General Case   The effect of adding a positive J_2 is to sharpen the tuning of the network. As illustrated in figure 13.6, for fixed values of J_0, Υ_c decreases with J_2 until it vanishes at $J_2 = 2$. This indicates that for larger values of J_2, even when Υ is zero, the system's activity profile is narrow (see section 13.4.4).

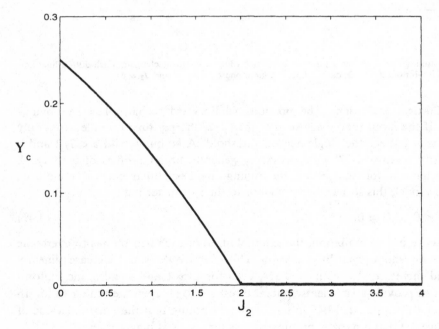

Figure 13.6
Υ_c as a function of the modulation J_2, for $J_0 = -2$.

13.4.4 Strongly Modulated Cortical Interactions

We now consider the parameter regime

$$J_2 > 2, \quad J_0 < J_C. \tag{13.52}$$

The upper bound on J_0, J_C, is a function of J_2 and Υ, as will be discussed below.

Homogeneous Input: Marginal Phase   In section 13.4.3, we analyzed the case where the external input is the only source of modulation of the cortical activity. In this section, we consider the question: can a narrow activity profile be generated by spatially modulated cortical interactions even in the absence of tuning in the external input? To study this question, we assume here

$$J_2 > 0, \quad \varepsilon = 0. \tag{13.53}$$

According to our previous analysis, the homogeneous state, characterized by eq. 13.29 is unstable. It is also clear that if the system possess an additional, inhomogeneous solution, this solution must be narrowly tuned because a broadly tuned profile obeys linear dynamics that does not poses more than one fixed point. Indeed, inspection of eq. 13.20 reveals that, for $\varepsilon = 0$, solutions with a narrow activity profile exist for $J_2 > 2$. The general stable solution is of the form

$$m(\theta) = M(\theta - \Psi). \tag{13.54}$$

The angle Ψ, which determines the peak in the population activity profile, is arbitrary because the external input is homogeneous. This means that there is a continuum of stable states. All the states have identical feature-tuned activity profiles, although the peaks of their profiles differ in location. Such a situation is termed a *marginal phase*, which indicates that the system relaxes to a line of fixed points rather than to one or several isolated fixed points. A marginal phase represents *spontaneous symmetry breaking*, that is, spontaneously generated spatial modulation of the activity in the network, and arises because spatial modulation of the cortical interactions, if sufficiently strong, destabilizes the homogeneous state. The stable state of the network is one where the activity is concentrated in a limited spatial range.

The shape of the activity profile in the marginal phase is still given by eq. 13.36. As for the width of the profile, inspection of eq. 13.38 reveals that when $\Upsilon = 0, \theta_C$ is given by

$$J_2 f_2(\theta_C) = 1, \tag{13.55}$$

which has a solution for $J_2 > 2$ (see figure 13.4). The gain in this limit is given by

$$G = \frac{1 - \cos(2\theta_C)}{f_0(\theta_C)} \left(\frac{1}{J_C - J_0} \right)$$ (13.56)

and

$$J_C = -\frac{\cos(2\theta_C)}{f_0(\theta_C)}, \quad \Upsilon \to 0.$$ (13.57)

Eqs. 13.36, 13.41, and 13.56, together with eq. 13.55, which determines θ_C, complete the solution for the activity profile. These equations imply that the amplitude of the external input determines the overall level of activity in the system, although the shape of the activity profile, in particular its width, is determined by the degree of spatial modulation of the cortical interactions.

It is clear from eq. 13.56 that for the marginal state to exist, J_0 has to be smaller than J_C (this condition can be also derived from a stability analysis presented in chapter appendix B). When J_0 approaches J_C, the system undergoes an amplitude instability similar to the instability that occurs at $J_0 = 1$ for the homogeneous state and $J_2 < 2$ (see eq. 13.32). The phase diagram for the stability of the various states in the case of a homogeneous stimulus is depicted in figure 13.7.

Tuned Input   We have considered a completely homogeneous input, for which the location of the peak of the activity profile is arbitrary. Because, however, we are primarily interested in how the system represents features present in external stimuli, we consider the solution of eqs. 13.36–13.42 in the parameter regime

$$0 < J_2 < 2, \quad \varepsilon > 0.$$ (13.58)

Solving eq. 13.38 shows that in most of this regime the tuning is largely independent of Υ, as illustrated in figure 13.5. This implies that the shape of the activity profile is determined essentially by the cortical interactions, eq. 13.55, and is barely affected by the presence of nonzero values of Υ. Thus the main effect of the inhomogeneity of the external input is to select among the continuum of possible states that state in which the peak in the activity matches the feature of the stimulus, that is

$$\Psi = \theta_0.$$ (13.59)

However, it will not greatly affect the shape of the tuning curve, as shown in figure 13.8. An exception is the case of low-intensity stimuli, characterized by C close to threshold T, that is, a large Υ. Once the single-neuron thresholding effect becomes

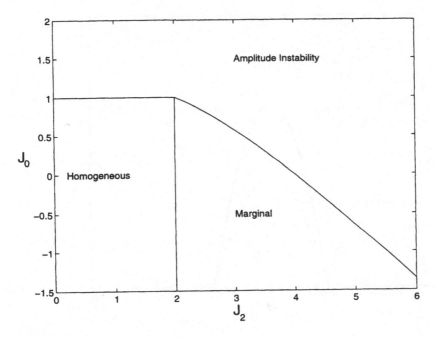

Figure 13.7
Phase diagram of the one-population rate model for $\varepsilon = 0$.

dominant, it sharpens the tuning curve beyond the sharpening provided by the cortical mechanisms. Another regime where the value of Υ is important is near the amplitude instability. This is because the critical value of J_0, J_C, depends on both J_2 and Υ, as shown in the phase diagram (figure 13.7). As Υ increases, the value of J_C decreses, expanding the regime where the fixed-point state is table.

Finally, we would like to point out the two main features that make the one-population model defined by eqs. 13.11–13.13 particularly simple. First, because the synaptic interaction, eq. 13.13, consists of only two Fourier components, the full dynamics can be reduced to a set of self-consistent equations involving a small number of order parameters, in our case, r_0, r_2, and Ψ. Second, as a consequence of the choice of threshold linear gain function, the dynamic equations in the regime of active population are linear equation. The only nonlinearity is the self-consistent equation for θ_C that results from matching the boundary between the active and quiescent populations.

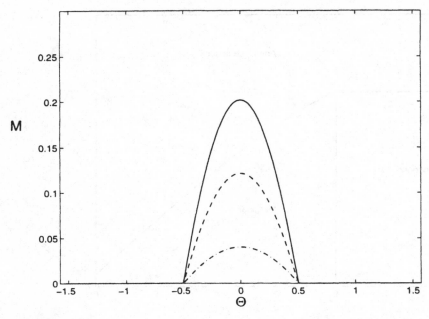

Figure 13.8
Activity profile of the one-population rate model in response to an homogeneous external input for different values of the intensity. $J_0 = -17.2$, $J_2 = 11.2$. Sold line: $C = 1.5$; dashed line: $C = 1.3$; dash-dotted line: $C = 1.1$.

13.5 Moving Activity Profiles

13.5.1 Response to Changing Stimulus Feature

Thus far, we have discussed the steady-state response to the onset of a stimulus with a time-independent feature value, θ_0. One of the most important consequences of the existence of the marginal phase is the dynamics of the system's response to perturbations. Consider the case where the system reaches a stable state located at the peak of weakly tuned input, and a weak transient perturbation is applied on it. Qualitatively, we expect that if the perturbation puts the system momentarily in a state unlike one of the attractor states, the system will quickly relax to the nearest stable profile. On the other hand, if the perturbation puts the system in a different state on the attractor, the system will relax to the original state, that is, the profile will move to its original location relatively slowly, and it will strongly depend on Υ, which represents the restoring force toward the original state. Indeed, for small perturbations, the relaxation times are the inverse of the eigenvalues of the stability matrix of the marginal phase (calculated in chapter appendix B). Eqs. 13.B15, 13.B16, and 13.B21 imply that whereas the relaxation times of the shape of the profile, which involves perturbation of r_0 and r_2, are short even in the marginal phase, the relaxation time of the perturbation to the position of the profile, namely, Ψ, is long and diverges in the limit of $\Upsilon \to 0$.

The slow dynamics of the marginal phase is manifest also in the response of the system to a time-dependent stimulus where θ_0 changes with time. In the present notation, such a stimulus is parametrized as

$$I^0(\theta, t) = I^0(\theta - \theta_0(t)) = C(1 - \varepsilon + \varepsilon \cos(2(\theta - \theta_0(t)))). \tag{13.60}$$

The dynamics of the network is described by eqs. 13.11–13.15, with time-dependent θ_0. The nature of their solution depends on the interaction parameters as well as on the stimulus-effective tuning parameter Υ. In general, if Υ is large, the response of the network may be dominated by the single-neuron dynamics, and the feedback effects will be minor. Here we will focus on the case of a *weakly tuned* input that *varies slowly* with time, where the network behavior may be quite different from that of an isolated neuron. In this regime, the dynamics of the network can be reduced to a simplified *phase model*, similar in some respects to phase descriptions of neuronal oscillatory systems. Our assumptions about the stimulus are formally expressed as

$$\left| \tau_0 \frac{d\theta_0}{dt} \right| = O(\Upsilon) \ll 1. \tag{13.61}$$

Under these conditions, after a long time compared to τ_0, the *shape* of the activity profile of the network becomes almost stationary and has the same form as that for a constant θ_0 and low Υ. The main effect of the motion of the stimulus is to initiate a translation of the activity profile across the network. Thus

$$m(\theta, t) = M(\theta - \Psi(t)), \tag{13.62}$$

where $M(\theta)$ has the same shape as in the stationary case at low Υ, which is given by eqs. 13.36, 13.56, and 13.55. The motion of the profile is conveniently described in terms of the difference between the instantaneous locations of the activity profile and the stimulus feature:

$$\Delta(t) = \Psi(t) - \theta_0(t). \tag{13.63}$$

In chapter appendix A, we show that, to leading order in ε, $\Delta(t)$ obeys the following equation:

$$\frac{d\Delta(t)}{dt} = -\frac{d\theta_0}{dt} + V_C \sin(2\Delta(t)),$$ (13.64)

where

$$\tau_0 V_C = \frac{\Upsilon}{2} f_0(\theta_C)(J_C - J_0) = \frac{\Upsilon(1 - \cos(2\theta_C))}{2G}$$ (13.65)

and where J_C is given in eq. 13.57. Note that $1/V_C$ is proportional to the large relaxation time of perturbations of Ψ, as seen in eq. 13.B21. We now discuss two applications of this equation.

Response to Sudden Change in Stimulus Feature–Virtual Rotation Consider the case where a stimulus with a feature value θ_1 is presented in the receptive field of the cells for a time sufficiently long that a stationary response to the stimulus that a stationary response to the stimulus has developed. Then at time $t = 0$ the stimulus feature is suddenly changed to the value θ_2. How will the cells respond to this change? We consider here separately the regimes of weak and strong cortical modulation.

To illustrate the transient response in the weak modulation regime, we consider the case of zero modulation of the cortical interactions, namely, $J_2 = 0$. In this case the evolution in time of $m(\theta, t)$ is given, according to eq. 13.11, by

$$\tau_0 \frac{d}{dt} m(\theta, t) = -m(\theta) + [I^0(\theta - \theta_2) + J_0 r_0 - T]_+, \quad t > 0,$$ (13.66)

where I^0 is the external input (eq. 13.14) corresponding to the second stimulus. This equation has to be solved with the initial condition $m(\theta, t = 0) = [I^0(\theta - \theta_1) - T]_+$. As will be shown below, the mean network activity r_0 is constant in time, hence the solution to eq. 13.66 is simply

$$m(\theta, t) = M(\theta - \theta_1)e^{-t/\tau_0} + M(\theta - \theta_2)(1 - e^{-t/\tau_0}), \quad t \geq 0,$$ (13.67)

where $M(\theta)$ is the stationary profile under constant stimulus with $\theta_0 = 0$. Thus the initial activity profile decays while the final one grows in amplitude, as shown in figure 13.9A, while intermediate columns remain inactive throughout this response. Note that r_0 indeed remains constant in time, as can be verified by spatial averaging of eq. 13.67. Thus the change in the stimulus redistributes the activity among the neurons within the network without affecting the mean activity level. For this reason, the network feedback $J_0 r_0$ does not modify the time constant associated with the buildup of activity around θ_2. Indeed, according to eq. 13.67, this time constant is the single-neuron time constant, τ_0.

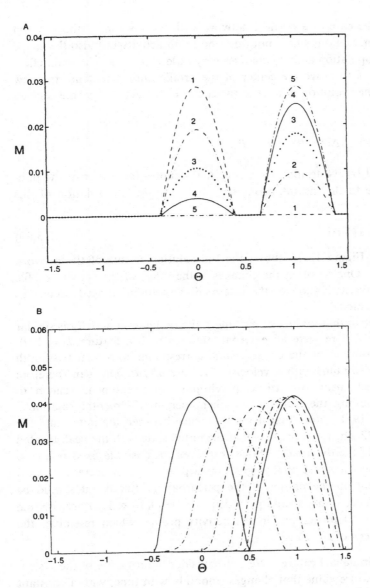

Figure 13.9
Evolution of the neuronal activity in response to a change in the stimulus orientation from an initial value $\theta_1 = 0^0$ to $\Theta_2 = 60^0$. The change occurs at $t = 0$. (A) Afferent mechanism with uniform inhibition. Parameters: $J_0 = -15.5$, $C = 1.1$, $\varepsilon = 0.5$. Times (units of τ_0): 0, 0.5, 1, 2, 6 (lines 1–5, respectively). (B) Virtual rotation in the marginal phase. The activity profile is moving toward θ_2. Parameters: $J_0 = -17.2$, $J_2 = 11.2$, $\varepsilon = 0.05$, $C = 2$. Times (left to right): 0 to $35\tau_0$ each $5\tau_0$.

We next consider the case of a cortical network with weakly tuned stimulus and strongly modulated interaction, where not only the mean activity but also the shape of the profile of the population activity changes very little with time. The main effect of the time evolution is to move the center of the profile until it matches the new stimulus feature θ_2. The evolution in time of the center of the activity profile is given by

$$\frac{d\Delta(t)}{dt} = -V_C \sin(2\Delta(t)), \quad \Delta(t=0) = \theta_1 - \theta_2, \tag{13.68}$$

where $\Delta(t) = \Psi(t) - \theta_0(t)$. Note that, for $t > 0$, $\Delta(t)$ denotes the center of the population profile relative to the instantaneous stimulus, here θ_2. The solution of this equation is

$$\Delta(t) = \arctan(A \exp(-2V_C t)), \tag{13.69}$$

where $A = \tan(\Delta(0))$. Figure 13.9B shows the full solution results of the network dynamics, for $\Upsilon = 0.1$. One sees that the changes in the shape of the activity profile are small and successive activation of the intermediate columns indeed occurs, as predicted by the phase model.

The above results mean that, at any given time t, the population activity is similar to what would occur if there were an external stimulus with a feature $\theta_0 = \Psi(t)$. Thus the temporal evolution of the cortical state corresponds to a virtual smooth change of an external stimulus with a velocity given by $d\Delta/dt$. This can therefore serve as a neural mechanism for various psychophysical phenomena related to apparent motion, including the well-studied phenomenon of "mental rotations" (Shepard and Metzler 1971). Note that if the difference between the initial and the final features equals $\pi/2$, eq. 13.68 predicts that the initial state with the peak located at θ_1 is a fixed point of the dynamics. This is, however, an unstable fixed point, so that slight perturbations will cause $\Psi(t)$ to grow toward $\theta_2 = \pi/2$ or decrease toward $-\theta_2 = -\pi/2$, depending on the nature of the perturbation. Finally, it should be noted that the result of eq. 13.68 is valid provided $V_C \tau_0 = O(\Upsilon) \ll 1$. Otherwise, the dynamics involve major deformations in the activity profile, which resembles the decay and growth pattern of eq. 13.67.

Locking to a Moving Stimulus Feature   We now consider the response of the system to a stimulus with a feature value that changes smoothly with time, with a constant velocity,

$$\theta_0(t) = Vt. \tag{13.70}$$

If the system encodes the instantaneous stimulus orientation by the location of the population activity profile, then this profile should be able to follow the change in the stimulus, which raises the following question. Can the population activity profile lock to the input? If so, what is the range of input velocities for which such locking occurs? For a stimulus that varies on time scales comparable to single-cell time constants, the answers to the above questions may depend strongly on the details of the single-cell microscopic dynamics. When, however, the temporal variation of the stimulus is slow and the direct coupling of the population profile to the changing stimulus relatively weak, cortical cooperative effects may be the dominant factor in determing the locking properties. We therefore focus here on the case of a weakly tuned ($\Upsilon \ll 1$) and slow time-dependent input, $\tau_0 V = O(\Upsilon)$. In weakly modulated cortical interactions, the network's responses to the moving stimulus will be essentially linear, similar to the broad profile in the stationary case. The motion of the stimulus will induce a small time-dependent component of the neuron's activity. The situation is qualitatively different in the parameter regime of the marginal phase, where the tuning of the network will be sharp, hence the response to the stimulus is highly nonlinear. In this limit, the changing stimulus generates a motion of the whole activity profiles without greatly affecting their shape. Hence the state of the system is given approximately by an activity profile whose shape is stationary but whose center moves with time. The motion of the population activity center relative to the stimulus, $\Delta(t)$, is given by eq. 13.64, with $\theta_0(t)$ of eq. 13.70:

$$\frac{d\Delta(t)}{dt} = -V - V_C \sin(2\Delta(t)). \tag{13.71}$$

The nature of the solution of this equation depends on the stimulus velocity, V, relative to the intrinsic velocity constant, V_C.

SLOW STIMULUS ($V < V_C$)   In this regime, eq. 13.71 has a stable fixed point:

$$\Delta = -\frac{1}{2}\arcsin(V/V_C). \tag{13.72}$$

This corresponds to a state in which the activity profile is locked to the stimulus and follows it with a constant phase lag. For $V \to V_C$, the phase lag between the excitatory population and the stimulus reaches $-\pi/4$. It should be emphasized that here, as opposed to the previous case, the locking is strong, involving the motion of a sharply tuned population profile. The positions of the population vectors and the stimulus in such a case are shown in figure 13.10A.

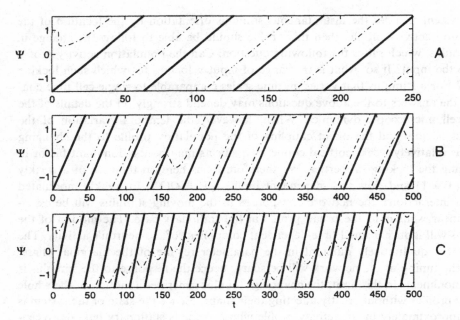

Figure 13.10
Response to a rotating stimulus in the marginal phase ($J_0 = -17.2, J_2 = 11.2, C = 1.1, \varepsilon = 0.05$). Bold lines are the feature of the stimulus, $\theta_0(t) = Vt$ as a function of time. Dash-dotted lines are the angle of the population vector. (A) Complete locking of the activity profile to the rotating stimulus at velocity $V = 0.05 \, \text{rad}/\tau_0$. (B) Partial locking in the case $V = 0.07 \, \text{rad}/\tau_0$. (C) No locking in the case $V = 0.15 \, \text{rad}/\tau_0$.

FAST STIMULUS ($V > V_C$) In this regime, eq. 13.71 does not have a fixed-point solution, and the activity profile is not locked to the rotating stimulus. The solution of the phase equation yields

$$\Delta(t) = \arctan\left\{\frac{V_C}{V} + \frac{W}{V}\tan(V(t - t_0))\right\}, \qquad (13.73)$$

where

$$\tau_0 W = \sqrt{V^2 - V_C^2} \qquad (13.74)$$

and t_0 is determined by the initial condition $\Delta(0) = \Delta_0$. The phase Δ is periodic in time with a period $P = 2\pi/W$. Thus the rotation of the population vector is quasi-periodic, with $\Psi(t) = Vt - \Delta(t)$. The average velocity of the population vector rotation is $V - W$, which is slower than the stimulus velocity, V. The behavior of $\Psi(t)$ for a value of V close to V_C is shown in figure 13.10B, and for a higher velocity in figure 13.10C. These results, obtained by numerical integration of the population dynamics, are in a good qualitative agreement with the predictions of the above phase equations, which are based on the limit of small ε and V.

13.5.2 Intrinsic Moving Profiles

Modeling Neuronal Adaptation One of the major limitations of the one-population model we have studied above is that, because of the symmetry of its connections (Hopfield 1984), it always settles into a stationary state when stimulated by a constant stimulus. Neuronal networks, on the other hand, quite often converge to an attractor that is not a fixed point, even when the stimulus is constant in time. A simple example is the appearance of stable temporal oscillations in the neuronal activity as a result of the network feedback (Wilson and Cowan 1972; Grannan, Kleinfeld, and Sompolinsky 1992). When the network architecture has spatial structure, as in our case, the time-dependent attractors are in general also spatially modulated. A simple class of such stable spatiotemporal patterns is a solution where a spatial activity profile rigidly moves across the network. Indeed, in the more complex architecture of a network comprising distinct excitatory and inhibitory populations, intrinsic moving profiles can appear, provided the internal spatial modulation of the inhibitory feedback is strong (this scenario has been studied in detail in Ben-Yishai, Hansel, and Sompolinsky 1997). Here we study a somewhat simpler scenario for generating such pattern, one that relies on neuronal adaptation, a ubiquitous phenomenon in excitatory cortical neurons (Connors, Gutnick, and Prince 1982; Connors and Gutnick 1990; Ahmed, Anderson, et al. 1994). Qualitatively, the movement of the activity profile is caused by the presence of strong, delayed negative feedback that is local in space. Such inhibitory feedback suppresses activity which develops in a localized region. The excitatory feedback, in turn, induces activity growth in nearby unadapted locations, thereby causing the propagation of the profile. We first present a simple way of incorporating adaptation in the population rate dynamics, and then study its effect on the network spatiotemporal state.

We incorporate adaptation by the following model:

$$\tau_0 \frac{d}{dt} m(\theta, t) = -m(\theta) + [I(\theta, t) - I_a(\theta, t) - T]_+, \tag{13.75}$$

where the total input $I(\theta, t)$ is given by eq. 13.12, and where the adaptation current $I_a(\theta, t)$ obeys a linear dynamical equation:

$$\tau_a \frac{dI_a(\theta, t)}{dt} = -I_a(\theta, t) + J_a m(\theta, t). \tag{13.76}$$

The parameter $J_a > 0$ measures the strength of the adaptation and τ_a is its time constant, which will be assumed to be large compared to τ_0. Note that the adaptation can be thought of as a slow local negative feedback, which we take to be linear.

In the absence of interaction between the neurons, and with a suprathreshold stimulus $(C > 1)$ constant in time, the fixed point of the dynamics is given by

$$m(\theta) = G(C - T) \tag{13.77}$$

$$I_a(\theta) = J_a m(\theta) \tag{13.78}$$

where the single-neuron gain G is given by

$$G = \frac{1}{1 + J_a}. \tag{13.79}$$

This fixed point is always stable. Thus, for an isolated neuron, the slow adaptation current does not generate persistent oscillation, and the only effect of the adaptation at the fixed point is simply to reduce the gain of the neuron by a factor $1 + J_a$. A reasonable value for the adaptation strength is $J_a = 1$. With this strength, the firing rates at large time are reduced by 50% compared to the situation without adaptation. This is compatible with experimental data concerning spikes adaptation of cortical neurons (Connors, Gutnick, Prince 1982; Ahmed, Anderson, et al. 1994).

The stationary solution of the network dynamic equations remains essentially the same as without adaptation. Here again, the only effect of the adaptation is to reduce the gain by the factor $1 + J_a$: the new fixed solution for $m(\theta)$ is as given above except that the parameters J_0, J_2, C, and T have to be divided by the factor $1 + J_a$. However, the presence of adaptation strongly affects the *stability* of this fixed-point solution, particularly when the spatial inhomogeneity of the stimulus is weak. For sufficiently strong adaptation, the fixed-point solution is unstable; instead, a new spatiotemporal solution appears as the system's attractor.

We first discuss the case of a homogeneous stimulus, $\Upsilon = 0$. The results of the stability analysis of the fixed point as a function of the interaction modulation and adaptation strength are summarized on the phase diagram of figure 13.11. The weak adaptation regime is marked by

$$J_a < \frac{\tau_0}{\tau_a}. \tag{13.80}$$

In this regime, the system's behavior is similar to that with no adaptation. When the

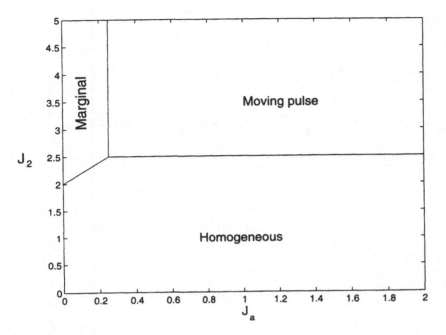

Figure 13.11
Phase diagram of the one-population rate model with firing adaptation, $\tau_a = 4\tau_0$.

modulation of the interaction J_2 is sufficiently small, the homogeneous state is stable. For a homogeneous input and $J_2 > 2(1 + J_a)$, the homogeneous state is unstable and a line of stationary attractors appears. As before, they correspond to stationary modulated activity profiles whose peaks are located at arbitrary positions. The shape of each activity profile can be deduced from the results of section 13.4 by normalizing the interactions J_0 and J_2 and the effective gain G by the factor $1/(1 + J_a)$.

In the strong adaptation regime

$$J_a > \frac{\tau_0}{\tau_a}, \tag{13.81}$$

the stationary homogeneous state is stable for $J_2 < 2(1 + \tau_0/\tau_a)$. Above this value, the state is destabilized in favor of a profile of activity that travels across the network (figure 13.12). The direction of the pulse movement depends on the initial conditions.

For $J_2 > 2(1 + \tau_0/\tau_a)$, the transition to a moving state as J_a increases above the value τ_0/τ_a (vertical line in figure 13.11) indicates the destabilization of the stationary

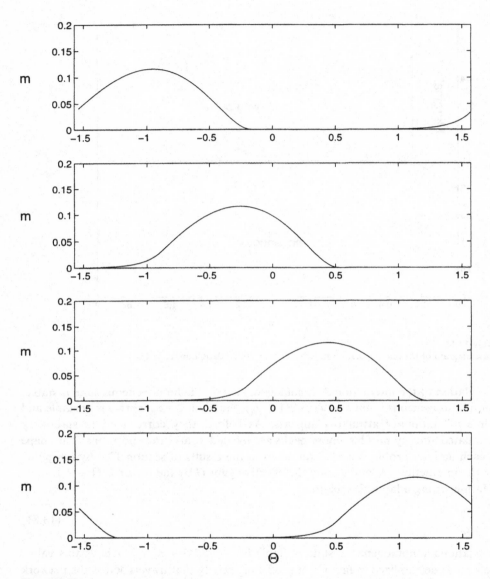

Figure 13.12
Traveling pulse of activity in the one-population rate model with adaptation. Parameters: $\tau_a = 4\tau_0$, $J_a = 1$, $J_0 = -2$, $J_2 = 6$, $C = 1.1$. Frames are for times $t = 0$, $5\tau_0$, $10\tau_0$, $15\tau_0$. Velocity of the pulse: $V = 0.1389\,\text{rad}/\tau_0$.

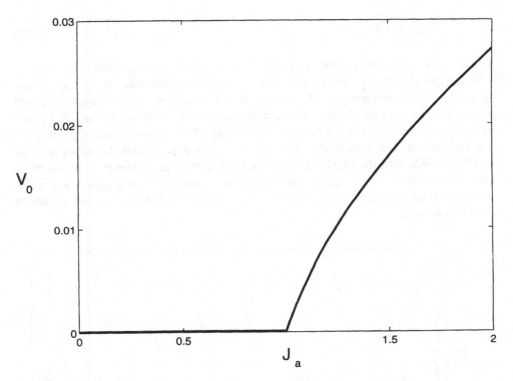

Figure 13.13
Velocity of the traveling pulse in the one-population rate model with adaptation against the adaptation strength J_a. Parameters: $\tau_a = 10\tau_0$, $J_0 = -2$, $J_2 = 6$, $C = 1.1$. Velocity in radians/τ_0.

inhomogeneous state is due to the appearance of an unstable transversal mode, which corresponds to the translation of the profile of activity across the network. Thus, on the right of the vertical line of figure 13.11, the network settles into a state where the activity profile moves without changing its shape. The velocity of the profile vanishes on the line as $J_a - \tau_0/\tau_a$. When J_a increases beyond this line, the velocity grows monotonically with J_a, as shown in figure 13.13.

For $J_a > \tau_0/\tau_a$, the destabilization of the stationary state as J_2 increases above $2(1 + \tau_0/\tau_a)$ (horizontal line in figure 13.11) corresponds to a pair of complex conjugate eigenvalues, whose real part becomes positive. This instability corresponds to a direct transition between the stationary homogeneous state and the traveling pulse. On this line, the half-width of the activity profile is $\pi/2$ and the velocity of the profile is

$$V_0 = \frac{1}{2\tau_a} \sqrt{J_a \frac{\tau_a}{\tau_0} - 1}. \tag{13.82}$$

The velocity is finite on the line except at $J_a = \tau_0/\tau_a$, where it vanishes.

When the stimulus is tuned, that is, $\varepsilon > 0$, three regimes exist depending on the value of ε. For ε sufficiently small ($\varepsilon < \varepsilon_1$), the hill of activity travels across the whole system but the velocity of the movement depends on the position of the hill. In particular, when the hill peak approaches the vicinity of the orientation of the stimulus, it is accelerated. For sufficiently large ε ($\varepsilon > \varepsilon_2$), one expects that the hill of activity will be pinned, with the maximum of activity located at the orientation of the stimulus. Finally, for $\varepsilon_1 < \varepsilon < \varepsilon_2$, the activity hill performs localized oscillations around the orientation of the stimulus. Figure 13.14 displays the behavior of the system in the three regimes.

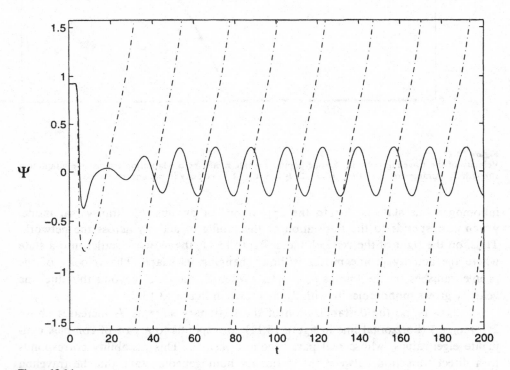

Figure 13.14
Pinning of the traveling pulse by the inhomogeneity of a tuned stimulus. Solid line: $\varepsilon = 0.2$; dash-dotted line: $\varepsilon = 0.06$. Same parameters as in figure 13.12.

13.6 Model with Short-Range Excitation

Until now, we have assumed a network architecture with space-dependent interactions whose range extended throughout the whole network (see eqs. 13.2 and 13.13). In this case, the strength of the spatial modulation of the cortical interactions is measured by the *amplitude* of their spatial modulation, for example, the parameter J_2 in eq. 13.13. In general, we expect that the range of the spatial modulation will also have an important effect on the spatial pattern of network activity. To study this issue, we consider in this section the case where the excitatory interactions decay exponentially with the distance between the interacting neurons. We will assume that the inhibitory interactions have significantly longer range than the excitatory interactions; hence we will approximate them by a global inhibition.

The exponential falloff of the excitatory interactions assumed here violates the periodic boundary conditions assumed until now. Periodic boundary conditions are appropriate for a network that processes angle variables such as orientation of an edge in the case of visual cortex, or representation of the direction of arm reaching movement in the case of motor cortex. For other features, such as tuning for spatial frequency in visual cortex or coding of place in hippocampus, such boundary conditions are not natural. Thus the present model will also illustrate to what extent the results we have obtained so far are sensitive to the idealized assumption about periodic boundary conditions and perfect translational symmetry.

Our model is a one-dimensional array of N neurons that code for a one-dimensional feature variable θ. The neurons are labeled by their PF, which is distributed uniformly in a range of size $2L$, that is, $-L < \theta < L$. The network dynamics are similar to those of the one-population rate model (eq. 13.11), with

$$I(\theta, t) = \sum_{\theta} J(\theta, \theta') m(\theta', t) + I^0(\theta - \theta_0). \tag{13.83}$$

The interaction between two neurons located at positions θ and θ' is of the form $J(\theta, \theta') = J(\theta - \theta')/N$, where

$$J(\theta - \theta') = \frac{2L}{\lambda}(-J_I + J_E \exp(-|\theta - \theta'|/\lambda)), \quad |\theta|, |\theta'| < L. \tag{13.84}$$

The parameter $J_I > 0$ represents a global inhibition. The second term with $J_E > 0$ is an exponentially decreasing excitation. The parameter J_E represents the amplitude of the spatial modulation of the cortical excitatory interactions, while the parameter λ denotes their spatial range. The external input has the form

$$I^0(\theta) = C(1 - 2\varepsilon + 2\varepsilon \exp(-|\theta|/\mu)). \tag{13.85}$$

The spatial dependence of the input is characterized by two parameters, namely, ε and μ. As in the case of the model investigated in section 13.3, ε is the amplitude of the spatial modulation of the input, generally defined as

$$\varepsilon = \frac{I^0_{max} - I^0_{min}}{2I^0_{max}}, \tag{13.86}$$

where $I^0_{max} = C$ is the maximum value of the external input and I^0_{min} is its minimum value. The parameter μ is the width of the input, which in the present model will be a free parameter.

We will assume that both λ and μ are on the scale of L but may be smaller than L. Thus, although the excitatory interactions are of a limited spatial range, each neuron (except at the boundaries) receives excitatory inputs from a sizable fraction λ/L of the N neurons. Thus, for large N, a continuum mean field description of the network dynamics is valid, yielding for the total input current at time t

$$I(\theta, t) = \int_{-L}^{+L} d\theta' \, J(\theta - \theta')m(\theta', t) + I^0(\theta - \theta_0). \tag{13.87}$$

The fixed-point state of the network is given by the following self-consistent equations:

$$m(\theta) = \left[\frac{-J_I}{\lambda}r_0 + \frac{J_E}{\lambda}\int_{-L}^{+L} d\theta' \exp(-|\theta - \theta'|/\lambda)m(\theta') + I^0(\theta - \theta_0) - T\right]_+, \tag{13.88}$$

where

$$r_0 = \int_{-L}^{+L} d\theta \, m(\theta). \tag{13.89}$$

Comparing eq. 13.88 with eqs. 13.16, 13.17, and 13.20, it is seen that the present model is more complex than our previous model. Because of the form of the present interaction function, the fixed-point equations cannot be reduced to a small number of global order parameters. Yet both models share the simplicity that within the *active* population the underlying equations are linear. In fact, differentiating eq. 13.88 twice with respect to θ in the regime where $m(\theta)$ is nonzero, we find that in this regime the activity profile obeys the following second-order linear differential equation:

$$\frac{d^2 m}{d\theta^2} + \frac{m}{\Lambda^2} = \frac{d^2 I^0}{d\theta^2} + \frac{1}{\lambda^2}\left(T + \frac{J_I}{\lambda}r_0 - I^0(\theta)\right), \tag{13.90}$$

where

$$\Lambda^2 = \frac{\lambda^2}{2J_E - 1}.$$ (13.91)

The above equation is supplemented with the following boundary conditions:

$$m(0) = -\frac{J_I r_0}{\lambda} + C - T + \frac{J_E}{\lambda} \int_{-L}^{L} \exp(-|\theta|/\lambda) m(\theta)\, d\theta$$ (13.92)

and

$$\frac{dm(0^{\pm})}{d\theta} = \frac{dI^0(0^{\pm})}{d\theta}.$$ (13.93)

Finally, r_0 has to be calculated self-consistently, using eq. 13.89. Eqs. 13.89–13.93 can be solved for broad and narrow profiles for the stimulus of the form given by eq. 13.85. We first consider the case of a homogeneous input, $\varepsilon = 0$.

13.6.1 Broad Activity Profile

The simplest solution to eqs. 13.91–13.94, for $I^0(\theta) = C$, that is, $d^2 I_0/d\theta^2 = 0$, is obtained assuming that the local fields on all the neurons are above threshold. The solution is of the form

$$m(\theta) = \begin{cases} (C - T)(A - B\cosh(\theta/\Lambda)) & J_E < \frac{1}{2} \\ (C - T)(A\cos(\theta/\Lambda) - B) & J_E > \frac{1}{2}. \end{cases}$$ (13.94)

The constants $A > B > 0$, determined by the boundary conditions and eq. 13.90, depend on the parameters J_I, J_E, L, and λ, as detailed in Hansel and Sompolinsky 1997. An example of the activity profile in this regime can be seen in figure 13.15, where the linear solution is unique and centered at $\theta = 0$. Contrary to the previous case, where the linear solution for homogeneous external inputs was uniform, here the corresponding solution is not uniform. The θ dependence of this solution is due to boundary effect: neurons close the boundaries receive less excitatory feedback; hence their level of activity is decreased.

13.6.2 Narrow Profiles and Marginal Phase

The above broad solution is valid, provided the $m(\theta)$ of eq. 13.94 is positive and does not vanish in the range $-L < \theta < +L$. Whether this condition holds depends on both J_E and λ. For $J_E < 1/2$, the broad solution is indeed a valid solution for all λ. For $J_E > 1/2$, however, the above solution is positive for all θ only for sufficiently

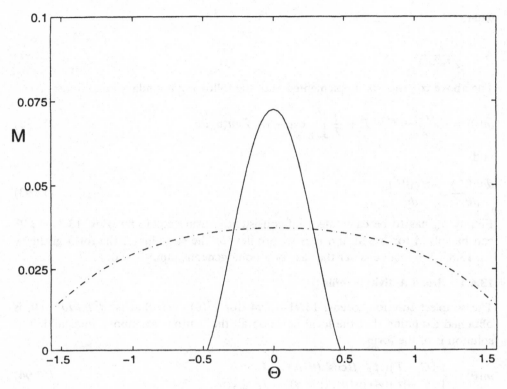

Figure 13.15
Profile of activity in the one-population rate model with short range excitation and open boundary conditions for $L = \pi, J_0 = -0.2, \lambda = 0.2, C = 1.01$. Dash-dotted line: broad profile for $J_2 = 0.45$; solid line: narrow profile for $J_2 = 1$.

large λ/L. If $\lambda < \lambda_c$, the above solution becomes negative, hence not valid. Instead, a solution with a narrow profile appears in which only part of the population is active. This solution is not unique. Because the active population does not receive inputs from neurons near the boundary, the activity of the neurons does not depend on their location relative to the boundary unless the activity profile is close to the boundary. Thus the narrow solution of eq. 13.90 (again, with $I^0(\theta) = C$) is of the form

$$m(\theta) = M(\theta - \Psi), \quad -L + \theta_C < \Psi < L - \theta_C, \tag{13.95}$$

where

$$M(\theta) = (C - T)A[\cos(\theta/\Lambda) - \cos(\theta_c/\Lambda)]_+. \tag{13.96}$$

The width of the profile is given by

$$\theta_C(J_E) = \Lambda(\pi - \arctan\sqrt{2J_E - 1}).$$ (13.97)

The constant A is related to the gain G through eq. 13.24. It can be shown that the gain of the narrow profile is

$$G = \frac{1 - \cos(\theta_C/\Lambda)}{f(\theta_C)(J_I - J_C)},$$ (13.98)

where

$$f(\theta_C) = \left(\frac{\theta_C}{\lambda} + 1\right)2\cos\left(\frac{\theta_c}{\Lambda}\right)$$ (13.99)

and

$$J_C = \frac{\tan^2\left(\frac{\theta_c}{\Lambda}\right)}{2\left(\frac{\theta_c}{\lambda} + 1\right)}.$$ (13.100)

Note the similarity between these equations and those of the marginal state in the periodic long-range model of section 13.4 (eqs. 13.55–13.57). The critical value of λ (or J_E) for which this phase exists is given by the condition that θ_C approaches the boundary, namely,

$$\theta_C = L$$ (13.101)

If L is large compared to the range of interactions λ, this marginal phase therefore exists for all λ as long as $J_E > 1/2$ (see figure 13.15). The phase diagram of the model is shown in figure 13.16. It should be noted that the shape of the activity profile is determined only by the modulated component of the interactions. However, as in the periodic system, the stability of all the above solutions depends also on the value of J_I.

In conclusion, the above results demonstrate the respective roles of the amplitude and the range of the cortical feedback excitation. The phase diagram (figure 13.16) shows that when the range of the excitatory interactions is small compared to the total extent of the network, namely, $\lambda \ll L$, the onset of the marginal phase and the associated emergence of narrow activity profiles in response to broadly tuned input depend on the amplitude of the spatial modulation of the cortical interactions and are insensitive to its range. On the other hand, the *width* of the narrow activity profile depends on both λ and J_E, as seen from eqs. 13.91 and 13.97.

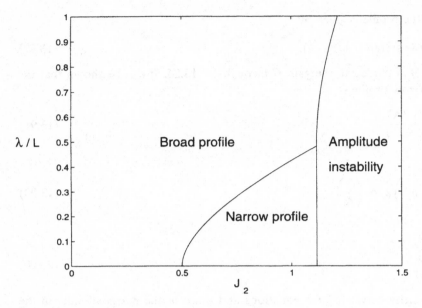

Figure 13.16
Phase diagram of the one-population rate model with short range excitation and open boundary conditions for $J_0 = -0.2$. The stimulus is homogeneous.

13.6.3 Tuned Input

Considering next the case of an input of the form of eq. 13.85, with $\varepsilon > 0$, we focus on the dependence of the resultant activity profile on the parameters C, ε, and μ of the external input. It is easy to see from the fixed-point equation that the profile of activity depends on C and ε through the *effective stimulus tuning* Υ defined by eq. 13.31. In particular, in the absence of cortical interactions, the resultant activity profile is the same as that of the input except for the thresholding effect. Thus, for strongly tuned input, defined by

$$\Upsilon > \tfrac{1}{2}, \tag{13.102}$$

the solution of eq. 13.88 has a narrow activity profile, with

$$m(\theta) \propto [\exp(-|\theta - \theta_0|/\mu) - \exp(-|\theta_C - \theta_0|/\mu)]_+, \quad \Upsilon > 1/2, \; J_I = J_E = 0, \tag{13.103}$$

where

$$\theta_C = -\mu \ln\left(1 - \frac{1}{2\Upsilon}\right).$$ (13.104)

This function is depicted in figure 13.17 for $\mu = 0.05$ and $\mu = 1.5$. When the stimulus tuning is weak, that is, $\Upsilon < 1/2$, the activity profile is broad, namely, all the neurons are above threshold.

We now consider the effect of the cortical excitation on the tuning of the network activity. We will focus on the parameter regime where the network possesses a marginal phase, namely,

$$J_E > 1/2, \quad J_I > J_C, \quad \lambda < \lambda_c.$$ (13.105)

As in our previous model the most important role of the tuned stimulus is to select from the continuum of fixed points (eq. 13.95) the profile

$$\Psi = \theta_0.$$ (13.106)

It can be shown that the general solution of the narrow profile in eq. 13.91 is of the form

$$m(\theta) = (C - T)[A\cos(\theta/\Lambda) - \Upsilon B|\sin(\theta/\Lambda)| + \Upsilon D\exp(-|\theta|/\mu) + F]_+.$$ (13.107)

Thus, for small Υ, the form of the activity profile is close to that for a uniform input (eq. 13.96). Note that despite the exponential shape of the external stimulus, the dominant part of the network activity profile is in this case of a cosine form. The cosine form of the activity profile in the marginal phase, predicted by eq. 13.36, is therefore not special to interactions with the cosine form such as eq. 13.13. Instead, the cosine form for the profile is quite general and is related to the fact that the instability to the formation of these patterns occurs first at long wavelength modes.

Recall that in the model of section 13.4, where both the excitatory interactions and the stimulus had long spatial range, the width of the activity profile was determined, in the marginal phase, by the cortical interactions and was rather insensitive to the effective stimulus tuning Υ. In the present model, however, the tuning of the network activity is in general a complicated function of both Υ and μ through the values of the constants A, B, D, and F (Hansel and Sompolinsky 1997). The qualitative behavior of the tuning width can be understood by considering narrow stimulus and broad stimulus limits.

Narrow Stimulus This case is defined as $\mu/\lambda \ll 1$, where the behavior depends on the effective stimulus tuning Υ.

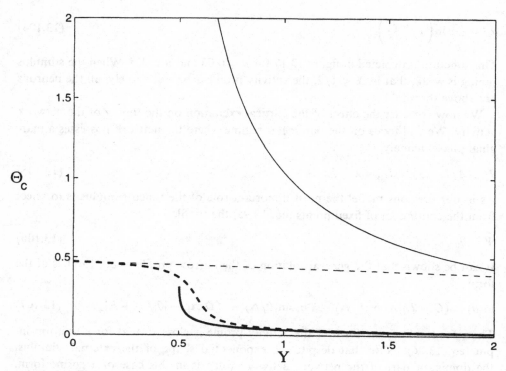

Figure 13.17
Width θ_c of the activity profile in the rate model with short range excitation and open boundary conditions; θ_c is plotted as a function of Υ. For $\mu = 1.5$, thin solid line: afferent mechanism; thin dashed line: marginal phase. For $\mu = 0.05$, thick solid line: afferent mechanism; thick dashed line: marginal phase. Parameters: $\lambda = 0.2, J_0 = -0.2, J_2 = 1$ for the marginal phase, and $J_0 = 0; J_2 = 0$ for the afferent mechanism.

STRONGLY TUNED INPUT   In the case $\Upsilon > 1/2$, we find that the width of the profile is

$$\theta_C \simeq -\mu \ln\left(1 - \frac{1}{2\,\Upsilon}\right), \quad \mu/\lambda \ll 1. \tag{13.108}$$

Thus the width of the tuning is the same as if there were no cortical interactions; namely, it is determined by the width of the input. This is expected because in this regime the tuning provided by the external input (of the order μ) is much sharper than that provided by the interactions (of the order λ).

WEAKLY TUNED INPUT   If $\Upsilon < 1/2$, we find that the tuning of the neuronal response is independent of the tuning of the input and is given by eq. 13.97. Therefore, in this limit, the shape of the activity profile is determined essentially by the cortical interactions; the main effect of inhomogeneity in the external input is to select among the continuum of possible states that state in which the peak in the activity matches the stimulus feature, namely, $\Psi = \theta_0$. The crossover between the two regimes occurs in the region $\Upsilon \simeq 1/2$. The size of the crossover region is a decreasing function of μ/λ.

Broad Stimulus   In the limit $\mu/\lambda \gg 1$, which corresponds to an input much broader than the excitatory interaction, the tuning of the input does not much affect the shape of the tuning curve; as in the previous case, its main effect is to select the state with $\Psi = \theta_0$. An exception is the case of a stimulus with intensity near threshold, namely, $\Upsilon \gg 1$: once the single-neuron thresholding effect becomes dominant, it sharpens the tuning curve beyond the sharpening provided by the cortical mechanisms.

Figure 13.17 shows θ_C for various stimulus parameters obtained by a full solution of the model with tuned input. In the case of μ/λ large, θ_C is determined by the cortical interactions, and Υ does not significantly affect it. On the other hand, when μ/λ is small, there is a pronounced decrease of θ_C when $\Upsilon \geq 1/2$, which agrees with the analysis above. Comparing these results with those of figure 13.5 (section 13.4), we see that figure 13.17 is similar to the cases $\mu/\lambda > 1$. The effect of the width of the stimulus is most pronounced in the regime of small μ/λ. Here, increasing Υ causes a sharp crossover from interaction-dominated tuning ($\Upsilon < 1/2$) to afferent-dominated tuning ($\Upsilon > 1/2$).

13.6.4   Intrinsic Moving Profiles

We now turn briefly to moving profiles with homogeneous external input. The addition of adaptation current to the present model, as in eqs. 13.75 and 13.76, tends to destabilize the stationary profile of the marginal phase and to induce moving activity profiles similar to those of the periodic system (as shown in "Instability of the Marginal Phase Due to Adaptation" in chapter appendix B). Although the boundaries do not affect the existence of stationary narrow solutions in the network's's interior, the situation is different in the case of moving solutions. The reason is that in the moving state all the neurons are active, hence they do feel the influence of the boundaries. The effect of the boundaries on the wave propagation depends on the amplitude of the adaptation current. For relatively low values of J_a (but sufficient to generate moving profiles), the boundaries act as reflecting walls. The profiles bounce between the two boundaries, as shown in figure 13.18A. On the other hand, for strong adaptation, the boundaries act as sinks; once the symmetry of the direction of movement is broken by the initial conditions, the profiles keep moving in the same direction, across the network, as shown in figure 13.18B. It is interesting to note that the boundaries act here like an inhomogenous external input peaked at the center in the periodic architecture, as in section 13.5.2; they distort the motion of the profile but do not reverse its direction of motion. On the other hand, in the case of relatively low adaptation, the boundaries act as relatively strong inhomogeneities that localize the moving profile, as shown figure 13.12.

13.7   Network Model with Conductance-Based Dynamics

13.7.1   Conductance-Based Dynamics of Point Neurons

This section describes a dynamic model based on the well-known Hodgkin and Huxley–type equations (see chapter 10, this volume) for a single space-clamped neuron and synaptic conductances opened after the occurance of action potential in the presynaptic neurons. The equation satisfied by the membrane potential of neuron θ of type α is

$$\frac{d}{dt} V^\alpha(\theta, t) = -G^\alpha_{leak}(V^\alpha(\theta, t) - V_{leak}) - I^\alpha_{gated}(\theta, t) + I^\alpha(\theta, t). \tag{13.109}$$

For simplicity, we assume the membranes' capacitance is 1. The first term on the right-hand side of eq. 13.109 corresponds to the contribution of the leak current, which has voltage-independent conductance G^α_{leak}. The current I^α_{gated} represents the voltage-gated ionic currents, which are in particular responsible for the generation of action potential. The last term of eq. 13.109 incorporates all the synaptic inputs converging on the neurons and consists of the three components described in eq. 13.1. Each of these components represents synaptic conductances,

A   B

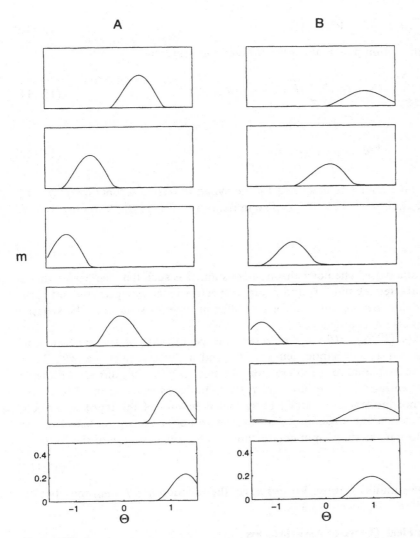

Figure 13.18
Traveling pulse in the short range model with open boundary conditions and adaptation. Parameters:
$L = \pi, J_0 = -0.2, J_2 = 1, \lambda = 0.2, C = 1.1, \tau_a = 10\tau_0$. (A) $J_a = 0.5$. The pulse is oscillating between the
boundaries. Times (top to bottom; in units of τ_0): $t = 0, 20, 30, 60, 80, 90$. (B) $J_a = 1$. The pulse is always
moving in the same direction. Times (top to bottom; in units of τ_0): $t = 0, 5, 15, 25, 30, 35$.

$$I^{\alpha\beta}(\theta, t) = g^{\alpha\beta}(\theta, t)(V^\beta - V^\alpha(\theta, t)), \tag{13.110}$$

triggered by the action potentials of the presynaptic neurons,

$$g^{\alpha\beta}(\theta, t) = \frac{1}{N_\beta} \sum_{i=1}^{N_\beta} g^{\alpha\beta}(\theta - \theta_i) \sum_{t_i} f^\beta(t - t_i), \quad \beta = E, I \tag{13.111}$$

$$g^{\alpha 0}(\theta, t) = \frac{1}{N_0} \sum_{i=1}^{N_0} g^{\alpha 0}(\theta, i) \sum_{t_i} f^0(t - t_i). \tag{13.112}$$

The synaptic time course is described by the synaptic response function $f^\beta(t - t_i)$, where t_i is the occurrence time for a spike in neuron i (of type β). A frequently used form is

$$f(t) = A(e^{-t/\tau_1} - e^{-t/\tau_2}), \quad t \geq 0, \tag{13.113}$$

and $f(t) = 0$ otherwise. The normalization constant A is such that the peak value of f is 1. The characteristic times τ_1 and τ_2 are, respectively, the synaptic rise and decay times, whose value may be different for the different types of synapses. The synaptic reversal potentials are denoted V_α.

The functions $(1/N_\beta)g^{\alpha\beta}(\theta - \theta')$ represent the peak value of the synaptic conductances between a presynaptic neuron, $\beta\theta'$, and a postsynaptic one, $\alpha\theta'$. These functions are proportional to the interaction functions $J^{\alpha,\beta}(\theta - \theta')$ introduced above. The spatial organization of the input from the stimulus is encoded in $g^{\alpha 0}(\theta, i)$. Because we are not modeling the architecture and dynamics of the input network in detail, we will assume the incoming spikes to a neuron obey Poisson statistics at rates that give rise to a fluctuating input conductance with a time average of the form

$$\langle g^{\alpha 0}(\theta, t) \rangle_{av} = g^{\alpha 0}(\theta - \theta_0), \tag{13.114}$$

where θ_0 is the stimulus feature. For instance, the function $g^{\alpha 0}(\theta - \theta_0)$ may be proportional to $I^{\alpha 0}(\theta - \theta_0)$ in eq. 13.3.

13.7.2   Mean Field Theory of Asynchronous States

In general, the network described above may develop complex dynamical behaviors that are hard to analyze. A particularly simple case is when the network settles in an asynchronous state, which may occur if the external input is statistically stationary and the temporal fluctuations of the inputs to different neurons are only weakly correlated. Under these conditions, if the network is large enough, it may settle into a state where the correlations between the activities of different neurons are weak, despite their interactions. In such a state, the total synaptic conductances on each neuron is constant in time, up to small fluctuations that vanish in the limit of a large network, $N_\alpha \to \infty$. Whether the network settles into a synchronous or asynchronous state depends on the network parameters (as described in detail in Hansel and Sompolinsky 1996).

In the asynchronous state, the feedback from the network on each neuron can be described in terms of constant currents and conductances, called "mean fields," which obey certain self-consistent equations. In our case, the total synaptic conductance from the α population on neuron θ is constant in time and is given by

$$g^{\alpha\beta}(\theta) = \int_{-\pi/2}^{+\pi/2} \frac{d\theta'}{\pi} J^{\alpha\beta}(\theta - \theta') m^\beta(\theta'), \quad \beta = E, I, \tag{13.115}$$

where $m^\alpha(\theta)$ is the time-average firing rate of neuron θ in the population α.

Taking into account the stationarity of the synaptic conductances, eq. 13.109 can be written as a single-neuron dynamic equation:

$$\frac{d}{dt} V^\alpha(\theta, t) = -(g^\alpha(\theta) + \delta g^{\alpha 0}(\theta, t)) V^\alpha(\theta, t) - I_{gated}(\theta, t) + I^\alpha(\theta), \tag{13.116}$$

with

$$g^\alpha(\theta) = G^\alpha_{leak} + g^{\alpha E}(\theta) + g^{\alpha I}(\theta) + g^{\alpha 0}(\theta - \theta_0) \tag{13.117}$$

$$I^\alpha(\theta) = (g^{\alpha E}(\theta) + g^{\alpha 0}(\theta - \theta_0)) V^E + g^{\alpha I}(\theta) V^I. \tag{13.118}$$

The term $\delta g^{\alpha 0}(\theta, t)$ represents the fluctuations in the input conductance due to the Poisson statistics of the incoming spikes. The currents I^α and conductances g^α themselves depend on the time-average activity profiles, $m^\alpha(\theta)$, of the neurons in the network through eq. 13.115. Thus to complete the solution, we have to calculate the time-average firing rates of single neurons obeying dynamics of the form of eq. 13.116. This results in self-consistent integral equations for the stationary activity profiles of the form $m^\alpha(\theta) = F(\theta, \{m^\beta(\theta')\})$. A similar approach can be used in principle to study the properties of the network in cases where the stimulus varies slowly with time.

In section we analyzed the network properties using simplified rate dynamics. Here we use numerical simulations to study the properties of a network with the same architecture as that of the rate model but with conductance-based dynamics. We first specify below the details of the model and then compare the numerical results with the theoretical prediction of the rate model.

13.7.3 Details of the Numerical Simulations

Single-Neuron Dynamics We have studied eq. 13.109 with voltage-gated current, I_{gated}, which incorporates sodium (I_{Na}) and potassium (I_K) currents, responsible for spike generation, as in the standard Hodgkin-Huxley model. It also includes a non-inactivating persistent sodium current, (I_{NaP}), and an A-current (I_A), known to be present in cortical and hippocampal cells (Llinás 1988; Stafstrom, Schwindt, and Crill 1982; Gustafsson et al. 1982; see also chapter 5, this volume). The first current enhances the excitability of the cells at voltages near threshold, leading to a frequency-current relationship that increases continuously from zero and thereby increases the dynamic range of the neurons. The A-current reduces the gain of the neurons, and thereby suppresses their maximal rate (Connor, Walter, and Mckown 1977; Rush and Rinzel 1994).

Below we will also study the effect of adaptation on the network state. Because regular spiking pyramidal cells in cortex display spike adaptation (Connors, Gutnick, and Prince 1982), but fast spiking neurons do not, we incorporate adaptation only in the excitatory population, which corresponds to the regular spiking pyramidal cells. This adaptation is introduced by adding to the single-neuron dynamics a slow potassium current with a relatively large time constant, chosen independently of the membrane potential for the sake of simplicity and in the range 10–100 msec in agreement with a recent study of firing adaptation (Ahmed, Anderson, et al. 1994).

The full kinetic equations of these currents are given in chapter appendix C, along with all the parameter values used in our simulations, which correspond to a cell with a resting potential, $V_{rest} = -71$ mV, and a membrane time constant at rest, $\tau_0 = 10$ msec. Typical values used below are $\tau = 60$ msec and $g_a = 10$ mS/cm^2. As illustrated in figure 13.19, this corresponds to a reduction in the firing rate on the order of 50%, which agrees with the experimental results. Traces of the membrane potentials of single, isolated excitatory and inhibitory neurons are shown in figure 13.20.

Network Architecture We have simulated a network with an equal number of excitatory and inhibitory neurons; within each population, the neurons have identical intrinsic and synaptic properties. The synaptic inputs are modeled according to eqs. 13.109–13.113. For the spatial modulation of the synaptic conductances $g^{\alpha\beta}(\theta - \theta')$ in eq. 13.111, we take a square function. All pairs of excitatory neurons whose PFs differ by an amount smaller in absolute value than a given value, $\delta\theta$, are connected with the same connection strength; if the difference is larger than this cutoff, the connection between them is zero. In the present simulations, we use $\delta\theta = 30°$ as the

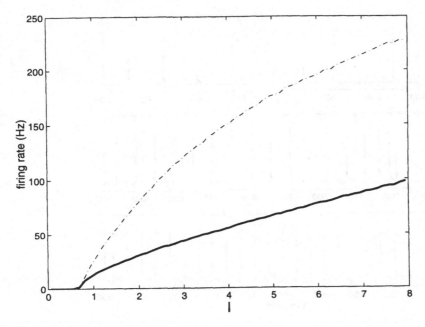

Figure 13.19
Firing rate of the neurons in the excitatory population in the spiking neuron network model (no inter-action). Solid line: firing rate at large time upon injection of a constant current; dash-dotted line: in-stantaneous firing rate from the first interspike interval after the injection of the current. The adaptation time constant is $\tau_a = 60\,\mathrm{msec}$. The adaptation maximal conductance is $g_a = 10\,\mathrm{mS/cm^2}$.

range of the excitatory interactions. The inhibition to inhibitory neurons is assumed to be global and homogeneous; each inhibitory neuron is assumed to inhibit all the excitatory neurons with the same maximal synaptic conductance (although the max-imal conductance of the inhibition to the inhibitory neurons can differ from that of the excitatory neurons). The synaptic action of the excitatory neurons on the in-hibitor neurons is also assumed to be global. For simplicity, propagation delays are not included in the model. The values of the synaptic strengths and time constants are give in table 13.1 (chapter appendix C).

Equation 13.112 for the external stimulus is implemented by assuming

$$g^{\alpha 0}(\theta,\, t) = g^0 \sum_{t_0} f^0(t - t_0), \qquad (13.119)$$

where t_0 is the arrival times of spikes generated by a Poisson process with a rate $C(1 - \varepsilon + \varepsilon \cos(2\theta - \theta_0))$. Here the stimulus intensity C is given in terms of the input

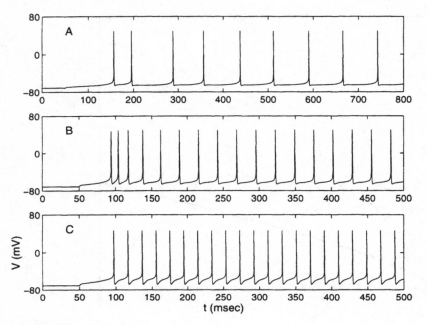

Figure 13.20
Membrane potential of the neurons in the spiking network model upon injection of a constant current I_0 (no interaction). (A) Excitatory neuron. Parameters are given in chapter appendix C. Adaptation parameters as in figure 13.19. $I_0 = 1\,\mu A/cm^2$. (B) Adaptation parameters as in panel A but with $I_0 = 2.5\,\mu A/cm^2$. (C) Inhibitory neuron. Parameters are given in table 13.1 (chapter appendix C). $I_0 = 2.5\,\mu A/cm^2$.

firing rate onto the maximally stimulated cortical neuron, which ranges between 400 Hz and 2,000 Hz. We assume that the characteristics of the afferent synapses are the same for all the neurons. The values of the strength g^0 and the time constant of the input conductance are given in table 13.1.

Below we present the results of the simulations with $N_E = N_I = 512$ neurons.

13.7.4   The Marginal Phase

Stationary Stimulus   In section 13.4.4 (see "Homogeneous Input, Marginal Phase"), it is predicted that if the orientation-dependent component of the cortical interactions is strong enough compared to the inverse gain of single neurons, then the system will exhibit a marginal phase where even in the absence of orientation-specific input it will spontaneously form a spatially inhomogeneous activity profile. In this *marginal phase*, and in the presence of weakly tuned stimulus, the orientation tuning of the system is strongly enhanced by the cortical feedback interactions. There is a range of parameters for which our model shows a similar enhancement of orientation tuning by the cortical feedback interactions. Indeed, we have found that for a sufficiently low value of g_a, a marginal phase appears (the results presented in this section were obtained for $g_a = 0 \, \text{mS/cm}^2$).

The network response to an homogeneous input ($C = 1,000 \, \text{Hz}$) is shown in figure 13.21A. The network settles spontaneously in an inhomogeneous state. The tuning curve of the neurons, as measured by averaging their activity between $t = 200 \, \text{msec}$ and $t = 400 \, \text{msec}$, is displayed in figure 13.21B; the width of this tuning curve is 50°. This response is the result of spontaneous symmetry breaking the translation invariance, as analyzed theoretically in "Homogeneous Input, Marginal Phase" (section 13.4.4). Note that the location of the activity profile displays random fluctuations. This is expected, since in the absence of a tuned stimulus, the noise in the network causes a slow random wandering of the profile along the marginal direction. Because this motion is a result of a coordinated change in the neuronal states, the time scale associated with it is proportional to $1/N$, where N is the number of neurons in the network.

Figure 13.22A shows the tuning curves of the neurons for different values of the tuning parameter ε. By comparing figures 13.21A and 13.22A, it can be seen that the system of figure 13.21A acts as if there were an external stimulus at a 30° orientation. The tuning width of the two figures is the same, indicating that it is determined by the cortical interactions. The weakly tuned stimulus fixes the position of the activity profile, selecting from among the set of attractors the one that best matches its own profile, namely, the one that peaks at the orientation column with the largest input. Figure 13.22A also shows that the width of the tuning curves of the neurons for different values of the tuning parameter ε remains almost the same, even for ε as large as 0.5. Indeed, in the presence of stimuli not too strongly tuned, it is almost independent of intensity even though the response of the neurons to stimuli at their preferred orientation can increase significantly when the intensity is increased (figure 13.22B). These properties of the tuning curve were predicted in the analytical solution of the rate model. Our simulations show that they remain valid in biophysically more realistic models that incorporate spikes.

Virtual Rotation   In our simplified model, the system's transient response to a step change in stimulus orientation was an indicator of the mechanism of orientation selectivity. If the alignment of the afferent LGN input is the main mechanism, then following a change in the stimulus orientation, the activity in previously stimulated columns will decay, while the activity of the columns with PFs close to the new stimulus orientation will increase. If, on the other hand, the spatial modulation of

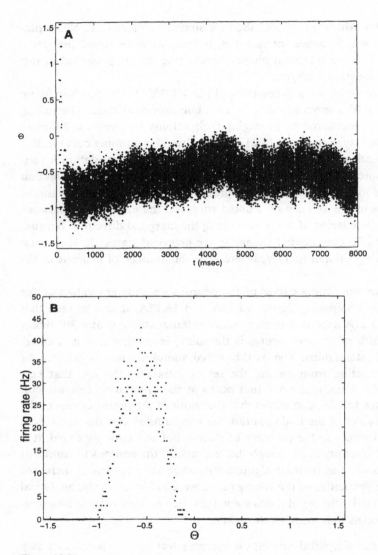

Figure 13.21
Response of the network to an homogeneous stimulus ($\varepsilon = 0$) in the marginal phase. Parameters are given in tables 13.1 and 13.2. Stimulus is presented at $t = 200$ msec. (A) Raster plot. (B) Activity profile averaged between $t = 200$ msec and $t = 400$ msec.

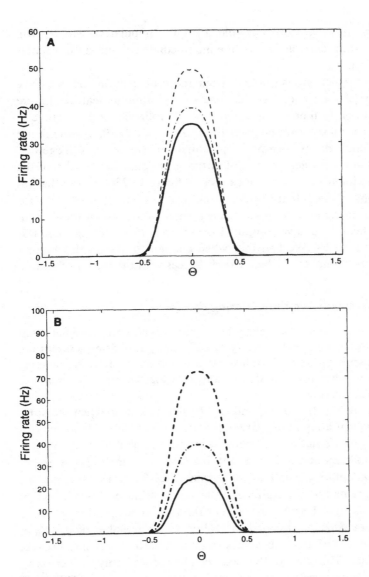

Figure 13.22
Marginal phase. Parameters are given in table 13.1 (chapter appendix C). (A) Tuning curve of a neuron $(\theta = 0^0)$ for $\varepsilon = 0.05$ (solid line) $\varepsilon = 0.1$ (dash-dotted line) and $\varepsilon = 0.2$ (dashed line). The intensity is $C = 1,000$ Hz. (B) Tuning curve of a neuron $(\theta = 0^0)$ for $C = 500$ Hz (solid line) $C = 1,000$ Hz (dash-dotted line) and $C = 2,000$ Hz (dashed line). The input tuning is $\varepsilon = 0.1$.

the cortical interactions plays a dominant role, then the population activity will move across the cortex, transiently activating the intermediate column until it settles in the new stable position.

To test whether this prediction also holds in our more realistic model, we have calculated the response of the system to changing of the stimulus feature. Figure 13.23A shows the evolution in time of the activity profile following a 60° change in the stimulus feature for a tuning parameter of the LGN input $\varepsilon = 0.1$, while figure 13.23B shows the evolution of the membrane potential for five neurons. Together, the figures clearly illustrate the phenomenon of virtual rotation. The velocity of the rotation depends on the input tuning, as we can see in figure 13.23C, where the trajectory of the maximum of the activity profile is plotted as a function of time, for different values of ε. To make a more quantitative comparison between these simulation results and our theory, we have computed the velocity V_C by fitting these trajectories according to eq. 13.69. We find that when ε is not too large, the angular velocity is inversely proportional to ε, which closely agrees with the theory of section 13.4.

13.7.5   Network with Adaptation-Intrinsic Moving Profiles

The theory of section 13.5.2 (see "Modeling Neuronal Adaptation") predicts that when single neurons display sufficiently strong or sufficiently fast firing adaptation, the response of the network to a weakly tuned input is a pulse of activity traveling across the network. Here we show that this result holds also in our more realistic network model of spiking neurons.

The raster plot of figure 13.24A corresponds to the network state when the stimulus is not tuned for typical adaptation parameters. It shows a pulse of activity of width $\theta_c = 30°$, which travels across the network at an angular velocity of $\omega = 9.2\,\text{rad/sec}$. For a given adaptation time constant, the velocity of the pulse decreases monotoncally with the adaptation maximal conductance (see figure 13.24B). For the corresponding set of parameters, the stationary state is destabilized for adaptation conductances as small as $g_a = 1.8\,\text{mS/cm}^2$, where the rate of adaptation is 5%, a value much smaller than what is observed in reality. For this value of g_a, $V_0 \approx 2.1\,\text{rad/sec}$. For small values of g_a, V_0 becomes small and hard to measure because of the noise in the network. The effect of this noise can be reduced only by increasing the network size. For instance, the result with the smallest g_a ($g_a = 1.8\,\text{mS/cm}^2$) in figure 13.24B was obtained in a network of $N_E = N_I = 2,048$ neurons by averaging the velocity of the pulse over 18 sec. Traveling pulses of activity exist for g_a as small as $1\,\text{mS/cm}^2$, but a quantitative evaluation of their velocity would have required even larger networks and longer time averaging.

Finally, we consider the effect input tuning has on these traveling pulses. For a sufficiently small value of ε, a pulse of activity can still propagate across the whole network. If we measure the tuning curve of neuron by averaging its response to stimuli with different features over different trials, we find it is extremely wide. For a sufficiently large value of ε, the traveling pulse is completely pinned around the column corresponding to the input feature (result not shown). This network state resembles what is obtained in the absence of adaptation. Finally, for intermediate values of ε, the profile of network activity performs oscillations around the angle corresponding to the stimulus feature (see figure 13.25). The tuning curve of the neurons, averaged over many trials, will show the right preferred feature but with a width greater than that of the network activity profile.

13.8 Discussion

We have studied how local excitatory and inhibitory feedback shapes the selective response of neurons to external stimuli. With regard to stationary states, we have found three qualitatively different regimes. In the first regime, the dominant feedback is afferent input; in the second, it is broad inhibition, which may, as a result, substantially sharpen the tuning of the neurons. Yet in both these regimes, the tuning width strongly depends on the *effective tuning* of the input, implying that decreasing the spatial modulation of the external input or increasing its overall intensity will broaden the tuning of the neuronal responses. As a corollary in both regimes, if the input is spatially homogeneous, the network activity will be uniform as well. The third, or marginal, regime is characterized by strong, spatially modulated excitatory feedback, leading to the emergence of an intrinsic line of stable states. Each of these states exhibits a single "hill" of activity whose width is determined by both the modulation amplitude and the spatial range of the cortical feedback, but whose height is linearly related to the stimulus intensity. Activating the network by a tuned input will select the profile whose peak coincides with that of the input. The width of the activity profile is substantially modified by the input only when the tuning provided by the afferent mechanism is significantly sharper than that of the intrinsic profile. Computationally, our work suggests a mechanism for generating a separable coding of several stimulus features (Salinas and Abbott 1996).

The intrinsic localized states in our models differ from those studied by Amari. In Amari's model (1977), the localized states appear exclusively as bistable where the stimulus is subthreshold and are characterized by a *saturated* activity of at least part of the network. In contrast, in our network, the stimulus is suprathreshold and all

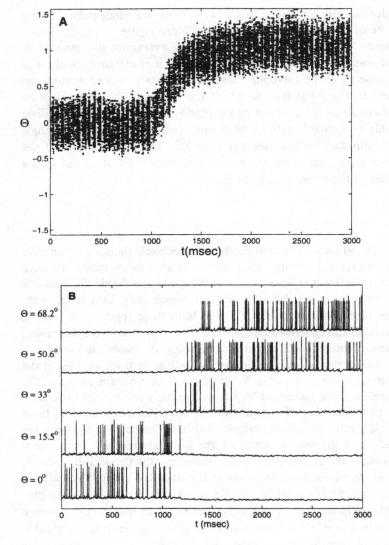

Figure 13.23
Virtual rotation in the marginal phase. Parameters are given in table 13.1 (chapter appendix C). The input intensity is $C = 1,000\,\text{Hz}$. The stimulus is at $\theta_1 = 0^0$ and is suddenly turned to $\theta_2 = \pi/3$ at $t = 1\,\text{sec}$. (A) Raster plot for $\varepsilon = 0.1$. (B) Trace of the membrane potentials of five neurons in the networks. (C) Trajectory of the population vector angle for $\varepsilon = 0.025$ and $\varepsilon = 0.2$.

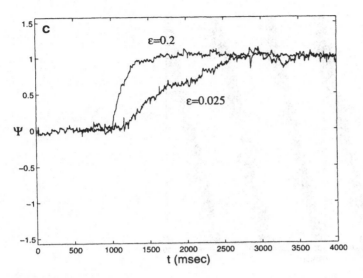

Figure 13.23 (continued)

the neurons are far below saturation, which leads to important differences in the properties of the localized states. In contrast to our network, in Amari's case, the width rather than the height of the activity profile depends strongly on the stimulus intensity. Another important difference is that in contrast to Amari's analysis, in our study stable states with multiple peaks do not exist. The reason for this is related to two features of our model: the above-mentioned unsaturated regime; and the long-range inhibition, which can stabilize a single hill of unsaturated neuronal activity, but not multiple hills.

The analytical work presented here used a one-population rate model, which contradicts the separation of excitation and inhibition in cortex. There are conditions, however, where the state of a two-population network can be exactly described by an equivalent one-population network. And even when these conditions are not met exactly, many qualitative properties of the stationary states may not differ, as is evident from our theoretical study of the full two-population model (Ben-Yishai, Hansel, and Sompolinsky 1997). The most important difference between these network types is that two populations may give rise to additional nonlinearities with respect to stimulus intensity. These effects may be functionally important. For instance, increasing stimulus intensity may suppress network activity. Also, in general, the invariance of the shape of the activity profile to changing the stimulus intensity

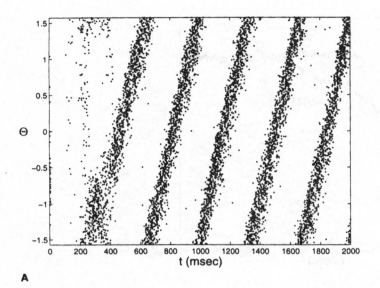

A

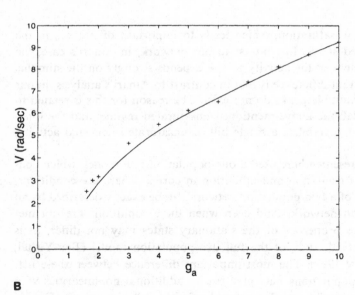

B

Figure 13.24
Traveling pulse of activity in the network model with spiking neurons. Parameters are given in table 13.1 (chapter appendix C). (A) Raster plot when the stimulus is homogeneous. Adaptation parameters: $g_a = 10 \, \text{mS/cm}^2$ and $\tau_a = 60 \, \text{msec}$. (B) Angular velocity of the wave as a function of the adaptation maximal conductance. Here $\tau_a = 60 \, \text{msec}$. The solid line is an interpolation of the simulation results.

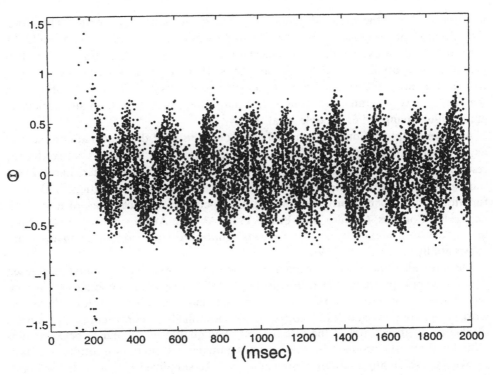

Figure 13.25
Pinning of the traveling pulse by inhomogeneous input. The parameters are as in figure 13.24A. The input tuning is $\varepsilon = 0.2$.

breaks down at low contrasts. Another important difference lies in the temporal do-main. Whereas the symmetry of the connections of the one-population model (without adaptation) precludes the appearance of temporal attractors, the two-population model may give rise to spatiotemporal attractors such as the above-mentioned moving hills and various other oscillatory states. Here, too, the threshold nonlinearities of the inhibitory population lead to potentially important dependence of the moving hill's velocity on the stimulus intensity (see Ben-Yishai, Hansel, and Sompolinsky 1997 for more details).

We have show that a substantial spike adaptation may give rise to intrinsic trav-eling waves in the form of activity pulses that move with constant velocity. In fact, neuronal adaptation can be viewed as a form of local inhibitory feedback (present in addition to explicit global inhibition). In this model, as in the two-population model mentioned above, the spatial dependence of the connections is symmetric. Therefore, the direction of propagation is determined by symmetry breaking, for example, by the initial conditions. An alternative mechanism for the generation of moving hills is provided by spatially asymmetric connections. If the pattern of connection is such that each neuron excites neighbors on its right more strongly than those on its left, the system may generate a traveling waves that always moves to the right. (Lukashin et al. 1996; Zhang 1996; Tsodyks et al. 1996)

Another simplification of our model is the description of the neuronal nonlinearity as a threshold linear gain function. This greatly simplifies the analytical study; the resultant dynamical equations are all linear except for one parameter, namely, the tuning width, whose value is given by an implicit nonlinear equation. This gain function is not a bad approximation of the rate-current characteristics of many cortical cells (Connors, Gutnick, and Prince 1982; Ahmed, Anderson, et al. 1994). Adding moderate nonlinearity to the neuronal suprathreshold gain function does not substantially change its behavior.

We have also analyzed the behavior of network models with conductance-based dynamics appropriate for cortical neurons. These models are too complex for a analytical study, we have nevertheless shown that under certain conditions these networks can in principle be described by a set of mean field self-consistent rate equations similar in spirit to those of the rate models. The qualitative similarity between simplified and realistic models is evident from the numerical simulation results. We have shown that the main qualitative predictions of the simplified rate models are manifest also in the realistic models, a conclusion also supported by the numerical simulations of Somers, Nelson, and Sur (1995), who have studied the role of cortical excitatory feedback in orientation selectivity in primary visual cortex using integrate-and-fire network models, with a more realistic modeling of the external input to the network. Earlier numerical investigations studied the role of cortical inhibition on orientation selectivity using integrate-and-fire network models (Wehmeier et al. 1989; Wörgötter and Koch 1991). One-dimensional networks of conductance-based neurons coding for the direction of movement have been simulated by Lukashin and Georgopoulos (1994). It should be emphasized, however, that all these models make similar simplifying assumptions about the local connectivity pattern in cortex; none incorporates potentially important synaptic dynamical properties such as short-term depression and facilitation.

We have limited our discussion to either stationary or coherent temporal behavior. In other studies (Ginzburg and Sompolinsky 1994; Ben-Yishai, Lev Bar-Or, and Sompolinsky 1995), it has been shown that the theory makes important predictions also with regard to the spatiotemporal spectrum of fluctuations in neuronal activities that can be tested by correlation measurements. Our numerical simulations have shown that these aspects can also be observed in the realistic networks (Hansel and Sompolinsky 1996). Thus the main spatiotemporal cooperative properties of these networks are the result of the architecture of connections rather than the details of the dynamics.

Line attractor neural networks have been also proposed as models of neural integrator circuits in the brainstem structures that control eye position (Robinson 1989; Seung 1996), where each state along the line represents one possible stable eye position. In the integrator models, it is proposed that the line attractor lies in a linearly marginally stable direction of the connection matrix. This mechanism relies on the system's being only weakly nonlinear. By contrast, the mechanism in our networks invokes the translational symmetry of the connections and is also present in strongly nonlinear regimes. Our study of the short-range model with open boundary conditions illustrates that the results are robust against boundary effects that break the symmetry. Nevertheless, it should be stressed that the existence of line attractor in both kinds of networks requires fine-tuning of some network parameters. In our networks, the existence of marginal phase is sensitive to local perturbations, such as nonuniform distribution of the representation of the preferred features (Zhang 1996; Lee et al. 1996; Tsodyks and Sejnowski 1995). Provided these perturbations are weak, however, the response of the system to an external stimulus may only be weakly affected, as long as the tuning bias generated provided by the stimulus is strong compared with those generated by the internal "imperfections." Ultimately, if line attractors are used for substantial computation, it is likely that their stability is maintained by an appropriate learning mechanism. Thus, even in sensory areas, the processing of stimuli may be intimately related to the short-term and long-term dynamics of the connections, an important topic outside the scope of this study.

Acknowledgments

This work is supported in part by the Fund for Basic Research of the Israeli Academy of Science and by the Centre National de la Recherche Scientifique: PICS "Dynamique neuronale et codage de l'information: Aspects physiques et biologiques." Most of the numerical simulations of section 13.7 have been performed on the supercomputers at the Institut de Développement et des Ressources en Informatique Scientifique; Orsay, France.

Many aspects of the work are based on research performed in collaboration with Rani Ben Yishai (see Ben-Yishai 1997) and Ruti Lev Bar-or (see Lev Bar-or 1993).

We have greatly benefited from many discussions with R. Ben Yishai, Sebastian H. Seung, and Carl van Vreeswijk. We acknowledge the hospitality of the Marine Biological Laboratory (Woods Hole, Mass.) during the summers of 1994, 1995, and 1996, where parts of this research were conducted. David Hansel acknowledges the very warm hospitality of the Racah Institute of Physics and the Center for Neural Computation of the Hebrew University.

Appendix A: Solution of the One-Population Rate Model

This appendix presents the details of the solution of the one-population model defined by eqs. 13.11–13.17.

General Time-Dependent Equations

We first consider the general case of stimulus with a time-varying feature $\theta_0(t)$. We write eq. 13.11 as

$$\tau_0 \frac{d}{dt} m(\theta, t) = -m(\theta, t) + [I_0(t) + I_2(t)\cos(2(\theta - \Phi(t)))]_+. \tag{13.A1}$$

By comparison with eq. 13.15, we obtain

$$I_0 = C(1 - \varepsilon) + J_0 r_0 - T \tag{13.A2}$$

$$I_2 = \varepsilon C \cos(2(\theta_0 - \Phi)) + J_2 r_2 \cos(2(\Psi - \Phi)), \tag{13.A3}$$

where, for simplicity, we have suppressed the time arguments. Note that, in general, r_0, θ_0, Ψ, and Φ are time-dependent. Phase Φ, the location at which the total input $I(\theta, t)$ (eq. 13.12) is maximum, is determined by the condition

$$0 = \varepsilon C \sin(2(\theta_0 - \Phi)) + J_2 r_2 \sin(2(\Psi - \Phi)). \tag{13.A4}$$

The case of broad-tuning where the input is above threshold for all θ and t is straightforward and will not be dealt with here. We focus on the case of narrow-tuning for which, by definition, there exists a value θ_C such that

$$I(\Phi \pm \theta_C, t) = I_0 + I_2 \cos(2\theta_C) = 0. \tag{13.A5}$$

Therefore, θ_C is given by

$$\theta_C = \frac{1}{2} \arccos(-I_0/I_2), \tag{13.A6}$$

and eq. 13.A1 can be written

$$\tau_0 \frac{d}{dt} m(\theta, t) = -m(\theta, t) + I_2(t)[\cos(2(\theta - \Phi(t))) - \cos(2(\theta_C(t)))]_+. \tag{13.A7}$$

Dynamical equations for the order parameters (eq. 13.16) are derived by Fourier-transforming eq. 13.A7, which yields

$$\tau_0 \frac{dr_0}{dt} = -r_0 + I_2 f_0(\theta_C) \tag{13.A8}$$

$$\tau_0 \frac{dr_2}{dt} = -r_2 + I_2 f_2(\theta_C)\cos(2(\Phi - \Psi)) \qquad (13.A9)$$

$$2r_2\tau_0 \frac{d\Psi}{dt} = I_2 f_2(\theta_C)\sin(2(\Phi - \Psi)), \qquad (13.A10)$$

where

$$f_0(\theta c) = \int_{-\pi/2}^{+\pi/2} \frac{d\theta}{\pi}[\cos(2\theta) - \cos(2\theta_C)]_+ \qquad (13.A11)$$

$$f_2(\theta_c) = \int_{-\pi/2}^{+\pi/2} \frac{d\theta}{\pi}\cos(2\theta)[\cos(2\theta) - \cos(2\theta_C)]_+. \qquad (13.A12)$$

Performing the integrals, we find the the functions given in eqs. 13.39 and 13.40.

Stationary State

In the case of a stimulus with a constant feature θ_0, the solution of the above equations converges at large time to a fixed point, which is obtained by substituting the time derivatives in all the above equations by zero. From eqs. 13.A4 and 13.A10 we find

$$\Phi = \Psi = \theta_0. \qquad (13.A13)$$

Another solution exists in which $\Phi = \Psi = \theta_0 + \pi$, but this solution is unstable, as can be seen from the next section. This means that in a stationary state the peaks of the profiles of both the total input and the output coincide with that of the stimulus. Thus eqs. 13.A2 and 13.A3 read

$$I_0 = C(1 - \varepsilon) + J_0 r_0 - T \qquad (13.A14)$$

$$I_2 = \varepsilon C + J_2 r_2. \qquad (13.A15)$$

Substituting this into eqs. 13.A8 and 13.A9 yields

$$r_0 = (C\varepsilon + J_2 r_2) f_0 \qquad (13.A16)$$

$$r_2 = (C\varepsilon + J_2 r_2) f_2. \qquad (13.A17)$$

$$(13.A18)$$

For $\varepsilon > 0$, the solution is

$$r_2 = \frac{C\varepsilon f_2(\theta_C)}{1 - J_2 f_2(\theta_C)} \qquad (13.A19)$$

$$r_0 = \frac{C\varepsilon f_0(\theta_C)}{1 - J_2 f_2(\theta_C)}. \qquad (13.A20)$$

Replacing r_0 and r_2 by these expressions in eq. 13.A6, we obtain the equation for the width of the activity profile. The stationary profile has the form of eq. 13.36, and the gain G is

$$G = I_2(1 - \cos(2\theta_C)), \qquad (13.A21)$$

yielding for the gain G the expression given in eq. 13.42.

For $\varepsilon = 0$, eq. 13.A17 always has a homogeneous solution, $r_2 = 0$, because the system is invariant by rotation. From eq. 13.A19, however, we see that an inhomogeneous solution ($r_2 \neq 0$) can also exist, provided that

$$1 = J_2 f_2(\theta_C). \tag{13.A22}$$

Eq. 13.A22, which corresponds to eq. 13.55, determines θ_C in the marginal phase and possesses a solution only if $J_2 > 2$. In this regime, r_0 and r_2 are determined by eq. 13.A6, 13.A14, and 13.A15, with $\varepsilon = 0$ and

$$r_0 = J_2 r_2 f_0. \tag{13.A23}$$

Substituting the results in eq. 13.A21 yields, finally, eq. 13.56.

Response to Moving Stimulus

We consider here the solution of the time-dependent eqs. 13.A8–13.A10 in the case of time-dependent stimulus feature $\theta_0(t)$. Eqs. 13.A10 and 13.A4 yield

$$\tau_0 \frac{d\psi(t)}{dt} = -V_C \sin(2(\theta_0(t) - \Phi(t))), \tag{13.A24}$$

where

$$\tau_0 V_C = \frac{\varepsilon C I_2 f_2(\theta_C)}{2 J_2 r_2^2}. \tag{13.A25}$$

Although, in general, V_C is itself a function of time, when $|\tau_0 \, d\theta_0/dt| = O(\Upsilon) \ll 1$, the time dependence of V_C introduces corrections of order Υ to V_C. To leading order, V_C is given by substituting the value of r_2 at order Υ, which in turn is given according to eq. 13.A9 (with $\Phi = \Psi$ and $dr_2/dt = 0$) by $r_2 = I_2 f_2$. Substituting this value yields $\tau_0 V_C = \varepsilon C/2 J_2 r_2$. Finally, using eqs. 13.55–13.57, we obtain eq. 13.65.

Appendix B: Stability of the Stationary States

This appendix presents the stability analysis for the stationary states of the one-population rate model with neuronal adaptation given by eqs. 13.75–13.76 and 13.12–13.14.

Stability of the Broad Profile

When the system has a broad profile, all the neurons are above threshold and the system operates in the linear regime. Thus small perturbations around the linear fixed point of eqs. 13.75 and 13.76 obey the linear equations

$$\tau_0 \frac{d}{dt} \delta m(\theta, t) = -\delta m(\theta, t) + J_0 \delta r_0 + J_2 \delta r_2 \cos(2\theta) + J_2 r_2 \sin(2\theta) \delta \Psi - \delta I_a(\theta, t) \tag{13.B1}$$

$$\tau_a \frac{d}{dt} \delta I_a(\theta, t) = -\delta I_a(\theta, t) + J_a \delta m(\theta, t). \tag{13.B2}$$

The solutions of these equations can be written in the form

$$\delta m(\theta, t) \propto e^{\gamma t} \tag{13.B3}$$

$$\delta I_a(\theta, t) \propto e^{\gamma t}. \tag{13.B4}$$

The homogeneous fixed point is stable if and only if $Re\,\gamma < 0$. Solving eq. 13.B2 for δI_a and substituting in eq. 13.B1 yields

$$(1 + \Gamma(\gamma)) \delta m(\theta, t) = J_0 \delta r_0 + J_2 \cos(2\theta) \delta r_2 + J_2 r_2 \sin(2\theta) \delta \Psi, \tag{13.B5}$$

where

$$\Gamma(\gamma) \equiv \gamma\tau_0 + \frac{J_a}{1 + \gamma\tau_a}. \tag{13.B6}$$

Fourier-transforming this equation gives

$$(1 + \Gamma(\gamma))\delta r_0 = J_0 \delta r_0 \tag{13.B7}$$

$$(1 + \Gamma(\gamma))\delta r_2 = \frac{J_2}{2}\delta r_2 \tag{13.B8}$$

$$(1 + \Gamma(\gamma))\delta\Psi = \frac{J_2}{2}\delta\Psi. \tag{13.B9}$$

(Eq. 13.B9 has to be considered only if $\varepsilon \neq 0$.) Thus the two Fourier modes of fluctuations are decoupled and the condition that δ_2 relaxes is identical to the condition for $\delta\Psi$ to relax.

The first mode corresponds to a homogeneous fluctuation of the neuron activity. Here γ is the solution of

$$1 + \Gamma(\gamma) = J_0. \tag{13.B10}$$

Therefore, in this mode, γ is determined by a second-order algebraic equation. Solving this equation, we see that, depending on the strength of the adaptation, the broad state may lose stability in two ways.

Case 1. $J_a < \tau_0/\tau_a$: γ is real and is negative only for $J_0 < 1 + J_a$. In particular, when there is no adaptation, we recover the result of eq. 13.34.

Case 2. $J_a > \tau_0/\tau_a$: γ is complex on the instability line which is given by

$$J_0 = 1 + \frac{\tau_0}{\tau_a}. \tag{13.B11}$$

On this instability line, the system enters into a global oscillatory state.

The second mode of instability corresponds to a spatial instability. For this mode, γ is determined by

$$1 + \Gamma(\gamma) = \frac{J_2}{2}. \tag{13.B12}$$

Here also, two cases have to be distinguished:

Case 1. $J_a < \tau_0/\tau_a$: γ is real on the instability line given by

$$J_2 = 2(1 + J_a). \tag{13.B13}$$

This instability corresponds to the fact that if $J_2 > 2(1 + J_a)$, the system prefers a narrowly tuned stationary state over the broadly tuned one, even when the input is homogeneous. In particular, for $J_a = 0$, we find eq. 13.35.

Case 2. $J_a > \tau_0/\tau_a$: γ is complex on the instability line given by

$$J_2 = 1 + \frac{\tau_0}{\tau_a}. \tag{13.B14}$$

This line is drawn in figure 13.11. For J_2 larger than this value, the system prefers a narrowly tuned state which, because γ is complex, is nonstationary and consists of a traveling pulse of activity. On the instability line, the velocity of the pulse is given by the imaginary part of γ, yielding eq. 13.83.

Stability of the Marginal Phase

We discuss here the stability of the narrow profile in the marginal phase. We first discuss the case of $\varepsilon = 0$ and $J_a = 0$. We linearize eqs. 13.A8–13.A10 about the fixed point of the marginal phase, eqs. 13.36 and 13.41 with eqs. 13.54–13.57, and we find

$$\tau_0 \frac{d\delta r_0}{dt} = -\left(1 - \frac{2J_0\theta_c}{\pi}\right)\delta r_0 + \frac{J_2}{\pi}\sin(2\theta_c)\delta r_2 \tag{13.B15}$$

$$\tau_0 \frac{d\delta r_2}{dt} = \frac{J_0}{\pi}\sin(2\theta_c)\delta r_0 - \left(1 - \frac{J_2}{\pi}\left(\theta_c + \frac{1}{4}\sin(4\theta_c)\right)\right)\delta r_2 \tag{13.B16}$$

$$\tau_0 \frac{d\delta\Psi}{dt} = -(1 - J_2 f_2(\theta_c))\delta\Psi = 0. \tag{13.B17}$$

In eq. 13.B17 we have used the relationship between θ_c and J_2 (eq. 13.55). This equation implies that the fluctuations keeping the shape of the activity profile but changing the position of its peak (also called "transverse fluctuations") are marginal, that is, they do not decay with time. The "longitudinal fluctuations," representing perturbations of the shape of the profile, evolve according to eqs. 13.B15–13.B16. Searching for a solution of the form δr_0, $\delta r_2 \propto e^{\gamma t}$, we find that γ satisfies the second-order algebraic equation

$$\gamma^2 + \left(3 - \frac{\theta_c}{\pi}(J_0 + J_2)\right)\gamma + \frac{J_2}{\pi}\sin(2\theta_c)f_0(\theta_c)(J_C - J_0) = 0, \tag{13.B18}$$

where J_C is given by eq. 13.57. Solving eq. 13.B18, we find that the instability occurs when γ is real and becomes positive, that is, on the line

$$J_C = J_0. \tag{13.B19}$$

This line is drawn in figure 13.7: it separates the marginal phase from the amplitude instability region.

The above stability analysis can be straightforwardly extended to include the case of inhomogeneous input. In particular, the transverse fluctuations still decouple from the longitudinal fluctuations; they evolve according to

$$\frac{d\delta\Psi}{dt} = -\frac{\delta\Psi}{\tau_\Psi}, \tag{13.B20}$$

where

$$\tau_\Psi = \frac{\tau_0}{\Upsilon}\frac{G}{(1 - \cos(2\theta_c))} > 0. \tag{13.B21}$$

Thus the external tuned input stabilizes the transverse fluctuations, whose relaxation time τ_Ψ is proportional to $1/\Upsilon$ and diverges as $\Upsilon \to 0$, in agreement with eq. 13.B17.

Instability of the Marginal Phase Due to Adaptation

We now extend the previous analysis to include adaptation. We will show that if $\varepsilon = 0$, the transverse fluctuation mode of the inhomogenous fixed point is unstable if

$$J_a > \frac{\tau_0}{\tau_a}. \tag{13.B22}$$

This condition corresponds to the vertical line drawn on figure 13.11. As will be shown, this result is general and independent of the form of interaction and the boundary conditions.

A narrow profile has the form

$$m(\theta) = \frac{I_a(\theta)}{J_a} = M(\theta - \Psi), \tag{13.B23}$$

where $M(\theta)$ satisfies

$$M(\theta) = \frac{1}{1 + J_a} \int_{-\theta_c}^{\theta_c} J(\theta - \theta') M(\theta') \, d\theta'. \tag{13.B24}$$

If we differentiate eq. 13.B24 with respect to θ and integrating by part the right-hand side, using $M(\theta_c) = M(-\theta_c) = 0$, we find

$$M'(\theta) = \frac{1}{1 + J_a} \int_{-\theta_c}^{\theta_c} J(\theta - \theta') M'(\theta') \, d\theta'. \tag{13.B25}$$

The fluctuations which maintain the shape of the profile but change its position have the form

$$\delta m(\theta, t) = M'(\theta - \Psi) \delta\Psi(t) \tag{13.B26}$$

$$\delta I_a(\theta, t) = J_a M'(\theta - \Psi) \delta\Psi_a(t) \tag{13.B27}$$

If we linearize the dynamical equations, using eq. 13.B25 and the fact that $M'(\theta) \neq 0$, we find that

$$\tau_0 \frac{d\delta\Psi}{dt} = J_a \delta\Psi - J_a \delta\Psi_a \tag{13.B28}$$

$$\tau_a \frac{d\Psi_a}{dt} = -\delta\Psi_a + \delta\Psi. \tag{13.B29}$$

These equations imply that the longitudinal mode is unstable if the condition given by eq. 13.B22 is satisfied. Note that this proof holds for any form of interaction and that it is also independent of the boundary conditions, hence it applies also to the short-range model of section 13.6. However, it crucially relies on the gain functions being semilinear.

Appendix C: Details of Conductance-Based Model

This appendix presents the details of the model, given by eqs. 13.1–13.4, we have used in our numerical simulations. The voltage-gated current in eq. 13.110 is of the form

$$I_{gated}^{\alpha}(\theta, t) = \sum_{l=1}^{n} G_l^{\alpha}(V^{\alpha}(\theta, t))(V^{\alpha}(\theta, t) - V_l^{\alpha}), \tag{13.C1}$$

where G_l and V_l are the voltage-gated conductances and the reversal potentials of the various ionic currents that contribute to I_{gated}, detailed below (see also table 13.1).

Sodium Current: $I_{Na} = g_{Na} m^3 h (V - V_{Na})$

The inactivation variable h follows the first-order relaxation equation

$$\frac{dh}{dt} = \Delta \frac{h_\infty(V) - h}{\tau_h(V)} \tag{13.C2}$$

$$h_\infty(V) = \frac{a_h(V)}{a_h(V) + b_h(V)} \tag{13.C3}$$

Table 13.1
Parameter and constant values for conductance-based cortical network model

	E	I		m
g_{N_a}	120	120	τ_1^e	3
g_K	10	20	τ_2^e	1
g_A	60	40	τ_1^i	7
g_{N_aP}	0.5	0.2	τ_2^i	1
g_l	0.1	0.1	g_{EE}	2
g_z	10	0	g_{EI}	1.3
V_{N_a}	55	55	g_{II}	0.8
V_K	-70	-70	g_{IE}	1
V_A	-75	-75	V_{syn}^e	0
V_I	-65	-65	V_{syn}^i	-75

$$\tau_h(V) = \frac{1}{a_h(V) + b_h(V)} \tag{13.C4}$$

$$a_h = 0.07\, e^{(-(V+55)/20)} \tag{13.C5}$$

$$b_h = 1/(1 + e^{(-(V+25)/10)}). \tag{13.C6}$$

To simplify the dynamics, we assume that the activation variable m is fast and equal to its instantaneous equilibrium value, given by

$$m_\infty(V) = \frac{a_m(V)}{a_m(V) + b_m(V)} \tag{13.C7}$$

$$a_m(V) = 0.1 \frac{(V + 30)}{1 - e^{(-(V+30)/10)}} \tag{13.C8}$$

$$b_m(V) = 4e^{(-(V+55)/18)}. \tag{13.C9}$$

The factor Δ has been introduced in order to tune the maximum firing rate to the desired high value. We use $\Delta = 4$.

Delayed-Rectifier Potassium Current: $I_K = g_K n^4 (V - V_K)$

The inactivation variable n satisfies

$$\frac{dn}{dt} = \Delta \frac{n_\infty(V) - n}{\tau_n(V)} \tag{13.C10}$$

$$n_\infty(V) = \frac{a_n(V)}{a_n(V) + b_n(V)} \tag{13.C11}$$

$$\tau_n(V) = \frac{1}{a_n(V) + b_n(V)} \tag{13.C12}$$

$$a_n = 0.01 \frac{(v+45)}{1 - e^{(-(V+45)/10)}} \tag{13.C13}$$

$$b_n = 0.125 e^{(-(V+55)/80)}. \tag{13.C14}$$

A-Current: $I_A = g_A ab(V - V_A)$

We assume activation is instantaneous and satisfies

$$a = a_\infty(V) = \frac{1}{1 + e^{(-(V+50)/4)}}. \tag{13.C15}$$

We further assume the relaxation time of the inactivation variable is independent of the membrane potential: $\tau_b = 10\,\text{msec}$, and satisfies

$$\frac{db}{dt} = \frac{b_\infty(V) - b}{\tau_b} \tag{13.C16}$$

$$b_\infty = \frac{1}{1 + e^{((V+70)/2)}}. \tag{13.C17}$$

Persistent Sodium Current: $I_{NaP} = g_{NaP} s_\infty(V)(V - V_{Na})$

The activation variables satisfies

$$s_\infty(V) = \frac{1}{1 + e^{(-0.3(V+50))}}. \tag{13.C18}$$

Slow Potassium Current: $I_z = g_z z(V - V_K)$

This currents is incorporated into the dynamics of the excitatory population. The activation variable z satisfies the relaxation equation

$$\frac{dz}{dt} = \frac{z_\infty(V) - z}{\tau_z}, \tag{13.C19}$$

where $\tau_z = 60\,\text{msec}$ is independent of the membrane potential and

$$z_\infty(V) = \frac{1}{1 + e^{(-0.7(V+30))}} \tag{13.C20}$$

Note that the sodium current and the potassium delayed rectifier have the same parameters as in the Hodgkin-Huxley model, except for a shift of the membrane potential by 55 mV. This shift ensures that the threshold to spike is in the range observed in cortical neurons. Membrane potential is measured in millivolts.

14 Numerical Methods for Neuronal Modeling

Michael V. Mascagni and Arthur S. Sherman

14.1 Introduction

In this chapter we will discuss some practical and technical aspects of numerical methods that can be used to solve the equations neuronal modelers frequently encounter. We will consider numerical methods for ordinary differential equations (ODEs) and for partial differential equations (PDEs) through examples. A typical case where ODEs arise in neuronal modeling would be in a single lumped-soma compartmental model used to describe a neuron. Arguably the most famous PDE system in neuronal modeling is Hodgkin and Huxley's phenomenological model of the squid giant axon (1952).

The difference between ODEs and PDEs is that ODEs involve the rate of change of an unknown function of a single variable, usually the derivative with respect to time, while PDEs involve the rates of change of the solution with respect to two or more independent variables, such as time and space. The numerical methods we will discuss for both ODEs and PDEs replace the derivatives in the differential equations with finite-difference approximations to these derivatives, which reduces the differential equations to algebraic equations. The two major classes of finite-difference methods we will discuss are characterized by whether the resulting algebraic equations explicitly or implicitly define the solution at the new time value. We will see that the method of solution for explicit and implicit methods will vary considerably, as will the properties of the solutions of the resulting finite-difference equations.

To simplify our exposition, we will use the Hodgkin-Huxley equations to illustrate the numerical methods. If a section of a squid giant axon is space-clamped, the membrane potential no longer depends on the spatial location within the clamped region. This reduces the original PDE to a system of ODEs, and leads us to model the membrane potential with the following system of ODEs:

$$C\frac{dV}{dt} = -\bar{g}_{Na}m^3h(V - E_{Na}) - \bar{g}_K n^4(V - E_K) - \bar{g}_{leak}(V - E_{leak}), \tag{14.1}$$

where

$$\frac{dm}{dt} = (1 - m)\alpha_m(V) - m\beta_m(V) \tag{14.2a}$$

$$\frac{dh}{dt} = (1 - h)\alpha_h(V) - h\beta_h(V) \tag{14.2b}$$

$$\frac{dn}{dt} = (1 - n)\alpha_n(V) - n\beta_n(V). \tag{14.2c}$$

In addition to this relation for current balance, Hodgkin and Huxley (1952) provided expressions for the rate functions $\alpha_m(V)$, $\alpha_h(V)$, $\alpha_n(V)$, $\beta_m(V)$, $\beta_h(V)$, and $\beta_n(V)$.

If instead of space-clamping the *Loligo* giant axon, the voltage across the membrane of the axon is allowed to vary with longitudinal distance along the axon, x, then the membrane potential satisfies a PDE. This PDE is similar to the space-clamped ODE case, except that eq. 14.1 is replaced with

$$C\frac{\partial V}{\partial t} = \frac{a}{2R}\frac{\partial^2 V}{\partial x^2} - \bar{g}_{Na}m^3h(V - E_{Na}) - \bar{g}_K n^4(V - E_K) - \bar{g}_{leak}(V - E_{leak}). \qquad (14.3)$$

Below we will consider the complete mathematical description, and numerical solution, of these two problems related to the squid giant axon. It is important to note that models based on the Hodgkin-Huxley equations are useful examples for numerical computation in two complementary ways. First, Hodgkin-Huxley models are very complex, and thus provide a realistic and challenging system to test our proposed numerical methods. Numerical methods that work on the Hodgkin-Huxley equations should work equally well on other equations the neuronal modeler may wish to explore. Second, the Hodgkin-Huxley equations are basic expressions of current conservation. Thus modification of our formulas for the numerical solution of the Hodgkin-Huxley equations to accommodate other neuronal models is straightforward, provided the models are also explicitly based on electrical properties of nerve, and provided the kinetics associated with the individual ionic currents can be described with first-order kinetic equations, as in eqs. 14.2a–14.2c

14.1.1 Numerical Preliminaries

We begin by dicussing sources of numerical error, both those which affect numerical calculations in general and those which arise specifically in solving differential equations. The fundamental reason for error (loss of *accuracy*) is the finite nature of computers, which limits their ability to represent inherently infinite processes. Irrational numbers, such as $\sqrt{2}$, transcendental numbers, such as π and e, and repeating decimals, such as .3333+, can only be represented to *finite precision*. Even exactly represented numbers are subject to *round-off error* when they are added or multiplied together. (For further discussion of these issues, consult a general numerical analysis text, such as Golub and Ortega 1992.) Numerical methods for ODEs and PDEs involve, in addition, finite approximations of the infinite limiting processes that define derivatives and integrals. These approximations introduce *truncation* or *discretization error*. Even if we solve the discretized problem exactly, the answer is still only an approximation to the original continuous problem.

Three concepts have been introduced, to analyze how the above sources of error are handled by particular numerical methods for ODEs and PDEs: *convergence*, *consistency*, and *stability*. The most fundamental is *convergence*, which means that the error between the numerical solution and the exact solution can be made as small as we please. We will be discussing finite-difference methods where space and time are discretized with a numerical time step, Δt, and a spatial mesh size, Δx. Thus demonstrating convergence for a finite-difference method means showing that the numerical solution differs from the exact solution by a term that goes to zero as Δt and Δx go to zero.

The concepts of consistency and stability have also emerged as fundamental in the establishment of general convergence theory. As the name implies, *consistency* of a numerical method ensures that the numerical solution solves a discrete problem that is the same as the desired continuous problem. For finite-difference methods, this amounts to determining whether the difference equations, when applied to the exact solution of the continuous problem, produce only a small approximation (truncation) error. If this truncation error goes to zero as Δt and Δx go to zero, then the numerical method is consistent. Although this definition for consistency sounds suspiciously like the definition for convergence, a method can be consistent and yet not convergent. Consistency demands only that the exact solution satisfy the finite-difference equations with a truncation error that formally goes to zero. By contrast, convergence demands that the numerical and exact solutions differ by an arbitrarily small amount at every point in time and space.

Filling the gap between consistency and convergence is the concept of stability. A finite-difference method is *stable* if the solution to the finite-difference equations remains bounded as the grid parameters go to zero. It is worth noting that some consistent finite-difference methods are not stable: the numerical solution may grow without bound even when the analytic solution to the same problem might actually be quite small. A method with this type of behavior is obviously not convergent. We should note that some stable finite-difference solutions can exhibit small oscillations about the exact solution and still be of great utility. We can therefore appreciate the importance of using finite-difference methods that give solutions that do not grow without bound.

One of the most remarkable results in the analysis of finite-difference methods for differential equations is the Lax equivalence theorem (Richtmyer and Morton 1967), which states that a finite-difference method for linear ODEs or PDEs is convergent if and only if it is both consistent and stable. Thus, for these linear problems, the two concepts of consistency and stability are complementary. Because of the elegant relationship between convergence, consistency, and stability for linear problems, numerical methods for nonlinear problems also discuss consistency and stability in the context of establishing numerical convergence, although there is no general Lax equivalence theorem in these nonlinear cases. (Technical treatments of this theory can be found in Isaacson and Keller 1966; Richtmyer and Morton 1967, and Sod 1985.)

14.2 Methods for Ordinary Differential Equations

The theory for the numerical solution of ODEs is very well established, and the rigorous analysis of many classes of numerical methods has an extensive literature (see, for example, Gear 1971a; Lambert 1973). We will distinguish numerical methods for ODEs based on a property of ODEs themselves, known as *stiffness*. Stiffness measures the difficulty of solving an ODE numerically, in much the same way the condition number of a matrix measures the difficulty of numerically solving the associated system of linear equations (see chapter appendix). Stiff systems are characterized by disparate time scales. Nonstiff systems can be solved by *explicit* methods that are relatively simple (i.e., can be coded by an amateur), while stiff systems require more complex *implicit* methods (usually from a professionally written package).

Methods can also be classified by how the accuracy depends on the step size, Δt, usually expressed in "big Oh" notation (Lin and Segel 1988, 112–113). For example, a method is $O((\Delta t)^2)$ accurate if the solution differs from the exact solution to the ODE by an amount that goes to zero like $(\Delta t)^2$, as Δt goes to zero. Thus, if we halve Δt, the error decreases by a factor of $(\frac{1}{2})^2$. Higher-order methods are more accurate, but are generally more complicated to implement than lower-order methods and require more work per time step. Thus a practical decision must be made, weighing the numerical accuracy requirement versus the overall cost of both implementing and using a particular method.

A more precise analysis leads to a distinction between *local* and *global* truncation errors. The *local truncation error* is the error between the numerical solution and the exact solution after a single time step; recalling the definition of consistency, it is the local truncation error that must go to zero as Δt goes to zero for a method to be consistent. We can generally compute the local truncation error from the Taylor series expansion of the solution. A method is called "p-order accurate" if the local truncation error is $O((\Delta t)^p)$. The *global truncation error* is the difference between the computed solution and the exact solution at a given time, $t = T = n\Delta t$; this is the error that must go to zero as Δt goes to zero for a method to be convergent. In general, we cannot merely use the Taylor series to calculate the global truncation error explicitly, but it can be shown that if the local truncation error is $O((\Delta t)^p)$, then the global truncation error of a convergent method will also be $O((\Delta t)^p)$ (Stoer and Bulirsch 1980).

We conclude with the mathematical setting and uniform notation for describing numerical methods. The Hodgkin-Huxley ODE model, eqs. 14.1 and 14.2, is a system of four first-order ODEs. We can define the four-dimensional vector of functions, $\vec{U} = (V, m, h, n)$, and rewrite eqs. 14.1 and 14.2 to obtain the single vector differential equation

$$\frac{d\vec{U}}{dt} = \vec{F}(\vec{U}, t). \tag{14.4}$$

Here $\vec{F}(\vec{U})$ is a vector-valued right-hand side corresponding to the right-hand sides in eqs. 14.1 and 14.2, with eq. 14.1 rewritten by dividing through by C. In general, it is always possible to rewrite any system of ODEs as a single system of first-order ODEs, even when we begin with ODEs that have second- or higher-order derivatives (Boyce and DiPrima 1992, 319–320). This is important because almost all numerical methods are designed to handle first-order systems.

Eq. 14.4 tells us only how the unknown functions change with time; to compute a particular solution, we must know the initial values of these functions. Together, the equations and initial conditions constitute an initial value problem (IVP), whose solution—given initial values—can be uniquely determined.

14.2.1 Runge-Kutta Methods

All ODE algorithms begin by discretizing time. Let $t^n = n\Delta t$ and $\vec{U}^n = \vec{U}(n\Delta t)$. Then the simplest method of all, which follows directly from the difference-quotient approximation to the derivative, is the forward Euler method:

$$\frac{\vec{U}^{n+1} - \vec{U}^n}{\Delta t} = \vec{F}(\vec{U}^n, t^n). \tag{14.5}$$

An alternative form of the difference quotient gives the backward Euler method:

$$\frac{\vec{U}^{n+1} - \vec{U}^n}{\Delta t} = \vec{F}(\vec{U}^{n+1}, t^{n+1}). \tag{14.6}$$

Both are examples of first-order Runge-Kutta methods. If we rewrite eq. 14.5 as $\vec{U}^{n+1} = \vec{U}^n + \Delta t\vec{F}(\vec{U}^n, t^n)$, we see that the forward Euler method gives us an explicit formula for $\vec{U}^{n+1}$ in terms of the known $\vec{U}^n$. If we rewrite eq. 14.6 with the known quantities on the right and the unknowns on the left, we get $\vec{U}^{n+1} - \Delta t \vec{F}(\vec{U}^{n+1}, t^{n+1}) = \vec{U}^n$, an equation whose solution implicitly defines $\vec{U}^{n+1}$. In general, some numerical method for solving nonlinear algebraic equations, such as Newton's method or functional iteration (Conte and de Boor 1980), must be used to advance to the next time step. Despite this distinct disadvantage, as we will see below, stability considerations often make implicit methods the methods of choice.

Forward Euler approximates the time derivative with its value at the beginning of the time step, and backward Euler at the end of the time step. By analogy to the trapezoidal rule for numerical quadrature, we can obtain second-order accuracy by using their average:

$$\vec{U}^{n+1} = \vec{U}^n + \frac{\Delta t}{2}[\vec{F}(\vec{U}^n, t^n) + \vec{F}(\vec{U}^{n+1}, t^{n+1})]. \tag{14.7}$$

This method is also implicit, and the following second-order Runge-Kutta method, also known as "Heun's method," is often used instead:

$$\vec{U}^{n+1} = \vec{U}^n + \frac{\Delta t}{2}[\vec{k}_1 + \vec{k}_2], \text{ where,}$$

$$\vec{k}_1 = \vec{F}(\vec{U}^n, t^n),$$
$$\vec{k}_2 = \vec{F}(\vec{U}^n + \Delta t \vec{k}_1, t^{n+1}). \tag{14.8}$$

Note that second-order accuracy is obtained at the cost of two evaluations of $\vec{F}$ per time step. By going to four function evaluations, we can get fourth-order accuracy:

$$\vec{U}^{n+1} = \vec{U}^n + \frac{\Delta t}{6}[\vec{k}_1 + 2\vec{k}_2 + 2\vec{k}_3 + \vec{k}_4], \text{ where,}$$

$$\vec{k}_1 = \vec{F}(\vec{U}^n, t^n),$$
$$\vec{k}_2 = \vec{F}(\vec{U}^n + \tfrac{1}{2}\Delta t \vec{k}_1, t^{n+1/2}),$$
$$\vec{k}_3 = \vec{F}(\vec{U}^n + \tfrac{1}{2}\Delta t \vec{k}_2, t^{n+1/2}),$$
$$\vec{k}_4 = \vec{F}(\vec{U}^n + \Delta t \vec{k}_3, t^{n+1}). \tag{14.9}$$

Heun's method can also be viewed as a *predictor-corrector* version of the trapezoidal rule, which first estimates $\vec{U}^{n+1}$ by taking a forward Euler step, then improves, or corrects, the estimate by taking a trapezoidal rule step. Further improvement can be made by correcting again, but it is usually preferable to reduce Δt if more accuracy is desired.

Because all these methods work well when stiffness is not an issue, the primary criterion in choosing between them is computational efficiency. There are no hard-and-fast rules for this, but here are a few rules of thumb. A measure of computational effort is the total number of evaluations of the right-hand-side functions. Suppose we wish to solve an IVP with initial conditions given at $t = 0$, up to a time $t = T$. If $M = T/\Delta t$ is the number of time steps, and K is the number of function evaluations per time step for a given numerical method, then the most efficient choice of numerical method minimizes the product MK. Higher-order methods reduce M but increase K. Unless $\vec{F}$ is very expensive to evaluate, the higher-order method generally turns out to be much more efficient. That fifth-order Runge-Kutta methods require *six* function evaluations, however, may partly explain the popularity of fourth-order methods. Also, as we shall see, achieving better than second-order accuracy is problematic for PDEs, and methods based on the trapezoidal rule are the norm.

14.2.2 Multistep Methods

The biggest weakness of Runge-Kutta methods is the cost of multiple function evaluations, whose results are never used again, at each time step. Multistep methods attempt to remedy this by approximating the derivative by a combination of the function values at several previous time steps. Defining $\vec{F}^k = \vec{F}(\vec{U}^k, t^k)$, the explicit, four-step Adams-Bashforth method has the form

$$\vec{U}^{n+1} = \vec{U}^n + \Delta t[c_0 \vec{F}^n + c_1 \vec{F}^{n-1} + c_2 \vec{F}^{n-2} + c_3 \vec{F}^{n-3}], \tag{14.10}$$

while the implicit, four-step Adams-Moulton method uses the function values at $t^{n+1}, \ldots, t^{n-2}$. The coefficients are chosen so as to interpolate $\vec{F}$ at the several time points with a polynomial (Golub and Ortega 1992), which is only valid if the solution is smooth.

The Adams-Bashforth and Adams-Moulton methods (Conte and de Boor 1980, Stoer and Bulirsch 1980) are often used as a predictor-corrector pair, efficiently attaining fourth-order accuracy with only two function evaluations per time step. One complication, however, is obtaining the initial time points to start the calculation. Generally, a few Runge-Kutta steps are used.

14.2.3 Methods with Adaptive Step Size

The efficiency of both Runge-Kutta and multistep methods can be enormously enhanced by using adaptive step size control. Adaptive methods exploit known formulas for the local truncation errors of given methods to estimate the global truncation error. By using this information as a criterion for either increasing or decreasing

Δt, a computation can be carried out to within a user-specified error tolerance with as large a step size as possible at each time step. In addition to efficiency, this also provides an estimate of the error in the solution.

A useful class of adaptive Runge-Kutta methods is based on the ideas of Fehlberg (see Press et al. 1992), who figured out how to combine the results of six function evaluations to obtain two Runge-Kutta methods. The Taylor series of the solution is matched by one of the methods to fourth order, and by the other to fifth order. The difference between the two extrapolated solutions is then the fifth term of the Taylor series of the solution, and serves as a good estimate for the error in the fourth-order method.

The increased efficiency is of particular value in studies of the long-time behavior of the system, which requires carrying out calculations until either periodic repetitive firing is observed or the system reaches a stable steady state. Also, many neurons are capable of bursting oscillations, characterized by alternating spiking and quiescent periods. An adaptive method will take small steps during the active phase and long steps during the silent phase. As a beneficial side effect, graphical display of the output will be adaptive as well because many data points are saved when the solution is varying rapidly and few when it is not.

14.2.4 Qualitative Analysis of Stiffness

A system of ODEs, or a single ODE, is said to be stiff if the solution contains a wide range of characteristic time scales. The problem with a wide range of time scales can be appreciated through a simple illustration. Suppose the fastest time scale in an ODE has duration τ, while the slowest has γ. If γ/τ is large, then a numerical time step, Δt, small enough to resolve phenomena on the τ time scale requires γ/τ steps to resolve phenomena on the γ time scale. This is not a problem if the phenomena on the τ time scale is of interest; however, if the τ time scale is of little interest, it would seem an obvious strategy to choose $\Delta t \approx \gamma$. For explicit methods, however, this is a numerical disaster. The inaccuracy in resolving the τ time scale leads to catastrophic instabilities, often resulting in wild oscillations in the computed solution.

We can gain insight here by examining the stability properties of some simple methods, applied to the trivial scalar equation

$$\frac{dU}{dt} = -kU, \tag{14.11}$$

with $k > 0$. The forward Euler iteration for this equation is

$$U^{n+1} = U^n(1 - k\Delta t). \tag{14.12}$$

In order for the numerical solution to decay, as does the true solution, we must have $-1 < 1 - k\Delta t < 1$. Therefore, Δt must satisfy

$$\Delta t < \frac{2}{k}. \tag{14.13}$$

Monotonic decay requires $1 - k\Delta t > 0$, or $\Delta t < \frac{1}{k}$. That is, Δt must be less than the time constant. For $\frac{1}{k} < \Delta t < \frac{2}{k}$, U^n is multiplied by a negative factor; the solution undergoes a damped oscillation. These constraints are reasonable but lead to problems when there are multiple time constants. Consider the general linear system of two equations with solution

$$\vec{U}(t) = \vec{A}e^{-100t} + \vec{B}e^{-t}, \tag{14.14}$$

where $\vec{A}$ and $\vec{B}$ are constant vectors that depend on the initial conditions. After a brief time, the first term contributes negligibly to the solution, but the forward Euler method must satisfy the condition of eq. 14.13 for the *fastest* rate constant, or the solution will explode.

In contrast, the backward Euler iteration for eq. 14.11,

$$U^{n+1} = U^n \frac{1}{1 + k\Delta t}, \tag{14.15}$$

decays monotonically for all $k > 0$. If Δt is chosen too large, the solution will be inaccurate, but it will not explode. Indeed, the solution will prematurely equilibrate to its steady-state value, 0, which is exactly the behavior we want when solving eq. 14.14. If Δt is chosen appropriate to the slow time scale, the fast component will be solved inaccurately (taken to steady state), but the total error of the solution will be small.

We can obtain second-order accuracy with the trapezoidal rule, which gives the iteration

$$U^{n+1} = U^n \frac{1 - k\Delta t}{1 + k\Delta t}. \tag{14.16}$$

This is also stable for all Δt, but we pay a price for the increased accuracy: the factor multiplying U^n approaches -1 as $k \to \infty$. For large k, the solution does not decay monotonically, but will exhibit damped ringing oscillations.

14.2.5 Methods for Stiff Systems

Although the space-clamped Hodgkin-Huxley ODE model is not particularly stiff, it is fairly easy to encounter extremely stiff ODEs simply related to eqs. 14.1 and 14.2.

If we incorporate the space-clamped Hodgkin-Huxley ODEs into a compartmental model of a neuron, the resulting multicompartment system will generally be stiff, its stiffness increasing with the number of compartments in the single-neuron model. The reason for this is the correspondence between compartmental models of neurons and the so-called method of lines for the numerical solution of PDE models for the same neurons. (This relationship between compartmental models and PDE models will be explained in detail in the chapter appendix, along with an explicit calculation of the stiffness of a compartmental model of passive dendritic cable.)

Stiffness can also occur in point neurons. A model of the bullfrog sympathetic ganglion cell includes ionic currents with the familiar millisecond time scale along with slow currents with time scales in the hundreds of milliseconds. Some bursting neurons, like R-15, have slow currents or other processes, such as Ca^{2+} accumulation, that vary on a time scale of seconds.

In general, explicit finite-difference methods are susceptible to stiffness, while implicit methods are not. Although the implicit versions of the ODE methods mentioned above, even backward Euler, are therefore viable candidates for integrating stiff ODEs, of even greater advantage is the Gear method (Gear 1971b; Lambert 1973), which is actually a family of methods of various orders, where both Δt and the order are varied to satisfy the error criteria most efficiently. The Gear methods are implicit multistep methods like Adams-Moulton, but are based on backward differentiation formulas, which use old values of $\vec{U}$, rather than $\vec{F}(\vec{U})$, and only evaluate $\vec{F}$ at the future time point. The qth-order method has the form

$$\vec{U}^{n+1} - a_0 \vec{U}^n - a_1 \vec{U}^{n-1} - \cdots - a_{q-1}\vec{U}^{n-(q-1)} = \Delta t b_q \vec{F}^{n+1}. \tag{14.17}$$

The implicit algebraic equations are solved by Newton's method, which requires information about the derivative of $\vec{F}$ (the Jacobian), either supplied by the user or approximated internally by the Gear solver, using finite differences.

Note that because these are variable-order methods, they do not have the starting problem of the Adams-Bashforth and Adams-Moulton methods. They begin with a one-step, first-order method and increase the order as time points are accumulated.

14.2.6 Boundary Value Problems

Another class of mathematical problems involving ODEs are boundary value problems (BVPs). To illustrate, we can get an idea of spatial effects while avoiding the full complexity of PDEs by letting the PDE settle down to a steady state, leaving space, x, as the sole independent variable. If we set all the time derivatives in eqs. 14.2 and 14.3 to zero, we obtain the following system of ODEs:

$$\frac{a}{2R}\frac{d^2V}{dx^2} = \bar{g}_{Na}m_\infty(V)^3 h_\infty(V)(V - E_{Na}) + \bar{g}_K n_\infty(V)^4(V - E_K) + \bar{g}_{leak}(V - E_{leak}),$$

where

$$m_\infty(V) = \alpha_m(V)/(\alpha_m(V) + \beta_m(V)), \tag{14.18}$$

and similarly for the other dimensionless variables, h_∞ and n_∞. The ∞ subscript indicates that they no longer obey differential equations but are instantaneous functions of membrane potential.

Suppose we want the steady-state solution for a Hodgkin-Huxley axon of length L. Initial conditions are no longer required, but we must now specify boundary conditions. A simple choice is

$$V(0) = V^0, \quad V(L) = V^L, \tag{14.19}$$

corresponding to a two-point voltage clamp, at $x = 0$ and $x = L$.

One approach to solving eqs. 14.18 and 14.19 is the *shooting method*, which converts the BVP to an IVP, with "time" running from 0 to L. Because eq. 14.18 is a second-order ODE, proper "initial" conditions are to specify $V(0)$ and $dV(0)/dx$. We know that $V(0) = V^0$, and we seek a value for $dV(0)/dx$ that will make $V(L) = V^L$. (See Conte and de Boor 1980, 412–416, for further details.)

Although more efficient methods would be used today, it is an interesting historical note that Hodgkin and Huxley solved the problem of determining the wave speed of the axon potential as a shooting problem. For a steadily progressing pulse of unvarying shape, the solution is a function of the variable $z = x - \theta t$, where θ is the wave speed. Hodgkin and Huxley therefore used the substitution $V(x, t) = \phi(z)$ to convert the PDE eq. 14.3 into a second-order ODE in z with boundary conditions $\phi(z) \to 0$ as $z \to \pm\infty$. This leads to an algorithm for determining the wave speed: for θ too small, ϕ diverges to ∞, for θ too large ϕ diverges to $-\infty$. Successive shooting trials allowed Hodgkin and Huxley to bracket the value of θ precisely. This recovery of the speed of the traveling pulse from space- and voltage-clamped currents was the capstone of their achievement that led to the Nobel prize.

More often, eqs. 14.18 and 14.19 are solved by the method of finite differences. We introduce a spatial grid with uniform width $\Delta x = L/N$, and with $x_0 = 0$ and $x_N = L$. Defining $V_i = V(i\Delta x)$, we use the Taylor series to derive a finite-difference approximation to the second spatial derivative:

$$V_{i\pm1} = V_i \pm \frac{dV}{dx}\Delta x + \frac{d^2V}{dx^2}\frac{(\Delta x)^2}{2} \pm \frac{d^3V}{dx^3}\frac{(\Delta x)^3}{3!} + \frac{d^4V}{dx^4}\frac{(\Delta x)^4}{4!} \pm \cdots, \tag{14.20}$$

where all the derivatives are evaluated at x_i. Combining the equations with $+$ and $-$ in 14.20, we solve for $\frac{d^2V}{dx^2}(x_i)$:

$$\frac{d^2V}{dx^2}(x_i) = \frac{V_{i-1} - 2V_i + V_{i+1}}{(\Delta x)^2} + O(\Delta x^2). \tag{14.21}$$

Using this $O((\Delta x)^2)$-accurate approximation, we replace eqs. 14.18 and 14.19 with the following nonlinear tridiagonal system of algebraic equations:

$$\frac{a}{2R} \frac{V_{i+1} - 2V_i + V_{i-1}}{(\Delta x)^2} = \bar{g}_{Na} m_\infty(V_i)^3 h_\infty(V_i)(V_i - E_{Na})$$

$$+ \bar{g}_K n_\infty(V_i)^4 (V_i - E_K) + \bar{g}_{leak}(V_i - E_{leak}),$$

$$V_0 = V^0, \quad V_N = V^L. \tag{14.22}$$

Methods for the solution of difference equations of this form will be treated in section 14.3, but note that with the boundary values V_0 and V_N given, eq. 14.22 completely defines $V_1, \ldots, V_{N-1}$.

The general problem of numerically solving BVPs for ODEs has many complications, including singular solutions, unstable solutions, and periodic and translational boundary conditions. A good resource is the monograph by Keller (1976).

14.2.7 Problems with Discontinuities

Discontinuities in solutions or their derivatives pose special challenges for numerical methods. Unfortunately, they occur naturally in simulations of voltage-clamping, applied current pulses, channel noise, and integrate-and-fire neurons. In the first two cases, the events are often imposed by the user and occur with modest frequency. Naive use of Adams-Bashforth and Adams-Moulton methods can fail here because they try to fit a smooth solution to the discontinuity. The remedy is to stop and restart the calculation at each event, which is clumsy and incurs extra overhead. Although robust implementations of the variable-order Gear algorithm can detect discontinuities and restart automatically with a first-order method, it is more efficient to instruct the solver explicitly to restart. Runge-Kutta methods with fixed step sizes sail through discontinuities, but accuracy may be reduced unless the jumps are arranged to occur at time step boundaries.

Channel noise and other stochastic simulations pose a harder problem because the transitions occur frequently and unpredictably. If events are constrained to time step boundaries, the simulation can only be first-order accurate, forcing use of small steps. Alternatively, we might use knowledge that transitions are, say, exponentially distributed to integrate from event to event (Clay and DeFelice 1983), although, if the population size is large, this will also result in small steps. We can then reformulate the problem as a continuous diffusion and solve the stochastic differential equations (Fox and Lu 1994). Special Runge-Kutta methods have been developed to solve these with second- or higher-order accuracy (Kloeden, Platen, and Schurz 1993).

Integrate-and-fire networks raise similar issues, with the additional complication that each element's firing can influence the other elements. Integration with fixed step sizes is again only first-order accurate, regardless of the accuracy between events, and can also artifactually synchronize the elements. The safest approach is to determine numerically or analytically when the next unit will fire, integrate up to that time, and calculate the interactions (Tsodyks, Mit'kov, and Sompolinsky 1993). It may be more efficient, however, to use second-order Runge-Kutta with linear interpolation to determine spike firing times (Hansel et al., in press). As for stochastic problems, we can smooth out the discontinuities for large networks by solving for the distribution of firing events (Kuramoto 1991).

14.2.8 Guide to Method Selection and Packages

For ODEs, stiffness is the critical factor to consider when choosing between alternative numerical methods. In general, because a compartmental model of a neuron will yield a rather stiff system of ODEs, an implicit method should be used to avoid numerical instabilities. Gear's adaptive time step method is particularly attractive. Popular public domain packages in FORTRAN include DDRIV and several variants of the subroutine LSODE. An updated version of LSODE, CVODE, is available in C. These packages can be downloaded from netlib. General commercial libraries, such as IMSL (Visual Numerics, Inc.), and NAGLIB (Numerical Algorithms Group Ltd.) also have FORTRAN and C routines for ODEs (and PDEs). A single source for information on all of these is the Guide to Available Mathematical Software (GAMS) maintained by the National Institutes of Standards and Technology. GAMS includes a problem decision tree and links to online documentation, example driver programs, and provider information.

Because, by contrast, small systems of ODEs, or a system of ODEs that does not have direct coupling between its domains, may not be very stiff, it may be computationally cheaper to use an explicit method, such as one of the Runge-Kutta methods. Although explicit second- or fourth-order methods that are easy for the user to write may be adequate, adaptive methods usually pay off handsomely and are well worth the effort to acquire or program. Public domain and commercial packages for both fixed- and variable-step Runge-Kutta methods can be obtained from the same sources as above. For do-it-yourselfers, Press et al. (1992) give a detailed explanation and code for Runge-Kutta-Fehlberg, as well as a number of other methods. Most Gear packages include options for Adams-Bashforth and Adams-Moulton methods and have well-tested heuristics for scaling variables and estimating errors, making them good general purpose solvers. Because the Adams implementations are also variable-order, hence self-starting and robust on discontinuities, and do not need to evaluate the Jacobian, they can be faster than Gear on nonstiff problems. Some packages (e.g., LSODA) attempt to automatically evaluate stiffness and switch between Gear and Adams.

If you are unsure about the stiffness of a particular ODE system whose numerical solution is required, it may be worthwhile to begin with a low-order explicit method, like the second-order Runge-Kutta method, and use it on a test problem where the solution's behavior is known. If the method produces good results, you may not need to look any further for a numerical method. If, however, the solution shows unexpected oscillatory behavior or requires, to avoid such instability, a time step much smaller than the time scale of interest, you should suspect stiffness.

Packages for boundary value problems can also be obtained from the sources listed above. In addition, the program AUTO (Doedel, Keller, and Kernévez 1991), designed primarily for bifurcation calculations (the study of how solutions change as parameters are varied), can also be used as a BVP solver.

Complete interactive programs that handle the allocation of memory, data input and output, and graphics are an increasingly popular solution. The user need only define the problem and choose an appropriate numerical method. Two programs available for Unix workstations are dstool (Back et al. 1992), which has a variable-step-size Runge-Kutta solver, and xpp, which has a Gear solver, allows automatic detection of and restarting at discontinuities, and features an interactive interface to AUTO, and which also can solve BVPs by the shooting method. Both dstool and xpp are general differential equation solvers and differ from the compartmental modeling programs described in section 14.3 in that they are equation-oriented, not object-oriented: the user must specify the problem in terms of equations, rather than in terms of channels and cable properties. DOS PC users can consider PHASER (Koçak 1989) or PHASEPLANE (Ermentrout 1990), a predecessor of xpp, and LOCBIF. Macintosh users can try MacMath (Hubbard and West 1992), for systems of two or three variables. General interactive mathematics packages such as MAPLE, MATHEMATICA, MATLAB, and MLAB, also have tools for solving differential equations with graphics. Details on the packages mentioned in this section and information on how to obtain them can be found at http://mrb.niddk.nih.gov/sherman.

We have downplayed the convergence of numerical methods for ODEs because the convergence theory for ODE methods is relatively straightforward. Even naive methods like forward Euler will converge for well-posed ODE problems, provided that Δt is chosen sufficiently small. As we will see in our discussion below, the issue of convergence for PDEs is a different matter altogether.

14.3   Methods for Partial Differential Equations

In general, numerical methods for PDEs are not as well understood as numerical methods for ODEs, largely because of the greater mathematical complexity of PDEs. In contrast to the numerical methods for ODEs, much of the intuition accumulated for understanding and choosing PDE methods has come from studying methods for solving linear PDEs. Thus we begin our discussion, not with the example of the Hodgkin-Huxley equations, but with its linear counterpart, the passive cable equation from dendritic modeling:

$$C\frac{\partial V}{\partial t} = \frac{a}{2R}\frac{\partial^2 V}{\partial x^2} - \bar{g}V, \tag{14.23}$$

where $\bar{g}$ is the passive membrane conductance per unit area.

14.3.1   Finite-Difference Methods

Two popular methods for numerically solving PDEs are finite-difference and finite-element methods. Finite-element methods in many cases reduce to finite-difference methods, especially for many neuronal models, where often only one spatial dimension is used in the PDEs. In cases where a model results in PDEs with more than one spatial dimension, however, finite-element methods and more advanced finite-difference methods should be considered. We describe only finite-difference methods in this chapter. As with ODEs, finite-difference methods for PDEs employ finite-difference approximations of the derivatives in the PDEs to reduce the differential equations to algebraic equations. The Hodgkin-Huxley equations and the linear cable equation are PDEs of the parabolic type; the methods we will discuss can generally be applied to other parabolic PDEs, such as heat and diffusion equations (Douglas 1961).

In treating parabolic PDEs, it is customary to first introduce the discretization of the spatial variables. This is called the "method of lines", and reduces the PDEs to a system of coupled ODEs (In the chapter appendix, we will see how conceptually close the method of lines for PDEs is to compartmental modeling). If we replace the continuous variable, x, with a uniformly spaced grid of length $\Delta x = L/N$ with $N + 1$ grid points over L spatial units, then the method of lines transforms eq. 14.23 into the following coupled system of ODEs:

$$C\frac{dV_i}{dt} = \frac{a}{2R}\frac{V_{i+1} - 2V_i + V_{i-1}}{(\Delta x)^2} - \bar{g}V_i, \quad i = 0, \ldots, N. \tag{14.24}$$

This system is stiff, its stiffness increasing with N. (Eq. 14.24 is the example we will use in the chapter appendix to explicitly compute the numerical stiffness of a simple compartmental model ODE formulation.)

Because eq. 14.24 is stiff, we should use an implicit method to solve it. Although we could use an ODE package described previously to solve such a system, such a package might or might not be able to solve the systems as efficiently as simple temporal discretization. Thus we will present three finite-difference methods for the numerical solution of these parabolic PDEs: (1) forward Euler, (2) backward Euler, and (3) Crank-Nicolson.

All three of these finite-difference methods use the $O((\Delta x)^2)$ finite-difference approximation to the second spatial derivative we have previously introduced. The methods differ only in the way they discretize the time derivative on the left-hand side of eq. 14.23. Let us now define the computational grid we will use with all the PDE finite-difference methods. The time variable will be replaced by a discrete set of time values with a uniform spacing of Δt. V_i^n refers to $V(i\Delta x, n\Delta t)$.

The forward Euler method uses the most naive time discretization. The typical form of this discretization is

$$C\frac{V_i^{n+1} - V_i^n}{\Delta t} = \frac{a}{2R}\frac{V_{i+1}^n - 2V_i^n + V_{i-1}^n}{(\Delta x)^2} - \bar{g}V_i^n. \tag{14.25}$$

If we define the constants $\sigma = a\Delta t/2RC(\Delta x)^2$ and $\gamma = \bar{g}\Delta t/C$, then eq. 14.25 can be rewritten as

$$V_i^{n+1} = \sigma V_{i+1}^n + (1 - 2\sigma - \gamma)V_i^n + \sigma V_{i-1}^n. \tag{14.26}$$

The error in using the forward Euler method is $O(\Delta t) + O((\Delta x)^2)$ (Isaacson and Keller 1966).

From eq. 14.26 we see that the forward Euler method is an explicit method; V_i^{n+1} is explicitly defined by the right-hand-side terms, which are known. Although the forward Euler method is also very easy to implement, it has numerical properties that are quite undesirable. As the worst of these, it is numerically unstable when $\sigma > 1/2$, which means that stability requires $\Delta t \le RC(\Delta x)^2/a$. If we wish to achieve higher spatial accuracy in our numerical solution by decreasing Δx by a factor of Q, we must also then decrease Δt by a factor of Q^2 to maintain numerical stability. The amount of work we must do is thus multiplied by Q^3 to achieve a spatial grid finer by a factor of Q.

If in eq. 14.15, the left-hand-side time difference is set equal to the right-hand side at time value $n + 1$, we obtain the backward Euler method

$$C\frac{V_i^{n+1} - V_i^n}{\Delta t} = \frac{a}{2R}\frac{V_{i+1}^{n+1} - 2V_i^{n+1} + V_{i-1}^{n+1}}{(\Delta x)^2} - \bar{g}V_i^{n+1}. \tag{14.27}$$

We can rewrite these equations as

$$-\sigma V_{i+1}^{n+1} + (1 + 2\sigma + \gamma)V_i^{n+1} - \sigma V_{i-1}^{n+1} = V_i^n. \tag{14.28}$$

Unlike eq. 14.26, eq. 14.28 does not explicitly define the values at that new time step in terms of the values at the old time step. Thus the backward Euler method is an implicit method; at each time step, a system of linear equations must be solved. Because the left-hand side of eq. 14.28 involves the unknown voltage and its two nearest neighbors on the grid, such a system is called a "tridiagonal linear system." (We discuss the numerical solution of tridiagonal linear systems in section 14.3.4, with special emphasis on efficiency.)

Even though it involves solving a tridiagonal linear system at each time step, the backward Euler method is considered superior to the forward for these types of PDE problems. Not only can we solve the tridiagonal system arising at each time step in the backward Euler method in $O(N)$ arithmetic operations, the same order of complexity as for the forward Euler method; more important, it does not suffer from numerical instability, as the forward Euler method does. Thus we can choose the grid parameters Δt and Δx independently and not have to worry whether some combination violates a stability inequality. Also, if the accuracy in one of the grid parameters is insufficient, we may refine that variable, without having to readjust the other grid parameter. One of the advantages of this independence in Δt and Δx for the backward Euler method is the possibility of using a rather large Δt to qualitatively explore the behavior of a system at little computational expense. When interesting behavior is noted, a smaller Δt can be used to reexamine the phenomena of interest, with greater numerical accuracy. We note that the backward Euler method has the same numerical accuracy as the forward, namely, $O(\Delta t) + O((\Delta x)^2)$.

The last method we present, the Crank-Nicolson method (Crank and Nicolson 1947), is related to both forward and backward Euler methods; its right-hand side is the average of the two Euler right-hand sides:

$$C \frac{V_i^{n+1} - V_i^n}{\Delta t}$$

$$= \frac{1}{2} \left(\frac{a}{2R} \frac{V_{i+1}^{n+1} - 2V_i^{n+1} + V_{i-1}^{n+1}}{(\Delta x)^2} - \bar{g} V_i^{n+1} + \frac{a}{2R} \frac{V_{i+1}^n - 2V_i^n + V_{i-1}^n}{(\Delta x)^2} - \bar{g} V_i^n \right).$$

$$(14.29)$$

Unlike the Euler methods, the Crank-Nicolson method has a numerical accuracy of $O((\Delta t)^2) + O((\Delta x)^2)$. The rationale for this is the same as described in the discussion of the trapezoidal rule for ODEs (section 14.2.1).

Let us rearrange eq. 14.29 by placing the values at the old time level on the right and the new values on the left:

$$-\frac{\sigma}{2} V_{i+1}^{n+1} + \left(1 + \sigma + \frac{\gamma}{2} \right) V_i^{n+1} - \frac{\sigma}{2} V_{i-1}^{n+1} = \frac{\sigma}{2} V_{i+1}^n + \left(1 - \sigma - \frac{\gamma}{2} \right) V_i^n + \frac{\sigma}{2} V_{i-1}^n,$$

$$(14.30)$$

where σ and γ are as previously defined. As with the backward Euler method, eq. 14.30 implicitly defines the new values as the solution to a tridiagonal system of linear equations. In addition, this method is unconditionally stable for any choice of the grid parameters, Δt and Δx. One subtle difference from the backward Euler method is that in some sense the Crank-Nicolson method is closer to numerical instability. This is observed in Crank-Nicolson numerical solutions where damped oscillations and over- or undershoot are seen although none are expected, even when large values of σ are used. This ringing is rarely seen with the backward Euler method, which is much more heavily damping than Crank-Nicolson, and is analogous to that described for the corresponding ODE methods (section 14.2.4; see especially eq. 14.16).

An interesting implementational detail exploits a useful relationship between the backward Euler and the Crank-Nicolson solutions. If V_i^{n+1} are the solution voltages to the backward Euler equations (eq. 14.28), starting with V_i^n, then $2V_i^{n+1} - V_i^n$ is the solution to the Crank-Nicolson equations, starting with V_i^n. Thus it is a trivial task to modify a computer program for the solution of these PDEs from an $O(\Delta t)$ backward Euler solver to an $O((\Delta t)^2)$ Crank-Nicolson solver by modifying a single line of code!

14.3.2 Boundary Conditions

Because PDEs involve derivatives with respect to more than one independent variable, specifying initial conditions is more complicated than for ODEs. Initial values must be given at all values of x, and boundary conditions at the endpoints of neuronal processes must also be specified. These types of initial-boundary value problems (IBVPs) have been shown rigorously to be well posed mathematically, meaning that their solutions are unique, depend continuously on the initial and boundary conditions, and remain bounded above and below for all time (Mascagni 1989a).

We have already encountered a common boundary condition in our discussion of BVPs for ODEs arising from steady-state computations for PDE problems. This first common type, called a "Dirichlet boundary condition," specifies the solution value at the end points, for example, eq. 14.19, which specifies the voltage at two ends of a neural cable. As we will see below, boundary conditions of the Dirichlet type are quite easy to incorporate into finite-difference methods for PDEs.

The second common type, called a "Neumann boundary condition", specifies the first spatial derivative of the solution at the end points. Neumann boundary conditions occur very naturally in neuronal modeling. Because $\partial V/\partial x$ is proportional to the longitudinal current through a cable, specifying a Neumann boundary conditions for neuronal cable models amounts to specifying the longitudinal current values at the end points. For example, the following Neumann boundary conditions for the Hodgkin-Huxley PDE system of eqs. 14.2 and 14.3,

$$\frac{\partial V(0)}{\partial x} = -\frac{RI}{\pi a^2}, \quad \frac{\partial V(L)}{\partial x} = 0, \tag{14.31}$$

biophysically correspond to injecting I microamps of current at $x = 0$, and demanding that no current pass out the $x = L$ end. The Neumann boundary condition at $x = L$ is commonly called a "no-leak" or "sealed-end" boundary condition" in neuronal modeling (Jack, Nobel, and Tsien 1983; zero–Dirichlet boundary conditions are also called "open" or "killed-end boundary conditions"). Neumann boundary conditions are more complicated than Dirichlet boundary conditions to incorporate into finite-difference methods for PDE IBVPs, but only slightly more.

Both the Dirichlet and Neumann boundary conditions are linear boundary conditions in the sense that linear PDEs with these boundary conditions obey a superposition property with respect to the boundary conditions. A more unusual type of linear boundary condition involves a linear combination of the Dirichlet and Neumann boundary conditions:

$$\alpha_0 \frac{\partial V(0)}{\partial x} + V(0) = \beta_0, \quad \alpha_L \frac{\partial V(L)}{\partial x} + V(L) = \beta_L, \tag{14.32}$$

which states that the voltage at the end points obeys a linear or ohmic current voltage relationship. The difficulty of implementing a finite-difference method for a PDE

IBVP with these mixed Dirichlet and Neumann boundary conditions is only slightly greater than handling simply a Neumann boundary condition. By making the coefficient α and β from eq. 14.32 nonlinear functions of the end point voltages, we can impose a nonlinear current voltage relationship at the end points, as did Baer and Tier (1986), who considered the effects of a Fitzhugh-Nagumo patch that formed the end of a dendritic cylinder as a model of an active membrane site within a passive dendrite. Li et al. (1995) used a similar approach to study the interaction of intracellular calcium handling with membrane ion channels and pumps, representing the former with a diffusion equation and the latter as a nonlinear boundary condition.

The Dirichlet boundary conditions, which directly prescribe the boundary values, are the simplest to incorporate into the finite-difference methods we have discussed. Thus in the forward Euler method, we use the known end point values, V_0 and V_N, in the equations for V_1^{n+1} and V_{N-1}^{n+1}. In the two implicit methods discussed, knowing V_0 and V_N allows us to reduce the number of equations to be solved from $N + 1$ to $N - 1$. We simply place the terms involving the known boundary values onto the right-hand sides of the equations for V_1^{n+1} and V_{N-1}^{n+1}, and solve the resulting tridiagonal system. For example, in the backward Euler case, the equation for V_1^{n+1} is

$$-\sigma V_2^{n+1} + (2\sigma + \gamma + 1)V_1^{n+1} - \sigma V_0^{n+1} = V_1^n.$$

Because V_0^{n+1} is known, we can rewrite this equation as

$$-\sigma V_2^{n+1} + (2\sigma + \gamma + 1)V_1^{n+1} = \sigma V_0^{n+1} + V_1^n.$$

We do the same for V_{N-1}^{n+1}. A similar manipulation can be used to incorporate Dirichlet boundary conditions into the Crank-Nicolson method.

It is only somewhat more difficult to incorporate Neumann boundary conditions. Here we ask that two properties of our numerical methods be preserved. First, because all of our numerical methods are $O((\Delta x)^2)$ spatially accurate, we ask that the boundary condition incorporation be at least this accurate. Second, we ask that the neat tridiagonal form of the linear equations arising from the implicit methods be maintained. Although these two requirements are in a sense competing, it is possible to achieve both through the following construction. Consider the Neumann boundary conditions from eq. 14.31 for the forward Euler method. A second-order-accurate finite-difference formula for the first derivative that involves only two points is the centered-difference approximation (Dahlquist and Bjorck 1974). If we wish to approximate the first derivative at $x = 0$ using the centered-difference formula, we need to know the value of V at $x = \pm \Delta x$; our computational grid does not, however, include the point at $x = -\Delta x$. If we pretend to know V at this point, we can achieve both of our requirements (Sod 1985; Cooley and Dodge 1966). Knowing both V_1 and V_{-1} gives us the centered-difference formula $(V_1 - V_{-1})/2\Delta x = \partial V(0)/\partial x$ up to $O((\Delta x)^2)$. Because the Neumann boundary condition specifies the value of $\partial V(0)/\partial x$, this can be used to write the unknown V_{-1} in terms of the given derivative value and V_1. Thus the equation for V_0^{n+1} for the forward Euler method can be rewritten as

$$V_0^{n+1} = \sigma V_1^n + (1 - 2\sigma - \gamma) V_0^n + \sigma V_{-1}^n \tag{14.33}$$

$$= \sigma V_1^n + (1 - 2\sigma - \gamma) V_0^n + \sigma \left(V_1^n + 2\Delta x \frac{\partial V(0)}{\partial x} \right). \tag{14.34}$$

With $\partial V(0)/\partial x$ specified in the boundary condition, the right-hand side is completely known. The same procedure can be followed for V_N^{n+1}.

We can use this same centered-difference approximation of $\partial V/\partial x$ to incorporate Neumann boundary conditions into the tridiagonal systems required by the implicit methods, solving for V_{-1}^{n+1} and V_{N+1}^{n+1}, then substituting these expressions into the V_0 and V_N equations. Because we use the centered-difference approximation to the derivative only at the two end points, this construction maintains the tridiagonal structure of the equations. For example, the first equation from the backward Euler system for the IBVP for eq. 14.23 with Neumann boundary conditions, eqs. 14.31, is

$$(1 + 2\sigma + \gamma) V_0^{n+1} - 2\sigma V_1^{n+1} = V_0^n + \frac{2RI\sigma\Delta x}{\pi a^2}. \tag{14.35}$$

The same problem discretized via Crank-Nicolson yields a first equation of

$$\left(1 + \sigma + \frac{\gamma}{2}\right) V_0^{n+1} - \sigma V_1^{n+1} = \left(1 - \sigma - \frac{\gamma}{2}\right) V_0^n + \sigma V_1^n + \frac{2RI\sigma\Delta x}{\pi a^2}. \tag{14.36}$$

Knowing how to incorporate both Dirichlet and Neumann boundary conditions into our three PDE methods, it is relatively easy to combine these techniques to allow mixed boundary conditions, as in eq. 14.32. Using the two extra grid points, V_{-1} and V_{N+1}, we can discretize eq. 14.32 up to $O((\Delta x)^2)$:

$$\alpha_0 \left(\frac{V_{-1} - V_1}{2\Delta x} \right) + V_0 = \beta_0, \quad \alpha_L \left(\frac{V_{N-1} - V_{N+1}}{2\Delta x} \right) + V_N = \beta_L. \tag{14.37}$$

We notice that both equations in eq. 14.37 involve the grid's end points and their two neighboring points. As with our treatment of the Neumann boundary conditions, these equations can be solved for the values at V_{-1} and V_{N+1} and the resulting expressions substituted into the equations for V_0 and V_N. This is elementary for the forward Euler method; for the two implicit methods, it is clear that a linear tridiagonal system of equations is again the final result.

14.3.3 Spatial Variation

Recall that the Hodgkin-Huxley PDE models the giant axon of the squid *Loligo*. A basic assumption is that the electrotonic properties of the squid's neuronal membrane are uniform and do not depend on the longitudinal location along the axon. While this is an adequate assumption for that preparation, we should be able to incorporate spatial variation of the neuronal membrane into PDE models. We now discuss how to express longitudinal variation in membrane properties in the linear cable PDE system, and how to incorporate this spatial variation into discretizations while preserving $O((\Delta x)^2)$ spatial accuracy.

In the linear cable model PDE, we can incorporate spatial variation in both the ionic conductance, $\bar{g}$, and the membrane capacitance, C, in the most trivial way, by making them functions of x. The hard part is what to do when the dentritic radius, a, and the specific axoplasmic resistivity, R, are functions of x. We cannot just make them functions of x in eq. 14.23, because that does not preserve the biophysical meaning of this equation. Eq. 14.23 is a statement of the instantaneous conservation of charge along the membrane, and the term $(a/2R)\partial^2 V/\partial x^2$ represents the total membrane current per unit area. This expression was originally obtained by using current conservation for an infinitesimal slice of dendrite and the differential form of Ohm's law. To see how to rewrite this term when a and R depend on x, we must go back to this derivation.

The expression for total membrane current per unit area can be written as

$$\frac{a}{2R}\frac{\partial^2 V}{\partial x^2} = \frac{1}{2\pi a}\frac{\partial}{\partial x}\left(\frac{\pi a^2}{R}\frac{\partial V}{\partial x}\right). \qquad (14.38)$$

The term in parentheses is the axial current. Eq. 14.38 restates conservation of charge by stating that the divergence of the axial current equals the total membrane current. The constants in this expression convert the axial current, which is per unit cross-sectional area, into the membrane current per unit membrane area. Using eq. 14.38, we can rewrite the linear cable equation, eq. 14.23, to allow spatial variation in all the cable parameters:

$$C(x)\frac{\partial V}{\partial t} = \frac{1}{2\pi a(x)}\frac{\partial}{\partial x}\left(\frac{\pi a^2(x)}{R(x)}\frac{\partial V}{\partial x}\right) - \bar{g}(x)V. \qquad (14.39)$$

By performing the analogous substitution with the Hodgkin-Huxley PDE model, eqs. 14.2 and 14.3, we can incorporate spatial variation in that case. Although, strictly speaking, we should replace the factor $a(x)$ in the denominator of eq. 14.39 by $a(x)\sqrt{1 + a'(x)^2}$ and make the corresponding change in eq. 14.40 to account for the increased membrane area of a tapered cable (see Jack, Noble, and Tsien 1983, 150), eq. 14.39 is usually quantitatively adequate because $a'(x)^2 \ll 1$.

Now we must consider how to convert these spatially varying continuous models into finite-difference equations with $O((\Delta x)^2)$ accuracy. In eq. 14.39, spatial dependence is only problematic when we try to discretize the term for the total membrane current per unit area. Because this term involves the derivative of a derivative, we proceed by discretizing the derivatives one at a time. A first-order approximation to the first derivative is $\partial V / \partial x = (V_{i+1} - V_i)/\Delta x$. Applying this expression twice to the total membrane current term in eq. 14.39 gives us

$$\frac{1}{2\pi a(x)} \frac{\partial}{\partial x} \left(\frac{\pi a^2(x)}{R(x)} \frac{\partial V}{\partial x} \right) \approx \frac{1}{2\pi a_i} \frac{\left(\frac{\pi a_{i+1/2}^2}{R_{i+1/2}} \left(\frac{V_{i+1} - V_i}{\Delta x} \right) - \frac{\pi a_{i-1/2}^2}{R_{i-1/2}} \left(\frac{V_i - V_{i-1}}{\Delta x} \right) \right)}{\Delta x}. \tag{14.40}$$

The value at grid point index $i + 1/2$ refers to the numerical value of the indexed function at $x + \Delta x/2$, while $i - 1/2$ refers to $x - \Delta x/2$. Even though the spatial grid does not include these points, it is reasonable to ask for the value of the continuously defined variables $a(x)$ and $R(x)$ at these points. If these intermediate values are not available, however, we can substitute the average of the values at the two flanking grid points in this discretization.

The spatial discretization of the troublesome second derivative term for the total membrane current given in eq. 14.40 can be shown to yield an $O((\Delta x)^2)$-accurate finite-difference approximation (Cooley and Dodge 1966). Thus we can use the discretization in eq. 14.39 to solve a spatially dependent problem with one of the finite-difference methods we have already described with the same numerical accuracy. These discretizations lead to the same types of equations as in the constant coefficient case. Because we can incorporate boundary conditions exactly as in the constant coefficient case, we can think of these spatially dependent coefficient problems as being no more complicated than their constant coefficient counterparts. Even so, we have yet to describe the solution of tridiagonal linear systems that arise in all our implicit discretizations.

14.3.4 Solving Tridiagonal Linear Systems

We will discuss only one algorithm for the solution of tridiagonal linear systems of equations, Gaussian elimination, also called "LU decomposition" and "forward elimination with back substitution." Gaussian elimination has many variants that are specialized for efficiency on specific classes of matrices (Golub and Van Loan 1985). A special variant, called the "Thomas algorithm," requires $O(M)$ mathematical operations to solve a tridiagonal system with M unknowns. The Thomas algorithm is numerically stable when the tridiagonal system has the property of diagonal dominance. Because all the tridiagonal systems that arise in finite-difference solution of the PDEs we have discussed are diagonally dominant, we can use the Thomas algorithm, which does not involve pivoting, to solve these systems. To say that a matrix is "diagonally dominant" means that the magnitude of the diagonal dominates the sum of the magnitudes of the off-diagonal elements in each row of the matrix. It is evident from eqs. 14.28 and 14.30 that for the finite-difference PDE approximations we have discussed, the tridiagonal systems that arise are diagonally dominant. In general, $O((\Delta x)^2)$ finite-difference approximations to well-posed parabolic PDEs will be diagonally dominant.

Let us denote our tridiagonal system as

$$L_i V_{i-1} + D_i V_i + U_i V_{i+1} = R_i, \quad 1 \leq i \leq M, \tag{14.41}$$

with $L_1 = U_M = 0$. The Gaussian elimination algorithm, without pivoting, proceeds by using adjacent equations in eq. 14.41 to eliminate the subdiagonal unknowns in a step known as "forward elimination." We may think of this procedure as sweeping through the equations and redefining the constants L_i, D_i, U_i, and R_i as follows:

$$D_1 = D_1, U_1 = U_1/D_1, R_1 = R_1/D_1,$$

$$D_i = D_i - L_i V_{i-1}, \quad i = 2, 3, \ldots, M,$$

$$R_i = (R_i - L_i V_{i-1})/D_i, \quad i = 2, 3, \ldots, M,$$

$$U_i = U_i/D_i, \quad i = 2, 3, \ldots, M - 1. \tag{14.42}$$

This forward elimination procedure succeeds in reducing the original tridiagonal system into an equivalent bidiagonal system, which can then be solved by a procedure called "backward substitution":

$$V_N = R_N, \tag{14.43}$$

$$V_i = R_i - U_i V_{i+1}, \quad i = M - 1, M, \ldots, 1. \tag{14.44}$$

We notice that this procedure requires only five arrays of length M, those for $L, D, U, R,$ and V. Because we overwrite these arrays with the Thomas algorithm, the coefficients for the tridiagonal systems must be recomputed for each time step.

And because the algorithm is defined with several "loops," each with a fixed number of arithmetic operations per iteration and with a length no more than M, it is obvious that this procedure requires $O(M)$ arithmetic operations.

14.3.5 Branching

Many of the models we use for individual neurons incorporate branching anatomical data. We consider two numerical methods for solving PDE neuronal models with branching. Because both assume that we employ an implicit finite-difference method to the PDEs, we will really be considering how to solve the tridiagonal-like linear systems that arise from these discretizations. The first method carefully numbers the unknowns on the branching structure to reduce the resulting linear system to what is essentially a single tridiagonal system. The second method uses the technique of domain decomposition to reduce the solution of the single system of equations on the entire branched structure to the solution of many smaller tridiagonal systems.

Hines (1984) describes an enumeration of the grid points in a branching cable structure that leads to direct solution of the resulting finite-difference equations, and that is equivalent in complexity to the Thomas algorithm. We illustrate with the example in figure 14.1, which is a diagram of a neuronal structure with six branches. We first choose a branch that is connected at only one end, and designate this as the "trunk." (A natural choice in a dendritic tree would be the most proximal branch to the soma.) The "trunk" will be the highest numbered branch; in our example, branch 6. The grid points in the "trunk" are ordered from the branch point toward the free end. We next number the branches connected to the "trunk." Those connected only to the "trunk" receive the highest numbers, while those with two connections are numbered lowest. The grid points in each branch are ordered toward the "trunk." Now we designate all branches connected at both ends as new "trunks" and continue the branch and grid point enumeration recursively.

Forward elimination in the branching case is exactly the same as in the nonbranching case except that we must also eliminate all the far off-diagonal elements associated with the several nearest neighbor grid points at a branch point. We proceed in order within the branches. Our chosen enumeration ensures that the only far subdiagonal element on a branch is associated with the last point. The order of elimination of the branches is also important for assuring that no new off diagonal elements are created. We must carry out forward elimination on all daughter branches before doing so on their parents. We therefore start with the lowest-numbered branches (the twigs), and sweep toward the trunk. With the numbering in our example, we can upper-triangularize the branches in order, from 1 to 6, although other orderings, such as 1, 2, 4, 5, 3, 6, are also permissible.

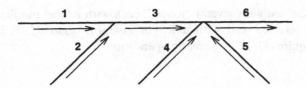

This enumeration yields the following matrix:

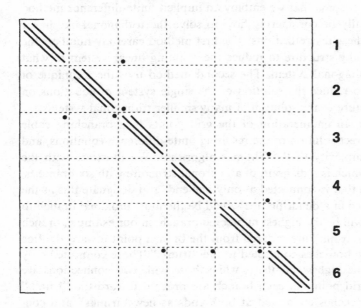

Figure 14.1
Example of a branch and grid point numbering of a branched neuronal structure and the resulting linear equation structure which arises with nearest-neighbor finite-difference discretization. After Hines 1984.

We then proceed to back substitution, marching backward through the unknowns along each branch. The only far superdiagonal elements are associated with the first point. The order of the branches in back substitution is essentially the reverse of their order in forward elimination: we must process each parent branch before its children. In our example, we can simply proceed in reverse order from 6 to 1, although again other orderings are permissible.

Because this method simply reworks Gaussian elimination without pivoting, it is obvious that $O(M)$ arithmetic operations and $O(M)$ storage are required to solve a branched structure with M grid points. If the rules above are observed, fill-in can be avoided; on the other hand, if the ordering along branch 1 is reversed, fill-in will result.

The second approach to branching is to solve small tridiagonal systems on the individual branches and form the solution on the entire branching structure out of a linear combination of these local solutions. This technique is known generally as "domain decomposition," the solution of a problem on one domain by solving smaller problems on subdomains and then building up the whole solution from these smaller parts (Mascagni 1991). Because we are solving a linear equation, we can exploit linear superposition. The simplest example of domain decomposition for a branching one-dimensional structure is illustrated in figure 14.2. Here we take a single cable and assume that an interior grid point is in fact a branch point. If we assume the value of the solution at the branch point V_{Br} is zero, we can solve the tridiagonal systems for the voltages on both branches. We call these solutions V_l^0 and V_r^0 for left and right. In general, the value at the branch point will not be zero. To take this into account, we call the solutions to the tridiagonal systems on each branch V_l^1 and V_r^1, with the right-hand side zero except for the contribution from $V_{Br} = 1$. By the principle of superposition, the solution on the left branch is $V_l^0 + V_{Br} V_l^1$, while $V_r^0 + V_{Br} V_r^1$ gives the solution on the right. A single equation for V_{Br} involves the nearest neighbors on the left and right branch, which gives us the value for V_{Br} and, via superposition, the complete solution on each branch.

The above procedure produces the solution on each branch even when a branch point is connected to more than two branches. In this case, the solution we seek is a linear combination of three tridiagonal solutions: the first with a normal right-hand side but with both branch end points zero; the second with a zero right-hand side and one branch point one; and the third with a zero right-hand side and the other branch point one. Thus we can use this domain decomposition method to solve the equations on any branching structure. Because we only solve several tridiagonal systems to obtain the overall solution, the arithmetic complexity for a structure with M unknowns is still $O(M)$.

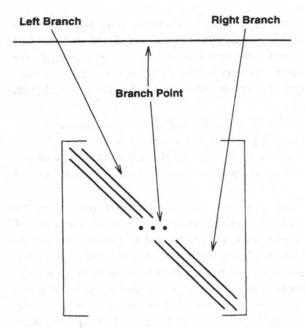

Figure 14.2
Example of domain decomposition for a branching one-dimensional structure using the simplest geometry.

14.3.6   Nonlinear Equations

Up to now, we have only considered finite-difference methods for linear PDEs. As we know, many of the most interesting PDE models in neuroscience are highly non-linear, for example, the Hodgkin-Huxley model. It is a trivial matter to use the forward Euler method on the Hodgkin-Huxley equations. We need only evaluate the nonlinear currents at the old time step value, which involves computing the dimensionless variables at the old time value. The forward Euler equation for m_i^{n+1} is simply

$$m_i^{n+1} = m_i^n + \Delta t[(1 - m_i^n)\alpha_m(V_i^n) - m_i^n\beta_m(V_i^n)]$$

$$= m_i^n[1 - \Delta t(\alpha_m(V_i^n) + \beta_m(V_i^n))] + \Delta t\alpha_m(V_i^n). \tag{14.45}$$

The expressions for h_i^{n+1} and n_i^{n+1} are analogous. The finite-difference equation for the voltage via the forward Euler method is then

$$V_i^{n+1} = \sigma(V_{i+1}^n + V_{i-1}^n) + (1 - 2\sigma - \gamma_i^n)V_i^n + \omega_i^n, \tag{14.46}$$

where $\sigma = a\Delta t/2RC(\Delta x)^2$, $\gamma_i^n = (\Delta t/C)(\bar{g}_{Na}(m_i^n)^3 h_i^n + \bar{g}_K(n_i^n)^4 + \bar{g}_{leak})$, and $\omega_i^n = (\Delta t/C)(\bar{g}_{Na}(m_i^n)^3 h_i^n E_{Na} + \bar{g}_K(n_i^n)^4 E_K + \bar{g}_{leak}E_{leak})$.

Generalizing the two implicit methods we have discussed to nonlinear equations raises more complicated issues. Because implicit methods require the solution of difference equations, when applied to nonlinear PDEs, nonlinear difference equations arise. The Hodgkin-Huxley equations have a property we will call "conditional linearity." Conditionally linear means that the PDE for the voltage, eq. 14.3, is a linear PDE if the values of the dimensionless variables are known. Similarly, the rate equations for the dimensionless variables, eqs. 14.2a–14.2c, are linear ODEs given values for V.

Although conditional linearity is a fairly generic property of nonlinear neuronal models, it is by no means universal. The nonlinearities in eq. 14.3 are associated with nonlinear ionic currents that are modeled as the product of a nonlinear ionic conductance and the difference between the membrane potential and the ionic reversal potential. Because the nonlinear ionic conductances are not directly functions of voltage, eq. 14.3 is conditionally linear. Therefore, if we can model our nonlinear ionic currents as the products of the difference between the membrane voltage and the ionic reversal potential and nonlinear ionic conductances not directly functions of the membrane conductance, we will have nonlinear PDE models of neurons that are conditionally linear.

What are the computational benefits of conditional linearity? Simply stated, the benefits are the separation of the complicated nonlinear problem into two simpler linear problems. This is ramified in different ways for the backward Euler and Crank-Nicolson methods. For the backward Euler method, separability gives us an algorithm for iterative solution of the nonlinear difference equations encountered at each time step via functional or Picard iteration. With Crank-Nicolson, separability reduces the nonlinear equations into a single set of linear equations that can be solved at each time step through a staggered-step procedure.

If we use the backward Euler method to discretize the Hodgkin-Huxley PDE, eq. 14.3, we arrive at the following system of nonlinear equations:

$$-\sigma V_{i+1}^{n+1} + (1 + 2\sigma + \gamma_i^{n+1})V_i^{n+1} - \sigma V_{i-1}^{n+1} = V_i^n + \omega_i^{n+1}, \qquad (14.47)$$

where the definition of γ_i and ω_i is as above. These nonlinear-difference equations must be solved for the values of V^{n+1}. To make matters worse, if we use the backward Euler discretization on the dimensionless variables as well, then eq. 14.47 must be solved in conjunction with the nonlinear-difference equations that arise. The equations for m are

$$m_i^{n+1} = \frac{m_i^n}{1 + \Delta t[\alpha_m(V_i^{n+1}) + \beta_m(V_i^{n+1})]} + \frac{\Delta t \alpha_m(V_i^{n+1})}{1 + \Delta t[\alpha_m(V_i^{n+1}) + \beta_m(V_i^{n+1})]}. \tag{14.48}$$

Equations for h and n are identical in form to eq. 14.48.

The backward Euler method for the Hodgkin-Huxley system requires the simultaneous solution of eq. 14.47 and three equations of the form of eq. 14.48 at each time step. We can hope to solve these nonlinear equations with the following iterative algorithm:

1. Solve eq. 14.47 with the previously known dimensionless variable values to give new voltage values.

2. Solve the dimensionless variable equations, eq. 14.48 and so on, using the new voltage values to give new dimensionless variable values.

3. Repeat steps 1 and 2 until voltage and dimensionless variable values have converged.

The starting values for this iterative procedure are the values of the unknowns at the previous time step. Because these equations are conditionally linear and hence separable, the equations to be solved in steps 1 and 2 will always be *linear*. The voltage equations become a single linear tridiagonal system, and the equations for the dimensionless variables are reduced to explicit expressions for the new values. This iterative procedure is sometimes called a "Picard", "fixed-point", or "functional" iteration. For the backward Euler method applied to the Hodgkin-Huxley equations, this iteration method has been proven to converge, provided that Δt is chosen sufficiently small (Mascagni 1987a).

As with the backward Euler method, the Crank-Nicolson method applied to the Hodgkin-Huxley equations leads to nonlinear equations:

$$-\frac{\sigma}{2} V_{i+1}^{n+1} + \left(1 + \sigma + \frac{\gamma_i^{n+1}}{2}\right) V_i^{n+1} - \frac{\sigma}{2} V_{i-1}^{n+1}$$

$$= \frac{\sigma}{2} V_{i+1}^n + \left(1 - \sigma - \frac{\gamma_i^n}{2}\right) V_i^n + \frac{\sigma}{2} V_{i-1}^n + \frac{\omega_i^{n+1} + \omega_i^n}{2}. \tag{14.49}$$

These must be solved concurrently with the difference equations for the dimensionless variables. If we wish to maintain an overall accuracy of $O((\Delta t)^2)$, we must use a method of at least second-order accuracy for the rate equations. Of course we know that the trapezoidal rule is second-order accurate and is the ODE analogue of the Crank-Nicolson method. Applying the trapezoidal rule to the equation for m

gives us

$$m_i^{n+1} = m_i^n \frac{1 - \Delta t/2[\alpha_m(V_i^{n+1/2}) + \beta_m(V_i^{n+1/2})]}{1 + \Delta t/2[\alpha_m(V_i^{n+1/2}) + \beta_m(V_i^{n+1/2})]}$$

$$+ \frac{\Delta t \alpha_m(V_i^{n+1/2})}{1 + \Delta t/2[\alpha_m(V_i^{n+1/2}) + \beta_m(V_i^{n+1/2})]}. \qquad (14.50)$$

We have used the values $V_i^{n+1/2}$ in the above expression to simplify the form of these difference equations while maintaining the desired second-order accuracy. We can use the average of the voltage at the nth and $(n+1)$th time step to estimate the value at time value $n + 1/2$, or we may use another method we discuss below.

Eqs. 14.49 and 14.50 and the analogous equations for h and n are a complicated set of simultaneous nonlinear equations. That these equations are conditionally linear can be exploited to give us an iterative algorithm for their simultaneous solution. Although there is no rigorous proof for the convergence of this method for the Crank-Nicolson method, it is believed that the techniques used in the proof of the backward Euler case can be easily extended to this case. The iterative solution method described for the backward Euler method can be used to solve the nonlinear equations we get with the Crank-Nicolson discretization; indeed, this method was used by Cooley and Dodge (1966), in a predictor-corrector variant of the method we described, to do the first systematic numerical simulation of the Hodgkin-Huxley equations.

Another approach to these equations, which exploits their conditional linearity and results in no iteration, is to use a previously mentioned implementational detail and the second-order accuracy of the trapezoidal rule. Recall that if V^{n+1} is the backward Euler solution to the linear cable equation, eq. 14.23, then $2V^{n+1} - V^n$ is the Crank-Nicolson solution. If we use eq. 14.47, with ω_i^{n+1} replaced by $\omega_i^{n+1/2}$, then $2V^{n+1} - V^n$ gives us a second-order-accurate solution to the Hodgkin-Huxley equations. Note that the definition of ω_i^n depends on the time level n only through the dimensionless variables. Thus we need only compute the values $m_i^{n+1/2}$, $h_i^{n+1/2}$, and $n_i^{n+1/2}$ to obtain $\omega_i^{n+1/2}$. This procedure requires values of the dimensionless variables at the midpoints of the time levels used in the voltage equations. If the dimensionless variable equations were solved at only the midpoint values, and the voltage values at the usual values, these could be combined to give an overall second-order method. This staggering of two time grids also simplifies the solution of the difference equations. Because the Hodgkin-Huxley equations are conditionally linear, this grid staggering leads to solving a single tridiagonal system for the voltage equation and evaluating the explicit equations for the dimensionless variables a single time to advance the solution Δt. One complication is the computation of the unknowns on the two time grids staggered by $\Delta t/2$. This can be accomplished by starting either the voltage or dimensionless variable equations with a $\Delta t/2$-sized time step and then proceeding as normal.

With the backward Euler and Crank-Nicolson discretizations of the Hodgkin-Huxley equations, we have shown two different ways conditional linearity can be exploited to simplify the numerical solution of these nonlinear systems. Because staggering is used to maintain $O((\Delta t)^2)$ accuracy in Crank-Nicolson, it is not required with the $O(\Delta t)$ backward Euler method. Thus, if we are content to use backward Euler, the minor complication of the staggered grids for Crank-Nicolson disappears, and we obtain an $O(\Delta t)$ implicit solution without iteration.

A warning must be made for users of the staggering method with Crank-Nicolson. Although this method is efficient and produces an $O((\Delta t)^2)$ solution to nonlinear problems without iteration, this is true only if the equations are conditionally linear. If a cable model is not conditionally linear, for example, if some ionic currents are explicitly nonlinear functions of the voltage, this method cannot assure an $O((\Delta t)^2)$ solution. On the other hand, the nonlinear equations arising from the implicit discretization can be solved using a functional (Picard) iteration or Newton's method. Alternatively, conditional linearity can be restored by expanding the nonlinear currents in a Taylor series and evaluating their first derivatives at the half time points, along with the conductances. An option based on this idea is included in Neuron.

Experience in computing solutions to the Hodgkin-Huxley PDEs has shown that the majority of the effort is spent in the evaluation of the α and β rate functions associated with the dimensionless variables. It is therefore considered prudent to use a lookup table to speed up the repeated evaluation of these functions. If you examine the equations for the advancement of the dimensionless variables, eqs. 14.45, 14.48, and 14.50, you will notice that they are all of the form $m^{n+1} = m^n K_1(V, \Delta t) + K_2(V, \Delta t)$. Thus we need only evaluate the two functions, K_1 and K_2, for each dimensionless variable at each time step. The functions K_1 and K_2, which involve combinations of the α and β functions, can be tabulated for the purpose of speed. If you do not plan to change the time step size, Δt, during a computation, the functions K_1 and K_2 can be tabulated once for all during the initialization of the computation.

It is most convenient to construct the lookup table over a wide range of possible voltage values using a uniform voltage increment. Experience has shown that the voltage range of -100 millivolts to 150 millivolts with a step of 0.1 millivolt will give sufficient accuracy for the Hodgkin-Huxley equations. Experience has also shown that, with piecewise quadratic interpolation, a step as large as 4.0 millivolts can be used with no degradation in the overall accuracy. (Interpolation with equally spaced points in a lookup table is handled quite well in Conte and de Boor 1980.)

Unlike linear PDEs, there is no neat Lax equivalence theorem for finite-difference methods applied to nonlinear PDEs. The analysis of these methods must instead proceed case by case. Fortunately, convergence of the backward Euler method for the Hodgkin-Huxley equations has been proven (Mascagni 1987a). In addition, there is a considerable body of results on the convergence of the Crank-Nicolson method for many classes of nonlinear parabolic PDEs (Douglas 1961; Lees 1959; Rose 1956). Although it appears that for both the backward Euler and Crank-Nicolson methods, no relationship between Δt and Δx need hold, it is known for the backward Euler method and likewise conjectured for the Crank-Nicolson method that convergence occurs for all values of Δt smaller than a certain maximal value (Mascagni 1987a).

14.3.7 Networks

Synthesizing the results of sections 14.3.1–14.3.6 gives us the ability to numerically simulate a single arbitrarily branched neuronal model with spatial variation and nonlinear ionic kinetics, already a significant capability. With new developments in computer technology, however, it is possible to solve problems of much greater complexity than merely a single neuron. The new technical capabilities provide us with the opportunity to model several hundred very complicated neurons that are synaptically connected to one another. The neuronal modeler should bear these new developments in mind when considering which questions to ask and which models to build.

The key to modeling a network of neurons is the selection of a model for synaptic conduction that is both biophysically satisfying and compatible with the finite-difference approach for the numerical solution of the nerve equations. To a large extent, this is a matter of personal taste. As a general rule, a deterministic model of synaptic conduction is most easily incorporated into a numerical scheme involving finite-difference approximations to nerve equations. For example, such a model might be the initiation of a characteristic postsynaptic conductance change in response to the presynaptic arrival of an action potential. This could be further embellished with a stochastic determination of the shape of the elicited postsynaptic conductance change. The types of models of this general form that cause numerical and implementational difficulties are those in which the repertoire of possible postsynaptic conductance time courses is large. In a computation that has many interacting neuronal elements, the accurate determination of the postsynaptic membrane

potential requires summation over the recent synaptic events. If these events can
assume many varied forms, a considerable amount of computer memory must be
used to implement the complicated bookkeeping task underlying the determination
of the postsynaptic membrane potential. In a network of p totally interconnected
neurons, $O(p^2)$ contributions to the postsynaptic potentials must be calculated at
each time step. This quadratic scaling with the number of neurons quickly dominates
the memory requirements of the computation, and it does so even more quickly
when a considerable amount of memory is required to store a single postsynaptic
event.

14.3.8   Concluding Remarks and Suggestions for PDEs

In deciding on one method over another for PDEs, considerations similar to those
discussed for choosing finite-difference methods for ODEs arise. In general, because
it takes no more computational work to use an implicit method than an explicit
method, you should use either the backward Euler or Crank-Nicolson method. The
backward Euler method with iteration has been used with great success for investigating certain problems (Mascagni 1987b), and the observed solutions remain
qualitatively correct for rather large values of Δt. The Crank-Nicolson method without iteration was first described in its entirety by Hines (1984). This method has also
been used with great success for certain computations (Mascagni 1989b). The
authors have observed that, because of ringing instabilities, you cannot use as large
values of Δt with the Crank-Nicolson method as you can with the backward Euler
method. This is true, for example, when modeling a voltage clamp step, which introduces high-frequency Fourier components into the solution. Where using a large
Δt is necessary and the modeler is willing to sacrifice quantitative accuracy, the
backward Euler method is preferable to the Crank-Nicolson method. On the other
hand, where accuracy is vital, it is recommended that the second-order-accurate
method be used, taking care to use Δt small enough to prevent ringing instabilities
from contaminating the computation. An alternative way to damp instabilities that
avoids the complication of implicit equations is the *exponential Euler* method, although it can be shown that the method converges only if $\Delta t/(\Delta x)^2 \rightarrow 0$, a condition
far more restrictive than the stability condition for forward Euler. Thus, while the
solutions do not explode, they may be highly inaccurate.

Users can also avail themselves of several neural simulation packages that include
solvers for compartmental or PDE models. These include GENESIS and NEURON
for Unix workstations and NODUS for Macintosh. NEURON is also available
for Windows. GENESIS and NEURON include the backward Euler and Crank-
Nicolson methods, and thus are efficient on stiff problems. While the time required

to learn these packages may be greater than writing a simple solver for a particular problem, they permit the user to define the problem in terms of objects natural to neural modeling, such as channels and geometrical features, rather than through equations. Also, once learned, these packages allow much flexibility to change the problem and to perform many numerical experiments. Finally, most of these packages have capabilities for producing highly useful graphical output. As for the ODE packages, further information can be found on the World Wide Web at URL: http://mrb.niddk.nih.gov/sherman.

A number of other problems may arise in neuronal modeling that produce PDEs for which we have not discussed methods of solution. Indeed, we have treated only one-dimensional parabolic PDE models. For those cases where more than one spatial dimension must be included in a PDE model, finite-element methods can be used, or extensions of the finite-difference methods presented here. Whether a finite-element or a finite-difference method is used, the resulting diagonally dominant system that arises from an implicit discretization is pentadiagonal in two dimensions and heptadiagonal in three. The diagonals are not contiguous, however, which introduces problems of fill-in that can ruin the sparsity of the matrices. While there are special variants of Gaussian elimination for the efficient solution of such problems, a particularly efficient method in the finite-difference case is the alternating direction implicit (ADI) method (Richtmyer and Morton 1967; Press et al. 1992). The ADI method produces an implicit solution to a two- or three-dimensional problem by solving several one-dimensional problems alternately in each of the dimensions.

There are also methods for solving PDEs that offer higher-order accuracy in space or time. Because methods that are higher-order in space complicate both the boundary conditions and the matrix equations that must be solved at each time step, they are seldom used. Methods that are higher-order in time can be obtained by using the method of lines with a high-order ODE solver. A version of the Gear algorithm, for example, may be appropriate where stiffness originates from the kinetics of the problem, rather than from the diffusion term of the PDE. It should be borne in mind, however, that all efforts to refine the temporal discretization are wasted if the spatial accuracy remains at $O((\Delta x)^2)$. Thus it is important to balance spatial and temporal accuracy when solving PDE neuronal models.

14.4 Final Comments

We have surveyed the current wisdom on the best solutions to what might be called the "easy problems" in neuronal modeling. Small systems of ODEs, even stiff ones, can be solved very efficiently to high accuracy. PDEs are naturally more difficult, but reasonable methods (i.e., second-order accurate; $O(N)$ work) are available for one-dimensional problems, including branched neurons. It is of course not difficult to come up with problems that will confound the best algorithms on the fastest computers, for example, any problem with stiff kinetics in two or three spatial dimensions. We have consciously avoided venturing into these areas, both because of our own limitations and those of computational mathematics as a whole.

In addition to the particular advice we have sprinkled throughout, we conclude here with some general observations that are relevant to problems on all scales of difficulty. Although some may have considerable artificial intelligence built into them, numerical methods are fallible. General dynamical systems theory can be very helpful in categorizing possible and impossible behaviors, but, in the end, there is no alternative to intimate knowledge of the particular physical problem on the part of the investigator.

There is no algorithm that solves all problems, and the user must know enough to adapt the tool to the job. It also pays to solve a problem by more than one method, which means supplementing numerical methods with analytical methods and also using more than one numerical method. In addition to catching routine errors, this may uncover very subtle ones. In one small but illuminating example that we know of, an instability in the dynamical system was sensitive to numerical error introduced by the Gear method, but not by Runge-Kutta, leading to discovery of a new class of phenomena (Sherman and Rinzel 1992). No computer program can be expected to anticipate such cases. Ultimately, computational science is isomorphic to all of science, and can no more ever be complete than all of science.

Acknowledgments

The authors would like to thank David Golomb, Larry Abbott, Misha Tsodyks, and David Hansel for discussions of integrate-and-fire problems, and Paul Smolen, Todd Geldon, and Mike Vanier for calculations with the exponential Euler method.

Appendix: Stiffness

Let us consider the PDE model of the squid axon, eqs. 14.2 and 14.3, to illustrate the method of lines and their relationship to compartmental models. In eq. 14.3, the right-hand side has a term involving a second spatial derivative. If we replace the continuous x-axis with a uniform grid of width Δx, and replace the term $\partial^2 V / \partial x^2$ with the familiar $O((\Delta x)^2)$ finite-difference approximation $(V_{i+1} - 2V_i + V_{i-1})/(\Delta x)^2$, the PDE is reduced to a system of coupled ODEs. This is the method of lines, where a single PDE is reduced to a system of ODEs by discretizing all but one of the independent variables in the PDE. The resulting method-of-lines ODE system for the Hodgkin-Huxley PDE model is stiff. This fact is well known from results for the method of lines for the PDE describing diffusion, $\partial V/\partial t = \partial^2 V/\partial x^2$, which displays the same qualitative stiffness properties.

A compartmental model that uses individual ODE models for each compartment and whose neighboring compartments are resistively coupled is equivalent to a method-of-lines discretization of some PDE model. This is easily seen by observing that we can rewrite our difference formula for the second derivative as

$$((V_{i+1} - V_i)/\Delta x - (V_i - V_{i-1})/\Delta x)/\Delta x.$$

Now assume that the spatial discretization is no longer uniform. If the distance between grid point $i + 1$ and i is denoted by Δx_1, while the distance between grid point i and $i - 1$ is denoted by Δx_2, then the second-order-accurate approximation to the second derivative on this nonuniform grid is given as

$$((V_{i+1} - V_i)/\Delta x_1 - (V_i - V_{i-1})/\Delta x_2)/((\Delta x_1 + \Delta x_2)/2).$$

This can be rewritten as $LV_{i-1} + DV_1 + UV_{i+1}$, where L, D, and U are constants. This is exactly the form we encounter in compartmental models whose nearest neighboring compartments are resistively coupled, where the ODE at one compartment depends on the voltage values of the central and the two flanking compartments.

In our above-mentioned example on the method of lines, eq. 14.24, we arrived at a system of coupled linear ODEs to describe the time evolution of a linear compartmental model. Because these ODEs came from a PDE model of a passive cable, we must impose certain boundary conditions to correctly specify the mathematical problem. For simplicity, let us assume that we desire the solution to eq. 14.24 with zero Dirichlet boundary conditions, namely, $V_0 = V_N = 0$. If we define the vector of voltages on the grid to be $\vec{V} = (V_1, V_2, \ldots, V_{N-1})$, we can rewrite eq. 14.24 as the following linear system of ODEs:

$$\frac{d\vec{V}}{dt} = \mathbf{A}\vec{V}. \tag{14.51}$$

The matrix $\mathbf{A}$ is a tridiagonal Toeplitz matrix (i.e., it has constant diagonals). Thus, if the elements of $\mathbf{A}$ are denoted as a_{ij}, then $a_{ij} = K_d$ whenever $i - j = d$ for $\mathbf{A}$ Toeplitz. Hence our Toeplitz, tridiagonal matrix $\mathbf{A}$ has $a/2RC(\Delta x)^2$ on both off diagonals and $-(a/RC(\Delta x)^2 + \bar{g}/C)$ along the main diagonal. Because eq. 14.51 is a linear system of ODEs, the general solution to this system can be expressed as a linear combination of exponential functions of the form $e^{\lambda t}$, where λ is an eigenvalue of the matrix $\mathbf{A}$. And because we are interested in computing the stiffness of this system, or the ratio of the largest to smallest time scale in the problem, we need only compute λ_{N-1}/λ_1, which is the ratio of the largest to the smallest eigenvalue of $\mathbf{A}$. It should be noted that this ratio of eigenvalues is exactly the l_2-norm condition number of this matrix (Stoer and Bulirsch 1980).

The eigenvalues of the tridiagonal Toeplitz matrix $\mathbf{A}$ are known to be (Isaacson and Keller 1966):

$$\lambda_k = \frac{2a}{RC(\Delta x)^2} \sin^2\left(\frac{k\pi}{2N}\right) + \frac{\bar{g}}{C}, \quad k = 1, \ldots, N - 1. \tag{14.52}$$

Thus the numerical stiffness is given by

$$\frac{\frac{2a}{RC(\Delta x)^2}\sin^2\left(\frac{(N-1)\pi}{2N}\right) + \frac{\bar{g}}{C}}{\frac{2a}{RC(\Delta x)^2}\sin^2\left(\frac{\pi}{2N}\right) + \frac{\bar{g}}{C}} = \frac{\sin^2\left(\frac{(N-1)\pi}{2N}\right) + \rho}{\sin^2\left(\frac{\pi}{2N}\right) + \rho}, \tag{14.53}$$

where $\rho = (2\bar{g}R(\Delta x)^2/a)$. The constant ρ is a parameter that measures the dissipation of this particular cable model. Large values of ρ mean the system relaxes much faster from dissipation than from diffusion.

With this explicit formula for the stiffness, we can ask what happens to the stiffness of our system as we vary certain parameters, namely, ρ and N. Since $0 \le \sin^2(x) \le 1$, if ρ is large, then eq. 14.53 has a numerical value close to 1, and thus the system is not in fact very stiff. If the system is very dissipative, it is numerically well behaved. On the other hand, if ρ is small, the stiffness is approximately the ratio of the sine terms in eq. 14.53. It can be shown that $\sin^2((N-1)\pi/2N)/\sin^2(\pi/2N) = O(N^2)$ as N gets large, which means that, for small values of ρ, the stiffness gets extremely large as we increase the number of compartments in our cable model. Indeed, it grows as the square of the number of compartments in our models. Compartmental models can therefore be very stiff when there is little dissipation via the membrane conductance. Paradoxically, this stiffness increases as we use smaller and smaller compartments to better resolve spatial details. This relationship of stiffness to the number of compartments is related to the inequality that must be satisfied for numerical stability of the forward Euler method for these PDEs (Lambert 1973).

References

Abbott, L. F., and Kepler, T. (1990). Model neurons: From Hodgkin-Huxley to Hopfield. In *Statistical mechanics of neural networks*, ed. L. Garrido, pp. 5–18. Berlin: Springer.

Abbott, L. F., and LeMasson, G. (1993). Analysis of neuron models with dynamically regulated conductances. *Neur. Comput.* 5: 823–842.

Abbott, L. F., Marder, E., and Hooper, S. L. (1991). Oscillating networks: Control of burst duration by electrically coupled neurons. *Neur. Comput.* 3: 487–497.

Abbott, L. F., Varela, J. A., Sen, K., and Nelson, S. B. (1997). Synaptic depression and cortical gain control. *Science.* 275: 220–224.

Abeles, M. (1990). *Corticonics: Neural circuits of the cerebral cortex.* Cambridge: Cambridge University Press.

Acerbo, P., and Nobile, M. (1994). Temperature dependence of multiple high-voltage-activated Ca^{2+} channels in chick sensory neurones. *Eur. Biophys. J.* 23: 189–195.

Adams, P. R., and Brown, D. A. (1982). Pharmacological inhibition of the M-current. *J. Physiol.* 332: 263–272.

Adams, P. R., Brown, D. A., and Constanti, A. (1982). M-currents and other potassium currents in bullfrog sympathetic neurones. *J. Physiol.* 330: 537–572.

Adams, P. R., Brown, D. A., and Constanti, A. (1982). Voltage clamp analysis of membrane currents underlying repetitive firing of bullfrog sympathetic neurons. In *Physiology and pharmacology of epileptogenic phenomena*, ed. M. R. Klee, pp. 175–187. New York: Raven Press.

Adams, P. R., Jones, S. W., Pennefather, P., Brown, D. A., Koch, C., and Lancaster, B. (1986). Slow synaptic transmission in frog sympathetic ganglia. *J. exp. Biol.* 124: 259–285.

Agmon-Snir, H. (1995). A novel theoretical approach to the analysis of dendritic transients. *Biophys. J.* 69: 1633–1656.

Agmon-Snir, H., and Segev, I. (1993). Signal delay and inputs synchronization in passive dendritic structures. *J. Neurophysiol.* 70: 2066–2085.

Agmon-Snir, H., and Segev, I. (1996). The concept of decision points as a tool in analyzing dendritic computation. In: *Computational neuroscience—Trends in research 1995*, ed. J. M. Bower, pp. 41–46. New York: Academic Press.

Aharon, S., Parnas, H., and Parnas, I. (1994). The magnitude and significance of Ca^{2+} domains for release of neurotransmitter. *Bull. Math. Biol.* 56: 1095–1119.

Ahmed, B., Anderson, J. C., Douglas, R. J., Martin, K. A. C., and Whitteridge, D. (1994). The current-discharge patterns of identified neurons in cat visual cortex.

Ahmed, B., Douglas, R. J, Martin, K. A. C., and Nelson, J. C. (1994). Map of the synapses formed with the dendrites of spiny stellate neurons in cat visual cortex. *J. Comp. Neurol.* 341: 16–24.

Aidley, D. J. (1991). *The physiology of excitable cells.* Cambridge: Cambridge University Press.

Albritton, M. L., Meyer, T., and Stryer, L. (1992). Range of messenger action of calcium ion and inositol 1,4,5-triphosphate. *Science* 258: 1812–1815.

Aldrich R. W., Corey, D. P., and Stevens, C. F. (1983). A reinterpretation of mammalian sodium channel gating based on single channel recording. *Nature* 306: 436–441.

Aldrich, R. W. (1981). Inactivation of voltage-gated delayed potassium current in molluscan neurons. *Biophys. J.* 36: 519–532.

Aldrich, R. W., and Stevens, C. F. (1987). Voltage-dependent gating of single sodium channels from mammalian neuroblastoma cells. *J. Neurosci.* 7: 418–431.

Alkon, D. L. (1984). Calcium-mediated reduction of ionic currents: A biophysical memory trace. *Science* 226: 1037–1045.

Allan, C., and Stevens, C. F. (1994). An evaluation of causes for unreliability of synaptic transmission. *Proc. Natl. Acad. Sci. U.S.A.* 91: 10380–10383.

Alonso, A., and Klink, R. (1993). Differential electroresponsiveness of stellate and pyramidal-like cells of medial entorhinal cortex layer II. *J. Neurophysiol.* 70: 128–143.

Alzheimer, C., Schwindt, P. C. and Crill, W. E. (1993). Modal gating of Na^+ channels as a mechanism of persistent Na^+ current in pyramidal neurons from rat and cat sensorimotor cortex. *J. Neurosci.* 13: 660–673.

Amari, S. (1977). Dynamics of pattern formation in lateral-inhibition-type neural fields. *Biol. Cybern.* 27: 77–87.

Amari, S., and Arbib, M. A. (1977). Competition and cooperation in neural nets. In *Systems neuroscience*, ed. J. Metzler, pp. 119–165. New York: Academic Press.

Amit, D. J. (1989). *Modeling brain function.* Cambridge: Cambridge University Press.

Amit, D. J, Gutfreund, H., and Sompolinsky, H. (1985). Spin-glass models of neural networks. *Physiol. Rev.* A2: 1007–1018.

Amitai, Y., Friedman, A., Connors, B. W., and Gutnick, M. J. (1993). Regenerative electrical activity in apical dendrites of pyramidal cells in neocortex. *Cerebral Cortex* 3: 26–38.

Anderson, J. C., Dehay, C., Friedlander, M. J., Martin, K. A. C., and Nelson, J. C. (1992). Synaptic connections of physiologically identified geniculocortical axons in kitten cortical area 17. *Proc. Roy. Soc. Lond.* B250: 187–194.

Anderson, J. C., Douglas, R. J., Martin, K. A. C., and Nelson, J. C. (1994). Map of the synapses formed with the dendrites of spiny stellate neurons of cat visual cortex. *J. Comp. Neurol.* 341: 25–38.

Anderson, T. W. (1994). *The statistical analysis of time series*, New York: J. Wiley.

Andreasen, M., and Lambert, J. D. (1995). The excitability of CA1 pyramidal cell dendrites is modulated by a local Ca^{2+}-dependent K^+ conductance. *Brain Res.* 698: 193–203.

Angelides, K. J., Elmer, L. W., Loftus, D., and Elson, E. (1988). Distribution and lateral mobility of voltage-dependent sodium channels in neurons. *J. Cell Biol.* 106: 1911–1924.

Angstadt, J. D., and Calabrese, R. L. (1991). Calcium currents and graded synaptic transmission between heart interneurons of the leech. *J. Neurosci.* 11: 746–759.

Antić, S., and Zečević, D. (1995). Optical signals from neurons with internally applied voltage-sensitive dyes. *J. Neurosci.* 15: 1392–1405.

Armstrong, C. M., and Bezanilla, F. (1977). Inactivation of the sodium channel: 1. Sodium current experiments; 2. Gating current experiments. *J. Gen. Physiol.* 70: 549–590.

Artola, A., and Singer, W. (1993). Long-term depression of excitatory synaptic transmission and its relationship to long-term potentiation. *Trends Neurosci.* 16: 480–487.

Augustine, G. J., and Charlton, M. P. (1986). Calcium dependence of presynaptic calcium current and post-synaptic response at the squid giant synapse. *J. Physiol.* 381: 619–640.

Augustine, G. J., Charlton, M. P., and Smith, S. J. (1985). Calcium entry and transmitter release at voltage-clamped nerve terminals of squid. *J. Physiol.* 367: 163–181.

Azouz, R., Jensen, M. S., and Yaari, Y. (1996). Ionic basis of spike after-depolarization and burst generation in adult rat hippocampal CA1 pyramidal cells. *J. Physiol.* 492: 211–223.

Back, A., Guckenheimer, J., Myers, M., Wicklin, F. and Worfolk, P. (1992). *dstool*: Computer-assisted exploration of dynamical systems. *Not. Am. Math. Soc.* 39: 303–309.

Baer, S. M., Rinzel, J., and Carrillo, H. (1995). Analysis of an autonomous phase model for neuronal parabolic bursting. *J. Math. Biol.* 33: 309–333.

Baer, S. M., and Tier, C. (1986). An analysis of a dendritic neuron model with an active membrane site. *J. Math. Biol.* 23: 137–161.

Bair, W., Koch, C., Newsome, W., and Britten, K. (1994). Power spectrum analysis of bursting cells in area MT in the behaving monkey. *J. Neurosci.* 14: 2870–2892.

Bal, T., Nagy, F., and Moulins, M. (1988). The pyloric central pattern generator in crustacea: A set of conditional neuronal oscillators. *J. Comp. Physiol.* 163: 715–727.

Bal, T., Nagy, F., and Moulins, M. (1994). Muscarinic modulation of a pattern-generating network: Control of neuronal properties. *J. Neurosci.* 14: 3019–3035.

Bal, T., von Krosigk, M., and McCormick, D. A. (1995a). Synaptic and membrane mechanisms underlying synchronized oscillations in the ferret lateral geniculate nucleus *in vitro*. *J. Physiol.* 483: 641–663.

Bal, T., von Krosigk, M., and McCormick, D. A. (1995b). Role of the ferret perigeniculate nucleus in the generation of synchronized oscillations *in vitro*. *J. Physiol.* 483: 665–685.

Baldi, P., Vanier, M. C., and Bower, J. M. (1996). On the use of Bayesian methods for evaluating compartmental neural models. Technical report, California Institute of Technology, ftp://achive.cis.ohiostate.edu/pub/neuroprose/baldi.comp.tar.Z.

Baluk, P. (1986). Scanning electron microscopic studies of bullfrog sympathetic neurons exposed by enzymatic removal of connective tissue elements and satellite cells. *J. Neurocytol.* 15: 85–95.

Banks, M. I., Haberly, L. B., and Jackson, M. B. (1996). Layer-specific properties of the transient K^+ current (I_A) in piriform cortex. *J. Neurosci.* 16: 3862–3876.

Banks, M. I., Haberly, L. B., and Jackson, M. B. (1996). Layer-specific properties of the transient K current (I_A) in piriform cortex. *J. Neurosci.* 16: 3862–3876.

Barchi, R. L. (1987). Sodium channel diversity: Subtle variations on a complex theme. *Trends Neurosci.* 10: 221–223.

Barkai, E., and Hasselmo, M. E. (1994). Modulation of the input/output function of rat piriform cortex pyramidal cells. *J. Neurophysiol.* 72: 644–658.

Barlow, H. B., Levick, W. R., and Yoon, M. (1971). Responses to single quanta of light in retinal ganglion cells of the cat. *Vis. Res. Supp.* 3: 87–101.

Barrett, J. N., and Crill, W. E. (1974a). Specific membrane properties of cat motoneurones. *J. Physiol.* 239: 301–324.

Barrett, J. N., and Crill, W. E. (1974b). Influence of dendritic location and membrane properties on the effectiveness of synapses on cat motoneurones. *J. Physiol.* 239: 325–345.

Barrett, J. N., Magleby, K. L., and Pallotta, B. S. (1982). Properties of single calcium-activated potassium channels in cultured rat muscle. *J. Physiol.* 331: 211–230.

Bartol, T. M., Land, B. R., Salpeter, E. E., and Salpeter, M. M. (1991). Monte Carlo simulation of miniature end-plate current generation in the vertebrate neuromuscular junction. *Biophys. J.* 59: 1290–1307.

Bartol, T. M., and Sejnowski, T. J. (1993). Model of the quantal activation of NMDA receptors at a hippocampal synaptic spine. *Soc. Neurosci. Abstr.* 19: 1515.

Bartol, T. M., Stiles, J. R., Salpeter, M. M., Salpeter, E. E., and Sejnowski, T. J. (1996). MCELL: Generalized Monte Carlo computer simulation of synaptic transmission and chemical signaling. *Soc. Neurosci. Abstr.* 22: 1742.

Baudry, M., and Davis, J. L., eds. (1994). *Long-term potentiation: A debate of current issues.* Cambridge, MA: MIT Press.

Baum, R. F. (1957). The correlation function of smoothly limited Gaussian noise. *IRE Trans. Inf. Th.* 3: 193–197.

Bayly, E. J. (1968). Spectral analysis of pulse frequency modulation in the nervous system. *IEEE Trans. Biomed. Eng.* 15: 257–265.

Bean, B. P. (1981). Sodium channel inactivation in the crayfish giant axon: Must channels open before inactivating? *Biophys. J.* 35: 595–614.

Bell, A. J. (1992). Self-organization in real neurons: Anti-Hebb in "channel space"? In *Advances in Neural information processing systems*, ed. J. Moody, S. Hanson, and R. Lippmann, pp. 59–66. Morgan Kaufmann, San Mateo.

Ben-Yishai, R. (1997). Cooperative properties of neuronal networks in visual cortex. Ph.D. diss., Hebrew University, Jerusalem.

Ben-Yishai, R., Hansel, D., and Sompolinsky, H. (1997). Traveling waves and processing of weakly tuned inputs in cortical module. *J. Comput. Neurosci.* 4: 57–77.

Ben-Yishai, R., Lev Bar-Or, R., and Sompolinsky, H. (1995). Theory of orientation tuning in visual cortex. *Proc. Natl. Acad. Sci. U.S.A.* 92: 3844–3848.

Bendat, J. S. (1990). *Nonlinear system analysis and identification from random data.* New York: Wiley.

Bernander, Ö., Douglas, R. J., Martin, K. A. C., and Koch, C. (1991). Synaptic background activity influences spatiotemporal integration in single pyramidal cells. *Proc. Natl. Acad. Sci. U.S.A.* 88: 11569–11573.

Bernander, Ö., Koch, C., and Douglas, R. J. (1994). Amplification and linearization of distal synaptic input to cortical pyramidal cells. *J. Neurophysiol.* 72: 2743–2753.

Berridge, M. J. (1993). Inositol triphosphate and calcium signalling. *Nature* 361: 315–325.

Bezprozvanny, I., Watras, J., and Ehrlich, B. E. (1991). Bell-shaped calcium-dependent curves of Ins (1,4,5)P3-gated and calcium-gated channels from endoplasmic reticulum of cerebellum. *Nature* 351: 751–754.

Bhalla, U. S. (1997). The network within: Signalling pathways. In *The Book of GENESIS.* 2d ed., ed. J. M. Bower and D. Beeman, pp. 169–192. New York: Springer.

Bhalla, U. S., and Bower, J. M. (1993). Exploring parameter space in detailed single neuron models: Simulations of the mitral and granule cells of the olfactory bulb. *J. Neurophysiol.* 69: 1948–1965.

Bialek, W., Rieke, F., de Ruyter van Steveninck, R. R., and Warland, D. (1991). Reading a neural code. *Science* 252: 1854–1857.

Biedenbach, M. A., and Stevens, C. F. (1969a). Electrical activity in cat olfactory cortex produced by synchronous orthodromic volleys, *J. Neurophysiol.* 32: 193–203.

Biedenbach, M. A., and Stevens, C. F. (1969b). Electrical activity in cat olfactory cortex as revealed by intracellular recording. *J. Neurophysiol.* 32: 204–214.

Birinyi, A., Antal, M., Wolf, E., and Szekely, G. (1992). The extent of the dendritic tree and the number of synapses in the frog motoneuron. *Eur. J. Neurosci.* 4: 1003–1012.

Black, J. A., Kocsis, J. D. and Waxman, S. G. (1990). Ion channel organization of the myelinated fiber. *Trends Neurosci.* 13: 48–54.

Blaustein, M. P., and Hodgkin A. L. (1969). The effect of cyanide on the efflux of calcium from squid axon. *J. Physiol.* 200: 497–527.

Blight, A. R. (1985). Computer simulation of action potentials and afterpotentials in mammalian myelinated axons: The case for a lower resistance myelin sheath. *Neurosci.* 15: 13–31.

Bliss, T. V. P., and Collingridge, G. L. (1993). A synaptic model of memory: Long-term potentiation in the hippocampus. *Nature* 361: 31–39.

Bloomfield, S. A., Hamos, J. E., and Sherman, S. M. (1987). Passive cable properties and morphological correlates of neurones in the lateral geniculate of the cat. *J. Physiol.* 383: 653–692.

Blumenfeld, H., Zablow, L., and Sabatini, B. (1992). Evaluation of cellular mechanisms for modulation of calcium transients using a mathematical model of fura-2 Ca^{2+} imaging in *Aplysia* sensory neurons. *Biophys. J.* 63: 1146–1164.

Borg-Graham, L. J. (1998). Interpretations of data and mechanisms for hippocampal pyramidal cell models In: *Cerebral cortex,* Vol. 12: *Cortical models,* eds. E. G. Jones, and P. S. Ulinski. New York: Plenum Press.

Borg-Graham, L. (1998). Interpretations of data and mechanisms for hippocampal pyramidal cell model. In: *Cerebral cortex.* Vol. 13: *Coctical models,* eds. P. S. Ulinski, E. G. Jones, and A. Peters. New York: Plenum.

Bormann, G., and De Schutter, E. (1996). Monte Carlo simulation of 3-D calcium diffusion in detailed neuronal models. *2nd Meeting Europ. Neurosci.* 13. Abstr. 9.21.

Borst, A., and Egelhaaf, M. (1994). Dendritic processing of synaptic information by sensory interneurons. *Trends Neurosci.* 17: 257–263.

Bower, J. M. (1990). Reverse engineering the nervous system: An anatomical, physiological, and computer based approach. In *An introduction to neural and electronic networks*, ed. S. F. Zornetzer, J. L. Davis and C. Lau, pp. 3–24. Academic Press.

Bower, J. M. (1995a). Constructing new models. In *The book of GENESIS: Exploring realistic neural models with the GEneral NEural SImulation System*, ed. J. M. Bower and D. Beeman, pp. 183–190. New York: Springer.

Bower, J. M. (1995b). Reverse engineering the nervous system: An *in vivo, in vitro*, and *in computo* approach to understanding the mammalian olfactory system. In *An introduction to neural and electronic networks*, ed. S. F. Zornetzer, J. L. Davis and C. Lau, 2d ed., pp. 3–28. New York: Academic Press.

Bower, J. M. (1996). What will save neuroscience? *Neuroimage* 4: S29–S33.

Bower, J. M., and Beeman, D. (1995). *The book of GENESIS: Exploring realistic neural models with the GEneral NEural SImulation System*. New York: Springer.

Bower, J. M., and Beeman, D. (1997). *The book of GENESIS*, 2nd edition. New York: TELOS.

Bower, J. M., and Haberly, L. B. (1986). Facilitating and nonfacilitating synapses on pyramidal cells: A correlation between physiology and morphology. *Proc. Natl. Acad. Sci. U.S.A.* 83: 1115–1119.

Boyce, W. E., and DiPrima, R. C. (1992). *Elementary differential equations and boundary value problems.* New York: Wiley.

Brazier, M. A. B. (1959). The historical development of neurophysiology. In: *Handbook of physiology (sect. 1). The nervous system. I. Cellular biology of neurons*, eds. Field, Magoun, and Hall, pp. 1–58. Washington, D.C.: American Physiology Society.

Bressler, S. L. (1984). Spatial organization of EEGs from olfactory bulb and cortex. *Electroencephalogr. and Clin. Neurophysiol.* 57: 270–276.

Britten, K. H., Shadlen, M. N., Newsome, W. T., and Movshon, A. (1992). The analysis of visual motion: A comparison of neuronal and psychophysical performance. *J. Neurosci.* 12: 4745–4765.

Brown, A. M., and Birnbaumer, L. (1990). Ionic channels and their regulation by G-protein subunits. *Ann. Rev. Physiol.* 52: 197–213.

Brown, A. M., Schwindt, P. C., and Crill, W. E. (1993). Voltage dependence and activation kinetics of pharmacologically defined components of the high-threshold calcium current in rat neocortical neurons. *J. Neurophysiol.* 70: 1530–1543.

Brown, A. M., Schwindt, P. C., and Crill, W. E. (1996). Different voltage dependence of transient and persistent Na$^+$ currents is compatible with modal-gating hypothesis for sodium channels. *J. Neurophysiol.* 71: 2562–2565.

Brown, D. A. (1990). G-proteins and potassium currents in neurons. *Ann. Rev. Physiol.* 52: 215–242.

Brown, T. H., and Johnston, D. (1983). Voltage-clamp analysis of mossy fiber synaptic input to hippocampal neuron. *J. Neurophysiol.* 50: 487–507.

Buchholtz, F., Golowasch, J., Epstein, I. R., and Marder, E. (1992). Mathematical model of an identified stomatogastric ganglion neuron. *J. Neurophysiol.* 67: 332–340.

Bunow, B., Segev, I., and Fleshman, J. W. (1985). Modeling the electrical properties of anatomically complex neurons using a network analysis program: Excitable membrane. *Biol. Cybern.* 53: 41–56.

Burgard, E. C., and Hablitz, J. J. (1993). NMDA receptor–mediated components of miniature excitatory synaptic currents in developing rat neocortex. *J. Neurophysiol.* 70: 1841–1852.

Burke, R. E., and Glenn, L. L. (1996). Horseradish peroxidase study of the spatial and electrotonic distribution of group Ia synapses on type-identified ankle extensor motoneurons in the cat. *J. Comp. Neurol.* 372: 465–485.

Burke, R. E., Fyffe, R. E. W., and Moschovakis, A. K. (1994). Electrotonic architecture of cat gamma motoneurons. *J. Neurophysiol.* 72: 2302–2316.

Busch, C., Sakmann, B. (1990). Synaptic transmission in hippocampal neurons: Numerical reconstruction of quantal IPSCs. *Cold Spr. Harb. Symp. Quant. Biol.* 55: 69–80.

Bush, P. C., and Sejnowski, T. J. (1991). Simulations of a reconstructed cerebellar Purkinje cell based on simplified channel kinetics. *Neur. Comput.* 3: 321–332.

Bush, P. C., and Sejnowski, T. J. (1993). Reduced compartmental models of neocortical pyramidal cells. *J. Neurosci. Meth.* 46: 159–166.

Bush, P., and Sejnowski, T. (1996). Inhibition synchronizes sparsely connected cortical neurons within and between columns in realistic network models. *J. Comput. Neurosci.* 3: 91–110.

Butera, R. J., Clark, J. W., and Byrne, J. H. (1996). Dissection and reduction of a modeled bursting neuron. *J. Comput. Neurosci.* 3: 199–223.

Butz, E. G., and Cowan, J. D. (1974). Transient potentials in dendritic systems of arbitrary geometry. *Biophys. J.* 14: 661–689.

Buzsaki, G., Penttonen, M., Nadasdy, Z., and Bragin, A. (1996). Pattern and inhibition-dependent invasion of pyramidal cell dendrites by fast spikes in the hippocampus *in vivo*. *Proc. Natl. Acad. Sci. U.S.A.* 93: 9921–9925.

Calabrese, R. L., and De Schutter, E. (1992). Motor pattern generating networks in invertebrates: Modeling our way toward understanding. *Trends Neurosci.* 15: 439–445.

Calvin, W., and Stevens, C. F. (1968). Synaptic noise and other sources of randomness in motoneuron interspike intervals. *J. Neurophysiol.* 31: 574–587.

Campbell, F. W., Cooper, G. F., and Enroth-Cugell, C. (1969). The spatial selectivity of the visual cells of the cat. *J. Physiol.* 203: 223–235.

Canavier, C. C., Baxter, D. A., Clark, J. W., and Byrne, J. H. (1993). Nonlinear dynamics in a model neuron provide a novel mechanism for transient synaptic inputs to produce long-term alterations of post-synaptic activity. *J. Neurophysiol.* 69: 2252–2257.

Cannon, S., Robinson, D., and Shamma, S. (1983). A proposed neural network for the integrator of the oculomotor system. *Biol. Cybern.* 49: 127.

Cao, B. J., and Abbott, L. F. (1993). A new computational method for cable theory problems. *Biophys. J.* 64: 303–313.

Carbone, E., and Lux, H. D. (1984). A low voltage activated fully inactivating Ca-channel in vertebrate sensory neurones. *Nature* 310: 501–502.

Carnevale, N. T., and Rosenthal, S. (1992). Kinetics of diffusion in a spherical cell: 1. No solute buffering. *J. Neurosci. Meth.* 41: 205–216.

Carnevale, N. T., Tsai, K. Y., and Hines, M. L. (1996). The electrotonic workbench. *Soc. Neurosci. Abstr.* 22: 1741. Abstract 687.1

Carter, G. C. (1987). Coherence and time delay estimation. In *Traitement du signal: Statistical signal processing*, eds. J. L. Lacoume, T. S. Durrani, and R. Stora, pp. 515–571. Les Houches Summer School in Theoretical Physics, XLV, Amsterdam: North Holland.

Cauller, L. J., and Connors, B. W. (1992). Functions of very distal dendrites: Experimental and computational studies of layer 1 synapses on neocortical pyramidal cells. In *Single neuron computation*, ed. T. McKenna, J. Javis, and S. F. Zarnetzer, pp. 199–229. Boston: Academic Press.

Cauller, L. J., and Connors, B. W. (1994). Synaptic physiology of horizontal afferents to layer 1 in slices of rat SI neocortex. *J. Neurosci.* 14: 751–762.

Celentano, J. J., and Wong, R. K. (1994). Multiphasic desensitization of the $GABA_A$ receptor in outside-out patches. *Biophys. J.* 66: 1039–1050.

Chad, J. E., and Eckert, R. (1984). Calcium domains associated with individual channels can account for anomalous voltage relations of Ca-dependent responses. *Biophys. J.* 45: 993–999.

Chad, J. E., and Eckert, R. (1986). An enzymatic mechanism for calcium current inactivation in dialysed helix neurones. *J. Physiol.* 378: 31–51.

Chagnac-Amitai, Y., Luhmann, H. J., and Prince, D. A. (1990). Burst generating and regular spiking layer 5 pyramidal neurons of rat neocortex have different morphological features. *J. Comp. Neurol.* 296: 598–613.

Chapman, B., Zahs, K. R., and Stryker, M. P. (1991). Relation of cortical cell orientation selectivity to alignment of receptive fields of the geniculocortical afferents that arborize within a single orientation column in ferret visual cortex. *J. Neurosci.* 11: 1347–1358.

Chay, T. R., and Keizer, J. E. (1983). Minimal model for membrane oscillations in the pancreatic β-cell. *Biophys. J.* 42: 181–190.

Christie, A. E., Skiebe, P., and Marder, E. (1995). Matrix of neuromodulators in neurosecretory structures of the crab *Cancer borealis. J. Exp. Biol.* 198: 2431–2439.

Christie, B. R., Eliot, L. S., Ito, K., Miyakawa, H., and Johnston, D. (1995). Different Ca^{2+} channels in soma and dendrites of hippocampal pyramidal neurons mediate spike-induced Ca^{2+} influx. *J. Neurophysiol.* 73: 2553–2557.

Christie, M. J. (1995). Molecular and functional diversity of K^+ channels. *Clin. Exp. Pharmacol. Physiol.* 22: 944–951.

Chung, S.-H., Raymond, S. A., and Lettvin, J. Y. (1970). Multiple meaning in single visual units. *Brain Behav. Evol.* 3: 72–101.

Claiborne, B. J. (1992). The use of computers for the quantitative, three-dimensional analysis of dendritic trees. In *Methods in neuroscience*, ed. P. M. Conn. Vol. 10, *Computers and computation in the neurosciences*, pp. 315–330. New York: Academic Press.

Clapham, D. E. (1995). Calcium signaling. *Cell* 80: 259–268.

Clarey, J., Barone, P., and Imig, T. (1992). Physiology of thalamus and cortex. In *The mammalian auditory pathway: Neurophysiology*, ed. D. Webster, A. Popper, and R. Fay, pp. 232–334. New York: Springer.

Clay, J. R., and DeFelice, L. J. (1983). Relationship between membrane excitability and single channel open-close kinetics.

Clements, J. D. (1996). Transmitter time course in the synaptic cleft: Its role into central synaptic function. *Trends Neurosci.* 19: 163–171.

Clements, J. D., Lester, R. A. J., Tong, G., Jahr, C. E., and Westbrook, G. L. (1992). The time course of glutamate in the synaptic cleft. *Science* 258: 1498–1501.

Clements, J., and Redman, S. (1989). Cable properties of cat spinal motoneurones measured by combining voltage clamp, current clamp and intracellular staining. *J. Physiol.* 409: 63–87.

Clements, J. D., Westbrook, G. L. (1991). Activation kinetics reveal the number of glutamate and glycine binding sites on the N-methyl-D-aspartate receptor. *Neuron* 258: 605–613.

Cohn, T. E., Green, D. G., and Tanner, W. P. (1975). Receiver operating characteristic analysis, application to the study of quantum fluctuation effects in optic nerve of *Rana pipiens. J. Gen. Physiol.* 66: 583–616.

Colbert, C. M., and Johnston, D. (1996). Axonal action potential initiation and Na^+ channel densities in the soma and axon initial segment of subicular pyramidal neurons. *J. Neurosci.* 16: 6676–6686.

Cole, K. S. (1968). *Membrane, ions and impulses: A chapter of classical biophysics.* Berkeley: University of California Press.

Cole, K. S., Guttman, R., and Bezanilla, F. (1970). Nerve excitation without threshold. *Proc. Natl. Acad. Sci. U.S.A.* 65: 884–891.

Colquhoun, D., Jonas, P., and Sakmann, B. (1992). Action of brief pulses of glutamate on AMPA/ Kainate receptors in patches from different neurons of rat hippocampal slices. *J. Physiol.* 458: 261–287.

Connor, J. A., Walter, D. and McKown, R. (1977). Neural repetitive firing: Modifications of the Hodgkin-Huxley axon suggested by experimental results from crustacean axons. *Biophys. J.* 18: 81–102.

Connors, B. W., and Gutnick, M. J. (1990). Intrinsic firing patterns of diverse neocortical neurons. *Trends Neurosci.* 13: 99–104.

Connors, B. W., Gutnick, M. J., and Prince, D. A. (1982). Electrophysiological properties of neocortical neurons in vitro. *J. Neurophysiol.* 48: 1302–1320.

Connors, J. A., and Stevens, C. (1971). Prediction of repetitive firing behavior from voltage clamp data on an isolated neurons soma. *J. Physiol.* 213: 31–53.

Constanti, A., and Galvan, M. (1983). M-current in voltage-clamped olfactory cortex neurones. *Neurosci. Lett.* 39: 65–70.

Constanti, A., and Galvan, M. (1983a). Fast-inward rectifying current accounts for anomalous rectification in olfactory cortex neurones. *J. Physiol.* 385: 153–178.

Constanti, A., and Galvan, M. (1983b). M-current in voltage-clamped olfactory cortex neurones. *Neurosci. Lett.* 39: 65–70.

Constanti, A., and Sim, J. A. (1987a). Calcium-dependent potassium conductance in guinea-pig olfactory cortex neurones *in vitro*. *J. Physiol.* 387: 173–194.

Constanti, A., and Sim, J. A. (1987b). Muscarinic receptors mediating suppression of the M-current in guinea-pig olfactory cortex neurones may be of the M_2-subtype, *Br. J. Pharmacol.* 90: 3–5.

Constanti, A., Galvan, M., Franz, P., and Sim, J. A. (1985). Calcium-dependent inward currents in voltage clamped guinea-pig olfactory cortex neurones. *Pflügers Arch.* 404: 259–265.

Constantine-Paton, M., Cline, H. T., and Debski, E. (1990). Patterned activity, synaptic convergence, and the NMDA receptor in developing visual pathways. *Ann. Rev. Neurosci.* 13: 129–154.

Conte, S. D., and de Boor, C. (1980), *Elementary numerical analysis: An algorithmic approach*. 3d ed. New York: McGraw-Hill.

Cooley, J. W., and Dodge, F. A. (1966). Digital computer solutions for excitation and propagation of the nerve impulse. *Biophys. J.* 6: 583–599.

Coombs, J. S., Curtis, D. R., and Eccles, J. C. (1957a). The generation of impulses in motoneurones. *J. Physiol.* 139: 232–249.

Coombs, J. S., Curtis, D. R., and Eccles, J. C. (1957b). The interpretation of spike potentials of motoneurones. *J. Physiol.* 139: 198–231.

Coombs, J. S., Eccles, J. C., and Fatt, P. (1955a). The electrical properties of the motoneurone membrane. *J. Physiol.* 130: 291–325.

Coombs, J. S., Eccles, J. C., and Fatt, P. (1955b). The specific ionic conductances and the ionic movements across the motoneurone membrane that produce the inhibitory post-synaptic potential. *J. Physiol.* 130: 326–373.

Coronado, R., Morrissette, J., Sukhareva, M., and Vaughan, D. M. (1994). Structure and function of ryanodine receptors. *Am. J. Physiol.* 266: C1485–C1504.

Cox, D. R. (1962). *Renewal theory*. London: Methuen.

Cox, D. R., and Isham, V. (1980). *Point processes*. London: Chapman and Hall.

Cox, D. R., and Lewis, P. A. W. (1966). *The statistical analysis of series of events*. London: Chapman and Hall.

Crank, J. (1975). *The mathematics of diffusion*. 2d ed. Oxford: Clarendon Press.

Crank, J., and Nicolson, P. (1947). A practical method for numerical evaluation of solutions of partial differential equations of the heat conduction type. *Proc. Camb. Philos. Soc.* 43: 50–67.

Crick, F., and Koch, C. (1990). Towards a neurobiological theory of consciousness. *Semin. Neurosci.* 2: 263–275.

Crill, W. E. (1996). Persistent sodium current in mammalian central neurons. *Ann. Rev. Physiol.* 58: 349–362.

Cullheim, S., Fleshman, J. W., Glenn, L. L., and Burke, R. E. (1987a). Three-dimensional architecture of dendritic trees in type-identified alpha-motoneurons. *J. Comp. Neurol.* 255: 82–96.

Cullheim, S., Fleshman, J. W., Glenn, L. L., and Burke, R. E. (1987b). Membrane area and dendritic structure in type-identified tricpes surae alpha-motoneurons. *J. Comp. Neurol.* 255: 68–81.

Cummins, T. R., Xia, Y., and Haddad, G. G. (1994). Functional properties of rat and human neocortical voltage-sensitive sodium currents. *J. Neurophysiol.* 71: 1052–1064.

Dahlquist, G., and Bjorck, A. (1974). *Numerical methods.* Englewood Cliffs, NJ: Prentice-Hall.

Dan, Y., Atick, J. J., and Reid, R. C. (1996). Efficient coding of natural scenes in the lateral geniculate nucleus: Experimental test of a computational theory. *J. Neurosci.* 16: 3351–3362.

Davies, C. H., Davies, S. N., and Collingridge, G. L. (1990). Paired-pulse depression of monosynaptic GABA-mediated inhibitory postsynaptic responses in rat hippocampus. *J. Physiol.* 424: 513–531.

Davis, L., Jr., and Lorente de Nó, R. (1947). Contribution to the mathematical theory of the electrotonous. *Studies from the Rockfeller Institute for Medical Research* 131: 442–496.

Davies, P. J., Ireland, D. R., and McLachlan, E. M. (1996). Sources of Ca^{2+} for different Ca^{2+}-activated K^+ conductances in neurones of the rat superior cervical ganglion. *J. Physiol.* 495: 353–366.

de Boer, A. E. (1973). On the principle of specific coding. *J. Dynam. Syst., Meas., and Contr.* 95: 265–273.

de Boer, A. E., and DeJongh, H. R. (1975). On cochlear encoding: Potentialities and limitations of the revese-correlation technique. *J. Acoust. Soc. Am.* 63: 115–135.

De Koninck, Y., and Mody, I. (1994). Noise analysis of miniature IPSCs in adult rat brain slices: Properties and modulation of synaptic $GABA_A$ receptor channels. *J. Neurophysiol.* 71: 1318–1335.

De Schutter, E. (1992). A consumer guide to neuronal modeling software. *Trends Neurosci.* 15: 462–464.

De Schutter, E. (1995). Dendritic calcium channels amplify the variability of postsynaptic responses. *Abstr. Soc. Neurosci.* 21: 586. Abstr. 240. 18

De Schutter, E., and Bower, J. M. (1993). Sensitivity of synaptic plasticity to the Ca^{2+} permeability of NMDA channels: A model of long-term potentiation in hippocampal neurons. *Neural Comput.* 5: 681–694.

De Schutter, E. and Bower, J. M. (1994a). An active membrane model of the cerebellar Purkinje cell. I. Simulation of current clamps in slice. *J. Neurophysiol.* 71: 375–400.

De Schutter, E. and Bower, J. M. (1994b). An active membrane model of the cerebellar Purkinje cell. II. Simulation of synaptic responses. *J. Neurophysiol.* 71: 401–419.

De Schutter, E. and Bower, J. M. (1994c). Simulated responses of cerebellar Purkinje cells are independent of the dendritic location of granule cell synaptic inputs. *Proc. Natl. Acad. Sci. U.S.A.* 91: 4736–4740.

De Schutter, E., Angstadt, J. D., and Calabrese, R. L. (1993). A model of graded synaptic transmission for use in dynamic network simulations. *J. Neurophysiol.* 69: 1225–1235.

De Young, G. W., and Keizer, J. (1992). A single-pool inositol-1,4,5-triphosphate-receptor-based model for agonist-stimulated oscillations in Ca^{2+} concentration. *Proc. Natl. Acad. Sci. U.S.A.* 89: 9895–9899.

DeAngelis, G. C., Ohzawa, I., and Freeman, R. D. (1993). Spatiotemporal organization of simple-cell receptive fields in the cat's striate cortex: 2. Linearity of temporal and spatial summation. *J. Neurophysiol.* 69: 1118–1135.

Decharms, R. C., and Merzenich, M. M. (1996). Primary cortical representation of sounds by the coordination of action potential timing. *Nature* 381: 610–613.

DeCoursey, T. E. (1990). State-dependent inactivation of K currents in rat type II alveolar epithelial cells. *J. Gen. Physiol.* 95: 617–646.

Delgotte, B. (1984). Speech coding in the auditory nerve: II. processing scheme, for vowel-like sounds. *J. Acoust. Soc. Am.* 75: 879–886.

Deng, L., Geisler, C. D., and Greenberg, S. (1988). A composite model of the auditory periphery for the processing of speech. *J. Phonet.* 16(1): 93–108.

Denk, W., Delaney, K. R., Gelperin, A., Kleinfeld, D., Strowbridge, B. W., Tank, D. W., and Yuste, R. (1994). Anatomical and functional imaging of neurons using 2-photon laser scanning microscopy. *J. Neurosci. Meth.* 54: 151–162.

Denk, W., Sugimori, M., and Llinás, R. R. (1995). Two types of calcium response limited to single spines in cerebellar Purkinje cells. *Proc. Natl. Acad. Sci. U.S.A.* 92: 8279–8282.

Denk, W., and Svoboda, K. (1997). Photon upmanship: Why multiphoton imaging is more than a gimmick. *Neuron* 18: 351–357.

Denk, W., Yuste, R., Svoboda, K., and Tank, D. W. (1996). Imaging calcium dynamics in dendritic spines. *Curr. Opin. Neurobiol.* 6: 372–378.

Deschênes, M., and Landry, P. (1980). Axonal branch diameter and spacing of nodes in the terminal arborization of identified thalamic and cortical neurons. *Brain Res.* 191: 538–544.

Destexhe, A. (1997). Conductance-based integrate and fire models. *Neur. Comput.* 9: 503–514.

Destexhe, A., Bal, T., McCormick, D. A., and Sejnowski, T. J. (1996). Ionic mechanisms underlying synchronized oscillations and propagating waves in a model of ferret thalamic slices. *J. Neurophysiol.* 76: 2049–2070.

Destexhe, A., Contreras, D., Sejnowski, T. J., and Steriade, M. (1994). A model of spindle rhythmicity in the isolated thalamic reticular nucleus. *J. Neurophysiol.* 72: 803–818.

Destexhe, A., Contreras, D., Steriade, M., Sejnowski, T. J., and Huguenard, J. R. (1996). *In vivo, in vitro,* and computational analysis of dendritic calcium currents in thalamic reticular neurons. *J. Neurosci.* 16: 169–185.

Destexhe, A., Mainen, Z. F., and Sejnowski, T. J. (1994). Synthesis of models for excitable membranes, synaptic transmission, and neuromodulation using a common kinetic framework. *J. Comput. Neurosci.* 1: 195–230.

Destexhe, A., Mainen, Z., and Sejnowski, T. J. (1994a). An efficient method for computing synaptic conductances based on a kinetic model of receptor binding. *Neur. Comput.* 6: 14–18.

Destexhe, A., McCormick, D. A., and Sejnowski, T. J. (1993). A model for 8–10 Hz spindling in interconnected thalamic relay and reticular neurons. *Biophys. J.* 65: 2473–2477.

Destexhe, A., and Sejnowski. T. J. (1995). G-protein activation kinetics and spill-over of GABA may account for differences between inhibitory responses in the hippocampus and thalamus. *Proc. Natl. Acad. Sci. U.S.A.* 92: 9515–9519.

DeValois, R., and DeValois, K. (1990). *Spatial vision.* Oxford, U.K.: Oxford University Press.

Devor, M. (1976). Fiber trajectories of olfactory bulb afferents in hamster, *J. Comp. Neurol.* 166: 31–48.

Dichiara, T. J., and Reinhart, P. H. (1995). Distinct effects of Ca^{2+} and voltage on the activation and deactivation of cloned Ca^{2+}-activated K^+ channels. *J. Physiol.* 489: 403–418.

Dickinson, P. S., Mecsas, C., and Marder, E. (1990). Neuropeptide fusion of two motor pattern generator circuits. *Nature* 344: 155–158.

Didday, R. L. (1976). A model of visuomotor mechanisms in the frog optic tectum. *Math. Biosci.* 30: 169–180.

DiFrancesco, D., and Noble, D. (1985). A model of cardiac electrical activity incorporating ionic pumps and concentration changes. *Philos. Trans. Roy. Soc. London* B 307: 353–398.

DiPolo, R., and Beauge, L. (1983). The calcium pump and sodium-calcium exchange in squid axons. *Ann. Rev. Neurosci.* 45: 313–332.

Dodge, F. A., and Cooley, J. W. (1973). Action potential of the motorneuron. *IBM J. Res. Develop.* 17: 219–229.

Dodt, H. U., and Zieglgansberger, W. (1994). Infrared videomicroscopy: A new look at neuronal structure and function. *Trends Neurosci.* 17: 453–458.

Doedel, E. J. (1981). *AUTO*: A program for the automatic bifurcation and analysis of autonomous systems. *Cong. Num.* 30: 265–284.

Doedel, E. J., Keller, H. B., and Kernévez, J. P. (1991). Numerical analysis and control of bifurcation problems. 1. Bifurcation in finite dimensions. *Int. J. Bifurc. and Chaos* 1: 493–520.

Dong, D. W. (1995). Statistics of natural time-varying images. *Network: Comput. Neur. Syst.* 6: 345–358.

Dong, D. W., and Atick, J. J. (1995). Temporal decorrelation: A theory of lagged and nonlagged responses in the lateral geniculate nucleus. *Network: Comput. Neur. Syst.* 6: 159–178.

Douglas, J., Jr. (1961). A survey of numerical methods for parabolic differential equations. In *Advances in computers*, vol. 2, ed. F. Alt, pp. 1–54. New York: Academic Press.

Douglas, R. and M. Mahowald (1995). A constructor set for silicon neurons. In *An introduction to neural and electronic networks*, ed. S. F. Zornetzer, J. L. Davis, C. Lau, and T. McKenna, 2 ed., pp. 277–296. San Diego: Academic Press.

Douglas, R. J., Koch, C., Mahowald, M., Martin, K., and Suarez, H. (1995). Recurrent excitation in neocortical circuits. *Science* 269: 981–985.

Douglas, R., Mahowald, M., and Mead, C. (1995). Neuromorphic analog VLSI. *Ann. Rev. Neurosci.* 18: 255–281.

Douglas, R., and Martin, K. (1993). Exploring cortical microcircuits: A combined anatomical, physiological, and computational approach. In *Single neuron computation*, ed. J. D. T. McKenna and S. Zornetzer, pp. 381–412. Orlando, FL: Academic Press.

Douglas, R., Martin, K., and Whitteridge, D. (1991). An intracellular analysis of the visual responses of neurones in cat visual cortex. *J. Physiol.* 440: 659–696.

Doupnik, C. A., Davidson, N., and Lester, H. A. (1995). The inward rectifier potassium channel family. *Curr. Opin. Neurobiol.* 5: 268–277.

Droulez, J. and Berthoz, A. (1991) A neural network model of sensoritopic maps with predictive short-term memory properties. *Proc. Natl. Acad. Sci. U.S.A.* 88: 9653–9657.

Durand, D. (1984). The somatic shunt cable model for neurons. *Biophys. J.* 46: 645–653.

Dutar, P., and Nicoll, R. A. (1988). A physiological role for $GABA_B$ receptors in the central nervous system. *Nature* 332: 156–158.

Eckert, R., and Chad, J. E. (1984). Inactivation of calcium channels. *Prog. Biophys. Molec. Biol.* 44: 215–261.

Edelstein-Keshet, L. (1988). *Mathematical models in biology. New York*: Random House.

Edmonds, B., and Colquhoun, D. (1993). Rapid decay of averaged single-channel NMDA receptor activations recorded at low agonist concentration. *Proc. Roy. Soc. Lond.* B250: 279–286.

Eichenbaum, H., Otto, T. A., Wible, C. G. and Piper, J. M. (1991). Building a model of the hippocampus in olfaction and memory. In *Olfaction: A model system for computational neuroscience*, ed. J. L. Davis and H. Eichenbaum, pp. 167–210. Cambridge, MA: MIT Press.

Eichler-West, R. M., and Wilcox, G. L. (1995). On the use of genetic algorithms for parameter optimization in compartmental models of hippocampal neurons. *Soc. Neurosci. Abstr.* 21: 1996. Abstr. 473.8

Eilers, J., Augustine, G. J., and Konnerth, A. (1995). Subthreshold synaptic Ca^{2+} signaling in fine dendrites and spines of cerebellar Purkinje neurons. *Nature* 373: 155–158.

Eilers, J., Plant, T., and Konnerth, A. (1996). Localized calcium signaling and neuronal integration in cerebellar Purkinje neurones. *Cell Calcium* 20: 215–226.

Eisen, J. S., and Marder, E. (1982). Mechanisms underlying pattern generation in lobster stomatogastric ganglion as determined by selective inactivation of identified neurons: 3. Synaptic connections of electrically coupled pyloric neurons. *J. Neurophysiol.* 48: 1392–1415.

Eisen, J. S., and Marder, E. (1984). A mechanism for the production of phase shifts in a pattern generator. *J. Neurophysiol.* 51: 1375–1393.

Ekerot, C. F., and Oscarsson, O. (1981). Prolonged depolarization elicited in Purkinje cell dendrites by climbing fibre impulses in the cat. *J. Physiol.* 318: 207–221.

Elias, J. G. (1993). Artificial dendritic trees. *Neur. Comput.* 5:648–664.

Epstein, I. R., and Marder, E. (1990). Multiple modes of a conditional neural oscillator. *Biol. Cybern.* 63: 25–34.

Ermentrout, B. (1990). *PhasePlane: The dynamical systems tool.* Pacific Grove, CA: Brooks/Cole.

Ermentrout G., and Cowan, J. (1980). Large-scale spatially organized activity in neural nets. *SIAM J. Appl. Math.* 38: 1–21.

Ermentrout, G. B. (1982). Asymptotic behavior of stationary homogeneous neural nets. In *Competitions and cooperation in: neural nets*, ed. S. Amari and M. A. Arbib. Lecture Notes in Biomathematics. Springer.

Ermentrout, G. B. (1996). Type I membranes, phase resetting curves, and synchrony. *Neur. Comput.* 8: 979–1002.

Ermentrout, G. B., and Kopell, N. (1991). Multiple pulse interactions and averaging in systems of coupled neural oscillators. *J. Math. Biology* 29: 195–217.

Eskandar, E. N., Richmond, B. J., and Optican, L. M. (1992). Role of inferior temporal neurons in visual memory: 1. Temporal encoding of information about visual images, recalled images and behavioral context. *J. Neurophysiol.* 68: 1277–1295.

Evans, J. D., Major, G., and Kember, G. C. (1995). Techniques for the application of the analytical solution to the multicylinder somatic shunt cable model for passive neurones. *Math. Biosci.* 125: 1–50.

Fariñas, I., and DeFelipe, J. (1991). Patterns of synaptic input on corticocortical and corticothalamic cells in the cat visual cortex: II. The axon initial segment. *J. Comp. Neurol.* 304: 70–77.

Fatt, P. (1957). Sequence of events in synaptic activation of a motoneurone. *J. Neurophysiol.* 20: 61–80.

Fatt, P., and Katz, B. (1953). The effect of inhibitory nerve impulses on a crustacean muscle fibre. *J. Physiol.* 121: 374–389.

Ferster, D. (1986). Orientation selectivity of synaptic potentials in neurons of cat primary visual cortex. *J. Physiol* 6: 1284–1301.

Ferster, D., and Koch, C. (1987). Neuronal connections underlying orientation selectivity in cat visual cortex. *Trends Neurosci.* 10: 487–492.

Fick, A. (1885). Über Diffusion. *Ann. Phys. Chem.* 94: 59–86.

Fields, R. D., Neale, E. A., and Nelson, P. G. (1990). Effects of patterned electrical activity on neurite outgrowth from mouse neurons. *J. Neurosci.* 10: 2950–2964.

Fierro, L., and Llano, I. (1996). High endogenous calcium buffering in Purkinje cells from rat cerebellar slices. *J. Physiol.* 496: 617–625.

FitzHugh, R. (1960). Thresholds and plateaus in the Hodgkin-Huxley nerve equations. *J. Gen. Physiol.* 43: 867–896.

FitzHugh, R. (1961). Impulses and physiological states in models of nerve membrane. *Biophys. J.* 1: 445–466.

FitzHugh, R. (1969). Mathematical models for excitation and propagation in nerve. In: *Biological engineering*, ed. H. P. Schwan, New York: McGraw Hill.

Flamm, R. E., and Harris-Warrick, R. M. (1986). Aminergic modulation in the lobster stomatogastric ganglion: 1. Effects on the motor pattern and activity of neurons within the pyloric circuit. *J. Neurophysiol.* 55: 847–865.

Fleshman, J. W., Segev, I., and Burke, R. E. (1988). Electrotonic architecture of type-identified alpha-motoneurons in the cat spinal cord. *J. Neurophysiol.* 60: 60–85.

Fletcher, C. A. J. (1991). *Computational techniques for fluid dynamics.* Vol. 1. Berlin: Springer.

Foster, W. R., Ungar, L. H. and Schwaber, J. S. (1993). Significance of conductances in Hodgkin-Huxley models. *J. Neurophysiol.* 70: 2502–2518.

Fox, R. F., and Lu, Y.-N. (1994). Emergent collective behavior in large numbers of globally coupled independently stochastic ion channels. *Phys. Rev.* E 49: 3421–3431.

Franceschetti, S., Guatteo, E., Panzica, F., Sancini, G. E. W., and Avanzini, G. (1995). Ionic mechanisms underlying burst firing in pyramidal neurons: Intracellular study in rat sensorimotor cortex. *Brain Res.* 696: 127–139.

Frank, K., and Fuortes, M. G. F. (1956). Stimulation of spinal motoneurone with intracellular electrodes. *J. Physiol.* 134: 451–470.

Franke, C., Hatt, H., and Dudel, J. (1987). Liquid filament switch for ultrafast exchanges of solutions at excised patches of synaptic membrane of crayfish muscle. *Neurosci. Lett.* 77: 199–204.

Frankenhaeuser, B. (1963). A quantitative description of potassium currents in mylenated nerve fibres of *Xenopus laevin. J. Physiol.* 169: 424–430.

Frankenhaeuser, B., and Hodgkin, A. L. (1956). The after effects of impulses in the giant nerve fibres of *Loligo. J. Physiol.* 131: 341–376.

Frankenhaeuser, B., and Huxley, A. F. (1964). Action potential in mylenated nerve fibre of *Xenopus laevis* as computed on the basis of voltage clamp data. *J. Physiol.* 171: 302–315.

Franklin, J., and Bair, W. (1995). The effect of a refractory period on the power spectrum of neuronal discharge. *SIAM J. Appl. Math.* 55: 1074–1093.

Franklin, J. L., Fickbohm, D. J., and Willard, A. L. (1992). Long-term regulation of neuronal calcium currents by prolonged changes of membrane potential. *J. Neurosci.* 12: 1726–1735.

Freeman, W. J. (1960). Correlation of electrical activity of prepyriform cortex and behavior in cat. *J. Neurophysiol.* 23: 111–131.

Freeman, W. J. (1968a). Effects of surgical isolation and tetanization on prepyriform cortex in cats. *J. Neurophysiol.* 31: 349–357.

Freeman, W. J. (1968b). Relations between unit activity and evoked potentials in prepyriform cortex of cats. *J. Neurophysiol.* 31: 337–348.

Freeman, W. J. (1975). *Mass action in the nervous system.* New York: Academic Press.

Freeman, W. J., and Schneider, W. (1982). Changes in spatial patterns of rabbit olfactory EEG with conditioning to odors. *Psychophysiol.* 19: 44–56.

French, C. R., Sah, P., Buckett, K. J., and Gage, P. W. (1990). A voltage-dependent persistent sodium current in mammalian hippocampal neurons. *J. Gen. Physiol.* 95: 1139–1157.

Fromherz, P., and Gaede, V. (1993). Exclusive-OR function of single arborized neuron. *Biol. Cybern.* 69: 337–344.

Fromherz, P., and Muller, C. O. (1994). Cable properties of a straight neurite of a leech neuron probed by a voltage-sensitive dye. *Proc. Natl. Acad. Sci. U.S.A.* 91: 4604–4608.

Fuortes, M. G. F., Frank, K., and Becker, M. C. (1957). Steps in the production of motoneuron spikes. *J. Gen. Physiol.* 40: 725–752.

Gabbiani, F. (1996). Coding of time-varying signals in spike trains of linear and half-wave rectifying neurons. *Network: Comput. Neur. Syst.* 7: 61–85.

Gabbiani, F., and Koch, C. (1996). Coding of time-varying signals in spike trains of integrate-and-fire neurons with random threshold. *Neur. Comput.* 8: 44–66.

Gabbiani, F., Metzner, W., Wessel, R., and Koch, C. (1996). From stimulus encoding to feature extraction in weakly electric fish. *Nature* 384: 564–567.

Gabbiani, F., Midtgaard, J., and Knöpfel, T. (1994). Synaptic integration in a model of cerebellar granule cells. *J. Neurophysiol.* 72: 999–1009.

Gabso, M., Neher, E., and Spira, M. E. (1997). Low mobility of the Ca^{2+} buffers in axons of cultured *Aplysia* neurons. *Neuron* 18: 473–481.

Gamble, E., and Koch, C. (1987). The dynamics of free calcium in dendritic spines in response to repetitive synaptic input. *Science* 236: 1311–1315.

Garrahan, P. J., and Rega, A. F. (1990). Plasma membrane calcium pump. In *Intracellular calcium regulation*, ed. F. Bronner, pp. 271–303. New York: Liss.

Gear, C. W. (1971a). *Numerical initial value problems in ordinary differential equations*. Englewood Cliffs, NJ: Prentice- Hall.

Gear, C. W. (1971b). The automatic integration of ordinary differential equations. *Commun. ACM* 14: 176–179.

Geiger, J. R., Melcher, T., Koh, D. S., Sakmann, B., Seeburg, P. H., Jonas, P., and Monyer, H. (1995). Relative abundance of subunit mR-NAs determines gating and Ca^{2+} permeability of AMPA receptors in principal neurons and interneurons in rat CNS. *Neuron* 15: 193–204.

Georgopoulos, A. P., Taira, M., and Lukashin, A. (1993). Cognitive neurophysiology of the motor cortex. *Science* 260: 47–52.

Gestri, G. (1971). Pulse frequency modulation in neural systems. *Biophys. J.* 11: 98–109.

Gestri, G., Masterbroek, H. A. K., and Zaagman, W. H. (1980). Stochastic constancy, variability and adaptation of spike generation: Performance of a giant neuron in the visual system of the fly. *Biol. Cybern.* 38: 31–40.

Getting, P. A. (1989). Emerging principles governing the operation of neural networks. *Ann. Rev. Neurosci.* 12: 185–204.

Getting, P. A., and Dekin, M. S. (1985a). *Tritonia* swimming: A model system for integration within rhythmic motor systems. In *Model neural networks and behavior*, ed. by A. I. Selverston, pp. 3–20. New York: Plenum Press.

Getting, P. A., and Dekin, M. S. (1985b). Mechanisms of pattern generation underlying swimming in *Tritonia*. IV. Gating of central pattern generator. *J. Neurophysiol.* 53: 466–480.

Ghosh, A., and Greenberg, M. E. (1995). Calcium signaling in neurons: Molecular mechanisms and cellular consequences. *Science* 268: 239–247.

Gilbert, C. D. (1992). Horizontal integration and cortical dynamics. *Neuron* 9: 1–13.

Ginzburg, I., and Sompolinsky, H. (1994). Theory of correlations in stochastic neural networks. *Phys. Rev. E50*: 3171–3191.

Glass, L., and Mackey, M. C. (1988). *From clocks to chaos: The rhythms of life*. Princeton: Princeton University Press.

Goddard, N., and Hood, G. (1997). Parallel genesis. In *The Book of GENESIS*. 2d ed., ed. J. M. Bower and D. Beeman, pp. 349–380. New York: Springer.

Goldbeter, A., Dupont, G., and Berridge, M. J. (1990). Minimal model for signal-induced Ca^{2+} oscillations and for their frequency encoding through protein phosphorylation. *Proc. Natl. Acad. Sci. U.S.A.* 87: 1461–1465.

Goldman, D. E. (1943). Potential, impedance, and rectification in membranes. *J. Gen. Physiol.* 27: 37–60.

Goldstein, S. A., Price, L. A., Rosenthal, D. N., and Rausch, M. H. (1996). ORK1, a potassium-selective leak channel with two pore domains cloned from *Drosophila melanogaster* by expression in *Saccharomyces cerevisiae*. *Proc. Natl. Acad. Sci. U.S.A.* 93: 13256–13261.

Goldstein, S. S., and Rall, W. (1974). Changes in action potential shape and velocity for changing core conductor geometry. *Biophys. J.* 14: 731–757.

Golomb, D., Guckenheimer, J., and Gueron, S. (1993). Reduction of a channel-based model for a stomatogastric ganglion LP neuron. *Biol. Cybern.* 69: 129–137.

Golowasch, J., Buchholtz, F., Epstein, I. R., and Marder, E. (1992). The contribution of individual ionic currents to the activity of a model stomatogastric ganglion neuron. *J. Neurophysiol.* 67: 341–349.

Golowasch, J., and Marder, E. (1992a). Ionic currents of the lateral pyloric neuron of the stomatogastric ganglion of the crab. *J. Neurophysiol.* 67: 318–331.

Golowasch, J., and Marder, E. (1992b). Proctolin activates an inward current whose voltage dependence is modified by extracellular Ca^{++}. *J. Neurosci.* 12: 810–817.

Golub, G. H., and Ortega, J. M. (1992). *Scientific computing and differential equations.* Boston: Academic Press.

Golub, G. H, and Van Loan, C. F. (1985). *Matrix computations.* Baltimore: Johns Hopkins University Press.

Gonzalez, J. E., and Tsien, R. Y. (1995). Voltage sensing by fluorescence resonance energy transfer in single cells. *Biophys. J.* 69: 1272–1280.

Graham, B., and Redman, S. (1994). A simulation of action potentials in synaptic boutons during presynaptic inhibition. *J. Neurophysiol.* 71: 538–549.

Gramoll, S., Schmidt, J., and Calabrese, R. L. (1994). Switching in the activity of an interneuron that controls coordination of the hearts in the medicinal leech (*Hirudo medicinalis*). *J. Exp. Biol.* 186: 157–171.

Grannan, E. R., Kleinfeld, D., and Sompolinsky, H. (1992). Stimulus-dependent synchronization of neuronal assemblies. *Neur. Comput.* 4: 550–569.

Gray, C. M. (1994) Synchronous oscillations in neuronal systems: Mechanisms and functions. *J. Comput. Neurosci.* 1: 11–38.

Gray, C. M., Konig, P., Engel, A. K., and Singer, W. (1989). Oscillatory responses in cat visual-cortex exhibit inter-columnar synchronization which reflects global stimulus properties. *Nature* 338: 334–337.

Green, D., and Swets, J. (1966). *Signal detection theory and psychophysics.* New York: Wiley.

Grinvald, A., Ross, W. N. and Farber, I. (1981). Simultaneous optical measurements of electrical activity from multiple sites on processes of cultured neurons. *Proc. Natl. Acad. Sci. U.S.A.* 78: 3245–3249.

Grossberg, S. (1976). Adaptive pattern classification and universal recoding: 1. Parallel development and coding of neural feature detectors. *Biol. Cybern.* 23: 121–134.

Gruol, D. L., Deal, C. R., Yool, A. J. (1992). Developmental changes in calcium conductances contribute to the physiological maturation of cerebellar Purkinje neurons in culture. *J. Neurosci.* 12: 2838–2848.

Gruol, D. L., Jacquin, T., and Yool, A. J. (1991). Single-channel K^+ currents recorded from the somatic and dendritic regions of cerebellar Purkinje neurons in culture. *J. Neurosci.* 11: 1002–1015.

Grynkiewicz, G., Poenie, M., and Tsien, R. Y. A. (1985). A new generation of Ca^{2+} indicators with greatly improved fluorescence properties. *J. Biol. Chem.* 260: 3440–3450.

Guckenheimer, J., Gueron, S., and Harris-Warrick, R. M. (1993). Mapping the dynamics of a bursting neuron. *Philos. Trans. Roy. Soc. Lond.* B341: 345–359.

Gurney, A. M., Tsien, R. Y., and Lester, H. A. (1987). Activation of a potassium current by rapid photochemically generated step increases of intracellular calcium in rat sympathetic neurons. *Proc. Natl. Acad. Sci, U.S.A.* 84: 3496–3350.

Gustafsson, B., Galvan, M., Grafe, P., and Wigstrom, H. (1982). Transient outward current in mammalian central neuron blocked by 4-aminopyridine. *Nature* 299: 252–254.

Gutfreund, Y., Yarom, Y., and Segev, I. (1995). Subthreshold oscillations and resonant frequency in guinea-pig cortical neurons: Physiology and modelling. *J. Physiol.* 483: 621–640.

Guttman, R., Lewis, S., and Rinzel, J. (1980). Control of repetitive firing in squid axon membrane as a model for a neuroneoscillator. *J. Physiol.* 305: 377–395.

Guyton, A. C. (1986). *Textbook of medical physiology.* Philadelphia: Saunders.

Györke, S., and Fill, M. (1993). Ryanodine receptor adaptation: Control mechanism of Ca^{2+}-induced Ca^{2+} release in heart. *Science* 260: 807–809.

Haag, J., and Borst, A. (1996). Amplification of high-frequency synaptic inputs by active dendritic membrane processes. *Nature* 379: 639–641.

Haberly, L. B. (1973a). Summed potentials evoked in opossum prepyriform cortex. *J. Neurophysiol.* 36: 775–788.

Haberly, L. B. (1973b). Unitary analysis of opossum prepyriform cortex. *J. Neurophysiol.* 36: 762–744.

Haberly, L. B. (1978). Application of collision testing to investigate properties of association axons originating from single cells in the piriform cortex of the rat. *Soc. Neurosci. Abstr.* 4: 75.

Haberly, L. B. (1983). Structure of the piriform cortex of the opossum: 1. Description of neuron types with Golgi methods. *J. Comp. Neurol.* 219: 448–460.

Haberly, L. B. (1990). Olfactory cortex. In *The synaptic organization of the brain*, ed. G. M. Shepherd, pp. 317–345. New York: Oxford University Press.

Haberly, L. B., and Behan, M. (1983). Structure of the piriform cortex of the opossum: 3. Ultrastructural characterization of synaptic terminals of association and olfactory bulb afferent fibers. *J. Comp. Neurol.* 219: 448–460.

Haberly, L. B., and Bower, J. M. (1984). Analysis of association fiber pathway in piriform cortex with intracellular recording and staining techniques. *J. Neurophysiol.* 51: 90–112.

Haberly, L. B., and Bower, J. M. (1989). Olfactory cortex: Model circuit for study of associative memory. *Trends Neurosci.* 12: 258–264.

Haberly, L. B., and Presto, S. (1986). Ultrastructural analysis of synaptic relationships of intracellularly stained pyramidal cell axons in piriform cortex. *J. Comp. Neurol.* 248: 464–474.

Halliwell, J. V. (1986). M-current in human neocortical neurones. *Neurosci. Lett.* 67: 1–6.

Hamill, O. P., Huguenard, J. R., and Prince, D. A. (1991). Patch-clamp studies of voltage-gated currents in identified neurons of the rate cerebral cortex. *Cerebral Cortex* 1: 48–61.

Hansel, D., Mato, G., and Meunier, C. (1993). Phase dynamics for weakly coupled Hodgkin-Huxley neurons. *Europhys. Lett.* 23: 367–372.

Hansel, D., Mato, G., and Meunier, C. (1995). Synchrony in excitatory neural networks. *Neur. Comput.* 7: 307–335.

Hansel, D., and Sompolinsky, H. (1996). Chaos and synchrony in a model of a hypercolumn in visual cortex. *J. Comput. Neurosci.* 3: 7–34.

Hansel, D., and Sompolinsky, H. (1997). Feature selectivity in a cortical module with short range excitation.

Hansel, D., Mato, G., Meunier, C., and Neltner, L. On numerical simulations of integrate-and-fire neural networks. *Neural Comput.*, in press.

Harris-Warrick, R. M., Coniglio, L. M., Barazangi, N., Guckenheimer, J., and Gueron, S. (1995a). Dopamine modulation of transient potassium current evokes phase shifts in a central pattern generator network. *J. Neurosci.* 15: 342–358.

Harris-Warrick, R. M., Coniglio, L. M., Levini, R. M., Gueron, S., and Guckenheimer, J. (1995b). Dopamine modulation of two subthreshold currents produces phase shifts in activity of an identified motoneuron. *J. Neurophysiol.* 74: 1404–1420.

Harris, K. M., Jensen, F. E., and Tsao, B. (1992). Three-dimensional structure of dendritic spines and synapses in rat hippocampus (CA1) at postnatal day 15 and adult ages: Implications for the maturation of synaptic physiology and long-term potentiation. *J. Neurosci.* 12: 2685–2705.

Harris, K. M., and Kater, S. B. (1994). Dendritic spines: Cellular specialization imparting both stability and flexibility to synaptic function. *Annu. Rev. Neurosci.* 17: 341–371.

Hartline, D. K. (1979). Pattern generation in the lobster (*Panulirus*) stomatogastric ganglion: 2. Pyloric network simulation. *Biol. Cybern.* 33: 223–236.

Hartline, D. K., and Graubard, K. (1992). Cellular and synaptic properties in the crustacean stomatogastric nervous system. In *Dynamic biological networks: The stomatogastric nervous system*, ed. R. M. Harris-Warrick, E. Marder, A. I. Selverston, and M. Moulins, pp. 31–86. Cambridge, MA: MIT Press.

Hartline, H. (1974). *Studies on excitation and inhibition in the retina*, ed. E. Ratliff. New York: Rockefeller University Press.

Harvey, R. J., and Napper, R. M. A. (1991). Quantitative studies of the mammalian cerebellum. *Prog. Neurobiol.* 36: 437–463.

Hasselmo, M. E., Wilson, M. A., Anderson, B. P., and Bower, J. M. (1990). Associative memory function in piriform (olfactory) cortex: Computational modeling and neuropharmacology. *Cold Spr. Harb. Symp. Quant. Biol.* 55: 599–610.

Hata, Y., Tsumoto, T., Sato, H., Hagihara, K., and Tamura, H. (1988). Inhibition contributes to orientation selectivity in visual cortex of cat. *Nature* 335: 815–817.

Haug, H. (1968). Quantitative elektronenmikroskopische Untersuchungen über den Markfaseraufbau in der Sehrinde der Katze. *Brain Res.* 11: 65–84.

Hausser, M., Stuart, G., Racca, C., and Sakmann, B. (1995). Axonal initiation and active dendritic propagation of action potentials in substantia nigra neurons. *Neuron* 15: 637–647.

Hayashi, H., and Ishizuka, S. (1992). Chaotic nature of bursting discharges in the *Onchidium* pacemaker neuron. *J. Theoret. Biol.* 156: 269–291.

Hearon, J. Z. (1963). Theorems on linear systems. *Ann. N. Y. Acad. Sci.* 108: 36–68.

Hebb, D. O. (1949). *The organization of behavior: A neuropsychological theory.* New York: Wiley.

Heimer, L. (1968). Synaptic distribution of centripetal and centrifugal nerve fibres in the olfactory system of the rat: An experimental anatomical study. *J. Anat.* 103: 413–432.

Hell, J. W., Westenbroek, R. E., Warner, C., Ahlijanian, M. K., Prystay, W., Gilbert, M. M., Snutch, T. P., and Catterall, W. A. (1993). Identification and differential subcellular localization of the neuronal class C and class D L-type calcium channel $\alpha 1$ subunits. *J. Cell Biol.* 123: 949–962.

Helmchen, F., Imoto, K., and Sakmann, B. (1996). Ca^{2+} buffering and action potential–evoked Ca^{2+} signaling in dendrites of pyramidal neurons. *Biophys. J.* 70: 1069–1081.

Hessler, N. A., Shirke, A. M. and Malinow, R. (1993). The probability of transmitter release at a mammalian central synapse. *Nature* 366: 569–572.

Hestrin, S. (1992). Activation and desensitization of glutamate-activated channels mediating fast excitatory synaptic currents in the visual cortex. *Neuron* 9: 991–999.

Hestrin, S. (1993). Different glutamate receptor channels mediate fast excitatory synaptic currents in inhibitory and excitatory cortical neurons. *Neuron* 11: 1083–1091.

Hestrin, S., and Sah, P., and Nicoll, R. A. (1990). Mechanisms generating the time course of dual component excitatory synaptic currents recorded in hippocampal slices. *Neuron* 5: 247–253.

Hill, A. V. (1910). A new mathematical treatment of changes of ionic concentration in muscle and nerve under the action of electric currents, with a theory as to their mode of excitation. *J. Physiol.* 40: 190–213.

Hille, B. (1992). *Ionic channels of excitable membranes.* 2d ed. Sunderland, MA: Sinauer.

Hines, M. (1984). Efficient computation of branched nerve equations. *Int. J. Bio-Med. Comput.* 15: 69–76.

Hines, M. (1993). NEURON: A program for simulation of nerve equations. In *Neural systems: Analysis and modeling*, ed. F. Eeckman, pp. 127–136. Norwell, MA: Kluwer Academic.

Hines, M. L., and Carnevale, N. T. (1997). The NEURON simulation environment. *Neural Comput.* 9: 1179–1209.

Hirsch, J. A., Alonso, J. M., and Reid, R. C. (1995). Visually evoked calcium action potentials in cat striate cortex. *Nature* 378: 612–616.

Hodgkin, A. L. (1948). The local electric changes associated with repetitive action in a non-medullated axon. *J. Physiol.* 107: 165–181.

Hodgkin A. L., and Huxley, A. F. (1952). A quantitative description of membrane current and its application to conduction and excitation in nerve. *J. Physiol.* 117: 500–544.

Hodgkin, A. L., and Katz, B. (1949a). The effect of sodium ions on the electrical activity of the giant axon of the squid. *J. Physiol.* 108: 37–77.

Hodgkin, A. L., and Katz, B. (1949b). The effect of temperature on the electrical activity of the giant axon of the squid. *J. Physiol.* 109: 240–249.

Hodgkin, A. L., and Rushton, W. A. H. (1946). The electrical constants of a crustacean nerve fiber. *Proc. Roy. Soc. Lond. B* 133: 444–479.

Hofer, A. M., and Machen, T. E. (1993). Technique for in situ measurement of calcium in intracellular inositol 1,4,5-triphosphate sensitive stores using the fluorescent indicator mag-fura-2. *Proc. Natl. Acad. Sci. U.S.A.* 90: 2598–2602.

Hoffman, J. A., Magee, J. C., Colbert, C. M., and Johnston, D. (1997). K^+ channels regulation of signal propagation in dendrites of hippocampal pyramidal neurons. *Nature* 387: 869–875.

Hoffman, D., Magee, J., and Johnston, D. (1996). Characterization of voltage-gated K^+ channels in the soma and dendrites of hippocampal CA1 pyramidal neurons. *Soc. Neurosci. Abstr.* 22: 793. Abstr.

Hoffman, W. H., and Haberly, L. B. (1989). Bursting induces persistent all-or-none EPSPs by an NMDA-dependent process in piriform cortex. *J. Neurosci.* 9: 206–215.

Hollingworth, S., Harkins, A. B., Kurebayashi, N., Konishi, M., and Baylor, S. M. (1992). Excitation-contraction coupling in intact frog skeletal muscle fibers injected with mmolar concentrations of fura-2. *Biophys. J.* 63: 224–234.

Holmes M., and Cole, J. (1984). Cochlear mechanics: Analysis for a pure tone. *J. Acoust. Soc. Am.* 76: 767–78.

Holmes, W. R. (1986). A continuous cable method for determining the transient potential in passive dendritic trees of known geometry. *Biol. Cybern.* 55: 115–124.

Holmes, W. R. (1995). Modeling the effect of glutamate diffusion and uptake on NMDA and non-NMDA receptor saturation. *Biophys. J.* 69: 1734–1747.

Holmes, W. R., and Levy, W. B. (1990). Insights into associative long-term potentiation from computational models of NMDA receptor-mediated calcium influx and intracellular calcium concentration changes. *J. Neurophysiol.* 63: 1148–1168.

Holmes, W. R., and Rall, W. (1992a). Electrotonic length estimates in neurons with dendritic tapering or somatic shunt. *J. Neurophysiol.* 68: 1421–1437.

Holmes, W. R., and Rall, W. (1992b). Estimating the electrotonic structure of neurons with compartmental models. *J. Neurophysiol.* 68: 1438–1452.

Holmes, W. R., and Rall, W. (1992c). Electrotonic models of neuronal dendrites and single neuron computation. In *Single neuron computation*, ed. T. McKenna, J. Davis, and S. F. Zornetzer, pp. 7–25. New York: Academic Press.

Holmes, W. R., Segev, I., and Rall, W. (1992). Interpretation of time constant and electrotonic length estimates in multicylinder of branched neuronal structures. *J. Neurophysiol.* 68: 1401–1420.

Holt, G., Softky, W., Koch, C., and Douglas, R. J. (1996). A comparison of discharge variability *in vitro* and *in vivo* in cat visual cortex neurons. *J. Neurophysiol.* 75: 1806–1814.

Honma, S. (1984). Functional differentiation in SB and SC neurons of toad sympathetic ganglia. *Jap. J. Physiol.* 20: 281.

Hooper, S. L. (1997a). Phase maintenance in the pyloric pattern of the lobster (*Panulirus interruptus*) stomatogastric ganglion. *J. Comput. Neurosci.* 4: 191–205.

Hooper, S. L. (1997b). The pyloric pattern of the lobster (*Panulirus interruptus*) stomatogastric ganglion comprises two phase maintaining subsets. *J. Comput. Neurosci.* 4: 207–219.

Hooper, S. L., and Marder, E. (1987). Modulation of the lobster pyloric rhythm by the peptide proctolin. *J. Neurosci.* 7: 2097–2112.

Hopfield, J. J. (1982). Neural networks and physical systems with emergent collective computational abilities. *Proc. Natl. Acad. Sci. U.S.A.* 79: 2554–2558.

Hopfield, J. J. (1984). Neurons with graded response have collective computational properties like those of two-state neurons. *Proc. Natl. Acad. Sci. U.S.A.* 81: 3088–3092.

Hopfield, J. J., and Tank, D. W. (1986). Computing with neural circuits: A model. *Science* 233: 625–633.

Hoppensteadt, F. (1986). *An introduction to the mathematics of neurons.* Cambridge: Cambridge University Press.

Horwitz, B. (1981). An analytical method for investigating transient potentials in neurons with branching dendritic trees. *Biophys. J.* 36: 155–192.

Horwitz, B. (1983). Unequal diameters and their effect on time-varying voltages in branched neuron. *Biophys. J.* 41: 51–66.

Hubbard, J. H., and West, B. (1992). *MacMath: A dynamical systems software package for the Macintosh.* New York: Springer-Verlag.

Hubel, D. H. (1988). *Eye, brain and vision.* New York: Freeman.

Hubel, D. H., and Wiesel, T. N. (1959). Receptive fields of single neurons in the cat's visual cortex. *J. Physiol.* 148: 574–591.

Hubel, D. H., and Wiesel, T. N. (1962). Receptive fields, binocular interaction and functional architecture in the cat's visual cortex. *J. Physiol.* 160: 106–154.

Hubel, D. H., and Wiesel, T. N. (1968). Receptive fields and functional architecture of monkey striate cortex. *J. Physiol.* 195: 215–243.

Hudspeth, A. J., and Lewis, R. S. (1988). A model for electrical resonance and frequency tuning in saccular hair cells of the bullfrog *Rana Catesbeiana. J. Physiol.* 400: 275–297.

Huguenard, J. R. (1996). Low-threshold calcium currents in central nervous system neurons. *Annu. Rev. Physiol.* 58: 329–348.

Huguenard, J. R., Hamill, O. P., and Prince, D. A. (1988). Developmental changes in Na^+ conductances in rat neocortical neurons: Appearance of a slowly inactivating component. *J. Neurophysiol.* 59: 778–794.

Huguenard, J. R., Hamill, O. P., and Prince, D. A. (1989). Sodium channels in dendrites of rat cortical pyramidal neurons. *Proc. Natl. Acad. Sci. U.S.A.* 86: 2473–2477.

Huguenard, J. R., and McCormick, D. A (1992). Simulation of the currents involved in rhythmic oscillations in thalamic relay neurons. *J. Neurophysiol.* 68: 1373–1383.

Huguenard, J. R., and Prince, D. A. (1994). Clonazepam suppresses $GABA_B$-mediated inhibition in thalamic relay neurons through effects in nucleus reticularis. *J. Neurophysiol.* 71: 2576–2581.

Huntley, G. W., Vickers, J. C., and Morrison, J. H. (1994). Cellular and synaptic localization of NMDA and non-NMDA receptor subunits in neocortex: Organizational features related to cortical circuitry, function and disease. *Trends Neurosci.* 17: 536–543.

Hutcheon, B., Miura, R. M., and Puil, E. (1996a). Models of subthreshold membrane resonance in neocortical neurons. *J. Neurophysiol.* 76: 698–714.

Hutcheon, B., Miura, R. M., and Puil, E. (1996b). Subthreshold membrane resonance in neocortical neurons. *J. Neurophysiol.* 76: 683–697.

Hutcheon, B., Segev, I., Carlen, P., and Yarom, Y. (1996). Resonance properties measured from soma and dendrites of layer 5 neocortical neurons. *Soc. Neurosci. Abstr.* 22: 792. Abstr. 315.12

Iansek, R., and Redman, S. J. (1973). An analysis of the cable properties of spinal motoneurones using a brief intracellular current pulse. *J. Physiol.* 234: 613–636.

Irvine, D. F. (1986). *The auditory brainstem. Sensory physiology*, vol. 7. Berlin: Springer.

Isaacson, E., and Keller, H. B. (1966). *Analysis of numerical methods*. New York: Wiley.

Isaacson, J. S., Solis, J. M., and Nicoll, R. A. (1993). Local and diffuse synaptic actions of GABA in the hippocampus. *Neuron* 10: 165–175.

Ishizuka, N., Cowan, W. M., and Amaral, D. G. (1995). A quantitative analysis of the dendritic organization of pyramidal cells in the rat hippocampus. *J. Comp. Neurol.* 362: 17–45.

Jack, J. J. B., Miller, S., Porter, R., and Redman, S. J. (1971). The time course of minimal excitatory postsynaptic potentials evoked in spinal motoneurones by group Ia afferent fibres. *J. Physiol.* 215: 353–380.

Jack, J. J. B., Noble, D., and Tsien, R. W. (1975). *Electric current flow in excitable cells*. Oxford, UK: Clarendon Press. (Reprinted in 1983.)

Jack, J. J. B., and Redman, S. J. (1971a). The propagation of transient potentials in some linear cable structures. *J. Physiol.* 215: 283–320.

Jack, J. J. B., and Redman, S. J. (1971b). An electrical description of the motoneurone, and its application to the analysis of synaptic transients. *J. Physiol.* 215: 321–352.

Jaeger, D., and Bower, J. M. (1996). The function of background synaptic input in cerebellar Purkinje cells explored with dynamic current clamping. *Soc. Neurosci. Abstr.* 22: 494.

Jaeger, D., De Schutter, E., and Bower, J. M. (1997). The role of synaptic and voltage-gated currents in the control of Purkinje cell spiking: A modeling study. *J. Neurosci.* 17: 91–106.

Jaffe, D. B., and Brown, T. H. (1994). Metabotropic glutamate receptor activation induces calcium waves within hippocampal dendrites. *J. Neurophysiol.* 72: 471–474.

Jaffe, D. B., Fisher, S. A., and Brown, T. H. (1994). Confocal laser scanning microscopy reveals voltage-gated calcium signals within hippocampal dendritic spines. *J. Neurobiol.* 25: 220–233.

Jaffe, D., Johnston, D., Lasser-Ross, N., Lisman, J. E., Miyakawa, H., and Ross, W. N. (1992). The spread of Na^+ spikes determines the pattern of dendritic Ca^{2+} entry into hippocampal neurons. *Nature* 21: 244–246.

Jafri, M. S., and Gillo, B. (1994). A membrane potential model with counterions for cytosolic calcium oscillations. *Cell Calcium* 16: 9–19.

Jahr, C. E. (1992). High probability of opening of NMDA receptor channels by L-glutamate. *Science* 255: 470–472.

Jahr, C. E., and Stevens, C. F. (1990a). A quantitative description of NMDA receptor-channel kinetic behavior. *J. Neurosci.* 10: 1830–1837.

Jahr, C. E., and Stevens, C. F. (1990b). Voltage dependence of NMDA-activated macroscopic conductances predicted by single-channel kinetics. *J. Neurosci.* 10: 3178–3182.

Jaslove, S. W. (1992). The integrative properties of spiny distal dendrites. *Neuroscience* 47: 495–519.

Jefferys, J. G. R., Traub, R. D., and Whittington, M. A. (1996). Neuronal networks for induced 40 Hz rhythms. *Trends Neurosci.* 19: 202–208.

Jensen, O., and Abbott, L. F. (1997). Self-assembling circuits of model neurons. In *Computational neuroscience: Trends in research*, ed. J. Bower, pp. 227–230. New York: Plenum.

John, F. (1952). On integration of parabolic differential equations by difference methods. *Commun. Pure and Appl. Math.* 5: 155–211.

John, F. (1982). *Partial differential equations*. 4th ed. Heidelberg: Springer.

Johnson, B. R., and Harris-Warrick, R. M. (1990). Aminergic modulation of graded synaptic transmission in the lobster stomatogastric ganglion. *J. Neurosci.* 10: 2066–2076.

Johnson, B. R., Peck, J. H., and Harris-Warrick, R. M. (1995). Distributed amine modulation of graded chemical transmission in the pyloric network of the lobster stomatogastric ganglion. *J. Neurophysiol.* 74: 437–452.

Johnston, D., Magee, J. C., Colbert, C. M., and Christie, B. R. (1996). Active properties of neuronal dendrites. *Annu. Rev. Neurosci.* 19: 165–186.

Johnston, D., and Wu, S. M. (1995). *Foundations of cellular neurophysiology*. Cambridge, MA: MIT Press.

Jonas, P., Major, G., and Sakmann, B. (1993). Quantal components of unitary EPSCs at the mossy fibre synapse on CA3 pyramidal cells of rat hippocampus. *J. Physiol.* 472: 615–663.

Jonas, P., Racca, C., Sakmann, B., Seeburg, P. H., and Monyer, H. (1994). Differences in Ca^{2+} permeability of AMPA-type glutamate receptor channels in neocortical neurons caused by differential GluR-B subunit expression. *Neuron* 12: 1281–1289.

Jones, J., and Palmer, L. (1987). The two-dimensional spatial structure of simple receptive fields in cat striate cortex. *J. Neurophysiol.* 58: 1187–1211.

Jones, E. G., and Powell, T. P. S. (1969). Synapses on the axon hillocks and initial segments of pyramidal cell axons in the cerebral cortex. *J. Cell Sci.* 5: 459–507.

Jones, O. T., Kunze, D. L., and Angelides, K. J. (1989). Localization and mobility of omega-conotoxin-sensitive Ca^{2+} channels in hippocampal CA1 neurons. *Science* 244: 1189–1193.

Jones, S. W. (1987). Sodium currents in dissociated bullfrog sympathetic neurons. *J. Physiol.* 389: 605–627.

Joyner, R. W., Sugiwara, H., and Tau, R. C. (1991). Unidirectional block between isolated rabbit ventricular cells coupled by a variable resistance. *Biophys. J.* 60: 1038–1045.

Jung, M. W., Larson, J., and Lynch, G. (1990). Role of NMDA and non-NMDA receptors in synaptic transmission in rat piriform cortex, *Exp. Brain Res.* 82: 451–455.

Kaczmarek, L. K., and Levitan, I. B., eds. (1987). *Neuromodulation: The biochemical control of neuronal excitability*. New York: Oxford University Press.

Kano, M., Garaschuk, O., Verkhratsky, A., and Konnerth, A. (1995). Ryanodine receptor–mediated intracellular calcium release in rat cerebellar Purkinje neurones. *J. Physiol.* 487: 1–16.

Kanter, E. D., and Haberly, L. B. (1990). NMDA-dependent induction of long-term potentiation in afferent and association fiber systems of piriform cortex *in vitro*. *Brain Res.* 525: 175–179.

Kao, J. P. Y., and Tsien, R. Y. (1988). Ca^{2+} binding kinetics of fura-2 and azo-1 from temperature-jump relaxation measurements. *Biophys. J.* 53: 635–639.

Kapicka, C. L., Carl, A., Hall, M. L., Percival, A. L., Frey, B. W., and Kenyon, J. L. (1994). Comparison of large-conductance Ca^{2+}-activated K^+ channels in artificial bilayer and patch-clamp experiments. *Am. J. Physiol.* 266: C601–C610.

Kargacin, G. J. (1994). Calcium signaling in restricted diffusion spaces. *Biophys. J.* 57: 262–272.

Kasai, H., and Petersen, O. H. (1994). Spatial dynamics of second messengers: IP_3 and cAMP as longe-range and associative messengers. *Trends Neurosci.* 17: 95–101.

Kater, S. B., and Mills, L. R. (1991). Regulation of growth cone behavior by calcium. *J. Neurosci.* 11: 891–899.

Kawato, M. (1984). Cable properties of a neuron model with non-uniform membrane resistivity. *J. Theor. Biol.* 111: 149–169.

Keener, J. (1983). Analogue circuitry for the FitzHugh-Nagumo equations. *IEEE Trans. Syst. Man and Cybern.* 13: 1010–1014.

Keller, H. B. (1976). *Numerical solution of two point boundary problems*. CMBS-NSF Regional Conference Series in Applied Mathematics, no. 24. Philadelphia: SIAM.

Kendall, J. M., Dormer, R. L., and Campbell, A. K. (1992). Targeting aequorin to the endoplasmic reticulum of living cells. *Biochem. and Biophys. Res. Commun.* 189: 1008–1016.

Kepler, T. B., Abbott, L. F., and Marder, E. (1992). Reduction of conductance-based neuron models. *Biol. Cybern.* 66: 381–387.

Ketchum, K. L., and Haberly, L. B. (1993a). Membrane currents evoked by afferent fiber stimulation in rat piriform cortex: Current source-density analysis. *J. Neurophysiol.* 69: 248–260.

Ketchum, K. L., and Haberly, L. B. (1993b). Membrane currents evoked by afferent fiber stimulation in rat piriform cortex. II. Analysis with a systems model. *J. Neurophysiol.* 69: 261–281.

Ketchum, K. L., and Haberly, L. B. (1993c). Synaptic events that generate fast oscillations in piriform cortex. *J. Neurosci.* 13: 3980–3985.

Kilmer, W. K., McCulloch, W. S., and Blum, J. (1969). A model of the vertebrate central command system. *Int. J. Man-Mach. Stud.* 1: 279–309.

Kim, H. G., and Connors, B. W. (1993). Apical dendrites of the neocortex: Correlation between sodium- and calcium-dependent spiking and pyramidal cell morphology. *J. Neurosci.* 13: 5301–5311.

Kirsch, G. E., and Brown, A. M. (1989). Kinetic properties of single sodium channels in rat heart and rat brain. *J. Gen. Physiol.* 93: 85–99.

Klee, M., and Rall, W. (1977). Computed potentials of cortically arranged populations of neurons. *J. Neurophysiol.* 40: 647–666.

Klee, R., Ficker, E., and Heinemann, U. (1995). Comparison of voltage-dependent potassium currents in rat pyramidal neurons acutely isolated from hippoampal regions CA1 and CA3. *J. Neurophysiol.* 74: 1982–1995.

Kloeden, P., Platen, E., and Schurz, H. (1993). *Numerical solution of stochastic differential equations through computer experiments.* Heidelberg: Springer.

Knight, B. (1972a). Dynamics of encoding in a population of neurons. *J. Gen. Physiol.* 59: 734–766.

Knight, B. (1972b). The relationship between the firing rate of a single neuron and the level of activity in a population of neurons. *J. Gen. Physiol.* 59: 767–778.

Kobayashi, T., Storrie, B., Simons, K., and Dotti, C. G. (1992). A functional barrier to movement of lipids in polarized neurons. *Nature* 359: 647–650.

Koçak, H. (1989) *Differential and difference equations through computer experiments.* New York: Springer.

Koch, C. (1997). Computation and the single neuron. *Nature* 385: 207–210.

Koch, C., Bernander, Ö., and Douglas, R. J. (1995). Do neurons have a voltage or a current threshold for action potential initiation? *J. Comput. Neurosci.* 2: 63–82.

Koch, C., and Poggio, T. (1985). A simple algorithm for solving the cable equation in dendritic trees of arbitrary geometry. *J. Neurosci. Meth.* 12: 303–315.

Koch, C., Poggio, T. (1987). Biophysics of computation: Neurons, synapses, and membranes, in: *Synaptic Function,* eds. Edelman, G. M., Gall, W. E., Cowan, W. M., A neurosciences institute publication, John Wiley and Sons, N.Y.

Koch, C., Poggio, T., and Torre, V. (1982). Retinal ganglion cells: A functional interpretation of dendritic morphology. *Philos. Trans. Roy. Soc. Lond. (Biol.)* 298: 227–264.

Koch, C., Poggio, T., and Torre, V. (1983). Nonlinear interactions in a dendritic tree: Localization, timing, and role in information processing. *Proc. Natl. Acad. Sci.* 80: 2799–2802.

Koch, C., and Zador, A. (1993). The function of dendritic spines: Devices subserving biochemical rather than electrical compartmentalization. *J. Neurosci.* 13: 413–422.

Kogan, A., Ross, W. N., Zecevic, D., and Lasser-Ross, N. (1995). Optical recording from cerebellar Purkinje cells using intracellularly injected voltage-sensitive dyes. *Brain Res.* 700: 235–239.

Koh, D. S., Geiger, J. R., Jonas, P., and Sakmann, B. (1995). Ca(2+)-permeable AMPA and NMDA receptor channels in basket cells of rat hippocampal dentate gyrus. *J. Physiol.* 485: 383–402.

Kopecz, K., and Schöner, G. (1995). Saccadic motor planning by integrating visual information and pre-information on neural, dynamic fields. *Biol. Cybern.* 73: 49–60.

Kopell, N. (1988). Toward a theory of modelling central pattern generators. In *Neural control of rhythmic movements in vertebrates,* ed. A. H. Cohen, S. Rossignol, and S. Grillner, pp. 369–413. New York: Wiley.

Kowalski, N., Depireux, D., and Shamma, S. (1996). Analysis of dynamic spectra in ferret primary auditory cortex: Characteristics of single unit responses to moving ripple spectra. *J. Neurophysiol.* 76: 3524–3534.

Krausz, H. I., and Friesen, W. O. (1977). The analysis of nonlinear synaptic transmission. *J. Gen. Physiol.* 70: 243–265.

Kuba, K., and Nishi, S. (1979). Characteristics of fast excitatory postsynaptic current in bullfrog sympathetic ganglion cells: Effects of membrane potential, temperature and Ca ions. *Pflügers Arch.* 378: 205–212.

Kuffler, S. W., and Sejnowski, T. J. (1983). Peptidergic and muscarinic excitation at amphibian sympathetic synapses. *J. Physiol.* 341: 257–278.

Kuramoto, Y. (1991). Collective synchronization of pulse-coupled oscillators and excitable units. *Physica D* 50: 15–30.

Lambert, J. D. (1973). *Computational methods in ordinary differential equations.* New York: Wiley.

Lancaster, B., and Adams, P. R. (1986). Calcium-dependent current generating the afterhyperpolarization of hippocampal neurons. *J. Neurophysiol.* 55: 1268–1282.

Lancaster, B., and Nicoll, R. A. (1987). Properties of two calcium-activated hyperpolarizations in rat hippocampal neurones. *J. Physiol.* 389: 187–203.

Lancaster, B., and Pennefather, P. (1987). Potassium currents evoked by brief depolarizations in bull-frog sympathetic gangliopn cells. *J. Physiol.* 387: 519–548.

Lancaster, B., and Zucker, R. S. (1994). Photolytic manipulation of Ca^{2+} and the time course of slow, Ca^{2+}-activated K^+ current in rat hippocampal neurones. *J. Physiol.* 475: 229–239.

Lapicque, L. (1907). Recherches quantitatives sur l'excitation électrique des nerfs traitée comme une polarisation. *J. Physiol. (Paris)* 9: 620–635.

Lapicque, L. (1926). *L'excitabilité en fonction du temps.* Paris: Presses Universitaires de France.

Larkman, A. U. (1991). Dendritic morphology of pyramidal neurones of the visual cortex of the rat: 3. Spine distributions. *J. Comp. Neurol.* 306: 332–343.

Lasser-Ross, N., and Ross, W. N. (1992). Imaging voltage and synaptically activated sodium transients in cerebellar Purkinje cells. *Proc. Roy. Soc. Lond.* B 247: 35–39.

Latorre, R., Oberhauser, A., Labarca, P., and Alvarez, O. (1989). Varieties of calcium-activated potassium channels. *Annu. Rev. Physiol.* 51: 385–399.

Laurent, G. (1996). Dynamical representation of odors by oscillating and evolving neural assemblies. *Trends Neurosci.* 19: 489–496.

Lee, D. D., Reis, B. Y., Seung, H. S., and Tank, D. W. (1996). Nonlinear network models of the oculomotor integrator. *Proceedings of the Computational Neuro Science 96 Conference, Boston.*

Lees, M. (1959). Approximate solution of parabolic equations. *J. SIAM* 7: 167–183.

LeMasson, G., Marder, E., and Abbott, L. F. (1993). Activity-dependent regulation of conductances in model neurons. *Science* 259: 1915–1917.

Lester, R. A. J., and Jahr, C. E. (1992). NMDA channel behavior depends on agonist affinity. *J. Neurosci.* 12: 635–643.

Lester, R. A. J., Clements, J. D., Westbrook, G. L., and Jahr, C. E. (1990). Channel kinetics determine the time course of NMDA receptor–mediated synaptic currents. *Nature* 346: 565–567.

Lev-Ram, V., Miyakawa, H., Lasser-Ross, N., and Ross, W. N. (1992). Calcium transients in cerebellar Purkinje neurons evoked by intracellular stimulation. *J. Neurophysiol.* 68: 1167–1177.

Lev Bar-Or, R. (1993). Statistical mechanics of a hypercolumn in primary visual cortex. M. S. thesis (in Hebrew), Hebrew University, Jerusalem.

Levay, S., and Gilbert, C. D. (1976). Laminar patterns of geniculocortical projection in the cat. *Brain Res.* 113: 1–19.

Li, M., Jia, M., Fields, R. D., Nelson, P. G. (1996). Modulation of calcium currents by electrical activity. *J. Neurophysiol.* 76: 2595–2607.

Li, M., West, J. W., Lai, Y., Scheuer, T., and Catterall, W. A. (1992). Functional modulation of brain sodium channels by cAMP-dependent phosphorylation. *Neuron* 8: 1151–1159.

Li, Y.-X., and Rinzel, J. (1994). Equations for InsP$_3$ receptor-mediated [Ca^{2+}]$_i$ oscillations derived from a detailed kinetic model: A Hodgkin-Huxley-like formalism. *J. Theoret. Biol.* 166: 461–473.

Li, Y. -X., Rinzel, J., Vergara, L., and Stojilković, S. S. (1995). Spontaneous electrical and calcium oscillations in unstimulated pituitary gonadotrophs. *Biophys. J.* 69: 785–795.

Lin, C. C., and Segel, L. A. (1988). *Mathematics applied to deterministic problems in the natural sciences.* Philadelphia: SIAM.

Linás, R., Steinberg, I. Z., and Walton, K., (1981). Presynaptic calcium currents in squid giant synapse. *Biophys. J.* 33: 289–322.

Ling, D. S. F., and Benardo, L. S. (1994). Properties of isolated GABA$_B$-mediated inhibitory postsynaptic currents in hippocampal pyramidal cells. *Neurosci.* 63: 937–944.

Linse, S., Helmersson, A., and Forsen, S. (1991). Calcium-binding to calmodulin and its globular domains. *J. Biol. Chem.* 266: 8050–8054.

Lipowsky, R., Gillessen, T., and Alzheimer, C. (1996). Dendritic Na$^+$ channels amplify EPSPs in hippocampal CA1 pyramidal cells. *J. Neurophysiol.* 76: 2181–2191.

Lisman, J. E. (1997). Bursts as a unit of neural information: Making unreliable synapses reliable. *Trends Neurosci.* 20: 38–43.

Liu, Z., Marder, E., and Abbott, L. F. (1997). A multicompartmental model of the AB neuron. Unpublished research.

Liu, Z., Golowasch, J., Marder, E., and Abbott, L. F. (1998). A model neuron with activity-dependent conductances regulated by multiple calcium sensors. *J. Neurosci.*, in press.

Ljung, L. (1987). *System identification theory for the user.* Upper Saddle River, NJ: Prentics Hall PTR.

Llano, I., DiPolo, R., and Marty, A. (1994). Calcium-induced calcium release in cerebellar Purkinje cells. *Neuron* 12: 663–673.

Llano, I., Dreessen, J., Kano, M., and Konnerth, A. (1991). Intradendritic release of calcium induced by glutamate in cerebellar Purkinje cells. *Neuron* 7: 577–583.

Llinás, R. R. (1988). The intrinsic electrophysiological properties of mammalian neurons: Insights into central nervous system function. *Science* 242: 1654–1664.

Llinás, R., Steinberg, I. Z., and Walton, K. (1981). Presynaptic calcium currents in squid giant synapse. *Biophys. J.* 33: 289–322.

Llinás, R. R., and Sugimori, M. (1980). Electrophysiological properties of *in vitro* Purkinje cell dendrites in mammalian cerebellar slices. *J. Physiol.* 305: 197–213.

Llinás, R. R., Sugimori, M., and Silver, R. B. (1992). Microdomains of high calcium concentration in a presynaptic terminal. *Science* 256: 677–679.

Logan, B. (1977). Information in the zero-crossings of band-pass signals. *Bell Sys. Tech. J.* 56: 510.

Lüscher, C., Streit, J. Lipp, P., and Lüscher, H. R. (1994a). Action potential propagation through embryonic dorsal root ganglion cells in culture: 2. Decrease of conduction reliability during repetitive stimulation. *J. Neurophsiol.* 72: 634–643.

Lüscher, C., Streit, J., Quadroni, R., and Lüscher, H. R. (1994b) Action potential propagation through embryonic dorsal root ganglion cells in culture: 1. Influence of the cell morphology on propagation properties. *J. Neurophysiol.* 72: 622–633.

Lüscher, H. R., and Shiner, J. S. (1990). Simulation of action potential propagation in complex terminal arborizations. *Biophys. J.* 58: 1389–1399.

Lukashin, A. V., Amirikian, B. R., Mozhaev, V. L., Wilcox, G. L., and Georgopoulos, A. P. (1996). Modeling motor cortical operations by an attractor network of stochastic neurons. *Biol. Cybern.* 74: 255–261.

Lukashin, A. V., and Georgopoulos, A. P. (1993). A dynamical neural network model for motor cortical activity during movement: Population coding of movement trajectories. *Biol. Cybern.* 69: 517–524.

Lukashin, A. V., and Georgopoulos, A. P. (1994). Directional operations in the motor cortex modeled by a neural network of spiking neurons. *Biol. Cybern.* 71: 79–85.

Luskin, M. B., and Price, J. L. (1983). The laminar distribution of intracortical fibers originating in the olfactory cortex of the rat. *J. Comp. Neurol.* 216: 292–302.

Lux, H.-D., Schubert, P., and Kreutzberg, G. W. (1970). Direct matching of morphological and electrophysiological data in cat spinal motoneurones. In *Excitatory synaptic mechanisms*, ed. P. Andersen, and J. K. S. Janse, pp. 189–198. Oslo: Universitetsforlaget.

Lyon, R., and Shamma, S. (1996). Auditory representation of timbre and pitch. In *Auditory computations*, ed. H. Hawkins, T. McMullen, A. Popper, and R. Fay, pp. 221–270. New York: Springer.

Lytton, J., Westlin, M., Burk, S. E., Shull, G. E., and MacLennan, D. H. (1992). Functional comparisons between isoforms of the sarcoplasmic or endoplasmic reticulum family of calcium pumps. *J. Biol. Chem.* 267: 14483–14489.

Lytton, W. W. (1996). Optimizing synaptic conductance calculation for network simulations. *Neur. Comput.* 8: 501–509.

Lytton, W. W., and Sejnowski, T. J. (1991). Simulations of cortical pyramidal neurons synchronized by inhibitory interneurons. *J. Neurophysiol.* 66: 1059–1079.

Ma, M., and Koester, J. (1995). Consequences and mechanisms of spike broadening of R20 cells in *Aplysia californica*. *J. Neurosci.* 15: 6720–6734.

Ma, M., and Koester, J. (1996). The role of potassium currents in frequency-dependent spike broadening in *Aplysia* R20 neurons: A dynamic clamp analysis. *J. Neurosci.* 16: 4089–4101.

MacLeod, K., and Laurent, G. (1996). Distinct mechanisms for synchronization and temporal patterning of odor-encoding neural assemblies. *Science* 274: 976–979.

Madison, D. V., and Nicoll, R. A. (1984). Control of repetitive discharges of rat CA1 pyramidal neurons *in vitro*. *J. Physiol.* 354: 319–331.

Magee, J. C., Christofi, G., Miyakawa, H., Christie, B., Lasser-Ross, N., and Johnston, D. (1995). Subthreshold synaptic activation of voltage-gated Ca^{2+} channels mediates a localized Ca^{2+} influx into the dendrites of hippocampal pyramidal neurons. *J. Neurophysiol.* 74: 1335–1342.

Magee, J. C., and Johnston, D. (1995a). Characterization of single voltage-gated Na^+ and Ca^{2+} channels in apical dendrities of rat CA1 pyramidal neurons. *J. Physiol.* 487: 67–90.

Magee, J. C., and Johnston, D. (1995b). Synaptic activation of voltage-gated channels in the dendrites of hippocampal pyramidal neurons. *Science* 268: 301–304.

Magee, J. C., and Johnston, D. (1997). A synaptically controlled, associative signal for Hebbian plasticity in hippocampal neurons. *Science* 275: 209–213.

Magleby, K. L., and Zengel, J. E. (1975). A quantitative description of stimulation-induced changes in transmitter release at the frog neuromuscular junction. *J. Gen. Physiol.* 80: 613–638.

Mahowald, M., and Douglas, R. (1991). A silicon neuron. *Nature* 354: 515–518.

Mainen, Z. F. (1996). Mechanisms of spike generation in neocortical neurons. Ph.D. diss., University of California, San Diego.

Mainen, Z. F., Carnevale, N. T., Zador, A. M., Claiborne, B. J., and Brown, T. H. (1996). Electrotonic architecture of hippocampal CA1 pyramidal neurons based on three-dimensional reconstructions. *J. Neurophysiol.* 76: 1904–1923.

Mainen, Z. F., Joerges, J., Huguenard, J. R., and Sejnowski, T. J. (1995). A model of spike initiation in neocortical pyramidal neurons. *Neuron* 15: 1427–1439.

Mainen, Z. F., and Sejnowski, T. J. (1995). Reliability of spike timing in neocortical neurons. *Science* 268: 1502–1506.

Mainen, Z. F., and Sejnowski, T. J. (1996). Influence of dendritic structure on firing pattern in model neocortical neurons. *Nature* 382: 363–366.

Major, G. (1992). The physiology, morphology and modelling of cortical pyramidal neurones. Ph.D. diss., University of Oxford.

Major, G. (1993). Solutions for transients in arbitrarily branching cables: 3. Voltage clamp problems [published erratum appears in *Biophys. J.* 65: 983]. *Biophys. J.* 65: 469–491.

Major, G., and Evans, J. D. (1994). Solutions for transients in arbitrarily branching cables: 4. Nonuniform electrical parameters. *Biophys. J.* 66: 615–633.

Major, G., Evans, J. D., and Jack, J. J. (1993a). Solutions for transients in arbitrarily branching cables: 1. Voltage recording with a somatic shunt [published errata appear in *Biophys. J.* 65: 982–983 and 2266]. *Biophys. J.* 65: 423–449.

Major, G., Evans, J. D., and Jack, J. J. (1993b). Solutions for transients in arbitrarily branching cables: 2. Voltage clamp theory [published erratum appears in *Biophys. J.* 65: 983]. Biophys. J. 65: 450–468.

Major, G., Larkman, A. U., Jonas, P., Sakmann, B., and Jack, J. J. B. (1994). Detailed passive cable models of whole-cell recorded CA3 pyramidal neurons in rat hippocampal slices. *J. Neurosci.* 14: 4613–4638.

Malenka, R. C., and Nicoll, R. A. (1993). MBDA-receptor-dependent synaptic plasticity: Multiple forms and mechanisms. *Trends Neurosci.* 16: 521–527.

Maletic-Savatic, M., Lenn, N. J., and Trimmer, J. S. (1995). Differential spatiotemporal expression of K^+ channel polypeptides in rat hippocampal neurons developing *in situ* and *in vitro*. *J. Neurosci.* 15: 3840–3851.

Manor, Y., Koch, C., and Segev, I. (1991). Effect of geometrical irregularities on propagation delay in axonal trees. *Biophys. J.* 60: 1424–1437.

Manor, Y., Nadim, F., Abbott, L. F., and Marder, E. (1997). Temporal dynamics of graded synaptic transmission in the lobster stomatogastric ganglion. *J. Neurosci.* 17: 5610–5621.

Marder, E. (1984). Roles for electrical coupling in neural circuits as revealed by selective neuronal deletions. *J. Exp. Biol.* 112: 147–167.

Marder, E., Abbott, L. F., Turrigiano, G. G., Liu, Z., and Golowasch, J. (1996). Memory from the dynamics of intrinsic membrane currents. *Proc. Natl. Acad. Sci. U.S.A.* 93: 13481–13486.

Marder, E., and Calabrese, R. L. (1996). Principles of rhythmic motor pattern generation. *Physiol. Rev* 76: 687–717.

Marder, E., Christie, A. E., and Kilman, V. L. (1995). Functional organization of cotransmission systems: lessons from small nervous systems. *Invert. Neurosci.* 1: 105–112.

Marder, E., and Hooper, S. L. (1985). Neurotransmitter modulation of the stomatogastric ganglion of decapod crustaceans. In *Model neural networks and behavior*, ed. A. I. Selverston, pp. 319–337. New York: Plenum Press.

Marder, E., Hooper, S. L., and Eisen, J. S. (1987). Multiple neurotransmitters provide a mechanism for the production of multiple outputs from a single neuronal circuit. In *Synaptic Function*, ed. G. M. Edelman, W. E. Gall, and M. W. Cowan, pp. 305–327. New York: Neuroscience Research Foundation, Wiley.

Marder, E., Jorge-Rivera, J. C., Kilman, V., and Weimann, J. M. (1997). Peptidergic modulation of synaptic transmission in a rhythmic motor system. In *The synapse: In development, health, and disease. Advances in Organ Biology*, vol 2, ed. B. W. Festoff, D. Hantai and B. A. Citron, pp. 213–233. Greenwich, CT: JAI Press.

Marder, E., and Selverston, E. (1992). Modeling the stomatogastric nervous system. In Dynamic biological networks: The stomatogastric nervous system, ed. R. M. Harris-Warrick, E. Marder, A. I. Selverston, and M. Moulins, pp. 161–196. Cambridge, MA: MIT Press.

Marder, E., and Weimann, J. M. (1992). Modulatory control of multiple task processing in the stomato-gastric nervous system. In *Neurobiology of motor programme selection: New approaches to mechanisms of behavioral choice*, ed. J. Kien, C. McCrohan, and W. Winlow, pp. 3–19. Oxford: Pergamon Press.

Markram, H., and Sakmann, B. (1994). Calcium transients in dendrites of neocortical neurons evoked by single subthreshold excitatory postsynaptic potentials via low-voltage-activated calcium channels. *Proc. Natl. Acad. Sci. U.S.A.* 91: 5207–5211.

Markram, H., and Tsodyks, M. V. (1996). Redistribution of synaptic efficacy between neocortical pyramidal neurons. *Nature* 382: 807–810.

Markram, H., Helm, P. J., and Sakmann, B. (1995). Dendritic calcium transients evoked by single back-propagating action potentials in rat neocortical pyramidal neurons. *J. Physiol.* 485: 1–20.

Markram, H., Lübke, J., Frotscher, M., and Sakmann, B. (1997). Regulation of synaptic efficacy by coincidence of postsynaptic APs and EPSPs. *Science* 275: 213–215.

Marmarelis. P. Z., and Marmarelis, V. Z. (1978). *Analysis of physiological systems: The white noise approach*. New York: Plenum Press.

Marom S., and Levitan, I. B. (1994). Cumulative inactivation of the Kv1.3 potassium channel. *Biophys. J.* 67: 579–589.

Marom, S., and Abbott, L. F. (1994). Modeling state-dependent inactivation of membrane currents. *Biophys. J.* 67: 515–520.

Marr, D. (1982). *Vision*. New York: Freeman.

Martin, K. A. C. (1988). From single cells to simple circuits in the cerebral cortex. *Quart. J. Exp. Physiol.* 73: 637–702.

Martone, M. E., Zhang, Y., Simpliciano, V. M., Carragher, B. O., and Ellisman, M. H. (1993). Three-dimensional visualization of the smooth endoplasmic reticulum in Purkinje cell dendrites. *J. Neurosci.* 13: 4636–4646.

Mascagni, M. (1987a). Negative feedback in neural networks. Ph.D. diss., New York University.

Mascagni, M. (1987b). Computer simulation of negative feedback in neurons. *Soc. Neurosci. Abstr.* 13: 375.4.

Mascagni, M. (1989a). An initial-boundary value problem of physiological significance for equations of nerve conduction. *Commun. Pure and Appl. Math.* 42: 213–227.

Mascagni, M. (1989b). Animation's role in modeling the nervous system. *Iris Universe* Winter: 6–18.

Mascagni, M. (1991). A parallelizing algorithm for computing solutions to arbitrarily branched cable neuron models. *J. Meth. Neurosci.* 36: 105–114.

Mason, A., and Larkman, A. U. (1990). Correlations between morphology and electrophysiology of pyramidal neurons in slices of rat visual cortex: 2. Electrophysiology. *J. Neurosci.* 10: 1415–1428.

Mason, A., Nicoll, A., and Stratford, K. (1991). Synaptic transmission between individual pyramidal neurons of the visual cortex *in vitro*. *J. Neurosci.* 11: 72–84.

Matsouka, K. (1985). Sustained oscillations generated by mutually inhibiting neurons with adaptation. *Biol. Cybern.* 52: 367–376.

Mayer, M. L., and Westbrook, G. L. (1987). Permeation and block of N-methyl-D-aspartic acid receptor channels by divalent cations in mouse cultured central neurones. *J. Physiol.* 394: 501–527.

McBain, C., and Dingledine, R. (1992). Dual-component miniature excitatory synaptic currents in rat hippocampal CA3 pyramidal neurons. *J. Neurophysiol.* 68: 16–27.

McBurney, R. N., and Neering, I. R. (1987). Neuronal calcium homeostasis. *Trends Neurosci.* 10: 164–169.

McCormick, D. (1990). Membrane properties and neurotransmitter actions. In *The synaptic organization of the brain*, ed. G. Shepherd, pp. 32–66. 3d ed. Oxford: Oxford University Press.

McCormick, D. A. (1992). Neurotransmitter actions in the thalamus and cerebral cortex and their role in neuromodulation of thalamocortical activity. *Prog. Neurobiol.* 39: 337–388.

McCormick, D. A., and Huguenard, J. R. (1992). A model of the electrophysiological properties of thalamocortical relay neurons. *J. Neurophysiol.* 68: 1384–1400.

McCormick, D. A., Connors, B. W., Lighthall, J. W. and Prince, D. A. (1985). Comparative electrophysiology of pyramidal and sparsely spiny stellate neurons of the neocortex. *J. Neurophysiol.* 54: 782–806.

McCormick, D. A., Huguenard, J. R., and Strowbridge, B. W. (1992). Determination of state-dependent procesing in thalamus by single neuron properties and neuromodulators. In *Single neuron computation*, ed. T. McKenna, J. Davis, and S. F. Zornetzer, pp. 259–290. Boston: Academic Press.

McKernan, R. M., and Whiting, P. J. (1996). Which GABA$_A$-receptor subtypes really occur in the brain? *Trends Neurosci.* 19: 139–143.

McLean, J., and Palmer, L. A. (1989). Contribution of linear spatiotemporal receptive field structure to velocity selectivity of simple cells in area 17 of cat. *Vis. Res.* 29: 675–679.

Mead, C. (1989). *Analog VLSI and neural systems.* Reading, MA: Addison-Wesley.

Mead, C. (1990). Neuromorphic electronic systems. *Proc. IEEE* 78: 1629–1636.

Mel, B. W. (1992). NMDA-based pattern discrimination in a modeled cortical neuron. *Neur. Comput.* 4: 502–516.

Mel, B. W. (1993). Synaptic integration in an excitable dendritic tree. *J. Neurophysiol.* 70: 1086–1101.

Mel, B. W. (1994). Information processing in dendritic trees. *Neur. Comput.* 6: 1031–1085.

Mel, B. W., Ruderman, D. L., and Niebur, E. (1996). Complex cell responses could arise directly from center-surround inputs: The surprising power of intra-dendritic computations. *Soc. Neurosci. Abstr.* 22: 1612. Abstr. 633.7.

Merzenich, M., Knight, P., and Roth, G. (1975). Representation of cochlea within primary auditory cortex in the cat. *J. Neurophysiol.* 28: 231–249.

Meumier, C. (1992). Two and three dimensional reduction of the Hodgkin-Huxley system: Separation of times scales and bifurcation schemes. *Biol. Cybern.* 67: 461–468.

Meyer, T., and Stryer, L. (1991). Calcium spiking. *Ann. Rev. Biophys. and Biophys. Chem.* 20: 153–174.

Meyrand, P., Simmers, J., and Moulins, M. (1991). Construction of a pattern-generating circuit with neurons of different networks. *Nature* 351: 60–63.

Meyrand, P., Simmers, J., and Moulins, M. (1994). Dynamic construction of a neural network from multiple pattern generators in the lobster stomatogastric nervous system. *J. Neurosci.* 14: 630–644.

Michaelis, L., and Menten, M. L. (1913). Die Kinetik der invertinwirkung. *Biochem. Z.* 49: 333–349.

Migliore, M. (1996). Modeling the attenuation and failure of action potentials in the dendrites of hippocampal neurons. *Biophys. J.* 71: 2394–2403.

Migliore, M., Alicata, F., and Ayala, G. F. (1995). A model for long-term potentiation and depression. *J. Comput. Neurosci.* 2: 335–343.

Milazzo, G. (1963). *Electrochemistry, theoretical principles and practical applications.* Amsterdam: Elsevier.

Miller, M., and Sachs, M. (1983). Representation of stop consonants in the discharge patterns of auditory-nerve fibers. *J. Acoust. Soc. Am.* 502–517.

Miller, J. P., and Selverston, A. I. (1979). Rapid killing of single neurons by an irradiation of intracellularly injected dye. *Science* 206: 702–704.

Miller, J. P., and Selverston, A. I. (1982a). Mechanisms underlying pattern generation in lobster stomatogastric ganglion as determined by selective inactivation of identified neurons: II. Oscillatory properties of pyloric neurons. *J. Neurophysiol.* 48: 1378–1391.

Miller, J. P., and Selverston, A. I. (1982b). Mechanisms underlying pattern generation in lobster stomatogastric ganglion as determined by selective inactivation of identified neurons: IV. Network properties of pyloric system. *J. Neurophysiol.* 48: 1416–1432.

Mills, L. R., Niesen, C. E., So, A. P., Carlen, P. L., Spigelman, I., and Jones, O. T. (1994). N-type Ca^{2+} channels are located on somata, dendrites, and a subpopulation of dendritic spines on live hippocampal pyramidal neurons. *J. Neurosci.* 14: 6815–6824.

Missiaen, L., Declerck, I., Droogmans, G., De Smedt, H., Raeymaekers, L., and Casteels, R. (1990). Agonist-dependent Ca^{2+} and Mn^{2+} entry dependent on state of filling of Ca^{2+} stores in aortic smooth muscle cells of the rat. *J. Physiol.* 427: 171–186.

Miyakawa, H., Lev-Ram, V., Lasser-Ross, N., and Ross, W. N. (1992a). Calcium transients evoked by climbing fiber synaptic inputs in guinea pig cerebellar Purkinje neurons. *J. Neurophysiol.* 68: 1178–1189.

Miyakawa, H., Ross, W. N., Jaffe, D., Callaway, J. C., Lasser-Ross, N., Lisman, J. E., and Johnston, D. (1992b). Synaptically activated increases in Ca^{2+} concentration in hippocampal CA1 pyramidal cells are primarily due to voltage-gated Ca^{2+} channels. *Neuron* 9: 1163–1173.

Moczydlowski, E., and Latorre, R. (1983). Gating kinetics of Ca^{2+} activated K^+ channels from rat muscle incorporated into planar lipid bilayers: Evidence for two voltage-dependent Ca^{2+}-binding reactions. *J. Gen. Physiol.* 82: 511–542.

Mody, I., De Koninck, Y., Otis, T. S., and Soltesz, I. (1994). Bridging the cleft at GABA synapses in the brain. *Trends Neurosci.* 17: 517–525.

Molinoff, P. B., Williams, K., Pritchett, D. B., and Zhong, J. (1994). Molecular pharmacology of NMDA receptors: Modulatory role of NR2 subunits. *Prog. Brain Res.* 100: 39–45.

Montalvo, F. S. (1975). Consensus versus competition in neural network: A cooperative analysis of three models. *Int. J. Man-Mach. Stud.* 7: 333–346.

Monyer, H., Burnashev, N., Laurie, D. J., Sakmann, B., and Seeburg, P. H. (1994). Developmental and regional expression in the rat brain and functional properties of four NMDA receptors. *Neuron* 12: 529–540.

Morishita, I., and Yajima, A. (1972). Analysis and simulation of networks of mutually inhibiting neurons. *Kybernetik* 11: 154–165.

Morissette, J. (1996). Plasticity in mammalian somatosensory cerebellar maps. Ph.D. diss., California Institute of Technology.

Morris, C., and Lecar, H. (1981). Voltage oscillations in the barnacle giant muscle fiber. *Biophys. J.* 35: 193–213.

Mosbacher, J., Schoepfer, R., Monyer, H., Burnashev, N., Seeburg, P. H., and Ruppersberg, J. P. (1994). A molecular determinant for submillisecond desensitization in glutamate receptors. *Science* 266: 1059–1062.

Moschovakis, A. K., Burke, R. E., and Fyffe, R. E. W. (1991). The size and dendritic structure of HRP-labeled gamma motoneurons in the cat spinal cord. *J. Comp. Neurol.* 311: 531–545.

Müller, J. W. (1974). Some formulae for a dead-time-distorted Poisson process. *Nucl. Inst. and Meth.* 117: 401–404.

Murphy, B. J., Rossie, S., DeJongh, K. S., and Catterall, W. A. (1993). Identification of the sites of selective phosphorylation and dephosphorylation of the rat brain Na^+ channel α-subunit by cAMP-dependent protein kinase and phosphoprotein phosphatases. *J. Biol. Chem.* 268: 27355–27362.

Murphy, T. H., Worley, P. F., Baraban, J. M. (1991). L-type voltage-sensitive calcium channels mediate synaptic activation of immediate early genes. *Neuron* 7: 625–635.

Murray, A., Hamilton, A., and Tarassenko, L. (1989). Programmable analog pulse-firing neural networks. In *Advances in neural information processing systems*, ed. D. S. Touretzky, vol. 1, pp. 712–719. San Mateo, CA: Kaufmann.

Murray, A., and Tarassenko, L. (1994). *Analogue neural VLSI*. London: Chapman and Hall.

Murray, J. D. (1989). *Mathematical biology*. New York: Springer.

Nadim, F., Olsen, Ø. H., De Schutter, E., and Calabrese, R. L. (1995). Modeling the leech heartbeat elemental oscillator: 1. Interactions of intrinsic and synaptic currents. *J. Comput. Neurosci.* 2: 215–235.

Nagumo, J. S., Arimato, S., and Yoshizawa, S. (1962). An active pulse transmission line simulating a nerve axon. *Proc. IRE* 50: 2061–2070.

Naraghi, M., Müller, T. H., Oheim, M., and Neher, E. (1995). Spatially resolved measurements of the endogenous calcium buffering capacity in adrenal chromaffin cells. *Soc. Neurosci. Abstr.* 21: 1090.

Neher, E., and Augustine, G. J. (1992). Calcium gradients and buffers in bovine chromaffin cells. *J. Physiol.* 450: 273–301.

Nelson, S., Toth, L., Sheth, B., and Sur, M. (1994). Orientation selectivity of cortical neurons during intracellular blockade of inhibition. *Science* 265: 774–777.

Nernst, W. (1888). Zur Kinetik der in Lösung befindlichen Körper: Theorie der Diffusion. Z. Phys. Chem. 3: 613–637.

Newsome, W. T., Britten, K. H., and Movshon, J. A. (1989). Neuronal correlates of a perceptual decision. *Nature* 341: 52–54.

Nicolelis, M. A. L., Baccala, L. A., Lin, R. C. S., and Chapin, J. K. (1995). Sensorimotor encoding by synchronous neural ensemble activity at multiple levels of the somatosensory system. *Science* 268: 1353–1358.

Nicoll, R. A. (1988). The coupling of neurotransmitter receptors to ion channels in the brain. *Science* 241: 545–551.

Niebur, E., Koch, C., and Rosin, C. (1993). An oscillation-based model for the neruonal basis of attention. *Vision Res.* 33: 2789–2802.

Nitzan, R., Segev, I., and Yarom, Y. (1990). Voltage behavior along the irregular dendritic structure of morphologically and physiologically characterized vagal motoneurons in the guinea pig. *J. Neurophysiol.* 63: 333–346.

Nowak, L., Bregestovski, P., Ascher, P., Herbet, A. and Prochiantz, A. (1984). Magnesium gates glutamate-activated channels in mouse central neurons. *Nature* 307: 462–465.

Nowycky, M. C., and Pinter, M. J. (1993). Time courses of calcium and calcium-bound buffers following calcium influx in a model cell. *Biophys. J.* 64: 77–91.

Nowycky, M. C., Fox, A. P., and Tsien, R. W. (1983). Three types of neuronal calcium channels with different calcium agonist sensitivity. *Nature* 316: 440–443.

Nunez, P. L. (1981). *Electric fields of the brain: The neurophysics of EEG.* Oxford: Oxford University Press.

Oguztoreli, M. (1979). Activity analysis of neural networks. *Biol. Cybern.* 34: 159–169.

Olsen, Ø. H., and Calabrese, R. L. (1996). Activation of intrinsic and synaptic currents in leech heart interneurons by realistic wave-forms. *J. Neurosci.* 16: 4958–4970.

Oppenheim, A., and Schafer, R. (1976). *Digital signal processing.* Englewood Cliffs, NJ: Prentice Hall.

Oppenheim, A. V., and Schafer, R. W. (1989). *Discrete signal processing.* Englewood Cliffs, NJ: Prentice Hall.

Orban, G. A. (1984). *Neuronal operations in the visual cortex.* Berlin: Springer.

Otis, T. S., and Mody, I. (1992). Modulation of decay kinetics and frequency of $GABA_A$ receptor-mediated spontaneous inhibitory postsynaptic currents in hippocampal neurons. *Neurosci.* 49: 13–32.

Otis, T. S., De Koninck, Y. and Mody, I. (1992). Whole-cell recordings of evoked and spontaneous $GABA_B$ responses in hippocampal slices. *Pharmacol. Commun.* 2: 75–83.

Otis, T. S., De Koninck, Y., and Mody, I. (1993). Characterization of synaptically elicited $GABA_B$ responses using patch-clamp recordings in rat hippocampal slices. *J. Physiol.* 463: 391–407.

Palay, S. L., and Chan-Palay, V. (1974). *Cerebellar cortex.* New York: Springer.

Palay, S. L., Sotelo, C., Peters, A., and Orkland, P. M. (1968). The axon hillock and the initial segment. *J. Cell Biol.* 37: 193–201.

Palm, G., and Poggio, T. (1977). The Volterra representation and the Wiener expansion: Validity and pitfalls. *SIAM J. Appl. Math.* 33: 195–217.

Palm, G., and Poggio, T. (1978). Stochastic identification methods for nonlinear systems: An extension of the Wiener theory. *SIAM J. Appl. Math.* 34: 524–534.

Parnas, H., Hovav, G., and Parnas, I. (1989). Effect of Ca^{2+} diffusion on the time course of neurotransmitter release. *Biophys. J.* 55: 859–874.

Parnas, I., Parnas, H., and Hochner, B. (1991). Amount and time course of release: The calcium hypothesis and the calcium-voltage hypothesis. *Ann. N. Y. Acad. Sci.* 635: 177–190.

Parnas, I., and Segev. I. (1979). A mathematical model for the conduction of action patentials along bifurcating axons. *J. Physiol.* 295: 323–343.

Patneau, D. K., and Mayer, M. L. (1991). Kinetic analysis of interactions between kainate and AMPA: Evidence for activation of a single receptor in mouse hippocampal neurons. *Neuron* 6: 785–798.

Pearce, R. A. (1993). Physiological evidence for two distinct $GABA_A$ responses in rat hippocampus. *Neuron* 10: 189–200.

Pei, X., Vidyasagar, T. R., Volgushev, M., and Creutzfeldt, O. D. (1994). Receptive field analysis and orientation selectivity of postsynaptic potentials of simple cells in cat visual cortex. *J. Neurosci.* 14: 7130–7140.

Peřina, J. (1985). *Coherence of light.* 2d ed. Dordrecht: Reidel.

Perkel, D. H., and Perkel, D. J. (1985). Dendritic spines: Role of active membrane in modulating synaptic efficiency. *Brain Res.* 325: 331–335.

Perkel, D. H., Mulloney, B., and Budelli, R. W. (1981). Quantitative methods for predicting neuronal behavior. *Neurosci.* 6: 823–837.

Perkel, D. H., Schulman, J. H., Bullock, T. H., Moore, G. P., and Segundo, J. P. (1964). Pacemaker neurons: Effects of regularly spaced synaptic input. *Science* 145: 61–63.

Perkins, K. L., and Wong, R. K. (1995). Intracellular QX-314 blocks the hyperpolarization-activated inward current I_q in hippocampal CA1 pyramidal cells. *J. Neurophysiol.* 73: 911–915.

Peters, A., and Jones, E. G. (1984). *Cerebral cortex.* Vol. 1, *Cellular components of the cerebral cortex.* New York: Plenum Press.

Peters, A., and Kaiserman-Abramof, I. R. (1970). The small pyramidal neuron of the rat cerebral cortex: The perikaryon, dendrites and spines. *Am. J. Anat.* 127: 321–355.

Peters, A., and Payne, B. R. (1993). Numerical relationships between geniculocortical afferents and pyramidal cell modules in cat primary visual cortex. *Cerebral Cortex* 3: 69–78.

Peters, A., Proskauer, C. C., and Kaiserman-Abramof, I. R. (1968). The small pyramidal neuron of the rat cerebral cortex: The axon hillock and the initial segment. *J. Cell Biol.* 39: 604–619.

Pinski, P. F., and Rinzel, J. (1994). Intrinsic and network rythmogenesis in a reduced Traub model for CA3 neurons. *J. Comput. Neurosci.* 1: 39–60.

Planck, M. (1890). Über die Erregung von Elektricität und Wärme in Elektrolyten. *Ann. Phys. Chem.* 39: 161–186.

Poggio, T., and Torre, V. (1977). A Volterra representation for some neuron models. *Biol. Cybern.* 27: 113–124.

Poggio, T. and Torre, V. (1978). A new approach to synaptic interactions. In *Lecture notes in biomathematics.* Vol. 21, *Theoretical approaches top complex systems,* eds. R. Heim, and G. Palm, pp. 89–115. Berlin: Springer.

Poggio, T., Torre, V., and Koch, C. (1985). Computational vision and regularization theory. *Nature* 317: 314–317.

Pongracz, F. (1985). The function of dendritic spines: A theoretical study. *Neuroscience* 15: 933–946.

Pongracz, F., Firestein, S., and Shepherd, G. M. (1991). Electrotonic structure of olfactory sensory neurons analyzed by intracellular and whole cell patch techniques. *J. Neurophysiol.* 65: 747–758.

Poor, H. V. (1994). *An introduction to signal detection and estimation.* 2d ed. New York: Springer.

Poznanski, R. R. (1987). Techniques for obtaining analytical solutions for the somatic shunt cable model. *Math. Biosci.* 85: 13–35.

Pozzan, T., Rizzuto, R., Volpe, P., and Meldolesi, J. (1994). Molecular and cellular physiology of intracellular calcium stores. *Physiol. Rev.* 74: 595–636.

Prakriya, M., Solaro, CR., and Lingle, C. J. (1996). $[Ca^{2+}]_i$ elevations detected by BK channels during Ca^{2+} influx and muscarine-mediated release of Ca^{2+} from intracellular stores in rat chromaffin cells. *J. Neurosci.* 16: 4344–4359.

Press, W. H., Flannery, B. P., Teukolsky, S. A., and Vetterling, W. T. (1986). *Numerical recipes: The art of scientific computing.* Cambridge, U.K.: Cambridge University Press.

Press, W. H., Teukolsky, S. A., Vetterling, W. T., and Flannery, B.P. (1992). *Numerical recipes in C: The art of scientific computing.* 2d ed. Cambridge: Cambridge University Press.

Price, R. (1958). A useful theorem for nonlinear devices having Gaussian inputs. *IRE Trans. Inform. Theory* 4: 69–72.

Prince, J. L. (1973). An autoradiographic study of complementary laminar patterns of termination of afferent fibers to the olfactory cortex. *J. Comp. Neurol.* 150: 87–108.

Protopapas, A., and Bower, J. M. (1995). Dynamics of cerebral cortical networks, In *The book of GENESIS: Exploring realistic neural models with the GEneral NEural SImulation System,* ed. J. M. Bower and C. Beeman, pp. 159–179. New York: Springer.

Protopapas, A., and Bower, J. M. (1997a). Piriform pyramidal cell response to physiologically plausible patterns of synaptic activity. In Preparation.

Protopapas, A., and Bower, J. M. (1997b). The responses of layer II pyramidal cells in piriform (olfactory) cortex to current injection: A combined *in vitro* and realistic modeling study. In Preparation.

Purves, D., and Lichtman, J. W. (1985). *Principles of neural development.* Sunderland, MA: Sinauer.

Qian, N., and Sejnowski, T. J. (1989). An electro-diffusion model for computing membrane potentials and ionic concentrations in branching dendrites, spines and axons. *Biol. Cybern.* 62: 1–15.

Qian, N., and Sejnowski, T. J. (1990). When is an inhibitory synapse effective? *Proc. Natl. Acad. Sci. U.S.A.* 87: 8145–8149.

Quadroni, R., and Knöpfel, T. (1994). Compartmental models of type A and type B guinea pig medial vestibular neurons. *J. Neurophysiol.* 72: 1911–1124.

Rall, W. (1957). Membrane time constant of motoneurones. *Science* 126: 454.

Rall, W. (1959). Branching dendritic trees and motoneuron membrane resistivity. *Exp. Neurol.* 1: 491–527.

Rall, W. (1960). Membrane potential transients and membrane time constant of motoneurons. *Exp. Neurol.* 2: 503–532.

Rall, W. (1962a). Theory of physiological properties of dendrites. *Annu. N.Y. Acad. Sci.* 96: 1071–1092.

Rall, W. (1962b). Electrophysiology of a dendritic neuron model. *Biophys. J.* 2: 145–167.

Rall, W. (1964). Theoretical significance of dendritic trees for neuronal input-output relations. In: *Neural theory and modeling,* ed. R. F. Reiss, pp. 73–94. Stanford, CA: Stanford University Press.

Rall, W. (1967). Distinguishing theoretical synaptic potentials computed for different soma-dendritic distributions of synaptic inputs. *J. Neurophysiol.* 30: 1138–1168.

Rall, W. (1969a). Time constants and electrotonic length of membrane cylinders and neurons. *Biophys. J.* 9: 1483–1508.

Rall, W. (1969b). Distributions of potential in cylindrical coordinates and time constants for a membrane cylinder. *Biophys. J.* 9: 1509–1541.

Rall, W. (1970). Dendritic neuron theory and dendrodendritic synapses in a simple cortical system. In: *The neurosciences: Second study program*, ed. F. O. Schmitt. New York: Rockfeller University Press.

Rall, W. (1977). Core conductor theory and cable properties of neurons. In: *Handbook of physiology (sect. 1). The nervous system. I. Cellular biology of neurons*, eds. E. R. Kandel, J. M. Brookhart, and V. B. Mountcastle, pp. 39–97. Bethesda, MD: American Physiology Society.

Rall, W. (1981). Functional aspects of neuronal geometry. In: *Neurones without impulses*, eds. B. M. H. Bush, and A. Roberts. Cambridge, U.K.: Cambridge University Press.

Rall, W., Burke, R. E., Holmes, W. R. Jack, J. J. B., Redman, S. J., and Segev, I. (1992). Matching dendritic neuron models to experimental data. *Physiol. Rev.* 72: S159–S186.

Rall, W., Burke, R. E., Nelson, P. G., Smith, T. G., and Frank, K. (1967). The dendritic location of synapses and possible mechanisms for the monosynaptic EPSP in motoneurons. *J. Neurophysiol.* 30: 1169–1193.

Rall, W., and Rinzel, J. (1973). Branch input resistance and steady attenuation for input to one branch of a dendritic neuron model. *Biophys. J.* 13: 648–688.

Rall, W., and Segev, I. (1985). Space-clamp problems when voltage clamping branched neurons with intracellular microelectrodes. In: *Voltage and patch clamping with microelectrodes*, eds. J. Thomas, G. Smith, H. Lecar, S. J. Redman, and P. W. Gage, pp. 191–215. Bethesda, MD: American Physiological Society.

Rall, W., and Segev, I. (1987). Functional possibilities for synapses on dendrites and dendritic spines. In: *Synaptic function*, eds. G. M. Edelman, W. F. Gall, and W. M. Cowan, pp. 605–636. New York: Neuroscience Research Foundation, Wiley and Sons.

Rall, W., and Shepherd, G. M. (1968). Theoretical reconstruction of field potentials and dendrodendritic synaptic interactions in olfactory bulb. *J. Neurophysiol.* 31: 884–915.

Rall, W., Shepherd, G. M., Reese, G. M., and Brightman, M. W. (1966). Dendro-dendritic synaptic pathway for inhibition in the olfactory bulb. *Exp. Neurol.* 14: 44–56.

Ramacher, U., and Ruckert, U. (1991). VLSI design of neural networks. Boston: Kluwer Academic.

Raman, I. M., and Trussell, L. O. (1992). The kinetics of the response to glutamate and kainate in neurons of the avian cochlear nucleus. *Neuron* 9: 173–186.

Raman, I. M., Zhang, S., and Trussell, L. O. (1994). Pathway-specific variant of AMPA receptors and their contribution to neuronal signaling. *J. Neurosci.* 14: 4998–5010.

Rand, R. H., and Armbruster, D. (1987). *Perturbation methods, bifurcation theory, and computer algebra*. Applied Mathematical Sciences, vol. 65. New York: Springer.

Randall, A., and Tsien, R. W. (1995). Pharmacological dissection of multiple types of Ca^{2+} channel currents in rat cerebellar granule neurons. *J. Neurosci.* 15: 2995–3012.

Rapp, M., Segev, I., and Yarom, Y. (1994). Physiology, morphology and detailed passive models of guinea-pig cerebellar Purkinje cells. *J. Physiol.* 474: 101–118.

Rapp, M., Yarom, Y., and Segev, I. (1992). The impact of parallel fiber background activity on the cable properties of cerebellar Purkinje cells. *Neur. Comput.* 4: 518–533.

Rapp, M., Yarom, Y., and Segev, I. (1996). Modeling back propagating action potential in weakly excitable dendrites of neocortical pyramidal cells. *Proc. Natl. Acad. Sci. U.S.A.* 93: 11985–11990.

Reale, R., and Imig, T. (1980). Tonotopic organization of auditory cortex in the cat. *J. Comp. Neurol.* 192: 265–291.

Redish, A. D., Elga, A. N., and Touretzky, D. S. (1996). A coupled attractor model of the rodent head direction system. *Network* 7: 671–685.

Redman, S. J. (1973). The attenuation of passively propagating dendritic potentials in a motoneurone cable model. *J. Physiol.* 234: 637–664.

Redman, S., and Walmsley, B. (1983). The time course of synaptic potentials evoked in cat spinal motoneurones at identified group Ia synapses. *J. Physiol.* 343: 117–133.

Reeves, J. P. (1990). Sodium-calcium exchange. In: *Intracellular calcium regulation*, ed. F. Bronner, pp. 305–347. New York: Liss.

Regehr, W. G., and Atluri, P. P. (1995). Calcium transients in cerebellar granule cell presynaptic terminals. *Biophys. J.* 68: 2156–2170.

Regehr, W. G., Connor, J. A., and Tank, D. W. (1989). Optical imaging of calcium accumulation in hippocampal pyramidal cells during synaptic activation. *Nature* 341: 533–536.

Regehr, W. G., Kehoe, J. S., Ascher, P., and Armstrong, C. (1993). Synaptically triggered action potentials in dendrites. *Neuron* 11: 145–151.

Reid, C. R., and Alonso, J.-M. (1995). Specificity of monosynaptic connections from thalamus to visual cortex. *Nature* 378: 281–284.

Reuter, H. (1996). Diversity and function of presynaptic calcium channels in the brain. *Curr. Opin. Neurobiol.* 6: 331–337.

Reuveni, I., Friedman, A., Amitai, Y., and Gutnick, M. J. (1993). Stepwise repolarization from Ca^{2+} plateaus in neocortical pyramidal cells: Evidence for nonhomogeneous distribution of HVA Ca^{2+} channels in dendrites. *J. Neurosci.* 13: 4609–4621.

Reyes, A. D., and Fetz, E. E. (1993). Two modes of interspike interval shortening by brief transient depolarizations in cat neorcortical neurons. *J. Neurophysiol.* 69: 1661–1672.

Reyes, A. D., Rubel, E. W., and Spain, W. J. (1996). In vitro analysis of optimal stimuli for phase-locking and time-delayed modulation of firing in avian nucleus laminaris neurons. *J. Neurosci.* 16: 993–1007.

Rhodes, P. A., and Gray, C. M. (1994). Simulations of intrinsically bursting neocortical pyramidal neurons. *Neur. Comput.* 6: 1086–1110.

Richardson, T. L., Turner, R. W., and Miller, J. J. (1987). Action-potential discharge in hippocampal CA1 pyramidal neurons: Current source-density analysis. *J. Neurophysiol.* 58: 981–996.

Richtmyer, R. D., and Morton, K. W. (1967). *Difference methods for initial-value problems.* 2d ed. New York: Wiley, Interscience.

Rieke, F., Warland, D., van Steveninck, R. R., and Bialek, W. (1996). *Spikes: Exploring the neural code.* Cambridge, MA: MIT Press.

Rinzel, J. (1978). On repetitive activity in nerve. *Federat. Proc.* 37: 2793–2802.

Rinzel, J. (1985). Excitation dynamics: insights from simplified membrane models, *Federat. Proc.* 44: 2944–2946.

Rinzel, J., and Ermentrout, G. B. (1989). Analysis of neural excitability and oscillations. In *Methods in neuronal modeling: From synapses to networks*, ed. C. Koch and I. Segev, pp. 135–169. Cambridge, MA: MIT Press.

Rinzel, J., and Keller, J. B. (1973). Traveling wave solutions of a nerve conduction equation. *Biophys. J.* 13: 1313–1337.

Rinzel, J., and Lee, Y. S. (1987). Dissection of a model for neuronal parabolic bursting. *J. Math. Biol.* 25: 653–675.

Rinzel, J., and Rall, W. (1974). Transient response in a dendritic neuronal model for current injected at one branch. *Biophys. J.* 14: 759–790.

Robinson, D. A. (1989). Integrating with neurons. *Ann. Rev. Neurosci.* 12: 33–45.

Robinson, H. P. C., and Kawai, N. (1993). Injection of digitally synthesized synaptic conductance transients to measure the integrative properties of neurons. *J. Neurosci. Meth.* 49: 157–165.

Roddey, J. C., and Jacobs, G. A. (1996). Information theoretic analysis of dynamical encoding by filiform mechanoreceptors in the cricket cercal system. *J. Neurophysiol.* 75: 1365–1376.

Rodriguez, R., and Haberly, L. B. (1989). Analysis of synaptic events in the opossum piriform cortex with improved current-source density techniques. *J. Neurophysiol.* 61: 702–718.

Ropert, N., Miles, R. and Korn, H. (1990) Characteristics of miniature inhibitory postsynaptic currents in CA1 pyramidal neurones of rat hippocampus. *J. Physiol.* 428: 707–722.

Rose, M. E. (1956). On the integration of nonlinear parabolic equations by implicit methods. *Quart. Appl. Math.* 15: 237–248.

Rose, P., Kierstead, S., and Vanner, S. (1985). A quantitative analysis of the geometry of cat motoneurons innervating neck and shoulder muscles. *J. Comp. Neurol.* 199: 191–203.

Rose, P., and Vanner, S. (1988). Differences in somatic and dendritic specific membrane resistivity of spinal motoneourons: An electrophysiological study of neck and shoulder motoneurons in the cat. *J. Neurophysiol.* 60: 149–166.

Ross, W. M. (1989). Changes in intracellular calcium during neuron activity. *Ann. Rev. Physiol.* 51: 491–506.

Russell, D. F., and Hartline, D. K. (1978). Bursting neural networks: A reexamination. *Science* 200: 453–456.

Rush, M. E., and Rinzel, J. (1994). The potassium A-current, low firing rates and rebound excitation in Hodgkin-Huxley models. *Bull. Math. Biol.* 57: 899–929.

Russell, D. F., and Hartline, D. K. (1984). Synaptic regulation of cellular properties and burst oscillations of neurons in gastric mill system of spiny lobster, *Panulirus interruptus. J. Neurophysiol.* 52: 54–73.

Sabatini, B. L., and Regehr, W. G. (1997). Control of neurotransmitter release by presynaptic waveform at the granule cell to Purkinje cell synapse. *J. Neurosci.* 17: 3425–3436.

Sachs, M. B. and Young, E. D. (1979). Encoding of steady state vowels in the auditory news: representation in terms of discharge rate. *J. Acoust. Soc. Am.* 66: 470–479.

Safri, S. M., and Keizer, J. (1995). On the roles of Ca^{2+} diffusion, Ca^{2+} buffers, and the endoplasmic reticulum in IP_3-induced Ca^{2+} waves. *Biophys. J.* 69: 2139–2153.

Sah, P. (1993). Kinetic properties of a slow apamin-insensitive Ca^{2+}-activated K^+ current in guinea pig vagal neurons. *J. Neurophysiol.* 69: 361–366.

Sah, P. (1995). Different calcium channels are coupled to potassium channels with distinct physiological role in vagal neurons. *Proc. Roy. Soc. Lond.* B260: 105–111.

Sah, P. (1996). Ca^{2+}-activated K^+ currents in neurones: Types, physiological roles and modulation. *Trends Neurosci.* 19: 150–154.

Sah, P., and Bekkers, J. M. (1996). Apical dendritic location of slow afterhyperpolarization current in hippocampal pyramidal neurons: Implications for the integration of longterm potentiation. *J. Neurosci.* 16: 4537–4542.

Sakai, H. M., Naka, K.-I., and Korenberg, J. (1988). White-noise analysis in visual neuroscience. *Vis. Neurosci.* 1: 287–296.

Sakmann, B., and Neher, E., eds. (1983). *Single channel recording.* New York: Plenum Press.

Sakmann, B., and Neher, E. (1995a). Geometric parameters of pipettes and membrane patches. In *Single channel recording,* ed. B. Sakmann and E. Neher, pp. 637–650. 2d ed. New York: Plenum Press.

Sakmann, B., and Neher, E. (1995b). *Single channel recording.* 2d ed. New York: Plenum Press.

Sakurai, T., Westenbroek, R. E., Rettig, J., Hell, J., and Catterall, W. A. (1996). Biochemical properties and subcellular distribution of the BI and rbA isoforms of $\alpha1A$ subunits of brain calcium channels. *J. Cell Biol.* 134: 511–528.

Sala, F., and Hernández-Cruz, A. (1990). Calcium diffusion modeling in a spherical neuron: Relevance of buffering properties. *Biophys. J.* 57: 313–324.

Saleh, B. E. A. (1978). *Photoelectron statistics.* New York: Springer.

Saleh, B. E. A., Tavolacci, J. T., and Teich, M. C. (1981). Discrimination of shot-noise-driven Poisson processes by external dead time: Application to radioluminescence from glass. *IEEE J. Quant. Electron.* 17: 2341–2350.

Saleh, B. E. A., and Teich, M. C. (1985). Multiplication and refractoriness in the cat's retinal-ganglion-cell discharge at low light levels. *Biol. Cybern.* 52: 101–107.

Salinas, E., and Abbott, L. F. (1996). A model of multiplicative neural responses in parietal cortex. *Proc. Nat. Acad. Sci U.S.A.* 93: 11956–11961.

Sargent, P. B. (1983). The number of synaptic boutons terminating on *Xenopus* cardiac ganglion cells is directly correlated with cell size. *J. Physiol.* 343: 85–104.

Satou, M., Mori, K., Tazawa, Y., and Takagi, S. F. (1982). Long-lasting disinhibition in pyriform cortex of the rabbit. *J. Neurophysiol.* 48: 1157–1163.

Saul, A. B., and Humphrey, A. L. (1990). Spatial and temporal response properties of lagged and nonlagged cells in cat lateral geniculate nucleus. *J. Neurophysiol.* 64: 206–224.

Scharf, L. L. (1991). *Statistical signal processing: Detection, estimation, and time series analysis.* New York: Addison-Wesley.

Schieg, A., Gerstner, W., Ritz, R., and van Hemmen, J. L. (1995). Intracellular Ca^{2+} stores can account for the time course of LTP induction: A model of Ca^{2+} dynamics in dendritic spines. *J. Neurophysiol.* 74: 1046–1055.

Schierwagen, A., and Werner, H. (1996). Saccade control through the collicular motor map: A two-dimensional neural field model. In: *Artificial neural neturachs—ICANN 96* (Lecture notes in computer science) Vol: 1112, eds. C. von der Malsburg, W. von Seelen, J. C. Vorbeaggen, B. Send hoff, pp. 439–444. Berlin: Springer.

Schiller, J., Helmchen, F., and Sakmann, B. (1995). Spatial profile of dendritic calcium transients evoked by action potentials in rat neocortical pyramidal neurones. *J. Physiol.* 487: 583–600.

Schmitt, F. O., ed. (1970). *The neurosciences: Second study program.* New York: Rockfeller University Press.

Schoepp, D. D., and Conn, P. J. (1993). Metabotropic glutamate receptors in brain function and pathology. *Trends Pharmacol. Sci.* 14: 13–20.

Schwartz, A. B. (1993). Motor cortical activity during drawing movements: Population representation during sinusoid tracing. *J. Neurophysiol.* 70: 28–36.

Schwarz, J. R., and Eikhof, G. (1987). Na^+ currents and action potentials in rat myelinated nerve fibres at 20 and 37 degrees celcius. *Pflügers Arch, Physiol.* 409: 569–577.

Schweizer, F. E., Betz, H., and Augustine, G. J. (1995). From vesicle docking to endocytosis: Intermediate reactions of exocytosis. *Neuron* 14: 689–696.

Schwindt, P. C., and Crill, W. E. (1995). Amplification of synaptic current by persistent sodium conductance in apical dendrite of neocortical neurons. *J. Neurophysiol.* 74: 2220–2224.

Schwindt, P. C., Spain, W. J. and Crill, W. E. (1989). Long-lasting reduction of excitability by a sodium-dependent potassium current neocortical neurons. *J. Neurophysiol.* 61: 233–244.

Schwindt, P. C., Spain, W. J. and Crill, W. E. (1992). Calcium-dependent potassium currents in neurons from cat sensorimotor cortex. *J. Neurophysiol.* 67: 216–226.

Schwindt, P. C., Spain, W. J., Foehring, R. C., Stafstrom, C. E., Chubb, M. C., and Crill, W. E. (1988). Multiple potassium conductances and their functions in neurons from cat sensorimotor cortex *in vitro*. *J. Neurophysiol.* 59: 424–449.

Schwob, J. E., and Price, J. L. (1978). The cortical projections of the olfactory bulb: Development in fetal and neonatal rats correlated with quantitative variations in adult rats. *Brain Res.* 151: 369–374.

Segal, M. (1995). Fast imaging of $[Ca]_i$ reveals presence of voltage-gated calcium channels in dendritic spines of cultured hippocampal neurons. *J. Neurophysiol.* 74: 484–488.

Segev, I. (1990). Computer study of presynaptic inhibition controlling the spread of action potentials into axonal terminals. *J. Neurophysiol.* 63: 987–998.

Segev, I. (1992). Single neuron model: Oversimple, complex and reduced. *Trends Neurosci.* 15: 414–421.

Segev, I. (1995). Dendritic processing. In *The handbook of brain theory and neuronal networks*, ed. M. A. Arbib, pp. 282–289. Cambridge, MA: MIT Press.

Segev, I., Fleshman, J. W., Miller, J. P., and Bunow, B. (1985). Modeling the electrical behavior of anatomically complex neurons using a network analysis program: Passive membrane. *Biol. Cybern.* 53: 27–40.

Segev, I. and Parnas, I. (1983). Synaptic integration mechanisms: Theoretical and experimental investigation of temporal postsynaptic interactions between excitatory and inhibitory inputs. *Biophys. J.* 41: 41–50.

Segev, I. and Rall, W. (1983). Theoretical analysis of neuron models with dendrites of unequal electrical length. *Soc. Neurosci. Abst.* 9: 102.20.

Segev, I., and Rall, W. (1988). Computational study of an excitable dendritic spine. *J. Neurophysiol.* 60: 499–523.

Segev, I., Rinzel, J., and Shepherd, G. M., eds. (1995). *The theoretical foundation of dendritic function: Collected papers of Wilfrid Rall with commentaries.* Cambridge, MA: MIT Press.

Sejnowski, T. (1977). Storing covariance with nonlinearly interacting neurons. *J. Math. Biol.* 4: 303–321.

Sellami, L. (1988). Vowel recognition in adaptive nerual networks. Master's thesis, University of Maryland, College Park.

Selverston, A. I., and Miller, J. P. (1980). Mechanisms underlying pattern generation in the lobster stomatogastric ganglion as determined by selective inactivation of identified neurons: I. Pyloric System. *J. Neurophysiol.* 44: 1102–1121.

Selverston, A. I., and Moulins, M. (1985). Oscillatory neural networks. *Ann. Rev. Physiol.* 47: 29–48.

Sen, K., Jorge-Rivera, J. C., Marder, E., and Abbott, L. F. (1996). Decoding synapses. *J. Neurosci.* 16: 6307–6318.

Seneff, S. (1984). Pitch and spectral estimation of speech based on auditory synchrony model. *Work. Pap. Ling.* MIT 4: 44.

Seung, H. S. (1996). How the brain keeps the eyes still. *Proc. Natl. Acad. Sci. U.S.A.* 93: 13339–13344.

Shadlen, M. N., and Newsome, W. T. (1994). Noise, neural codes and cortical organization. *Curr. Opin. Neurobiol.* 4: 569–579.

Shamma, S., and Versnel, H. (1995). Ripple analysis in the ferret primary auditorycortex: 2. Prediction of unit responses to arbitrary spectral profiles. *J. Audit. Neurosci.* 1: 255–270.

Shamma, S. (1985a). Speech processing in the auditory system: 1. Representation of speech sounds in the responses of the auditory nerve. *J. Acoust. Soc. Am.* 78: 1612–1621.

Shamma, S. (1985b). Speech processing in the auditory system: 2. Lateral inhibition and the processing of speech-evoked activity in the auditory nerve. *J. Acoust. Soc. Am.* 78: 1622–1632.

Shamma, S. (1986). Encoding the acoustic spectrum in the spatio-temporal responses of the auditory nerve. In *Auditory frequency selectivity*, ed. B. C. J. Moore and R. Patterson, pp. 289–298. U.K.: Cambridge, Plenum Press.

Shamma, S., Chadwick, R., Wilbur, J., Rinzel J., and Moorish, K. (1986). A biophysical model of cochlear processing: Intensity dependence of pure tone responses. *J. Acoust. Soc. Am.* 80: 133–145.

Shamma, S., Versnel, H., and Kowalski, N. (1995). Ripple analysis in the ferret primary auditory cortex: 1. Response characteristics of single units to sinusoidally rippled spectra. *J. Audit. Neurosci.* 1: 233–254.

Sharp, A. A. (1994). Single neuron and small network dynamics explored with the dynamic clamp. Ph.D. Diss., Brandeis University.

Sharp, A. A., Abbott, L. F., and Marder, E. (1992). Artificial electrical synapses in oscillating networks. *J. Neurophysiol.* 67: 1691–1692.

Sharp, A. A., O'Neil, M. B., Abbott, L. F., and Marder, E. (1993a). The dynamic clamp: Computer-generated conductances in real neurons. *J. Neurophysiol.* 69: 992–995.

Sharp, A., O'Neil, M. B., Abbott, L. F., and Marder, E. (1993b). The dynamic clamp: Artificial conductances in biological neurons. *Trends Neurosci.* 16: 389–394.

Sharp, A. A., Skinner, F. K., and Marder, E. (1996). Mechanisms of oscillation in dynamic clamp constructed two-cell half-center circuits. *J. Neurophysiol.* 76: 867–883.

Sheinberg, D. L., and Logothetis, N. K. (1997). The role of temporal cortical areas in perceptual organization. *Proc. Natl. Acad. Sci. U.S.A.* 94: 3408–3413.

Shelton, D. P. (1985). Membrane resistivity estimated for the Purkinje neuron by means of a passive computer model. *Neurosci.* 14: 111–131.

Sheng, M., Tsaur, M. L., Jan, Y. N., and Jan, L. Y. (1992). Subcellular segregation of two A-type K^+ channel proteins in rat central neurons. *Neuron* 9: 271–284.

Sheng, M., Tsaur, M. L., Jan, Y. N., and Jan, L. Y. (1994). Contrasting subcellular localization of the Kv1.2 K^+ channel subunit in different neurons of rat brain. *J. Neurosci.* 14: 2408–2417.

Shepard, R. N., and Metzler, J. (1971). Mental rotation of three-dimensional objects. *Science* 171: 701–703.

Shepherd, G. M. (1996). The dendritic spines: A multifunctional integrative unit. *J. Neurophysiol.* 75: 2197–2210.

Shepherd, G. M., and Brayton, R. K. (1979). Computer simulation of a dendro-dendritic synaptic circuit for self- and lateral inhibition in the olfactory bulb. *Brain. Res.* 175: 377–382.

Shepherd, G. M., and Brayton, R. K. (1987). Logic operations are properties of computer-simulated interactions between excitable dendritic spines. *Neuroscience* 21: 151–165.

Shepherd, G. M., Brayton, R. K., Miller, J. P., Segev, I., Rinzel, J., and Rall, W. (1985). Signal enhancement in distal cortical dendrites by means of interactions between active dendritic spines. *Proc. Natl. Acad. Sci. U.S.A.* 82: 2192–2195.

Sherman, A., and Rinzel J. (1992). Rhythmogenic effects of weak electrotonic coupling in neural models. *Proc. Natl. Acad. Sci. U.S.A.* 89: 2471–2474.

Sherman, A., Keizer, J., and Rinzel, J. (1990). Domain model for Ca^{2+} inactivation of Ca^{2+} channels at low channel density. *Biophys. J.* 58: 985–995.

Siebert, W. M. (1970). Frequency discrimination in the auditory system: Place or periodicity mechanisms? *Proc. IEEE* 58: 723–730.

Siegel, M., Marder, E., and Abbot, L. F. (1994). Activity dependent current distributions in model neurons. *Proc. Natl. Acad. Sci. U.S.A.* 91: 11308–11312.

Sigworth, F. J., and Zhou, J. (1992). Ion channels: Analysis of nonstationary single-channel currents. *Meth. Enzymol.* 207: 746–762.

Sillito, A. M. (1977). Inhibitory process underlying the directional specificity of simple, complex and hypercomplex cells in cat's visual cortex. *J. Physiol.* 271: 699–720.

Sillito, A. M., Kemp, J. A., Milson, J. A., and Berardi, N. (1980). A re-evaluation of the mechanisms underlying simple cell orientation selectivity. *Brain Res.* 194: 517–520.

Simon, S., and Llinás, R. (1985). Compartmentalization of submembrane calcium activity during calcium influx and its significance in transmitter release. *Biophys J.* 48: 559–569.

Sinex, D., and Geisler, C. (1983). Responses of auditory-nerve fibers to consonant-vowel syllables. *J. Acoust. Soc. Am.* 73: 602–615.

Singer, W., and Gray, C. M. (1995). Visual feature integration and the temporal correlation hypothesis. *Ann. Rev. Neurosci.* 18: 555–586.

Sloper, J. J., and Powell, T. P. S. (1978). A study of the axon initial segment and the proximal axon of neurons in the primate motor and somatic sensory cortices. *Philos. Trans. Roy. Soc. Lond.* B 285: 173–197.

Smith, G. D. (1985). *Numerical solutions of partial differential equations: Finite difference methods.* 3d ed. Oxford: Clarendon Press.

Sneyd, J., Charles, A. C., and Sanderson, M. J. (1994). A model for the propagation of intracellular calcium waves. *Am. J. Physiol.* 266: C293–C302.

Sneyd, J., Wetton, B. T. R., Charles, A. C., and Sanderson, M. J. (1995). Intercellular calcium waves mediated by diffusion of inositol triphosphate: A two-dimensional model. *Am. J. Physiol.* 268: C1537–C1545.

Snowden, R. J., Treue, S., and Andersen, R. A. (1992). The response of neurons in areas V1 and MT of the alert rhesus monkey to moving random dot patterns. *Exp. Brain Res.* 88: 389–400.

Snyder, D. L. (1975). *Random point processes.* New York: Wiley.

Sod, G. A. (1985). *Numerical methods in fluid dynamics: Initial and initial boundary-value problems.* Cambridge: Cambridge University Press.

Softky, W. (1994). Sub-millisecond coincidence detection in active dendritic trees. *Neurosci.* 58: 13–41.

Softky, W. R., and Koch, C. (1993). The highly irregular firing of cortical cells is inconsistent with temporal integration of random EPSPs. *J. Neurosci.* 13: 334–350.

Somers, D., and Kopell, N. (1993). Rapid synchronization through fast threshold modulation. *Biol. Cybern.* 68: 393–407.

Somers, D., Nelson, S., and Sur, M. (1995). An emergent model of orientation selectivity in cat visual cortical simple cells. *J. Neurosci.* 15: 5448–5465.

Somogyi, P., Freund, T. F., and Cowey, A. (1982). The axo-axonic interneuron in the cerebral cortex of the rat, cat and monkey. *Neuroscience* 11: 2577–2607.

Spain, W. J., Schwindt, P. C., and Crill, W. E. (1990). Post-inhibitory excitation and inhibition in layer 5 pyramidal neurons from cat sensorimotor cortex. *J. Physiol.* 434: 609–626.

Sparks, D. L., and Mays, L. E. (1990). Signal transformations required for the generation of saccadic eye movements. *Ann. Rev. Neurosci.* 13: 309–336.

Spencer, W. A., and Kandel, E. R. (1961). Electrophysiology of hippocampal neurons: 4. Fast prepotentials. *J. Neurophysiol.* 24: 272–285.

Spruston, N., and Johnston, D. (1992). Perforated patch-clamp analysis of the passive membrane properties of three classes of hippocampal neurons. *J. Neurophysiol.* 67: 508–529.

Spruston, N., and Stuart, G. (1996). Voltage attenuation and intracellular resistivity in neocortical pyramidal neurons. *Soc. Neurosci. Abstr.* 22: 792. Abstr. No. 315.10.

Spruston, N., Jaffe, D. B., and Johnston, D. (1994). Dendritic attenuation of synaptic potentials and currents: The role of passive membrane properties. *Trends Neursoci* 17: 161–166.

Spruston, N., Jaffe, D. B., Williams, S. H., and Johnston, D. (1993). Voltage- and space-clamp errors associated with the measurement of electrotonically remote synaptic events. *J. Neurophysiol.* 70: 781–802.

Spruston, N., Jonas, P., and Sakmann, B. (1995). Dendritic glutamate receptor channels in rat hippocampal CA3 and CA1 pyramidal neurons. *J. Physiol.* 482: 325–352.

Spruston, N., Schiller, Y., Stuart, G., and Sakmann, B. (1995). Activity-dependent action potential invasion and calcium influx into hippocampal CA1 dendrites. *Science* 268: 297–300.

Srinivasan, R., and Chiel, H. J. (1993). Fast calculation of synaptic conductances. *Neur. Comput.* 5: 200–204.

Srinivasan, Y., Elmer, L., Davis, J., Bennett, V., and Angelides, K. (1988). Ankyrin and spectrin associate with voltage-dependent sodium channels in barin. *Nature* 333: 177–180.

Stafstrom, C. E., Schwindt, P. C., and Crill, W. E (1982). Negative slope conductance due to a persistent subthreshold sodium current in cat neocortical neurons in vitro. *Brain Res.* 236: 221–226.

Staley, K. J., Otis, T. S., and Mody, I. (1992). Membrane properties of dentate gyrus granule cells: Comparison of sharp microelectrode and whole-cell recordings. *J. Neurophysiol.* 67: 1346–1358.

Staley, K. J., Soldo, B. L., and Proctor, W. R. (1995). Ionic mechanisms of neuronal excitation by inhibitory GABA$_A$ receptors. *Science* 269: 977–981.

Standley, C., Ramsey, R. L., and Usherwood, P. N. R. (1993). Gating kinetics of the quisqualate-sensitive glutamate receptor of locust muscle studied using agonist concentration jumps and computer simulations. *Biophys. J.* 65: 1379–1386.

Stein, R. B. (1967a). The frequency of nerve action potentials generated by applied currents. *Proc. Roy. Soc. Lond.* B167: 64–86.

Stein, R. B. (1967b). Some models of neuronal variability. *Biophys. J.* 7: 37–68.

Stein, R., Leung, K., Oguztoreli M., and Williams D. (1974). Properties of small neural networks. *Kybernetik* 14: 223–230.

Steinberg, I. Z. (1996). On the analytic solution of electrotonic spread in branched passive trees. *J. Comput. Neurosci.* 3: 301–311.

Stephenson, D. G., Wendt, I. R., and Forrest, Q. G. (1981). Non-uniform ion distribution and electrical potential in sarcoplasmic regions of skeletal muscle fiber. *Nature* 289: 690–692.

Steriade, M., McCormick, D. A., and Sejnowski., T. J. (1993). Thalamocortical oscillations in the sleeping and aroused brain. *Science* 262: 679–685.

Stevens, C. F. (1978). Interactions between intrinsic membrane protein and electric field. *Biophys. J.* 22: 295–306.

Stevens, C. F., and Wang, Y. (1995). Facilitation and depression at single central synapses. *Neuron* 14: 795–802.

Stiles, J. R., Van Helden, D., Bartol, T. M., Salpeter, E. E., and Salpeter, M. M. (1996). Miniature endplate current rise times less than 100 microseconds from improved dual recordings can be modeled with passive acetylcholine diffusion from a synaptic vesicle. *Proc. Natl. Acad. Sci. U.S.A.* 93: 5747–5752.

Stoer, J., and Bulirsch, R. (1980). *Introduction to numerical analysis.* Heidelberg: Springer.

Storm, J. F. (1987). Action potential repolarization and a fast after-hyperpolarization in rat hippocampal pyramidal cells. *J. Physiol.* 385: 733–759.

Storm, J. F. (1988). Temporal integration by a slowly inactivating K^+ current in hippocampal neurons. *Nature* 336: 379–381.

Storm, J. F. (1989). An after-hyperpolarization of medium duration in rat hippocampal pyramidal cells. *J. Physiol.* 409: 171–190.

Storm, J. F. (1990). Potassium currents in hippocampal pyramidal cells. *Prog. Brain Res.* 83: 161–187.

Strassberg, A. F., and DeFelice, L. J. (1993). Limitations of the Hodgkin-Huxley formalism: Effects of single channel kinetics on transmembrane voltage dynamics. *Neur. Comput.* 5: 843–855.

Stratford, K., Mason, A., Larkman, A., Major, G., and Jack, J. J. B. (1989). The modelling of pyramidal neurones in the visual cortex. In *The computing neuron*, ed. R. Durbin, C. Miall, and G. Mitchison, pp. 296–321. London: Addison-Wesley.

Strehler, B. L., and Lestienne, R. (1986). Evidence on precise time-coded symbols and memory of patterns in monkey cortical neuronal spike trains. *Proc. Natl. Acad. Sci. U.S.A.* 83: 9812–9816.

Stricker, C., Field, A. C., and Redman, S. J. (1996). Statistical analysis of amplitude fluctuations in EPSCs evoked in rat CA1 pyramidal neurones *in vitro. J. Physiol.* 490: 419–441.

Strogatz, S. H. (1994). *Nonlinear dynamics and chaos.* With application to physics, biology, chemistry and engineering. Reading MA: Addison-Wesley.

Stryer, L., Biochemistry, 4th ed., W. H. Freeman and Company, New York (1995) pp. 192–193.

Stühmer, W., Methfessel, C., Sakmann, B., Noda, M., and Numa, S. (1987). Patch, clamp characterization of sodium channels expressed from rat brain cDNA. *Eur. Biophys. J.* 14: 131–138.

Stuart, G., Dodt, H. U., and Sakmann, B. (1993). Recordings from the soma and dendrites of neurones in brain slices using infrared video microscopy. *Pflügers Arch. Physiol.* 423: 511–518.

Stuart, G., and Sakmann, B. (1994). Active propagation of somatic action potentials into neocortical pyramidal cell dendrites. *Nature* 367: 69–72.

Stuart, G., and Sakmann, B. (1995). Amplification of EPSPs by axosomatic sodium channels in neocortical pyramidal neurons. *Neuron* 15: 1065–1076.

Stuart, G., and Sakmann, B. (1996). Action potential initiation in neocortical pyramidal neurons—revisited. *Soc. Neurosci. Abstr.* 22: 794. Abstr. 316.6.

Stuart, G., and Spruston, N. (1995). Probing dendritic function with patch pipettes. *Curr. Opin. Neurobiol.* 5: 389–394.

Sutor, B., and Hablitz, J. J. (1993). Influence of barium on rectification in rat neocortical neurons. *Neurosci. Lett.* 157: 62–66.

Svoboda, K., Denk, W., Kleinfeld, D., and Tank, D. W. (1997). *In vivo* dendritic calcium dynamics in neocortical pyramidal neurons. *Nature* 385: 161–165.

Takei, K., Stukenbrok, H., Metcalf, A., Mignery, G. A., Südhof, T. C., Volpe, P., and De Camilli, P. (1992). Ca^{2+} stores in Purkinje neurons: Endoplasmic reticulum subcompartments demonstrated by the heterogeneous distribution of the InsP$_3$ receptor, Ca^{2+}-ATPase, and calsequestrin. *J. Neurosci.* 12: 489–505.

Tang, A. C., Bartels, A. M., and Sejnowski, T. J. (1997). Cholinergic modulation preserves spike timing under physiologically realistic fluctuating input. In *Advances in neural information-processing systems: Natural and synthetic*, ed. M. Mozer, M. Jordan, and T. Petshce. Vol. 9, pp. 111–117. Cambridge, MA: MIT Press.

Taxi, J. (1976). In *Frog neurobiology*, eds. R. Llinas, and W. Precht, pp. 95–150. Heidelberg: Springer.

Taylor, R. E. (1963). Cable theory. In: *Physical techniques in biological research*, vol. 6, ed. W. L. Natsuk, pp. 219–262. New York: Academic Press.

Teich, M. C. (1981). Role of the doubly stochastic Neyman type-A and Thomas counting distributions in photon detection. *Appl. Optics* 20: 2457–2467.

Teich, M. C. (1989). Fractal character of the auditory neural spike train. *IEEE Trans. Biomed. Eng.* 36: 150–160.

Teich, M., Turcott, R. G., and Siegel, R. M. (1996). Temporal correlation in cat striate-cortex neural spike trains. *IEEE Eng., Med. and Biol.* 15: 79–87.

Tempia, F., Kano, M., Schneggenburger, R., Schirra, C., Garaschuk, O., Plant, T., and Konnerth, A. (1996). Fractional calcium current through AMPA-receptor channels with a low calcium permeability. *J. Neurosci.* 16: 456–466.

Terasaki, M., Slater, N. T., Fein, A., Schmidek, A., and Reese, T. S. (1994). Continuous network of endoplasmic reticulum in cerebellar Purkinje neurons. *Proc. Natl. Acad. Sci. U.S.A.* 91: 7510–7514.

Thayer, S. A., and Miller, R. J. (1990). Regulation of the intracellular free calcium concentration in single rat dorsal root ganglions *in vitro*. *J. Physiol.* 425: 85–115.

Theander, S., Fahraeus, C., and Grampp, W. (1996). Analysis of leak current properties in the lobster stretch receptor neurone. *Acta Physiol. Scand.* 157: 493–509.

Theunissen, F., Roddey, J. C., Stufflebeam, S., Clague, H., and Miller, J. P. (1996). Information-theoretic analysis of dynamical encoding by four identified primary sensory interneurons in the cricket cercal system. *J. Neurophysiol.* 75: 1345–1364.

Thibos, L. N., Levick, W. R., and Cohn, T. E. (1979). Receiver operating characteristic curves for Poisson signals. *Biol. Cybern.* 33: 57–61.

Thompson, S. M. (1994). Modulation of inhibitory synaptic transmission in the hippocampus. *Prog. Neurobiol.* 42: 575–609.

Thompson, S. M., and Gähwiler, B. H. (1992). Effects of the GABA uptake inhibitor tiagabine on inhibitory synaptic potentials in rat hippocampal slice cultures. *J. Neurophysiol.* 67: 1698–1701.

Thomson, A. M., and Deuchars, J. (1994). Temporal and spatial properties of local circuits in neocortex. *Trends Neurosci.* 17: 119–126.

Tierney, A. J., and Harris-Warrick, R. M. (1992). Physiological role of the transient potassium current in the pyloric circuit of the lobster stomatogastric ganglion. *J. Neurophysiol.* 67: 599–609.

Timmermann, M. P., and Ashley, C. C. (1986). Fura-2 diffusion and its use as an indicator of transient free calcium changes in single striated muscle cells. *Fed. Eur. Biochem. Soc. Lett.* 209: 1–8.

Traub, R. D. (1979). Neocortical pyramidal cells: A model with dendritic calcium conductance reproduces repetitive firing and epileptic behavior. *Brain Res.* 173: 243–257.

Traub, R. D. (1982). Simulation of intrinsic burdsting in CA3 hippocampal neurons. *Neurosci.* 7: 1233–1242.

Traub, R. D., Dudek, F. E., Taylor, C. P., and Knowles, W. D. (1985). Simulation of hippocampal after discharges synchronized by electrical interactions. *J. Neurosci.* 4: 1033–1038.

Traub, R. D., Jefferys, J. G. R., Miles, R., Whittington, M. A. and Tóth, K. (1994). A branching dendrite model of a rodent CA3 pyramidal neurone. *J. Physiol.* 481: 79–95.

Traub, R. D., and Llinás, R. (1977). The spatial distribution of ionic conductances in normal and axotomized motoneurons. *Neuroscience* 2: 829–850.

Traub, R. D., and Llinás, R. (1979). Hippocampal pyramidal cells: Significance of dendritic ionic conductances for neuronal function and epileptogenesis. *J. Neurophysiol.* 42: 476–496.

Traub, R. D., and Miles, R. (1991) *Neuronal networks of hippocampus.* Cambridge: Cambridge University Press.

Traub, R. D., Whittington, M. A., Stanford, I. M., and Jefferys, J. G. R. (1996). A mechanism for generation of long-range synchronous fast oscillations in the cortex. *Nature* 383: 621–624.

Traub, R. D., Wong, R. K. S., Miles, R., and Michelson, H. (1991). A model of a CA3 hippocampal pyramidal neuron incorporating voltage-clamp data on intrinsic conductances. *J. Neurophysiol.* 66: 635–650.

Tuckwell, H. C. (1985). Some aspects of cable theory with synaptic reversal potentials. *J. Theoret. Neurobiol.* 4: 113–127.

Troyer, T. W., and Miller, K. D. (1997). Physiological gain leads to high ISI variability in a simple model of a cortical regular spiking cell. *Neur. Comput.* 9: 971–983.

Ts'o, D. Y., Gilbert, C. D., and Wiesel, T. N. (1986). Relationship between horizontal interactions and functional architecture in cat striate cortex as revealed by cross-correlation analysis. *J. Neurophysiol.* 6: 1160–1170.

Tseng, G., and Haberly, L. B. (1986). A synaptically mediated K$^+$ potential in olfactory cortex: Characterization and evidence for interneuronal origin. *Soc. Neurosci. Abstr.* 12: 667.

Tseng, G., and Haberly, L. B. (1988). Characterization of synaptically mediated fast and slow inhibitory processes in piriform cortex in an *in vitro* slice preparation. *J. Neurophysiol.* 59: 1352–1376.

Tseng, G., and Haberly, L. B. (1989). Deep neurons in piriform cortex: 2. Membrane properties that underlie unusual synaptic responses. *J. Neurophysiol.* 62: 386–400.

Tsien, R. W., Lipscombe, D., Madison, D. V., Bley, K. R., and Fox, A. P. (1988). Multiple types of neuronal calcium channels and their selective modulation. *Trends Neurosci.* 11: 431–438.

Tsodyks, M. V., and Markram, H. (1996). The neural code between neocortical pyramidal neurons depends on neurotransmitter release probability. *Proc. Natl. Acad. Sci. U.S.A.* 94: 719–723.

Tsodyks, M., and Sejnowski, T. J. (1995). Associative memory and hippocampal place cells. *Int. J. Neur. Syst.* (Supplementary Issue: *Proceedings of the Third Workshop on Neural Networks: From Biology to High Energy Physics*) 6: 81–86.

Tsodyks, M. V., Mit'kov, I., and Sompolinsky, H. (1993). Pattern of synchrony in inhomogeneous networks of oscillators with pulse interactions. *Phys. Rev. Lett.* 71: 1280–1283.

Tsodyks, M., Skaggs, W., Sejnowski, T. J., and McNaughton, B. (1996). Population dynamics and theta rhythm phase precession of hippocampal place cell firing: A spiking neuron model. *Hippocampus* 6: 271–280.

Tsubokawa, H., and Ross, W. N. (1996). IPSPs modulate spike backpropagation and associated $[Ca^{2+}]_i$ changes in the dendrites of hippocampal CA1 pyramidal neurons. *J. Neurophysiol.* 76: 2896–2906.

Tsumoto, T., Eckart, W., and Creutzfeldt, O. D. (1979). Modification of orientation selectivity of cat visual cortex neurons by removal of GABA-mediated inhibition. *Exp. Brain Res.* 34: 351–363.

Tuckwell, H. C. (1988). *Introduction to theoretical neurobiology.* Vol. 2, *Nonlinear and stochastic theories.* Cambridge: Cambridge University Press.

Turner, R. W., Maler, L., Deerinck, T., Levinson, S. R., and Ellisman, M. H. (1994). TTX-sensitive dendritic sodium channels underlie oscillatory discharge in a vertebrate sensory neuron. *J. Neurosci.* 14: 6453–6471.

Turner, R. W., Meyers, D. E., and Barker, J. L. (1993). Fast pre-potential generation in rat hippocampal CA1 pyramidal neurons. *Neuroscience* 53: 949–959.

Turner, R. W., Meyers, D. E., Richardson, T. L., and Barker, J. L. (1991). The site for initiation of action potential discharge over the somatodendritic axis of rat hippocampal CA1 pyrmaidal neurons. *J. Neurosci.* 11: 2270–2280.

Turrigiano, G., Abbott, L. F., and Marder, E. (1994). Activity-dependent changes in the intrinsic properties of cultured neurons. *Science* 264: 974–977.

Turrigiano, G., LeMasson, G., and Marder, E. (1995). Selective regulation of current densities underlies spontaneous changes in the activity of cultured neurons. *J. Neurosci.* 15: 3640–3652.

Turrigiano, G., Marder, E., and Abbott, L. F. (1996). Cellular short-term memory from a slow potassium conductance. *J. Neurophysiol.* 75: 963–966.

Ulrich, D., and Huguenard, J. R. (1996). GABA$_B$-dependent burst-firing in thalamic neurons: A dynamic clamp study. *Proc. Natl. Acad. Sci. U.S.A.* 93: 13245–13249.

Ulrich, D., Quadroni, R., and Lüscher, H.-R. (1994). Electrotonic structure of motoneurons in spinal cord slice cultures: A comparison of compartmental and equivalent cylinder models. *J. Neurophysiol.* 71: 861–871.

Usher, M., Stemmler, M., Koch, C., and Olami, Z. (1994). Network amplification of local fluctuations causes high spike rate variability, fractal firing patterns and oscillatory local field potentials. *Neur. Comput.* 6: 795–836.

van Egeraat, J. M., and Wikswo, J. P., Jr. (1993). A model for axonal propagation incorporating both radial and axial ionic transport. *Biophys. J.* 64: 1287–1298.

van-Pelt, J. (1992). A simple vector implementation of the Laplace-transformed cable equations in passive dendritic trees. *Biol. Cybern.* 68: 15–21.

van Ooyen, A., and van Pelt, J. (1994). Activity-dependent outgrowth of neurons and overshoot phenomena in developing neural networks. *J. Theoret. Biol.* 167: 27–44.

van Vreeswijk, C., Abbott, L. F., and Ermentrout, G. B. (1994). When inhibition not excitation synchronizes neuronal firing. *J. Comput. Neurosci.* 1: 313–321.

van Vreeswijk, C., and Sompolinksy, H. (1996). Chaos in neuronal networks with balanced excitatory and inhibitory activity. *Science* 274: 1724–1726.

Vandenberg, C. A., and Bezanilla, F. (1991). A sodium channel gating model based on single channel, macroscopic ionic, and gating currents in the squid giant axon. *Biophys. J.* 60: 1511–1533.

Vanier, M. C., and Bower, J. M. (1996). A comparison of automated parameter-searching methods for neural models in *Computational Neuroscience: Trends in Research 1995*, ed. J. M. Bower (pp. 477–482). San Diego Academic Press.

Varela, J., Sen, K., Gibson, J., Fost, J., Abbott, L. F., and Nelson, S. B. (1997). A quantitative description of short-term plasticity at excitatory synapses in layer 2/3 of rat primary visual cortex. J. Neurosci. 17: 7926–7940.

Versnel, H., Shamma, S., and Kowalski, N. (1995). Ripple analysis in the ferret primary auditory cortex: 3. Topographic and columnar distribution of ripple response parameters. *J. Audit. Neurosci.* 1: 271–285.

Victor, J. D. (1987). The dynamics of the cat retinal X cell centre. *J. Physiol.* 386: 219–246.

Victor, J. D. (1988). The dynamics of the cat retinal Y cell subunit. *J. Physiol.* 405: 289–320.

Victor, J. D., and Shapley, R. (1980). A method of nonlinear analysis in the frequency domain. *Biophys. J.* 29: 459–484.

Vogels, R., and Orban, G. A. (1990). How well do response changes of striate neurons signal differences in orientation? A study in the discriminating monkey. *J. Neurosci.* 10: 3543–3558.

Vogels, R., Spileers, W., and Orban, G. A. (1989). The response variability of striate cortical neurons in the behaving monkey. *Exp. Brain Res.* 77: 432–436.

von der Malsurg, C., and Schneider, W. (1986). A neural cocktail-party processor. *Biol. Cybern.* 54: 29–40.

Wagner, J., and Keizer, J. (1994). Effects of rapid buffers on Ca^{2+} diffusion and Ca^{2+} oscillations. *Biophys. J.* 67: 447–456.

Wall, P. D. (1995). Do nerve impulses penetrate terminal arborizations? A pre-presynaptic control mechanism. *Trends Neurosci.* 18: 99–103.

Wandell, B. A. (1995). *Foundations of vision.* Sunderland, MA: Sinauer.

Wang, K., and Shamma, S. (1994). Self-normalization and noise-robustness in early auditory representations. *IEEE Trans. Speech and Aud. Proc.* 2: 421–435.

Wang, K., and Shamma, S. (1995). Representation of spectral profiles in the primary auditory cortex. *IEEE Trans. Speech and Aud. Proc.* 3: 382–395.

Wang, H., Kunkel, D. D., Schwartzkroin, P. A., and Tempel, B. L. (1994). Localization of Kv1.1 and Kv1.2, two K^+ channel proteins, to synaptic terminals, somata and dendrites in the mouse brain. *J. Neurosci.* 14: 4588–4599.

Wang, M., and Zhang, C. N. (1996). Single neuron local rational arithmetic revealed in phase space of input conductances. *Biophys. J.* 71: 2380–2393.

Wang, S. S.-H., and Augustine, G. J. (1995). Confocal imaging and local photolysis of caged compounds: Dual probes of synaptic function. *Neuron* 15: 755–760.

Wang, X.-J., and Rinzel, J. (1992). Alternating and synchronous rhythms in reciprocally inhibitory model neurons. *Neur. Comput.* 4: 84–97.

Wang, X.-J., and Rinzel, J. (1995). Oscillatory and bursting properties of neurons. In *Handbook of brain theory and neural networks*, ed. M. A. Arbib, pp. 689–691. Cambridge, MA: MIT Press.

Warman, E. N., Durand, D. M., and Yuen, G. L. (1994). Reconstruction of hippocampal CA1 pyramidal cell electrophysiology by computer simulation. *J. Neurophysiol.* 71: 2033–2045.

Wathey, J. C., Lytton, W. W., Jester, J. M. and Sejnowski, T. J. (1992). Computer simuations of EPSP-to-spike (E-S) potentiation in hippocampal CA1 pyramidal cells. *J. Neurosci.* 12: 607–618.

Waxman, S. G. (1975). Integrative properties and design principles of axons. *Int. Rev. Neurobiol.* 18: 1–40.

Waxman, S. G., Kocsis, J. D., and Stys, P. K., eds. (1995). *The axon: Structure, function and pathophysiology.* New York: Oxford University Press.

Waxman, S. G., and Melker, R. J. (1971). Closely spaced nodes of Ranvier in the mammalian brain. *Brain Res.* 32: 445–448.

Waxman, S. G., and Ritchie, J. M. (1993). Molecular dissecution of the myelinated axon. *Ann. Neurol.* 33: 121–136.

Webster, D. (1992). Overview of mammalian auditory pathways with emphasis on humans. In *The mammalian auditory pathway: Neuroanatomy*, ed. D. Webster, A. Popper, and R. Fay, pp. 1–22. New York: Springer.

Wehmeier, U., Dong, D., Koch, C., and van Essen, D. (1989). Modeling the mammalian visual system. In *Methods in neuronal modeling*, ed. C. Koch and I. Segev, pp. 335–359. Cambridge, MA: MIT Press.

Wehr, M., and Laurent, G. (1996). Odor encoding by temporal sequences of firing in oscillating neural assemblies. *Nature* 384: 162–166.

Weimann, J. M., Marder, E., Evans, B., and Calabrese, R. L. (1993). The effects of SDRNFLRFamide and TNRNFLRFamide on the motor patterns of the stomatogastric ganglion of the crab *Cancer borealis*. *J. exp. Biol.* 181: 1–26.

Weiser, M., Bueno, E., Sekirnjak, C., Martone, M. E., Baker, H., Hillman, D., Chen, S., Thornhill, W., Ellisman, M., and Rudy, B. (1995). The potassium channel subunit KV3.1b is localized to somatic and axonal membranes of specific populations of CNS neurons. *J. Neurosci.* 15: 4298–4314.

Weiss, T. F. (1996). *Cellular biophysics.* Vol. 2, *Electrical properties.* Cambridge, MA: MIT Press.

Wessel, R., Koch, C., and Gabbiani, F. (1996). coding of time-varying electric field amplitude modulations in a wave-type electric fish. *J. Neurophysiol.* 75: 2280–2293.

Westenbroek, R. E., Ahlijanian, M. K., and Catterall, W. A. (1990). Clustering of L-type calcium ion channels at the base of major dendrites in hippocampal pyramidal neurons. *Nature* 347: 281–284.

Westenbroek, R. E., Hell, J. W., Warner, C., Dubel, S. J., Snutch, T. P. and Catterall, W. A. (1992). Biochemical properties and subcellular distribution of an N-type calcium channel $\alpha 1$ subunit. *Neuron* 9: 1099–1115.

Westenbroek, R. E., Merrick, D. K., and Catterall, W. A. (1989). Differential subcellular localization of the R_I and R_{II} Na$^+$ channel subtypes in central neurons. *Neuron* 3: 695–704.

Westenbroek, R. E., Sakurai, T., Elliott, E. M., Hell, J. W., Starr, T. V. B., Snutch, T. P., and Catterall, W. A. (1995). Immunochemical identification and subcellular distribution of the $\alpha 1A$ subunits of brain calcium channels. *J. Neurosci.* 15: 6403–6418.

Westerman, L. A., and Smith, R. L. (1984). Rapid and short term adaptation in auditory nerve responses. *Hear. Res.* 15: 249–260.

Westrum, L. E. (1970). Observations on the initial segments of axons in the prepyriform cortex of the rat. *J. Comp. Neurol.* 139: 337–356.

White, E. L., and Rock, M. P. (1980). Three-dimensional aspects of synaptic relationship of a Golgi-impregnated spiny stellate cell reconstructed from serial thin sections. *J. Neurocytol.* 9: 615–636.

White, J. A., Manis, P. B., and Young, E. D. (1992). The parameter identification problem for the somatic shunt model. *Biol. Cybern.* 66: 307–318.

White, J. A., Sekar, N.S., and Kay, A. R. (1995). Errors in persistent inward currents generated space-clamp errors: A modeling study. *J. Neurophysiol.* 73: 2369–2377.

Whittington, M. A., Traub, R. D. and Jefferys, J. G. R. (1995). Synchronized oscillations in interneuron networks driven by metabotropic glutamate receptor activation. *Nature* 373: 612–615.

Williams, S., and Johnston, D. (1991). Kinetic properties of two anatomically distinct excitatory synapses in hippocampla CA3 neurons. *J. Neurophysiol.* 66: 1010–1020.

Wilson, C. J. (1984). Passive cable properties of dendritic spines and spiny neurons. *J. Neurosci.* 4: 281–297.

Wilson, C. J. (1995). Dynamic modification of dendritic cable properties and synaptic transmission by voltage-gated potassium channels. *J. Comput. Neurosci.* 2: 91–115.

Wilson, C. J., and Kawaguchi, Y. (1996). The origin of two-state spontaneous membrane potential fluctuations of neostriatal spiny neurons. *J. Neurosci.* 16: 2397–2410.

Wilson, H. R., and Cowan, J. D. (1972). Excitatory and inhibitory interactions in localized populations of model neurons. *Biophys. J.* 12: 1–24.

Wilson, M. A. (1990). An analysis of olfactory cortical behavior and function using computer simulation techniques. Ph.D. diss., California Institute of Technology.

Wilson, M. A., Bhalla, U.S., Uhley, J. D., and Bower, J. M. (1989). GENESIS: A system for simulating neural networks. In *Advances in neural information processing systems,* ed. D. Touretzky, pp. 485–492. San Mateo, CA: Kaufmann.

Wilson, M. A., and Bower, J. M. (1987). A computer simulation of a three-dimensional model of piriform cortex with functional implications for storage and recognition of spatial and temporal olfactory patterns. *Soc. Neurosci. Abstr.* 13: 1401.

Wilson, M. A., and Bower, J. M. (1989). The simulation of large-scale neural networks. In *Methods in neuronal modeling*, ed. C. Koch and I. Segev, pp. 291–333. Cambridge, MA: MIT Press.

Wilson, M. A., and Bower, J. W. (1991). A computer simulation of oscillatory behavior in primary visual cortex. *Neur. Comput.* 3: 498–509.

Wilson, M. A., and Bower, J. M. (1992). Cortical oscillations and temporal interactions in a computer simulation of piriform cortex. *J. Neurophysiol.* 67: 981–995.

Winfree, A. T. (1980). *The geometry of biological time*. Biomathematics, vol. 8. New York: Springer.

Winslow, R. L., Duffy, S. N., and Charlton, M. P. (1994). Homosynaptic facilitation of transmitter release in crayfish is not affected by mobile calcium chelators: Implications for the residual ionized calcium hypothesis from electrophysiological and computational analysis. *J. Neurophysiol.* 72: 1769–1793.

Wörgötter, F., and Koch, C. (1991). A detailed model of the primary visual pathway in the cat: Comparison of afferent excitatory and intracortical inhibitory connection schemes for orientation selectivity. *J. Neurosci.* 11: 1959–1979.

Wollner, D. A., and Catterall, W. A. (1986). Localization of sodium channels in axon hillocks and initial segments of retinal ganglion cells. *Proc. Natl. Acad. Sci. U.S.A.* 83: 8424–8428.

Wong, R. K., Prince, D. A., and Basbaum, A. I. (1979). Intradendritic recordings from hippocampal neurons. *Proc. Natl. Acad. Sci. U.S.A.* 76: 986–990.

Xiang, Z., Greenwood, A. C., and Brown, T. (1992). Measurement and analysis of hippocampal mossy-fiber synapses. *Soc. Neurosci. Abstr.* 18: 1350.

Yamada, W. M., and Zucker, R. S. (1992). Time course of transmitter release calculated from simulations of a calcium diffusion model. *Biophys. J.* 61: 671–682.

Yamada, W., Koch, C., and Adams, P. R. (1988). Modelling electrical excitability in the cell body and axon of type B bullfrog sympathetic ganglion cells. *Soc. Neurosci. Abst.* 14: Abstract 118.11.

Yamada, W., Koch, C., and Adams, P. (1989). Multiple channels and calcium dynamics. In *Methods in neuronal modeling: From synapses to networks*, ed. C. Koch and I. Segev, pp. 97–134. Cambridge: MIT Press.

Yang, C. R., Seamans, J. K., and Gorelova, N. (1996). Electrophysiological and morphological properties of layers 5–6 principal pyramidal cells in rat prefrontal cortex *in vitro*. *J. Neurosci.* 16: 1904–1921.

Yang, X., Wang, K., and Shamma, S. (1992). Auditory representations of acoustic signals. *IEEE Trans. Inform. Theory* 38: 824–839.

Yokoyama, C. T., Westenbroek, R. E., Hell, J. W., Soong, T. W., Snutch, T. P., and Catterall, W. A. (1995). Biochemical properties and subcellular distribution of the neuronal class E calcium channel $\alpha 1$ subunit. *J. Neurosci.* 15: 6419–6432.

Young, E., and Sachs, M. (1979). Representation of steady-state vowels in the temporal aspects of the discharge patterns of populations of auditory nerve fibers. *J. Acoust. Soc. Am.* 66: 1381–1403.

Yuste, R., and Denk, W. (1995). Dendritic spines as basic functional units of neuronal integration. *Nature* 375: 682–684.

Yuste, R., and Tank, D. W. (1996). Dendritic integration in mammalian neurons: A century after Cajal. *Neuron* 16: 701–716.

Yuste, R., Gutnick, M. J., Saar, D., Delaney, R. D., and Tank, D. W. (1994). Ca^{2+} accumulations in dendrites of neocortical pyramidal neurons: An apical band and evidence for two functional compartments. *Neuron* 13: 23–43.

Zador, A. M., Agmon-Snir, H., and Segev, I. (1995). The morphoelectrotonic transform: A graphical approach to dendritic function. *J. Neurosci.* 15: 1669–1682.

Zador, A. M., Claiborne, B. J., and Brown, T. H. (1992). Nonlinear pattern separation in single hippocampal neurons with active dendritic membrane. In *Advances in neural information-processing systems*, ed. J. Moody, S. Hanson, and R. Lippmann, San Mateo, pp. 51–58. Kaufmann.

Zador, A., and Koch, C. (1994). Linearized models of calcium dynamics: Formal equivalence to the cable equation. *J. Neurosci.* 14: 4705–4715.

Zador, A., Koch, C., and Brown, T. H. (1990). Biophysical model of a Hebbian synapse. *Proc. Natl. Acad. Sci. U.S.A.* 87: 6718–6722.

Zečević, D. (1996). Multiple spike-initiation zones in single neurons revealed by voltage-sensitive days. *Nature* 381: 322–325.

Zeevi, Y. Y., and Bruckstein, A. M. (1977). A Note on single signed integral pulse frequency modulation. *IEEE Trans. Syst., Man, and Cybern.* 7: 875–877.

Zengel, J. E., and Magleby, K. L. (1982). Augmentation and facilitation of transmitter release. *J. Gen Physiol.* 80: 583–611.

Zhang, K. (1996). Representation of spatial orientation by the intrinsic dynamics of the head-direction cell ensemble: A theory. *J. Neurosci.* 16: 2112–2126.

Zhang, S., and Trussell, L. O. (1994). Voltage clamp analysis of excitatory synaptic transmission in the avian nucleus magnocellularis. *J. Physiol.* 480: 123–136.

Zhou, Z., and Neher, E. (1993). Mobile and immobile calcium buffers in bovine adrenal chromaffin cells. *J. Physiol.* 469: 245–273.

Zukin, R. S., and Bennett, M. V. (1995). Alternatively spliced isoforms of the NMDARI receptor subunit. *Trends Neurosci.* 18: 306–313.

Contributors

Larry Abbott
Volen Center and Department of
Biology
Brandeis University
Waltham, Massachusetts

Paul R. Adams
Department of Neurobiology and
Behavior
State University of New York at Stony
Brook
Stony Brook, New York

Hagai Agmon-Snir
Mathematical Research Branch
National Institutes of Health
Bethesda, Maryland

James M. Bower
Division of Biology
California Institute of Technology
Pasadena, California

Robert E. Burke
Laboratory of Neural Control
National Insitute of Neurological
Disorders and Stroke
National Institutes of Health
Bethesda, Maryland

Eric De Schutter
Born Bunge Foundation
University of Antwerp–UIA
Antwerp, Belgium

Alain Destexhe
Department of Physiology
Laval University School of Medicine
Quebec, Canada

Rodney Douglas
Institute of Neuroinformatics
ETH/UNIZ
Zürich, Switzerland

Bard Ermentrout
Department of Mathematics
University of Pittsburgh
Pittsburgh, Pennsylvania

Fabrizio Gabbiani
Division of Biology
California Institute of Technology
Pasadena, California

David Hansel
Centre de Physique Théorique
École Polytechnique
Palaiseau, France

Michael Hines
Department of Computer Science
Yale University
New Haven, Connecticut

Christof Koch
Division of Biology
California Institute of Technology
Pasadena, California

Misha Mahowald
Institute of Neuroinformatics
ETH/UNIZ
Zürich, Switzerland

Zachary F. Mainen
Cold Spring Harbor Laboratory
Cold Spring Harbor, New York

Eve Marder
Volen Center and Department of
Biology
Brandeis University
Waltham, Massachusetts

Michael V. Mascagni
Director, Doctoral Program in Scientific
Computing
University of Southern Mississippi
Hattiesburg, Mississippi

Alexander Protopapas
Division of Biology
California Institute of Technology
Pasadena, California

Wilfrid Rall
Mathematical Research Branch
National Institutes of Health
Bethesda, Maryland

John Rinzel
New York University
Center for Neural Science and Courant
Institute of Mathematical Sciences
New York, New York

Idan Segev
Department of Neurobiology and
Center for Neural Computation
Institute of Life Sciences
Hebrew University
Jerusalem, Israel

Terrence J. Sejnowski
The Howard Hughes Medical Institute
The Salk Institute
La Jolla, California

Shihab Shamma
Department of Electrical Engineering
University of Maryland
College Park, Maryland

Arthur S. Sherman
National Institutes of Health
Bethesda, Maryland

Paul Smolen
Department of Neurobiology and
Anatomy
University of Texas Medical School
Houston, Texas

Haim Sompolinksy
Racah Institute of Physics and Center
for Neural Computation
Hebrew University
Jerusalem, Israel

Michael Vanier
Computation and Neural Systems
California Institute of Technology
Pasadena, California

Walter M. Yamada
Department of Electrical Engineering
and Computer Science
University of California–Berkeley
Berkeley, California

Index

Printed in the United States
By Bookmasters